ACSM'S
RESOURCE MANUAL FOR
GUIDELINES
FOR
EXERCISE TESTING
AND
PRESCRIPTION

Editors:

J. Larry Durstine, Ph.D., F.A.C.S.M.
Associate Professor
Department of Exercise Science
The University of South Carolina
Columbia, South Carolina

Abby C. King, Ph.D.
Assistant Professor of Health Research & Policy and Medicine
Stanford University School of Medicine
Palo Alto, California

Patricia L. Painter, Ph.D., F.A.C.S.M.
Director of Transplant Rehabilitation
University of California at San Francisco
San Francisco, California

Jeffrey L. Roitman, Ed.D., F.A.C.S.M.
Director of Cardiac Rehabilitation
Research Medical Center
Kansas City, Missouri

Linda D. Zwiren, Ph.D., F.A.C.S.M.
Department of Health, Physical Education and Recreation
Department of Biology
Hofstra University
Hempstead, New York

Contributing Editor:
W. Larry Kenney, Ph.D., F.A.C.S.M.
Associate Professor of Applied Physiology
The Pennsylvania State University
University Park, Pennsylvania

ACSM'S RESOURCE MANUAL FOR GUIDELINES FOR EXERCISE TESTING AND PRESCRIPTION

Second Edition

AMERICAN COLLEGE OF SPORTS MEDICINE

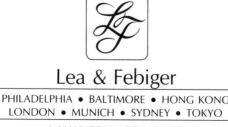

Lea & Febiger

PHILADELPHIA • BALTIMORE • HONG KONG
LONDON • MUNICH • SYDNEY • TOKYO
A WAVERLY COMPANY
1993

Lea & Febiger
Box 3024
200 Chester Field Parkway
Malvern, Pennsylvania 19355-9725
U.S.A.
(215) 251-2230

American College of Sports Medicine™
P.O. Box 1440
401 W. Michigan St.
Indianapolis, Indiana 46202-3233
U.S.A.
(317) 637-9200

Executive Editor—Matthew Harris
Development Editor—Lisa Stead
Production Manager—Robert N. Spahr
Manuscript Editor—Jessica Howie Martin
ACSM Group Publisher—D. Mark Robertson

First Edition, 1988
Second Edition, 1993

Library of Congress Cataloging-in-Publication Data

American College of Sports Medicine.
    ACSM's resource manual for Guidelines for exercise testing and
prescription / American College of Sports Medicine : editors, J.
Larry Durstine . . . [et al.].—2nd ed.
        p.   cm.
    Rev. ed. of: Resource manual for Guidelines for exercise testing
and prescription / American College of Sports Medicine : editors,
Steven N. Blair . . . [et al.]. 1988.
    Includes bibliographical references and index.
    ISBN 0-8121-1589-9
    1. Exercise therapy. 2. Exercise tests. I. Durstine, J. Larry.
II. Guidelines for exercise testing and prescription. III. Resource
manual for Guidelines for exercise testing and prescription.
IV. Title.
    [DNLM: 1. Exercise Test. 2. Exercise Therapy. WE 103 A5125g
1991 Suppl.]
RM725.R42   1993
615.8′24—dc20
DNLM/DLC
for Library of Congress   92-48810
                                                     CIP

PRINTED IN THE UNITED STATES OF AMERICA

Print number: 5   4   3   2   1

Reprints of chapters may be purchased from Lea & Febiger in quantities of 100 or more.
Contact Sally Grande in the Sales Department.

Foreword

It is with great pride that I recommend to the reader this Second Edition of the American College of Sports Medicine's *Resource Manual for Guidelines for Exercise Testing and Prescription*. This thoroughly updated volume presents, in concise and readable form, the core material that must be mastered by candidates for the ACSM's various certifications in preventive and rehabilitative exercise programming. Therefore, at the most practical level, this book should be seen as an invaluable resource for students and in-service professionals who seek to enhance their credentials in the field of clinical exercise programming.

However, I believe that this *Resource Manual* should be seen as much more than a study guide for certification candidates. As we approach the year 2000, it seems clear that the twentieth century will be known as an era of many triumphs in public health but also as a period during which many new health problems emerged. One of the most virulent of these new public health problems is physical inactivity. This problem, once confined to a small, affluent segment of society, has been transmitted to the masses as a side effect of technologic advancement. In my view, this book symbolizes society's effort to respond to the physical inactivity epidemic that is evident in contemporary culture.

There are signs that, in recent decades, we have made some progress in promoting physically active lifestyles. But all surveys indicate that we have a long way to go. It is my view that our best weapon in the battle to make our society more physically active is *knowledge*—knowledge of the health implications of exercise, knowledge of the clinical applications of exercise and, perhaps most critically, knowledge of the effective strategies for promotion of active lifestyles. This book represents ACSM's commitment to dissemination of the rapidly expanding body of knowledge concerning exercise and health. Those who master the material in this volume will be prepared to advance the public health in a most powerful way.

President
American College
of Sports Medicine
1993–1994

Russell R. Pate, Ph.D., F.A.C.S.M.

Mission Statement

The American College of Sports Medicine promotes and integrates scientific research, education, and practical applications of sports medicine and exercise science to maintain and enhance physical performance, fitness, health, and quality of life.

Preface

The American College of Sports Medicine certification programs began in 1975 with the publication of *ACSM's Guidelines for Graded Exercise Testing and Exercise Prescription* (referred to as *Guidelines*) and subsequent examinations of certification candidates. The *Guidelines* presented behavioral objectives for the several certification tracks. Candidates were expected to master these objectives and be able to pass written and oral examinations on the content. In the early years of the certification process, candidates were given no assistance in finding educational materials to provide the necessary information relative to the objectives. For this reason, *ACSM's Resource Manual for Guidelines for Exercise Testing and Prescription* (referred to as the *Resource Manual*) was developed.

The *Resource Manual* was developed to provide certification candidates with appropriate information relative to the behavioral objectives found in the *Guidelines*. The Resource Manual addresses a broad array of topics. Although no single source provides all available information on exercise testing and exercise prescription, the Resource Manual is a comprehensive and authoritative book. After completion of the fourth edition of the *Guidelines*, all behavioral objectives therein were reviewed. Chapters in the first edition of the *Resource Manual* have been updated to include new objectives and new topics that were considered by the reviewers to be important to exercise practitioners. Effort was particularly placed on including information relevant to those working in nonmedical settings.

The material presented in each chapter includes key information relevant to the behavioral objectives on the chapter's topic. The authors were asked to distill their knowledge into a few main points, yet provide sufficient detail to avoid a superficial treatment of the topic. Similar objectives appear in the different certification levels; however, the expected depth of knowledge differs among certification levels. For example, the exercise test technologist and the exercise program director are expected to be able to describe the effects of different drugs on heart rate and blood pressure. The exercise program director, however, must also be able to describe the mechanism of action of a drug and know its major side effects. Behavioral objectives for both of these examples are presented in a single chapter in the *Resource Manual*, providing a coherent theme and being useful to all levels of certification. Candidates should thus read the material and use it at whatever level they are preparing for. For example, the health fitness instructor certification candidates will encounter information in the *Resource Manual* that is more advanced than they need, but the information they do need is present.

We do not expect the *Resource Manual* to provide answers to all examination questions, but it is an authoritative source, and candidates who know the material therein will do well on the examination. The primary value of the *Resource Manual* is that it provides a great deal of information on the behavioral objectives in one place. It should be used as a starting point, and when more in-depth information is needed, candidates should seek references presented in the chapters here.

The Editorial Committee hopes that this book will prove useful to ACSM certification candidates and other students of exercise science. We hope that this book makes your study of exercise science exciting and interesting, and wish you the best of luck with your studies.

Editorial Committee

Acknowledgments

The editors thank these individuals who contributed to this book by reviewing manuscripts and providing editorial assistance:

Reviewers

Donald M. Cummings, M.S.
Susan J. Hall, Ph.D., F.A.C.S.M.
George Havenith, Drs.
W. Larry Kenney, Ph.D., F.A.C.S.M.
Patricia M. Kenney, M.S.
James A. Pawelczyk, Ph.D.
Susan M. Puhl, Ph.D.
Neil B. Vroman, R.P.T., Ph.D., F.A.C.S.M.
Maureen Smith-Plombon, R.D., M.S.
James Davis, Ph.D., F.A.C.S.M.
Ann Ward, Ph.D., F.A.C.S.M.
Fredrick Pashkow, M.D., F.A.C.S.M.
Glenn Porter, Ph.D., F.A.C.S.M.
William Dafoe, M.D.
Janet P. Wallace, Ph.D., F.A.C.S.M.
Cedric X. Bryant, Ph.D.
Theresa Foti, Ph.D.
Walter Thompson, Ph.D., F.A.C.S.M.
Scott Powers, Ph.D., F.A.C.S.M.
Kathy Berra, B.S.N.
Tony G. Babb, Ph.D., F.A.C.S.M.
Neil F. Gordon, M.D., Ph.D., M.P.H., F.A.C.S.M.
William L. Haskell, Ph.D., F.A.C.S.M.

William G. Herbert, Ph.D., F.A.C.S.M.
Robert G. Holly, Ph.D., F.A.C.S.M.
Lyle J. Micheli, M.D., F.A.C.S.M.
Henry S. Miller, M.D., F.A.C.S.M.
Ray Shepherd, Ph.D., F.A.C.S.M.
L. Kent Smith, M.D.
Paul Thompson, M.D., F.A.C.S.M.
Steven Van Camp, M.D., F.A.C.S.M.
Ami M. Drimmer, Ph.D.
Sheryl T. Zigon, Ph.D.
Robert W. Patton, Ph.D., F.A.C.S.M.
Elizabeth Holford, J.D., Ph.D.
Martha Livingston, R.N., M.B.A.
Michael D. Wolfe, Ph.D.
Richard J. Sabbath, Ed.D.
David Letterman
Oded Bar-Or, M.D., F.A.C.S.M.
Patricia Dubbert, Ph.D.
Bess Marcus, Ph.D.
Penny Kris-Etherton, Ph.D.
Sally Mackey, M.S., R.D.
Janet Walberg-Rankin, Ph.D., F.A.C.S.M.
Barbara Newman, M.S.
Marcia Ward, Ph.D.

Contributors

Steven N. Blair, P.E.D., F.A.C.S.M.
Director, Division of Epidemiology
Institute for Aerobics Research
Dallas, TX

Susan Bloomfield, Ph.D.
University of Iowa
Department of Physical Education
Iowa City, IA

Tommy Boone, Ph.D.
Professor, Exercise Physiology
University of Southern Mississippi
School of Human Performance and
    Recreation
Hattiesburg, MS

J. David Branch, M.S.
Department of Exercise Science
The University of South Carolina
Columbia, SC

Kelly D. Brownell, Ph.D.
Professor of Psychology
Department of Psychology
Yale University
New Haven, CT

Maria Lonnett Burgess, Ph.D
Medical School at the University of South
    Carolina
Columbia, SC

Carl J. Caspersen, Ph.D.
Cardiovascular Health Branch
Division of Chronic Disease Control and
    Community Intervention
National Center for Chronic Disease
    Prevention and Health Promotion
Centers for Disease Control
Atlanta, GA

Edward F. Coyle, Ph.D., F.A.C.S.M.
Director, Human Performance Laboratory
College of Education
The University of Texas at Austin
Department of Physical and Health Education
Austin, TX

Nicholas Cucuzzo, Ph.D.
Department of Nutrition, Food, and
    Movement Sciences
The Florida State University
Tallahassee, FL

Donald M. Cummings
Assistant Professor
Department of Professional Physical
    Education
East Stroudsburg University
East Stroudsburg, PA

Ami M. Drimmer, Ph.D.
Research Associate
Institute for Aerobics Research
Dallas, TX

J. Larry Durstine, Ph.D., F.A.C.S.M.
Associate Professor
Department of Exercise Science
The University of South Carolina
Columbia, SC

Robert S. Eliot, M.D., F.A.C.C.
Institute of Stress Medicine
Denver, CO
Clinical Professor of Medicine
University of Nebraska Medical Center
Omaha, NE

Darlene Fink-Bennett, M.D.
Vice Chief, Nuclear Medicine
Department of Medicine, Division of
    Cardiology
William Beaumont Hospital
Royal Oak, MI

Robert H. Fitts, Ph.D., F.A.C.S.M.
Professor of Biology
Department of Biology
Marquette University
Milwaukee, WI

Terry A. Fortin, M.S.
Research Assistant
Brockton/West Roxbury
Department of Veterans Affairs
West Roxbury, MA

Barry A. Franklin, Ph.D., F.A.C.S.M.
Program Director, Cardiac Rehabilitation and
  Exercise Laboratories
Department of Medicine, Division of
  Cardiology
William Beaumont Hospital
Royal Oak, MI

Larry R. Gettman, Ph.D., F.A.C.S.M.
Vice President, Research and Development
National Health Enhancement Systems, Inc.
Phoenix, AZ

Neil F. Gordon, M.D., Ph.D., F.A.C.S.M.
Director, Exercise Physiology
The Cooper Institute for Aerobics Research
Dallas, TX

Andrew M. Gottlieb, Ph.D.
Clinical Psychologist
Stanford University Medical Center
Stanford, CA

Daniel G. Graetzer, Ph.D.
Assistant Professor
Human Performance Laboratory
University of Montana
Missoula, MT

William C. Grantham, M.S.
General Manager
Little Rock Athletic Club
Little Rock, AR

Carlos M. Grilo, Ph.D.
Department of Psychology
Yale University
New Haven, CT

Linda K. Hall, Ph.D., F.A.C.S.M.
Director, Cardiac Rehabilitation
Allegheny General Hospital
Pittsburgh, PA

Susan J. Hall, Ph.D., F.A.C.S.M.
Associate Professor
Department of Kinesiology
California State University at Northridge
Northridge, CA

Peter Hanson, M.D.
Professor of Medicine
Director, Preventive Cardiology
University of Wisconsin Clinical Science
  Center
Madison, WI

William L. Haskell, M.D., F.A.C.S.M.
Associate Professor of Medicine
Division of Cardiology
Stanford University
Stanford, CA

George Havenith, Drs.
TNO Institute for Perception
Soesterburg, The Netherlands

Gregory W. Heath, D.H.Sc., M.P.H.,
  F.A.C.S.M.
Health Intervention and Translation Branch
Division of Chronic Disease Control and
  Community Intervention
National Center for Chronic Disease
  Prevention and Health Promotion
Centers for Disease Control
Atlanta, GA

David L. Herbert, J.D.
Attorney
The Belpar Law Center
Canton, OH

William G. Herbert, Ph.D., F.A.C.S.M.
Professor, Health, Physical Education and
  Recreation
Virginia Tech University
Blacksburg, VA

Robert G. Holly, Ph.D., F.A.C.S.M.
Department of Physical Education
University of California–Davis
Davis, CA

Edward T. Howley, Ph.D., F.A.C.S.M.
Professor, Human Performance and Sport
  Studies
University of Tennessee
Knoxville, TN

Bruce H. Jones, M.D., M.P.H., M.A.,
  F.A.C.S.M.
Chief, Occupational Medicine Division
U.S. Army Research Institute of
  Environmental Medicine
Natick, MA

W. Larry Kenney, Ph.D., F.A.C.S.M.
Associate Professor of Applied Physiology
Pennsylvania State University
Laboratory for Human Performance Research
University Park, PA

Abby C. King, Ph.D.
Assistant Professor of Health Research and
   Policy and Medicine
Stanford University School of Medicine
Stanford, CA

Jamil A. Kirdar, M.D.
Director, Cardiac Rehabilitation
Instructor in Medicine
Harvard Medical School
Boston, MA
Department of Veterans Affairs
West Roxbury, MA

Julia M. Lash, Ph.D.
Assistant Professor
Department of Physiology and Biophysics
Indiana University School of Medicine
Indianapolis, IN

Wendell Liehmon, Ph.D.
Professor of Exercise Science
Department of Human Performance and
   Sport Studies
University of Tennessee-Knoxville
Knoxville, TN

Paul J. Lloyd, Ph.D.
Professor, Chairperson
Department of Psychology
Southeast Missouri State University
Cape Girardeau, MO

John E. Martin, Ph.D.
Professor of Psychology
San Diego State University
San Diego, CA

Mike McGahan, M.D.
Emergency Physicians Networks
St. Elizabeth Hospital
Lincoln, NE

Kevin M. McIntyre, M.D., J.D.
Staff Cardiologist
Assistant Clinical Professor of Medicine
Harvard Medical School
Boston, MA
Brockton/West Roxbury
Department of Veterans Affairs
West Roxbury, MA

Patricia J. McSwegin, Ph.D., F.A.C.S.M.
Associate Professor
Chair, Department of Physical Education
University of Missouri at Kansas City
Kansas City, MO

Stephen P. Messier, Ph.D., F.A.C.S.M.
Professor
Department of Health and Sport Science,
   Wake Forest University
Winston-Salem, NC

Nancy Houston Miller, R.N.
Department of Cardiology
Stanford University Medical Center
Stanford, CA

Brenda S. Mitchell, Ph.D., F.A.C.S.M.
Director, Behavioral Science and Health
   Promotion
The Cooper Institute for Aerobics Research
Dallas, TX

Jere H. Mitchell, M.D., F.A.C.S.M.
Professor
Harry S. Moss Heart Center
Departments of Internal Medicine and
   Physiology
University of Texas Southwestern Medical
   Center
Dallas, TX

Robert J. Moffatt, Ph.D.
Department of Nutrition, Food, and
   Movement Sciences
The Florida State University
Tallahassee, FL

Michael P. Moore, M.D.
Rehabilitation and Physical Medicine
Tennessee Orthopaedics
Lebanon, TN

Barbara R. Newman, M.S.
Center for Research in Disease Prevention
Stanford University
Stanford, CA

Patricia L. Painter, Ph.D., F.A.C.S.M.
Director, Transplant Rehabilitation
University of California at San Francisco
San Francisco, CA

Diane Panton Lapsley, M.S., R.N., C.S.
Cardiovascular Clinical Specialist/Research
　Nurse
Brockton/West Roxbury
Department of Veterans Affairs
West Roxbury, MA

Russell R. Pate, Ph.D., F.A.C.S.M.
Professor
Department of Exercise Science
The University of South Carolina
Columbia, SC

Gregory Pavlides, M.D.
Director, Invasive Echocardiography
Department of Medicine, Division of
　Cardiology
William Beaumont Hospital
Royal Oak, MI

Cynthia L. Pemberton, Ph.D.
Associate Professor
Department of Physical Education
University of Missouri at Kansas City
Kansas City, MO

Scott K. Powers, Ph.D., Ed.D., F.A.C.S.M.
Professor and Co-Director, Center for
　Exercise Science
Departments of Exercise and Sport Science
　and Physiology
University of Florida
Gainesville, FL

Katy L. Reynolds, M.D.
Research Medical Officer
Occupational Medicine Division
U.S. Army Research Institute of
　Environmental Medicine
Natick, MA

Paul B. Rock, D.O., Ph.D.
Flight Surgeon, Altitude Physiology and
　Medicine Division
U.S. Army Research Institute of
　Environmental Medicine
Natick, MA

Jeffrey L. Roitman, Ed.D., F.A.C.S.M.
Director of Cardiac Rehabilitation
Research Medical Center
Kansas City, MO

Deborah Brown Rupp, M.S.
Georgia State University
Atlanta, GA

David P. L. Sachs, M.D.
Clinical Assistant Professor of Medicine
Stanford University School of Medicine
Director, Center for Pulmonary Disease
　Prevention
Director, Smoking Cessation Research
　Institute
Stanford, CA

Robert D. Safian, M.D.
Director, Interventional Cardiology
Department of Medicine, Division of
　Cardiology
William Beaumont Hospital
Royal Oak, MI

Vicky Savas, M.D.
Academic Attending Cardiologist
Department of Medicine, Division of
　Cardiology
William Beaumont Hospital
Royal Oak, MI

J. P. Schaman, M.D.
Medical Director
Rehabilitation and Sports Medicine
Ontario Aerobics Centre
Breslau, Ontario, Canada

Brian J. Sharkey, Ph.D., F.A.C.S.M.
Professor
Human Performance Laboratory
University of Montana
Missoula, MT

Roy J. Shephard, M.D., Ph.D., D.P.E.,
　F.A.C.S.M.
Professor of Applied Physiology
School of Physical and Health Education
University of Toronto
Toronto, Ontario, Canada

W. Michael Sherman, Ph.D., F.A.C.S.M.
Associate Professor
Exercise Physiology Laboratory
School of Health, Physical Education, and
　Recreation
The Ohio State University
Columbus, OH

Wesley E. Sime, M.P.H., Ph.D.
Departments of Health and Human
　Performance and Counseling Psychology
University of Nebraska
Lincoln, NE

Michael L. Smith, Ph.D.
Assistant Professor
Department of Medicine
Case Western Reserve University
Cleveland, OH

Ray W. Squires, Ph.D., F.A.C.S.M.,
    F.A.A.C.V.P.R.
Associate Professor of Medicine, Mayo
    Medical School
Director, Cardiovascular Health Clinic and
    Exercise Electrocardiography Laboratory
Consultant in the Division of Cardiovascular
    Diseases and Internal Medicine
Mayo Clinic and Foundation
Rochester, MN

Suzanne Nelson Steen, M.S., R.D.
Sports Nutritionist
University of Pennsylvania
School of Medicine
Philadelphia, PA

William E. Strauss, M.D.
Assistant Professor of Medicine
Harvard Medical School
Boston, MA
Director, Preventive Cardiology
Brockton/West Roxbury
Department of Veterans Affairs
West Roxbury, MA

C. Barr Taylor, M.D.
Professor of Psychiatry
Stanford University School of Medicine
Stanford, CA

Paul D. Thompson, M.D., F.A.C.S.M.
Director, Preventive Cardiology
University of Pittsburgh Heart Institute
Pittsburgh, PA

James A. Vogel, Ph.D., F.A.C.S.M.
Director, Occupational Health and
    Performance
U.S. Army Research Institute of
    Environmental Medicine
Natick, MA

Neil B. Vroman, R.P.T., Ph.D., F.A.C.S.M.
Associate Professor
Department of Physical Education
University of New Hampshire
Durham, NH

Steven P. Van Camp, M.D., F.A.C.S.M.
Professor
College of Professional Studies
San Diego State University
Alvarado Medical Group
San Diego, CA

William L. Williams, M.D.
Associate Professor of Medicine
University of Ottawa Heart Institute
Ottawa, Ontario, Canada

Linda D. Zwiren, Ph.D., F.A.C.S.M.
Department of Health, Physical Education
    and Recreation
Department of Biology
Hofstra University
Hempstead, NY

Contents

Section VII: Human Development and Aging
Abby C. King, Ph.D., Section Editor

Section VIII: Human Behavior/Psychology
Abby C. King, Ph.D., Section Editor

Section IX: Administrative Concerns
Jeffrey Roitman, Ed.D., Section Editor

Section I

APPLIED ANATOMY

Chapter 1

SURFACE ANATOMY FOR EXERCISE PROGRAMMING

Tommy Boone and Linda D. Zwiren

ANATOMIC SITES FOR THE LIMB AND CHEST LEADS

Impulse formation and conduction throughout the heart produce electric currents, which are conveyed through tissues to the surface of the skin by salts dissolved in the body fluids.[1] The electrocardiogram (ECG or EKG) is a graphic record of these electric currents of the heart. The usefulness of the ECG depends on a knowledge of the anatomic landmarks where electrodes are placed, producing the various ECG lead configurations as well as appropriate electrode site preparation. The standard ECG recording system is the 10-electrode combination that permits recording of the standard 12-lead ECG.[2] Of six frontal plane (limb) leads in the 12-lead ECG, three are bipolar (I, II, and III) and three are unipolar (aVR, aVL, and aVF). Bipolar leads represent a difference of electric potential between two sites, whereas unipolar leads measure the electric potential at a specific site. The remaining six leads are unipolar precordial (chest) leads (V_1 through V_6). The frontal plane is represented by the anterior surface of the thorax (chest). The precordial leads form a roughly horizontal plane through the thorax and perpendicular to the frontal plane (Fig. 1–1).

Electrodes may be in a standard or modified placement. Standard placement is most appropriate for recording resting ECGs in the supine patient before exercise testing. Because standard conditions exist, this ECG is a point of comparison for all other preceding and succeeding standard ECGs obtained in this or any other setting. Modified electrode placement is appropriate in the exercise setting because the focus is on obtaining a quality ECG tracing during exercise with an emphasis on ST segments and rhythm changes.

The commonly accepted modification of electrode placement for exercise is the Mason-Likar placement.[3] For this hook-up, the axis of lead I extends from the right shoulder (RA), which is the negative electrode, to the left shoulder (LA), which is the positive electrode (Fig. 1–1). For exercise (not supine rest, in which the wrists and ankles are used), the negative or RA electrode of lead I is positioned in the right infraclavicular fossa. This site is located on the upper right aspect of the chest-shoulder region just below the distal end of the right clavicle. Anatomically, this site is described as the anterior surface of the thorax between the superior margin of the right fan-shaped pectoralis major muscle and the medial border of the right anterior deltoid muscle. The positive or LA electrode of lead I is placed in the left infraclavicular fossa, which is located on the upper left aspect of the chest-shoulder region just inferior to the distal end of the left clavicle. Anatomically, this site is located on the anterior surface of the thorax between the superior border of the left pectoralis major muscle and the medial border of the left anterior deltoid. The axis of lead II extends from the right shoulder, which is the negative electrode, to the left leg (LL), which is the positive electrode. The positive electrode of lead II is positioned on the lower left anterior surface of the external oblique muscle. This site is just above the iliac crest at the level of the navel on the outer third of the anterior surface of the abdomen. The axis of lead III is the difference of potential between the LL and the LA electrodes. The negative electrode is on the LA and the positive electrode is on the LL. The placement of the right leg (RL) electrode, which is the ground electrode, is consistent with the procedure outlined for the LL electrode except that it is placed on the anterior surface of the right external

3

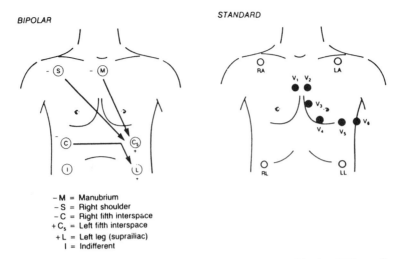

BIPOLAR

STANDARD

− M = Manubrium
− S = Right shoulder
− C = Right fifth interspace
+ C$_s$ = Left fifth interspace
+ L = Left leg (suprailiac)
 I = Indifferent

Fig. 1–1. Electrocardiographic (ECG) leads used in exercise testing. Bipolar ECG configurations (left) are variations of V$_5$, using sternal (CS-5) or manubrial (CM-5) lead placements along with an indifferent reference lead. The 10-electrode (Mason-Likar) placement (right) permits standard 12-lead ECG tracings during exercise. (Modified from Chaitman B et al.: *Am J Cardiol 47*:1335–1349, 1981.) With permission from *ACSM's Guidelines for Exercise Testing and Prescription.* Philadelphia: Lea & Febiger, 1991.

oblique muscle. The LL and RL positions may need to be modified to avoid motion artifact caused by the electrode box belt rubbing on the electrode or excessive suprailiac fat deposition. If the electrodes are moved, care should be taken to avoid placement on the rib cage, which significantly affects vectors and masks inferior myocardial infractions.

The three unipolar limb leads are aVR, aVL, and aVF. The letter "a" refers to augmented or increased voltage. The "R," "L," and "F" indicate the location of the positive electrode: R indicates the RA (right arm) position, L indicates the LA (left arm) position, and F denotes the foot (actually, LL, left leg) position.[4] The three augmented unipolar leads are recorded from the same electrodes as leads I, II, and III.

Although the precordial ("V") electrodes are positioned predominantly on the left side of the anterior chest wall, the precordial electrode site for V$_1$ is the fourth intercostal space on the right border of the sternum.[5] This space (between the fourth and fifth ribs) may be identified by locating the proximal end of the clavicle (at the root of the neck) and sliding the fingers inferiorly (caudal) alongside of the sternum into the first intercostal space. Continue to slide the fingers over the ribs into the intercostal

spaces until reaching the fourth space. V$_2$ is also positioned in the fourth intercostal space, but on the left sternal border. V$_4$ is located in the fifth intercostal space at about the midpoint of the clavicle. Electrode placement for V$_3$ is equidistant (midway) between V$_2$ and V$_4$. The electrode site for V$_5$ is horizontal to V$_4$ in the anterior axillary line. V$_6$ is lateral to and at the same level as V$_5$ in the midaxillary line.[6] Note that V$_4$, V$_5$, and V$_6$ are on the same level and do not curve upward to follow the fifth intercostal space (refer to Fig. 1–1).

In some instances, particularly during exercise testing of obese individuals or women with large breasts, moving a precordial lead to a lower intercostal space may be necessary, such as positioning V$_4$ or V$_5$ in the sixth intercostal space. In women, the wearing of an undergarment to support the breasts during exercise might help to reduce motion artifacts leading to extremely poor quality ECG recordings. If electrodes are moved from the standard exercise positions, this should be noted on the test results.

Single-lead ECG recording during exercise, although not ideal, is not uncommon. Modified lead placements are usually utilized. Leads CC$_5$ or CM$_5$, which are anterolateral leads, similar to the unipolar precordial V_5 lead, are the best choices for a single-lead recording. Lead CC_5 places the negative electrode on the right clavicle and the positive electrode at the same site as V_5. Lead CM_5 places the negative electrode of the manubrium and the positive electrode at the same site as V_5.

"Mixed" lead systems include some combination of the 12 leads normally used. One common combination is Lead II (aVF), V_1, and V_5 which allows frontal and horizontal plane views of inferior, lateral and anterior leads (see Fig. 1–1).

Proper preparation of the anatomic skin-electrode sites is especially important. The overall quality of the site for electrode placement is improved first by shaving hair if necessary, second by removing surface body oil and dirt with a fat solvent such as isopropyl alcohol or acetone, and third by removing the superficial layer of the skin by abrading with fine-grain emery paper, dental burr, gauze, or other appropriate material. Abrasion should result in an erythema (reddening) of the skin at the electrode site, but should not result in bleeding. The goal of the electrode site preparation is to reduce impedance to 5000 ohms or less, which can be verified before the exercise test with an inexpensive AC impedance meter driven at 10 Hz. Do not use a DC meter because it can polarize the electrodes. Each electrode is tested against a common electrode with the ohm meter, and when 5000 ohms or less is not achieved, the electrode must be removed and skin preparation repeated. This maneuver saves time by obviating the need to interrupt a test because of noisy tracings.[7,8]

Excessive motion artifact resulting from movement of the chest electrodes during exercise can be minimized or even avoided in individuals with oily skin or who sweat excessively by using an additional adhesive (such as tincture of bezoin) to increase the stickiness of the electrodes. The lead wires can also be looped and taped on the torso to minimize pull on the electrode.

ANATOMIC SITES FOR MEASUREMENT OF BLOOD PRESSURE

A stethoscope and a sphygmomanometer are used in the indirect measurement (auscultation) of systematic arterial blood pressure, which is the force exerted by the blood against the walls of blood vessels. A sphygmomanometer includes an inflatable cuff connected by rubber tubes to a manometer (either mercury or aneroid) and a rubber bulb to regulate air during inflation and deflation of the cuff (Fig. 1–2).

The deflated cuff is wrapped snugly around the upper arm, centering the bladder over the brachial artery. The lower margin of the cuff should be about 1 inch (2.5 cm) above the antecubital fossa.[9] Palpate the brachial artery (located on the medial aspect of the antecubital fossa), and then fit the diaphragm of the stethoscope firmly (with light pressure) over the brachial pulse point during cuff inflation. Anatomically, the brachial artery courses in the groove between the biceps brachii (anterior arm muscle) and the triceps brachii (posterior arm muscle) just at the inner surface of the elbow (antecubital fossa). (See

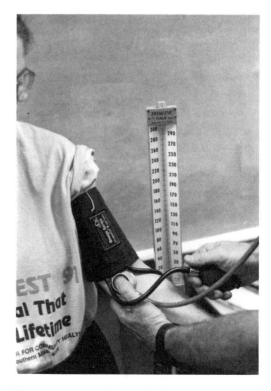

Fig. 1–2. Anatomic site for the measurement of blood pressure. The sphygmomanometer consists of an inflatable cuff connected by rubber tubes to a manometer and a rubber bulb to regulate air during the auscultation of blood pressure by a stethoscope.

Appendix 1 for complete description of the technique used in measuring blood pressure.)

ANATOMIC SITES IN DETERMINING THE PERIPHERAL PULSES

Carotid Pulse: The common carotid arteries on both sides of the neck have similar anatomic landmarks. The common carotid pulse can be found in the neck bounded by the body of the mandible (lower jawbone), the sternocleidomastoid muscle, and the larynx ("Adam's apple") (Fig. 1–3). The carotid arterial pulses are palpated by gently compressing inward and backward along the anterior border of the sternocleidomastoid muscle at the level of the thyroid cartilage.[10,11]

The carotid pulses are palpated singly (i.e., one carotid artery at a time) by placing the first two fingers (not the thumb) lightly on, for example, the right carotid artery (refer to Fig. 1–3). Although this method is commonly used to estimate exercise heart rate after exercise is stopped, reports have shown that carotid artery palpation may produce bradycardia (slowing of the heart rate) in some individuals[12,13] but have little to no effect on heart rate at rest or during exercise and recovery in other individuals.[14,15] This method would be inappropriate in patients who have various forms of vascular disease that affect the sensitivity of the carotid sinus.[16]

Radial Pulse: The radial artery descends on the lateral (thumb) side of the forearm to become quite superficial at the distal (lower) end of the radius.[17] It is at this point that the pulse is usually taken by gently compressing the artery against the anterior surface of the distal end of the radius (Fig.1–4). The pulse (i.e., the pressure wave that expands the arterial walls) is felt in the radial artery at the wrist about 0.1 second after the peak of systolic ejection into the aorta.[18]

Lower Extremity Pulses: Some information about cardiac function can be revealed from assessment of the peripheral pulses. The information is valuable, particularly with respect to peripheral perfusion. In the cardiac subject, palpation of the dorsalis pedis artery and posterior tibial artery must be gentle to avoid further marked reduction in arterial flow. In that the pulses may be either difficult to palpate or congenitally absent, bilateral comparison is frequently necessary.

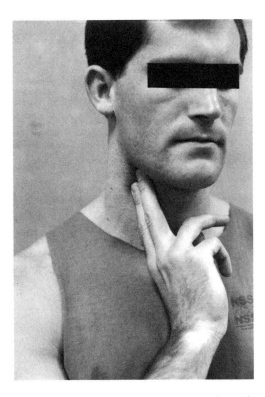

Fig. 1–3. Anatomic site for palpating the right carotid artery. Note that one side is palpated at a time. Avoid massaging or applying too much pressure on the carotid sinus, which is located at the level of the thyroid cartilage just below the angle of the jaw.

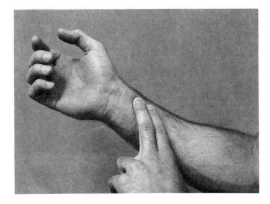

Fig. 1–4. Anatomic site for palpating the right radial artery, which is located on the flexor surface of the wrist laterally.

The inguinal ligament runs from the anterior superior iliac spine (the uppermost and largest anatomic landmark of the ilium) to the pubic symphysis (where the two pubic bones articulate).[19] The femoral artery enters the anterior thigh posterior to the inguinal ligament approximately midway between the anterior superior iliac spine and pubic symphysis. This location is the point at which the femoral artery is readily palpated, because it can be pressed posteriorly against the pectineus muscle and the superior ramus of the pubic bone (Fig. 1–5).

The popliteal artery lies deep within the popliteal fossa (a diamond-shaped area behind the distal end of the femur).[20] The knee joint should be flexed to relax the deep fascia and related muscle. Then the pulse may be determined as the fingertips press deeply into the popliteal fossa (Fig. 1–6).

To locate the posterior tibial artery, the fingers should be placed about halfway between the medial malleolus (distal end of the tibia) and the medial aspect of the tendo calcaneus (Achilles' tendon). The artery is palpated by positioning the fingers between the tendons of the flexor hallucis longus and flexor digitorum longus muscles (Fig. 1–7).

With the foot in dorsiflexion to obviate tension on the artery, the pulsations of the dorsalis pedis artery can be felt between the tendons of the extensor hallucis longus and the extensor digitorum longus muscles (Fig. 1–8). Even though this artery is typically located on the dorsum (top) of the foot between the two malleoli, clinically insignificant congenital absence or variation in the arteries to the foot may result in only one pedal pulse or no dorsal pedal pulses.[21–23]

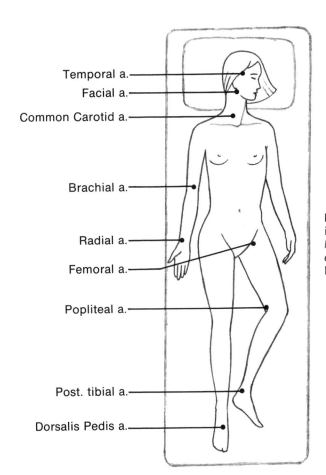

Temporal a.
Facial a.
Common Carotid a.
Brachial a.
Radial a.
Femoral a.
Popliteal a.
Post. tibial a.
Dorsalis Pedis a.

Fig. 1–5. Anatomic site for palpating various pulses. Redrawn with permission from Marieb EN: *Human Anatomy and Physiology*. Redwood, CA: Benjamin/Cummings Publishing Co., Inc., 1992, p. 636.

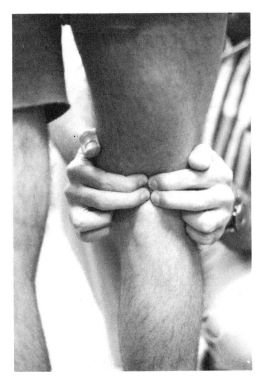

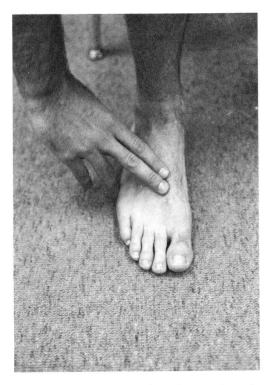

Fig. 1–6. Anatomic site for palpating the right popliteal artery, which is a continuation of the femoral artery and is located behind the knee.

Fig. 1–8. Anatomic site for palpating the right dorsalis pedis artery, which is felt in the groove between the first two tendons on the medial side of the dorsum (top) of the foot.

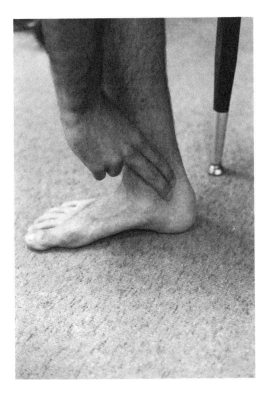

ANTHROPOMETRIC MEASUREMENTS

Basic human anthropometry includes standing height, body weight, girths, bone widths, and skin fold measurements. These measurements can be placed into regression equations to estimate percentage of body fat and the general external morphologic structure of the body.[24] Commonly used anthropometric measures are described below. *However, if anthropometric measures are to be used in specific regression equations not cited in this chapter, measurements must be taken precisely as described for the equation being used.*

Standing Height: An individual's height should be measured against a vertical upright (such as a wall). Heel, buttocks, and upper back should be touching the vertical upright. The chin should be level and not

Fig. 1–7. Anatomic site for palpating the right posterior tibial artery, which is located behind and below the medial malleolus.

lifted. The individual should be barefoot (or wearing thin socks) and wear limited clothing so that positioning of the body can be seen. A horizontal headboard should be used to contact the most superior point of the head. Record height to the nearest 0.1 cm or to the nearest $\frac{1}{4}$ of an inch.[25,26]

Body Weight: Body weight should be measured while the individual is standing on a leveled platform scale with a beam and movable weights. Light clothing should be worn, excluding shoes, long trousers, sweaters, or sweat shirts. Note the individual's dress if it is not lightweight clothing. Record body weight in pounds (nearest $\frac{1}{4}$ lb.) and/or in kilograms (to the nearest 100 grams).[26]

Girth or Circumference: Girth or circumference measurement requires use of a tape measure. The tape should be flexible but inelastic (nonstretchable), should preferably have only one ruling on a side (i.e., metric or English) and should be about 0.7 cm wide. If the tape has a spring-retractable mechanism at its end, it should be held so that retraction spring tension does not affect the measurement.

The tension applied to the tape by the measurer affects the validity and reliability of the measurements. The tape is held snugly around the body part, but not tightly enough to compress the subcutaneous adipose tissue (check that the tape is not indenting the skin or that there are gaps between the tape and the skin). Whenever possible, take measurements on bare skin.

Measurement of selected sites is described as follows, so that standardization and precision can be increased (Fig. 1–9).

Abdomen: With the subject's abdomen relaxed, a horizontal measure is taken at the level of the umbilicus.

Calf: With the subject standing erect, a horizontal measure is taken at the level of *maximum* circumference between the knee and the ankle.

Forearm: With the subject standing erect with arms hanging downward but slightly away from the trunk and palms facing forward, the measure is taken perpendicular to the long axis of the forearm at the level of *maximum* circumference.

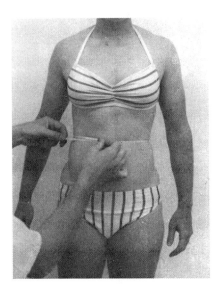

A. Measurement of waist circumference.

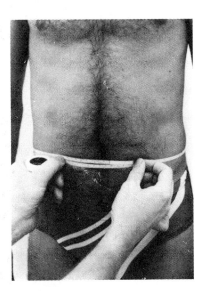

B. Measurement of abdominal circumference.

Fig. 1–9. Locations for circumference measurement with permission from Lohman TG, Roche AF, Martorell R (Eds.): *Anthropometric Standardization Reference Manual.* Champaign, IL: Human Kinetics Publishers, 1988, pp. 45–53.

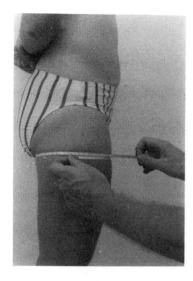

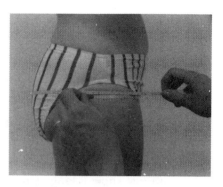

D. Measurement of buttocks (hip).

C. Measurement of proximal thigh.

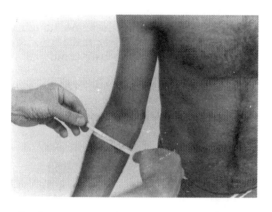

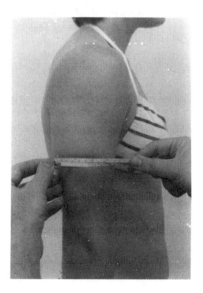

E. Measurement of forearm circumference.

F. Measurement of arm circumference.

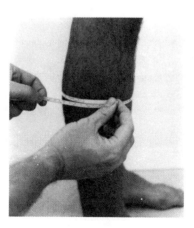

G. Measurement of calf circumference.

Fig. 1–9. (*Continued*)

Hip/Buttocks: With the subject standing erect naturally, a horizontal measure is taken at the *maximum* circumference. (The individual should be wearing a thin swimsuit or briefs.) The measurer should squat at the side of the individual so that maximum extension of the buttocks can be seen.

Arm: With the subject's arm to the side of the body, a horizontal measure is taken midway between the acromion and olecranon processes.

Waist: With the subject's abdomen relaxed, a horizontal measure is taken at the level of the narrowest part of the torso.

Thigh: With the subject's legs slightly apart, a horizontal measure is taken at the maximum circumference, just below the gluteal fold.

For the abdomen and hip/buttocks measurements, because the placement of the measurer is at the individual's side, an assistant on the opposite side would be helpful to ensure that the tape is level.

Skin-fold Measurements: The following subcutaneous skin fold sites are described for use in determining body composition with the Jackson and Pollack[27] and Jackson, Pollack, and Ward[28] equations (Fig. 1–10).

Abdominal: A vertical fold taken at a distance of 2 cm to the right side of the umbilicus.

Biceps: A vertical fold on the anterior aspect of the arm over the belly of the biceps muscle; 1 cm above the level used to mark the triceps.

Chest/Pectoral: A diagonal fold taken one half of the distance between the anterior axillary line and the nipple (men) and one third of the distance between the anterior axillary line and the nipple (women).

Medial Calf: A vertical fold at a level of the maximum circumference of the calf on the midline of the medial border.

Midaxillary: A vertical fold taken on the midaxillary line at the level of the xiphoid process of the sternum. (An alternative method is a horizontal fold taken at the level of the xiphoid/sternal border in the midaxillary line.)[26]

Subscapular: An angular fold taken at a 45-degree angle 1 to 2 cm below the inferior angle of the scapula.

Suprailium: An oblique fold taken in line with the natural angle of the iliac crest taken in the anterior axillary line immediately superior to the iliac crest.

Thigh: A vertical fold on the anterior midline of the thigh, midway between the proximal border of the patella and the inguinal crease (hip).

Triceps: A vertical fold on the posterior midline of the upper right arm, halfway between the acromion and the olecranon processes, with the arm held freely to the side of the body.

Bone Widths: Bone diameters (body breadths) are often used as indices of body frame or in somatotyping. Body breadth sites are typically defined by bony landmarks. Therefore, it is important to be able to palpate the bony landmarks. If this cannot be done (e.g., in obese individuals), selection of an alternative site is appropriate. Body breadths are typically measured by special calipers that have narrow or broad blades that slide open and closed (anthropometers). The biacromial, bi-iliac, and knee breadth measurements are described below. Measurements are recorded to the nearest 0.1 cm.

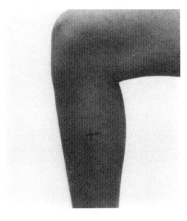

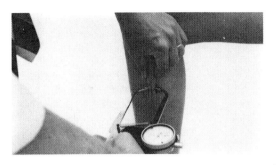

B.   Measurement of medial calf skinfold.

A.   Foot placed on platform or box for location of medial calf skinfold site.

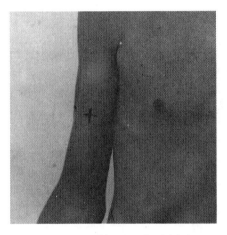

C.   Location of biceps skinfold site.

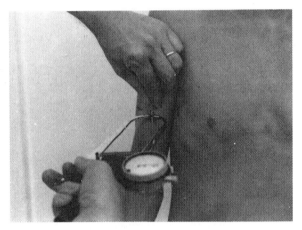

D.   Measurement of biceps skinfold.

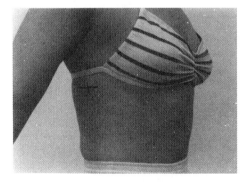

E.   Subject position for midaxillary skinfold measurement.

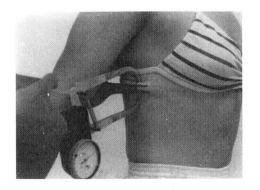

F.   Measurement of midaxillary skinfold.

Fig. 1–10.   (*Legend on p. 14*)

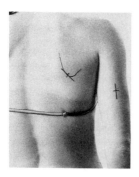

G. Location of scapula skinfold.

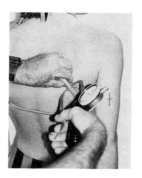

H. Measurement of scapula skinfold.

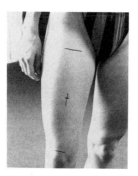

I. Location of thigh skinfold.

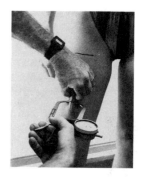

J. Measurement of thigh skinfold.

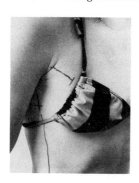

K. Location of pectoral skinfold.

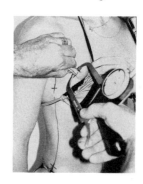

L. Measurement of pectoral skinfold.

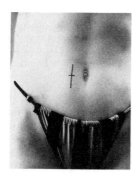

M. Location of abdominal skinfold.

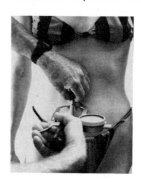

N. Measurement of abdominal skinfold.

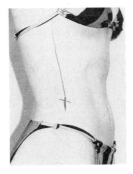

O. Location of hip skinfold.

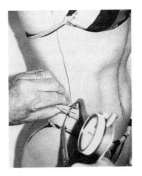

P. Measurement of hip skinfold.

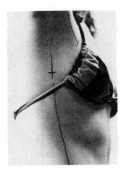

Q. Location of axilla skinfold.

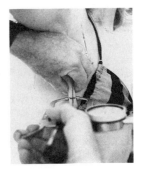

R. Measurement of axilla skinfold.

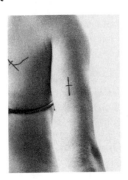

S. Location of tricep skinfold.

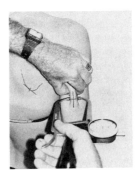

T. Measurement of tricep skinfold.

Fig. 1–10. Locations for skinfold measurements. **A** through **F** with permission from Lohman TG, Roche AF, Martorelli R (Eds.): *Anthropometric Standardization Reference Manual.* Champaign, IL: Human Kinetics Publishers, 1988, pp. 59, 66, 67. **G** through **S** with permission from Golding LA, Meyers CR, Sinning WE (Eds.): *Y's Way to Physical Fitness.* Champaign, IL: Human Kinetics Publishers, 1989, pp. 86–88.

BIACROMIAL BREADTH. The measurer should stand behind the individual so that the acromial processes can be located easily. The individual is standing with heels together and arms hanging at the side. Measurement should be taken on the skin. The individual is relaxed, with shoulders downward and slightly forward so that the reading is maximal. The measurer runs his or her hands from the base of the neck outward to the tips of the shoulders. The most lateral borders of the acromial processes are palpated and the blades of the anthropometer are applied firmly to the most lateral borders of the acromial processes (Fig. 1–11).[26]

BI-ILIAC BREADTH. The measurement is made from the rear with the individual to

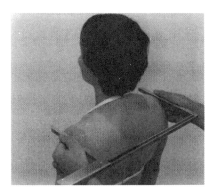

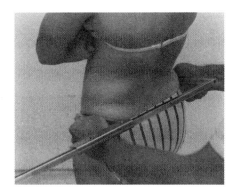

A. Anthropometer in place for biacromial breadth measurement.

B. Anthropometer in place for bi-iliac breadth measurement.

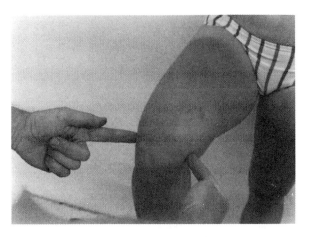

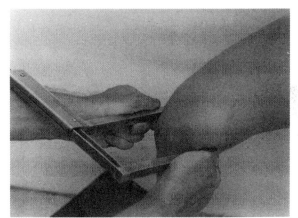

C. Location of lateral aspects of femoral condyles.

D. Caliper in place for knee breadth measurement.

Fig. 1–11. Locations for measurement of body breadths: Biacromial, bi-iliac, knee. With permission from Lohman TG, Roche AF, Martorelli R (Eds.): *Anthropomorphic Standardization Reference Manual.* Champaign, IL: Human Kinetics Publishers, 1989, pp. 29, 32, 34.

be measured standing with the feet slightly apart and arms folded across the chest. The anthropometer blades are applied at a downward angle of 45 degrees with firm pressure on the iliac crests. Maximum breadth is recorded (Fig. 1–11).[26]

KNEE BREADTH. This is the distance between the most medial and most lateral aspects of the femoral epicondyles. The individual is seated with the leg flexed 90 degrees, or can be standing with the leg flexed at the hip and knees and the foot resting on a platform. The measurer stands in front, facing the individual. The anthropometer is held diagonally downward and toward the subject. The blades are placed firmly on the most lateral point of the lat-

eral epicondyle and the most medial aspect of the medial epicondyle (Fig. 1–11).[26]

SURFACE ANATOMY OF THE STERNUM

The sternum (Fig. 1–12) is located in the midline of the chest. The sternum consists of three parts. The most superior part, the manubrium, is shaped like a necktie knot. Laterally, the manubrium articulates with the clavicles and the first two pairs of ribs. The body (midportion) forms the bulk of the sternum. The third to seventh ribs articulate with the body of the sternum. The xiphoid process forms the inferior part of the sternum and does not articulate with any ribs.

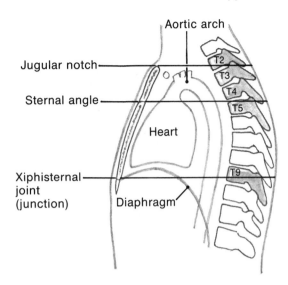

Fig. 1-12. Left lateral view of the thorax, illustrating the relationship of the surface anatomical landmarks of the thorax to the vertebral column (thoracic portion). Redrawn with permission from Marieb EN: *Human Anatomy and Physiology.* Redwood, CA: Benjamin/Cummings Publishing Co., Inc., 1992, p. 201.

The sternum has three major surface anatomic landmarks. The jugular (suprasternal) notch (the superior aspect of the manubrium) is an easily felt indentation at the base of the neck. The jugular notch is generally in line with the intervertebral disk between the second and third thoracic vertebrae and overlies the point where the left common carotid artery exits from the aorta.[29] Traveling slightly down the sternum from the jugular notch, a horizontal ridge or prominence can be felt. This is the sternal angle, the point at which the manubrium joins the sternum. The second rib is found lateral to the sternal angle. Therefore, the sternal angle is a reference point for finding the second rib and for counting the other ribs and intercostal spaces.

The xiphoid process articulates only with the body of the sternum and sometimes projects backwards. If compressed sharply, the xiphoid has the potential to be pushed into the heart or liver.[29]

Therefore, during cardiopulmonary resuscitation (CPR), it is important that compressions be done on the body of the sternum and not over the xiphoid process. To find the appropriate placement of the hands for CPR compression (while kneeling next to the individual), take the index and middle fingers (of the hand that is toward the stomach) and follow the lower border of the rib cage toward the midline until you feel the notch where the ribs meet. Keeping the middle finger on the notch, place the index finger down. The heel of the other hand should be placed next to and above (i.e., toward the head) the index finger.[30]

REFERENCES

1. Previte JJ: *Human Physiology.* New York: McGraw-Hill, 1983.
2. Hanson P: Clinical exercise testing. In *Sports Medicine.* Edited by RH Strauss. Philadelphia: W.B. Saunders, 1984.
3. Froelicher VF: *Exercise and the Heart: Clinical Concepts.* Yearbook Medical Publishers: 1987, pp. 17–27.
4. Conover MH, Zalis EG: *Understanding Electrocardiography: Physiological and Interpretive Concepts.* 2nd Ed. St. Louis: C.V. Mosby, 1976.
5. Woods SL: Electrocardiography, vectorcardiography, and polarcardiography. In *Cardiac Nursing.* Edited by SL Underhill, SL Woods, ES Sivarajan, and CJ Halpenny. Philadelphia: J.B. Lippincott, 1982.
6. Adamovich DR: *The Heart.* New York: Sports Medicine Books, 1984.
7. Ellestad MH: *Stress Testing: Principles and Practice.* Philadelphia: F.A. Davis, 1986.
8. Froelicher VF: *Exercise and the Heart: Clinical Concepts.* Chicago: Year Book, 1986.
9. American Heart Association (AHA): Recommendations for human blood pressure determination by sphygmomanometers. Report of the Special Task Force, 1987.
10. Hamilton WJ: *Textbook of Human Anatomy.* 2nd Ed. St. Louis: C.V. Mosby, 1976.
11. Snell RS: *Atlas of Clinical Anatomy.* Boston: Little, Brown and Co., 1978.
12. Boone T, Frentz KL, Boyd NR: Carotid palpation at two exercise intensities. *Med Sci Sports Exerc, 17:*705, 1985.

13. White JR: EKG changes using carotid artery for heart rate monitoring. *Med Sci Sports, 9:*88, 1977.
14. Couldry W, Corbin C, Wilcox A: Carotid vs. radial pulse counts. *Phys Sportsmed, 10:* 67, 1982.
15. Gardner GW, Danks DI, Scharfsienin L: Use of carotid pulse for heart rate monitoring. *Med Sci Sports, 11:*111, 1979.
16. McArdle WD, Katch FI, Katch VL: *Exercise Physiology: Energy, Nutrition, and Human Performance.* Philadelphia, PA: Lea & Febiger, 1991.
17. Spence AP: *Basic Human Anatomy.* Reading, MA: The Benjamin/Cummings Publishing Co., 1982.
18. Ganong WF: *Review of Medical Physiology.* 11th Ed. Los Altos, CA: Lange, 1983.
19. Silverstein A: *Human Anatomy and Physiology.* New York: John Wiley & Sons, 1980.
20. Hoppenfeld S: *Physical Examination of the Spine and Extremities.* New York: Appleton-Century-Crofts, 1976.
21. Snell RS: *Atlas of Clinical Anatomy.* Boston: Little, Brown and Co., 1978.
22. Craven RF: Disorders of the peripheral vascular system. In *Cardiac Nursing.* Edited by SL Underhill, SL Woods, ES Sivarajan, and CJ Halpenny. Philadelphia: J.B. Lipppincott, 1982.
23. Malasanos L, Barkauskas V, Moss M, Stoltenberg-Allen K: *Health Assessment.* St. Louis: C.V. Mosby, 1977.
24. Reid JG, Thomson JM: *Exercise Prescription for Fitness.* Englewood Cliffs, NJ: Prentice-Hall, 1985.
25. Golding LA, Meyers CR, Sinning WE (Eds.): *Y's Way to Physical Fitness.* Champaign, IL: Human Kinetics Publishers, 1989.
26. Lohman TG, Roche AF, Martorell R (Eds): *Anthropometric Standardization Reference Manual.* Champaign, IL: Human Kinetics Publishers, 1988.
27. Jackson AS, Pollack ML. Generalized equations for predicting body density of men. *Brit J Nutr 40:*497–504, 1978.
28. Jackson AS, Pollack ML, Ward A: Generalized equation for predicting body density of women. *Med Sci Sport Exerc 12:*175–182, 1980.
29. Marieb EN: *Human Anatomy and Physiology.* Redwood, CA: Benjamin/Cummings Publishing Co., Inc., 1992.
30. American Red Cross Community CPR Workbook. American National Red Cross. 1988, p. 91.

Chapter 2

FUNDAMENTALS OF CARDIORESPIRATORY ANATOMY

Donald M. Cummings

A fundamental knowledge of gross cardiac and pulmonary anatomy is essential for the practitioner who wishes to understand cardiopulmonary diagnostic testing (i.e., ECG, echocardiography, etc.), acute cardiorespiratory responses during an exercise session, and cardiorespiratory adaptations caused by chronic exposure to exercise. This knowledge provides a solid base for developing a comprehensive program in either preventive or rehabilitative exercise settings. This chapter discusses these two organ systems as they specifically relate to exercise.

CARDIOVASCULAR ANATOMY

The cardiovascular system consists of the heart, blood vessels, and blood. The heart serves as a muscular pump that circulates the blood and each of its components (i.e., oxygen, nutrients, etc.) to all tissue and organ systems of the body by way of the tubular structure of the blood vessels. This section provides a basic anatomic description of these three structures.

The Heart

". . . the heart is no more than the transport system pump; the delivery routes are the hollow blood vessels." (Anderson JE: *Grant's Atlas of Anatomy.* 8th Ed. Baltimore: Williams & Wilkins, 1983, p. 604)

Overview

The heart is a muscular pump. Its walls are made up of three layers: an inner lining (endocardium), an outer protective layer (epicardium), and a middle layer of muscle (myocardium). The myocardium is made up of cells similar to skeletal muscle. The heart is encased in a protective, loose-fitting, tough sac (pericardium).

The heart has four chambers. The upper receiving chambers are called the atria and the lower pumping chambers are the ventricles. The right and left sides of the heart are completely separated by a thick muscle wall called the septum. On each side of the heart, the atrium and ventricle are separated by valves (the atrioventricular valves).

The heart is really a double-close system pump. The left side of the heart (systemic circuit) pumps blood through the aorta to the entire body to supply each cell with oxygen and nutrients and to pick up carbon dioxide and other waste products. Deoxygenated blood returning from the cells of the body is returned (by way of the superior and inferior vena cava) to the right atrium. Blood passes into the right ventricle. The right ventricle of the heart (pulmonary circuit) pumps blood through the pulmonary arteries to the lungs to reoxygenate the blood and to get rid of the carbon dioxide. Blood with high levels of oxygen and low levels of carbon dioxide is returned to the left atrium (by way of pulmonary veins) and flows into the left ventricle to be pumped around the body. Ensuring that blood flows in one direction, and does not fall back into the ventricles when the ventricles are not contracting, is the job of the semilunar valves (located between the ventricles and the large arteries that carry blood away from the heart). See Figure 2–1 for an overview of the flow of blood in the body and in the heart.

The heart chambers contract (systole) and relax (diastole) in a coordinated pattern so that blood continues to flow in the above described direction. This coordinated pattern of contraction is mainly the responsibility of the heart's own internal electrical conducting system. This "in-house" conduction system initiates an action potential (impulse) and makes sure that the heart muscle depolarizes (contracts) in a smooth coordinated fashion.

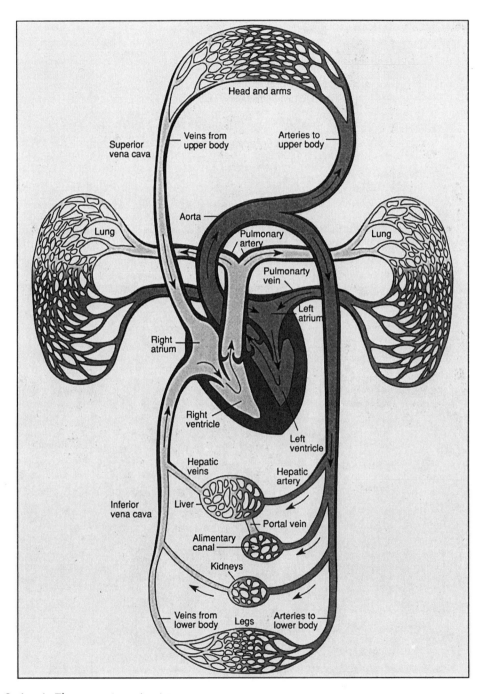

Fig. 2–1.   A. The systemic and pulmonary circuits. The left side of the heart is the systemic pump; the right side is the pulmonary circuit pump. (Although there are two pulmonary arteries, one each to the right and left lung, only one is shown for simplicity.) From McArdle W. D., Katch F. I., and Katch V. L.: *Exercise Physiology*. Philadelphia: Lea & Febiger, 1991, p 293.

Deoxygenated blood returning from the body via Superior & Inferior Vena Cava
↓
RIGHT ATRIUM
↓
tricuspid valve
↓
RIGHT VENTRICLE
↓
semilunar valve
↓
PULMONARY ARTERIES
↓
PULMONARY CAPILLARY BED
↓
PULMONARY VEINS
↓
LEFT ATRIUM
↓
mitral valve
↓
LEFT VENTRICLE
↓
semilunar valve
↓
AORTA
↓

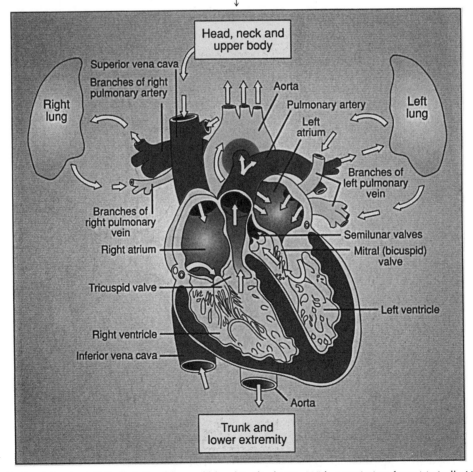

Fig. 2–1. (*Continued*) B. Details of flow of blood in the heart. With permission from McArdle W. D., Katch F. I. and Katch V. L.: *Exercise Physiology*. Philadelphia: Lea & Febiger, 1991, p 294.

The heart is situated in an area of the chest (thoracic cavity) known as the middle mediastinum and is partially overlapped by the lungs. Anteriorly, it is covered by the sternum and the third, fourth, and fifth ribs. About two thirds of the heart mass lies to the left of chest's midline as it rests on the diaphragm. It is conical in shape and is described as having a base and an apex. The base is made up largely of the left atrium and part of the right atrium, and lies primarily at the right sternal border at the level of the third and fourth ribs. The apex is made up of the left ventricle and points downward, toward the left, as well as forward. The apex rests at the level of the fourth or fifth intercostal space where the apical impulse can be felt (palpated). Therefore, if you place your fingers between the fifth and sixth ribs, you can easily feel the beating of your heart where the apex touches the chest wall.

The weight and size of the heart vary according to age, sex, body size, etc. It is approximately the size of a fist and weighs an average of 310 ± 75 grams in men and 255 ± 75 grams in women.[8]

External Structure

Externally, the heart is divided into sections by grooves called sulci. These grooves, visible on the heart surface, identify the boundaries of the four chambers. The atria can be distinguished from the ventricles by the atrioventricular (coronary) sulcus. The left and right ventricles are delineated by the posterior and anterior interventricular sulci. The point at which the coronary sulcus meets the posterior interventricular sulcus is known as the crux. The surface of the heart that lies below the crux is known as the diaphragmatic or inferior area of the heart. These sulci act as channels for the coronary arteries, which supply the heart muscle with oxygen and nutrients (Fig. 2–2).

Structure of the Heart

The infrastructure of the heart is constructed on a framework of dense cartilaginous tissue that consists of four rings and is known as the fibrous skeleton. This structure acts as: (1) the anchor for the heart valves, (2) the origin and instruction points

for the cardiac muscle fibers, and (3) the separation of the atria from the ventricles.

The walls of the heart enclose four hollow interior chambers referred to as the atria and the ventricles. Figure 2–3 represents a cross-sectional view of the internal structures of the heart. Superiorly, the two small "receiving" chambers, the right and left atria (RA and LA), have relatively thin walls and are separated by the interatrial septum. Inferiorly, the two large "pumping" chambers, the right and left ventricles (RV and LV), have considerably thicker walls than the atria to enable them to pump against a greater resistance. Furthermore, the left ventricular walls are three times as thick as those of the right ventricle because of the higher resistance it must pump against. The ventricles are separated by the thick, muscular interventricular septum, which contracts in conjunction with the left ventricle.

The walls of the heart are composed of three distinctive layers. The innermost layer, the endocardium, is a thin layer of endothelial cells supported by underlying connective tissue. It repeatedly folds on itself to form the valves of the heart and is continuous with the innermost layer of the large blood vessels (tunica intima) that enter and exit from the heart. Four valves are attached to the fibrous skeleton and ensure one-way flow of blood through the heart. Two atrioventricular (AV) valves between the atria and ventricles prevent backflow from the ventricles to the atria during ventricular contraction (systole). They are composed of leaflets from the endocardium and their names indicate the number of leaflets in each valve. The right side is separated by the tricuspid valve and the left by the bicuspid (mitral) valve. The free edges of the AV valves are located in their respective ventricles and are prevented from encroaching into the atria during ventricular contraction by their attachment to the chordae tendineae and papillary muscles (see below). The two other valves, known as semilunar valves, are composed of three cusps each from the endocardium, and control the backflow of blood from their respective great arteries to the ventricles during diastole. Because of their anatomic structure, the free edges do not need anchoring by chordae tendineae. The pul-

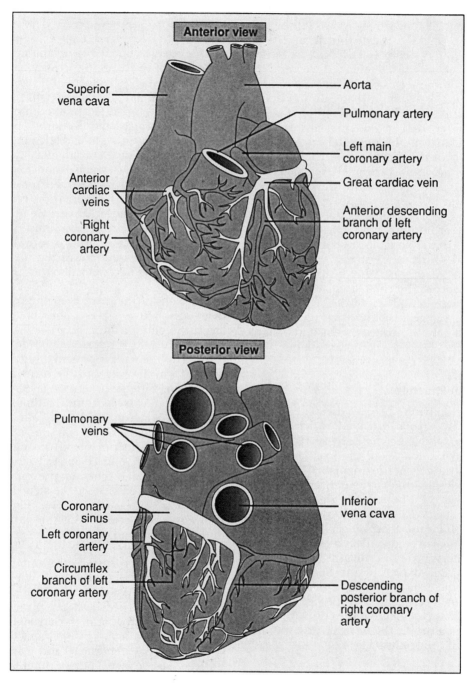

Fig. 2–2. The coronary circulation. Arteries are shaded dark, and veins are unshaded. With permission from McArdle, W. D., Katch, F. I. and Katch V. L. *Exercise Physiology: Energy Nutrition, and Human Performance.* Philadelphia, Lea & Febiger, 1991, p. 306.

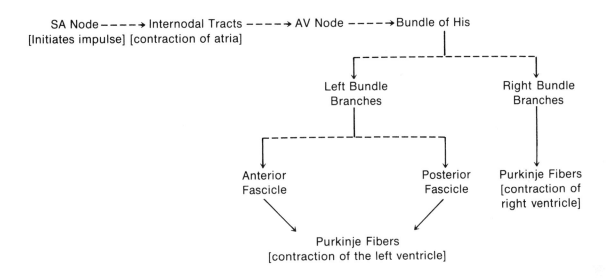

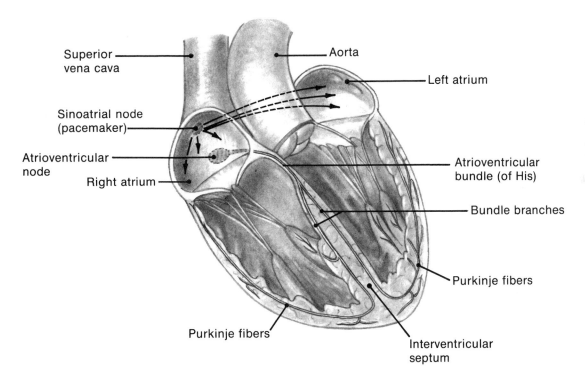

Fig. 2–3. The intrinsic conduction system of the heart and succession of the action potential through areas of the heart during one heartbeat. Redrawn with permission from Marieb, E. N.: *Human Anatomy and Physiology*. Redwood, CA: Benjamin/Cummings, 1992.

monic valve lies between the RV and the pulmonary artery. The aortic valve lies between the LV and the aorta. Behind each cusp of the aortic valve is a bulging of the wall of the aorta. This sac-like area is known as the sinus of Valsalva and houses the openings (ostia) of the major coronary arteries.

The middle layer, the myocardium, is the contractile layer of the heart and is composed primarily of cardiac muscle fibers and comprises 75% of the heart's total mass.[3] Cardiac muscle contains unique structures, intercalated discs, which transmit the depolarization wave (the electrical impulses of the heart that initiate contraction of the myocardium) from one fiber to the next, ensuring that all the muscle fibers depolarize (contract) with only one electrical stimulus. Internally, the myocardium forms ridges, trabeculae carneae, on the surface of the ventricles. These ridges give rise to muscular projections known as papillary muscles. The papillary muscles are attached to the free edges of the atrioventricular valves by means of tendon-like structures (chordae tendineae) "heart strings" and serve as a valvular anchor during contraction. When the ventricles contract, the atrioventricular (AV) valves are closed by the force of the blood pushing upward. This closing of the AV valves prevents the blood from flowing back into the atrium. The chordae tendinae and papillary muscles prevent the valves from being inverted back into the atrium (comparable to a gust of wind inverting an umbrella).

The outer layer, the epicardium, is a thin membrane that encases the myocardium, and is the root of the great vessels. The epicardium is also called the visceral pericardium. The epicardium turns back on itself to encase the whole heart in a sac known as the parietal (serous) pericardium. These two pericardial layers are separated and lubricated by approximately 10 to 20 mL of a thin pericardial fluid, which reduces friction during myocardial contraction.[8]

Coronary Circulation

Although the chambers of the heart are continuously filled with blood, this blood supplies very little nourishment to the ma-jority of the heart muscle. The coronary arteries provide the majority of blood to the epicardium and myocardium and are found on the outer surface of the heart (Fig. 2–2). The endocardium is nourished directly from the blood in the chambers of the heart. The left and right coronary arteries arise from the sinus of Valsalva (located at the base of the aorta just above the semilunar valves) and encircle the heart in the atrioventricular sulcus (groove). Immediately upon exiting the aorta, the left coronary artery runs toward the left side of the heart and divides into the left anterior descending (LAD) and the circumflex artery (CxA). The LAD (also known as anterior intraventricular artery) follows the anterior interventricular sulcus and supplies blood to the interventricular septum and anterior walls of both ventricles.[8] The CxA travels left in the atrioventricular sulcus and supplies blood to the left atrium and the lateral left ventricle. Therefore, these two coronary arteries (LAD and CxA) give rise to numerous branches, which supply blood to the anterior and lateral surfaces of the ventricle as well as to the left atrium. The right coronary artery (RCA) travels to the right, encircles the heart in the atrioventricular sulcus, and gives rise to numerous branches that supply anterior and lateral surfaces of the right ventricle as well as the right atrium. Posteriorly, the RCA merges (anastomoses) with the circumflex artery. As the RCA travels around the heart to the crux (the anterior lateral surface of the heart below the right atrium where the coronary sulcus meets the posterior interventricular sulcus), the artery turns inferiorly (downward) and gives rise to the posterior descending artery (PDA), which travels along the posterior interventricular sulcus and supplies blood to the posterior areas of both right and left ventricles.[8] (The PDA is also known as the posterior interventricular artery). The branches of the LAD and PDA anastomose (merge) near the apex of the heart. There is considerable variation in the arterial supply of the heart. For example, 10% of the time, the CxA gives rise to the PDA.[8]

All coronary arteries are paired with veins that transport the blood back to the right atrial chamber by way of the coronary sinus. The coronary sinus is obvious on the posterior aspect of the heart. Three large tributaries bring returning blood to the coronary sinus: the great cardiac vein (travelling in the anterior interventricular sulcus), the middle cardiac vein (in the posterior interventricular sulcus), and the small cardiac vein (travelling in the heart's right inferior margin). Additionally, several anterior cardiac veins empty directly into the right atrium.

Any blockage of the coronary circulation is a matter of concern. Blood flow to the heart cells can be temporarily reduced in a narrowed coronary vessel (atherosclerotic vessel) when under increased physical demand. This temporary deficiency in blood delivery can result in angina pectoris (pain in the chest or "choked chest"). This results in a temporary lack of oxygen to the heart cells. If a clot becomes lodged in an atherosclerotic vessel, a coronary blockage occurs which can lead to a myocardial infarction (MI, commonly called a "heart attack"). An MI indicates that a part of the heart is not receiving blood, and heart cells die. The severity of the MI depends on the extent of the blockage and which part of the heart is denied blood flow. Damage to the left ventricle is most serious. A person may also have minimal damage to the heart if there is collateral circulation. This is when the branches of the main coronary arteries anastomose and a fused network of bypasses is formed. This way, if the main road is blocked, blood can still reach the cells by way of the small back roads.

Conduction System

The heart contains "special" noncontractile cardiac cells that have the ability to generate an electrical impulse (action potential) and conduct (distribute) the impulses throughout the heart, so that the myocardium depolarizes and contracts in an orderly, sequential manner from atria to ventricle. These "special" cells, in conjunction with the intercalated discs, make up the heart's intrinsic conduction system. Figure 2–3 depicts the structures of this conduction system and the direction of a normal depolarization wave. Identified are the sinoatrial (SA) node, also known as the "pacemaker" of the heart. It is a group of cells located in the right atrium just inferior to the entrance of the superior cava, and its rate of spontaneous depolarization is normally the fastest of all the cells comprising the conduction system. Therefore, it is the primary determinant of the heart rate. Once the SA node initiates an electrical impulse, it is rapidly conducted throughout both atria by way of internodal tracts. These tracts converge at the inferior septal portion of the right atrium (just above the tricuspid valve) to form the atrioventricular (AV) node, which is responsible for initiating the signal for the ventricles to contract. The depolarization wave cannot spread to the ventricles because the fibrous skeleton separating atria from ventricles contains no conducting cells. The AV node delays the electrical impulse to allow the atria to contract and propel blood through the AV valves to the ventricles. When the AV node fires, the impulse is then conducted through the fibrous skeleton by a small band of conducting cells known as the bundle of His. At the superior edge of the right side of the interventricular septum, the bundle of His divides into two branches. A right bundle branch (RBB) travels down the right side of the interventricular septum and spreads throughout the right ventricle. A left bundle branch perforates the interventricular septum to the left ventricle and further divides into an anterior and posterior fascicle which spreads throughout the left ventricle. Both the RBB and the LBB deliver the electrical impulse to thousands of Purkinje fiber cells, which transmit the action potential to ventricular muscle cells, resulting in ventricular contraction.

The heart is innervated extrinsically by both the parasympathetic and sympathetic nervous systems. The former predominantly innervates the atria and exerts its primary effect of slowing the heart rate (chronotropic). The sympathetic nervous system innervates both the atria and ventricles. Its effect is both chronotropic, increasing heart rate by increasing the automaticity and conduction velocity of the conduction system; and inotropic, increasing the force of contraction of the heart muscle.

Blood Vessels

The blood is carried away from the heart by a series of diverging vessels known as arteries. The major arteries diverge into smaller arterioles which, in turn, diverge into small single-cell layer cells known as capillaries. Capillaries bring blood in close contact with other tissues of the body so that an exchange of gases, nutrients, and metabolites may take place. The capillaries converge into venules, which in turn converge into veins that carry blood back to the heart (see Fig. 2–1).

All capillaries, arteries, and veins have a lining of a single layer of squamous cells (endothelial) and supporting connective tissue known as the tunica intima. Capillaries have exceedingly thin walls consisting only of a thin tunica intima so that exchange with cells can take place easily. Arteries and veins are very similar in their remaining structure, with a middle layer of smooth muscle and supporting tissue known as the tunica media (muscularis) and an outer layer of connective and elastic tissue called the tunica adventitia. The smooth muscle layer, being stimulated by the autonomic nervous system, can contract to make the opening (lumen) of the vessel smaller (vasoconstriction); or can relax to widen the lumen (vasodilate). The primary difference between arteries and veins is the amount of muscle, connective, and elastic tissue each possesses. Arteries have greater amounts of smooth muscle and elastic tissue to allow them to withstand the higher pressures and to maintain blood pressure and continuous blood flow. The veins are thinner and more compliant, allowing them to store up to 70% of the blood at any time,[2] and thus are christened the capacitance vessels. Because the blood pressure in veins is low, veins have special anatomic adaptations (valves), which prevent backflow of the blood and help blood continue to flow toward the heart. Venous valves are formed from folds of the tunica intima and resemble semilunar valves of the heart. Valves are most abundant in the veins of legs, where upward flow of blood is opposed by gravity.

Blood

Fifty-five percent of a person's 5 to 6 liter blood volume is composed of a complex liquid, plasma, which also acts as a suspension for the blood cells. Plasma, which is 90% water, contains many organic solutes such as proteins, nutrients, and metabolic end products. In addition, it contains a large variety of electrolytes. It should be noted that plasma serves many functions other than merely that of a transport vehicle.

Blood cells account for the remaining 45% of the blood volume and are known as erythrocytes or red blood cells (RBC),[12] leukocytes or white blood cells (WBC), and platelets. RBCs make up 99% of the total blood cell volume, and their primary importance is the presence of the protein, hemoglobin, which carries oxygen and the enzyme carbonic anhydrase, which facilitates the transport of carbon dioxide. Leukocytes comprise less than 1% of the total blood cell volume[7] and use the plasma as vehicle for transport to damaged or infected areas. Many types of leukocytes confer their functions on infected or damaged areas in a variety of different ways to defend the tissues against insult or injury. Platelets are not complete cells and lack a nucleus. They act as containers for numerous granules (i.e., epinephrine, serotonin, growth factor, ADP, etc.), which they transport to sites of insult or damage to blood vessels. Once at the site of injury, the platelets adhere to the injured site obstructing the injury and releasing its granules to aid in the control of the loss of blood.

RESPIRATORY ANATOMY

Every cell of the body needs constantly to receive oxygen and get rid of carbon dioxide. Because the cells of the body are not all exposed to the atmospheric air, it is the responsibility of the respiratory system to exchange gases with the atmospheric (ambient) air, so that blood, high in levels of oxygen and low in levels of carbon dioxide, can be pumped to all cells of the body. Therefore, the respiratory system is designed to bring atmospheric air into the lungs and to allow gas exchange to take place between the alveoli (sacs at the end of the bronchial tree of the lungs) and the very extensive capillary network surrounding the alveoli (Figure 2–4). (In fact, alveolar tissue has the largest blood supply of any organ in the body). There are

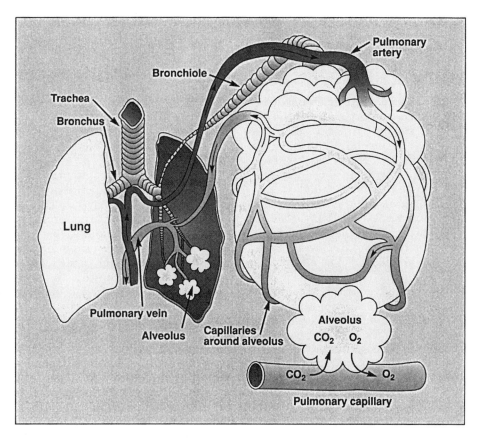

Fig. 2–4. Pulmonary system. With permission from McArdle W. D., Katch F. I., and Katch, V. L.: *Exercise Physiology: Energy, Nutrition, and Human Performance.* Philadelphia: Lea & Febiger, 1991, p 236.

hundreds of millions of alveoli, which are elastic, thin-walled sacs. If all alveolar sacs were opened and spread out, the area covered would be about half a tennis court. Thus, the alveoli are anatomically designed to provide a large surface area for rapid gas exchange.

The process of bringing atmospheric air into the lungs and down to the alveoli sacs where gas exchange with pulmonary capillaries can take place is called pulmonary ventilation. Air enters the body through the nose and/or the mouth, and travels down the passageways of the pharynx (throat), larynx (voice box), and trachea (windpipe); down the large tubes that go to the right and left lungs (bronchi); and into the numerous branching smaller tubes (bronchioles) that end in the alveolar sacs. Because air being brought down to the alveoli is relatively high in oxygen and low in

carbon dioxide (compared to the gas concentration in the blood *entering* the pulmonary capillaries, which has just returned from all cells of the body), a pressure gradient is established. Therefore, gas will diffuse across the lining (membranes) of the alveoli and the capillaries from an area of high concentration to an area of lower concentration. In other words, at the alveoli, oxygen diffuses (passes) from the alveoli into the capillaries, while carbon dioxide diffuses from the pulmonary capillaries into the alveoli. As a result, blood *leaving* the pulmonary capillaries to return to the heart (left atrium) is ready to be pumped to the cells of the body replenished with oxygen and with low levels of carbon dioxide.

The secondary functions of the respiratory system are to humidify, warm or cool, and filter the inspired (inhaled) air, assist in the development of sound, and assist in the acid-base balance (through increasing elimination of carbon dioxide).

Components of the Respiratory System

The nasal airway is the primary entry site of air into the respiratory system. The air is warmed or cooled by the blood in the nasal tissues. The mucous cells and tiny hair-like projections (cilia) in nasal passage moisturize and filter the inspired air. The oral cavity can be used as a secondary passage to move atmospheric air into the lungs. It also possesses the ability to moisturize and warm or cool the air, but has a limited capacity for filtration. When large amounts of air are needed to be moved into the lungs, the air will have to enter the passageways by way of the nose and mouth.

The pharynx acts as a common pathway for both respiratory and digestive passages. Sections of the pharynx are named for their locations. The nasopharynx lies posterior to the oral cavity. At the inferior (lower) end of the pharynx, just above the voicebox, it is known as the laryngopharynx, then extends downward and becomes the larynx anteriorly and the esophagus posteriorly. The larynx is a short, cartilaginous tube that contains the thyroid cartilage, commonly known as the "Adam's apple," the vocal cords for sound production, and connects the laryngopharynx with the trachea. A leaf-shaped piece of cartilage, the epiglottis, covers the opening of the larynx during swallowing to allow food to enter the esophagus and not the trachea.

The trachea (windpipe), also a cartilaginous tube, is the distal continuation of the larynx that descends through the neck and into the thorax for a distance of approximately 10–12 cm.[7] The trachea bifurcates (divides) into the right and left primary bronchi, with one bronchus serving each lung respectively. The right primary bronchus is the shorter of the two as it deviates slightly from the orientation of the trachea and trifurcates into three secondary (lobar) bronchi that enter each of the three lobes of the right lung. The left primary bronchus deviates more severely off the trachea and bifurcates into two secondary (lobar) bronchi that enter the two lobes of the left lung. The branching continues as the secondary bronchi subdivide into tertiary bronchi, which divide into smaller bronchioles that subsequently split into smaller tubules called alveolar ducts. These ducts terminate into approximately 200 to 300 million alveoli with a total surface area of 70 to 80 m^2.[7] The alveoli are thin-walled, epithelial structures surrounded by capillaries and are the site of the exchange of respiratory gases between the blood and the lungs.

The lungs are composed primarily of all the structures mentioned above from the lobar bronchi to the alveoli. They are located in the thoracic cavity and are separated by the mediastinum. The lungs extend from the clavicles superiorly, known as the apex of the lung, to the inferior border of the rib cage, known as the base. They are enclosed in two layers of membranous tissue, pleura, similar to the structure of the pericardium. The layer closest to the lung is the visceral pleura, which turns back on itself and becomes the second layer, the parietal pleura. The parietal pleura is attached to the chest wall and is separated from its counterpart by a thin layer of lubricating fluid. This arrangement makes the lungs "stick" to the walls of the thoracic cavity and causes the lungs to follow the movement of the cavity. The lungs remain in an semi-expanded state at the end of expiration because of the subatmospheric pressure in the pleural cavity.

Breathing (i.e., movement of air in and out of the lungs and passageways) is accomplished by making the thoracic cavity larger or smaller. As the thoracic cavity increases in size (increases its volume), the air pressure deceases inside the chest cavity (application of gas laws). Therefore, because the air pressure is higher outside the cavity, air rushes into the passageways. (As the thoracic cavity increases in size, so do the lungs.) Because of the previously described anatomic arrangement, the lungs adhere to the ribs and the diaphragm relaxes and rises up into the thoracic cavity. The lungs recoil and the thoracic cavity and lung volume decrease, air pressure inside increases, and air is pushed out of the respiratory system. The lung tissue itself does not contain muscle cells. Therefore, ventilation depends on muscles to change the size of the thoracic cavity. During quiet inhalation, the diaphragm contracts and lowers (flattens out toward the abdominal cavity) and increases the size of the thoracic cavity. When *more* air is needed to be moved into the lungs (i.e., during exercise), the ribs and sternum move upward (expanding the front-to-back diameter of the cavity) by contraction of the external intercostals, sternocleidomastoid, and scalene muscles.

During quiet exhalation, no muscle action is needed. The diaphragm simply relaxes and bulges up into the thoracic cavity. During exercise, however, greater volumes of air must be expired. The internal intercostals contract to force the ribs downward, and the abdominal muscles contract to push the internal organs up into the diaphragm. These actions cause a further reduction in the size of the thoracic cavity. Because more muscles are called into action when rapid, deep breathing is needed, the energy cost or breathing increases with an increase in exercise intensity.

REFERENCES

1. Anderson JE: *Grant's Atlas of Anatomy.* 8th Ed. Baltimore: Williams & Wilkins, 1983.

2. Berne RN, Levy MN: *Cardiovascular Physiology.* 5th Ed. St. Louis: C.V. Mosby, 1986.

3. Creager JG: *Human Anatomy and Physiology.* Belmont, CA: Wadsworth, 1983.

4. Gardener ED: *Gardener-Gray-O'Rahilly Anatomy: A Regional Study of Human Structure.* 5th Ed. Philadelphia: W.B. Saunders, 1986.

5. Gray H: *Anatomy of the Human Body.* Philadelphia: Lea & Febiger, 1985.

6. Hole JW, Jr: *Human Anatomy and Physiology.* 2nd Ed. Dubuque: William C. Brown, 1981.

7. Hollinshead WH, Rosse C: *Textbook of Anatomy.* 4th Ed. Philadelphia: Harper & Row, 1985.

8. Hurst JW, et al.: *The Heart.* 7th Ed. New York: McGraw-Hill, 1990.

9. Jacob SW: *Structure and Function in Man.* Philadelphia: W.B. Saunders, 1982.

10. Marieb, EN: *Human Anatomy and Physiology.* Redwood City, CA: Benjamin/Cummings Publishing Co., 1992.

11. McArdle WD, Katch FI, Katch VL: *Exercise Physiology, Energy, Nutrition and Human Performance.* Philadelphia: Lea & Febiger, 1991.

12. Steen EB: *Anatomy and Physiology.* 2nd Ed. New York: Barnes & Noble, 1985.

Chapter 3

FUNDAMENTALS OF MUSCULOSKELETAL ANATOMY

Neil B. Vroman and Linda D. Zwiren

Exercise, like any other physical activity, involves movement. Movement mainly results when muscular tension created by our muscles (by means of contraction) pulls on a system of levers (i.e., bones) across a joint, thereby moving the muscle's insertion closer to its origin (concentric action). Some movements in the body are the result of muscles developing force to control the lowering of resistance against gravity (eccentric action). For example, when lowering a barbell in a bicep curl, the biceps and other elbow flexors are developing force while the muscle is actually getting longer (lengthening). Movement occurs in both concentric and eccentric action; therefore, these actions are called dynamic. In some cases, muscles develop force (tension) while no movement occurs (isometric action). Isometric (static) tension would be developed in the biceps when trying to curl a barbell that is much too heavy. The biceps would tighten, but the whole muscle does not get any shorter, and the barbell does not move. Muscles that act primarily to hold the body upright (postural muscles) and to hold joints in stationary positions are referred to as isometric.

This chapter discusses the basic principles of anatomy of bones, muscles, and other structures that comprise the musculoskeletal system. In addition, fundamental principles of human movement and the major anatomic structures involved are discussed.

BASIC ANATOMY

The skeletal system provides the structural framework of the body, in addition to providing protection for vital soft tissue areas such as the brain, heart and lungs. Bone, the major tissue component of the skeleton, is a living, dynamic group of cells that secrete a specialized extracellular matrix, composed of calcium salts, that provides structural integrity.

Adjacent bones are moved relative to each other through the tension created by the contraction of skeletal muscle. Muscle comprises the largest portion of the body's total mass. Even the simplest of human movements is a complex, coordinated effort of activation (contraction) of certain muscles (agonists), deactivation (relaxation) of others (antagonists), or a co-contraction of both agonists and antagonists. For example, when one is lifting the barbell in a bicep curl, the muscles most involved (agonists or prime movers) are the elbow flexors (biceps brachii and brachioradialis). The antagonist muscle (triceps brachii) will relax to allow the elbow to bend. Antagonist muscles also act to control the movement of the prime movers. When you want to slow down or stop bending the elbow, the triceps will generate force to control elbow flexion. Some muscles act as guiding muscles (synergists) to rule out undesired motion. When making a firm fist, both the extensors and flexors co-contract isometrically to neutralize the tendency of the other to move the wrist. Some muscles contract to stabilize (or fixate) a joint or bone so that another body part can exert force against a fixed point. The trapezius contracts to stabilize the scapula so that the deltoid muscle can raise the upper arm out to the side.

Figure 3–1 depicts the "macro" and "micro" anatomic arrangement of skeletal muscle. Individual skeletal muscles (like the bicep's brachii muscle) are composed of muscle cells called fibers (contractile units) and connective tissue (protective and structural units). Skeletal muscle fibers are made up of many parallel bundles of contractile filaments (actin and myosin), which in turn are arranged into sarcomere units. When a muscle contracts, the thin filaments (actin) slide over the thick (myosin)

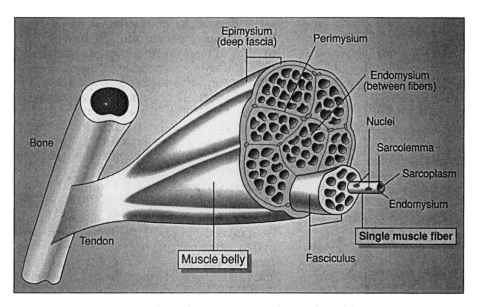

Fig. 3–1. Macroscopic anatomy of muscle. Cross section of a muscle and the arrangement of connective tissue wrappings. The individual fibers are covered by the endomysium. Groups of fibers called fasciculi are surrounded by the perimysium, and the entire muscle is wrapped in a fibrous sheath of connective tissue, the epimysium. The sarcolemma is a thin, elastic membrane that covers the surface of each muscle fiber. From McArdle WD, Katch FI, & Katch VL: *Exercise Physiology: Energy, Nutrition, and Human Performance*. Philadelphia: Lea & Febiger, 1991, p. 349.

filaments shortening the length of the sarcomere (see Chap. 10 for complete description). Because sarcomeres are arranged in series along the length of the muscle fiber, the whole muscle fiber will shorten. Each muscle fiber is wrapped in a fine layer of connective tissue (endomysium); groups of muscle fibers are surrounded by another connective tissue (perimysium) to form bundles (fasciculi); and a connective tissue (perimysium) surrounds all muscle bundles. These connective sheaths continue beyond the length of the muscle fibers to form the dense, strong connective tissue of the tendons. Tendons are, therefore, the fibrous extensions of skeletal muscle, which anchors the ends (origins and insertions) of muscle to bone. Tendons and ligaments (tough fibrous connective tissue connecting bone to bone) are partially composed of the proteins collagen and elastin.

Figure 3–1 also illustrates the concept that muscle strength (or the tension that can produced by a particular muscle across a joint) is, in large part, determined by the number of parallel bundles in the muscle, which determines its cross-sectional area.

Cartilage, another type of specialized connective tissue, provides smooth and protective bony end surfaces in a joint. This is especially crucial at the weight-bearing joints (i.e., vertebrae, hips, knees, ankles).

Bones of the Body

The 206 bones of the human skeleton are divided into axial and appendicular skeletons. The axial skeleton includes the skull, the vertebral column, and the rib cage. The appendicular skeleton consists of the bones of the upper and lower limbs and the girdles (shoulder bones and hip bones) that attach the limbs to the axial skeleton. See Figure 3–2 for the names of the major bones of the body.

Muscles of the Body

The names of the superficial skeletal muscles appear in Figure 3–3. Muscles can be named for their location (brachii-upper arm); size (maximus); direction of fibers (rectus-strength); number of origins (biceps, triceps); shape (deltoid-triangle); bone of origin or insertion (sternocleidomastoid); action (supinator). Often several

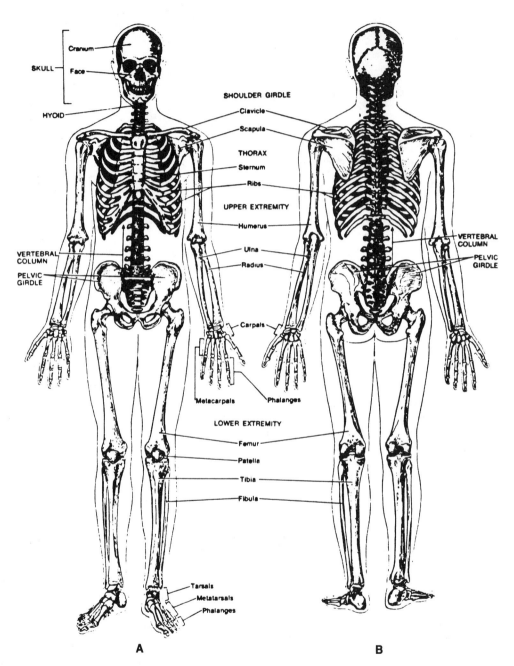

Fig. 3–2.   Divisions of the skeletal system. **A.** Anterior view. **B.** Posterior view. (Courtesy of Tortora GJ: *Principles of Human Anatomy.* 2nd Ed. New York: Harper & Row, 1986.)

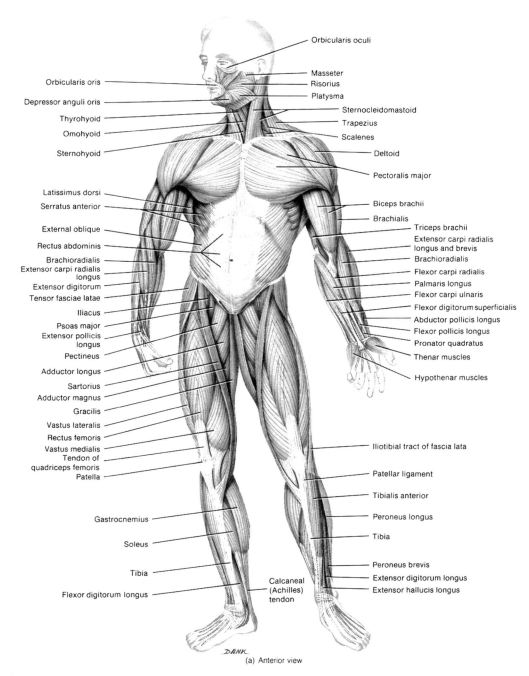

Fig. 3–3. **A.** Diagrammatic anterior view of superficial muscles of the body. With permission from Tortora GJ: *Principles of Human Anatomy*. 6th Ed. New York: Harper-Collins, 1992, p 242.

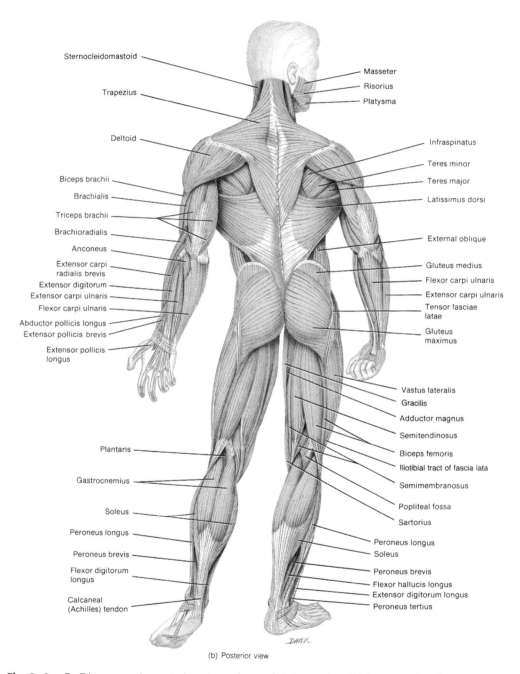

Sternocleidomastoid

Trapezius

Deltoid

Biceps brachii

Brachialis

Triceps brachii

Brachioradialis

Anconeus

Extensor carpi
radialis brevis

Extensor digitorum

Extensor carpi ulnaris

Flexor carpi ulnaris

Abductor pollicis longus

Extensor pollicis brevis

Extensor pollicis
longus

Plantaris

Gastrocnemius

Soleus

Peroneus longus

Peroneus brevis

Flexor digitorum
longus

Calcaneal
(Achilles) tendon

Masseter

Risorius

Platysma

Infraspinatus

Teres minor

Teres major

Latissimus dorsi

External oblique

Gluteus medius

Flexor carpi ulnaris

Extensor carpi ulnaris

Tensor fasciae
latae

Gluteus
maximus

Vastus lateralis

Gracilis

Adductor magnus

Semitendinosus

Biceps femoris

Iliotibial tract of fascia lata

Semimembranosus

Popliteal fossa

Sartorius

Peroneus longus

Soleus

Peroneus brevis

Flexor hallucis longus

Extensor digitorum longus

Peroneus tertius

(b) Posterior view

Fig. 3–3. B. Diagrammatic posterior view of superficial muscles. With permission from Tortora GJ: *Principles of Human Anatomy.* 6th Ed. New York: Harper-Collins, 1992, p 243.

criteria are used in the naming of muscles (rectus abdominis, extensor digitorium longus, latissimus dorsi).

PRINCIPLES OF HUMAN MOVEMENT

Table 3–1 lists the terms used to describe the different motions of the various joints of the body. Precise, appropriate use of these terms is important when performing an analysis of joint movements of a particular human activity, and in describing the actions of the major muscle groups involved in that activity. The anatomic position serves as the reference position for movements (Figures 3–2 and 3–3 show the body in the anatomic position).

Joints (articulations) are the sites where two or more bones meet. Some joints are immovable (synarthrodial), such as the rigid joints of the skull. Some joints have only limited movement (amphiarthrodial). In human movement, we are mainly concerned with joints that are freely movable (diarthrodial or synovial articulations). The ends of the two joining bones are covered with cartilage. Surrounding and holding the ends of the bones making up a diarthrodial joint is a fibrous connective tissue sleeve (articular capsule). This arrangement of the bones and capsule forms a cavity within the joint (synovial cavity). This cavity is filled with slippery synovial fluid allowing movement within the joint with minimal friction. The different types of diarthrodial joints are listed in Table 3–2.

Bursae, which are sacs filled with synovial fluid, are located between the tendons,

Table 3–1. Movement Terms

Flexion:	Decreasing the angle between two bones; bending the elbow or knee (at the shoulder flexion of the upper arm is when one raises the arm parallel to the body, i.e., raising the hand in the saggital plane)
Extension:	Increasing the joint angle between 2 bones; straightening the knee or elbow
Hyperextension:	Movement of any joint beyond the joint's normal position of extension (during a swan-dive, the cervical and lumbar spine are in hyperextension)
Abduction:	Moving away from the midline in the frontal plane (raising the arms out to the side)
Adduction:	Moving toward the midline in the frontal plane (returning laterally raised arms to side of the body)
Horizontal-adduction (-flexion):	Movement at shoulder of bringing upper arm toward the midline in the transverse (horizontal) plane (moving arms that are raised out to side to front of body)
Horizontal-abduction (-extension):	Movement at shoulder of bringing upper arm away from midline in transverse plane
Pronation:*	Moving forearm palms up to palms down (i.e. rotation of radius around ulna turning palms turn down or back)
Supination:*	Moving forearm palms down to palms up
Dorsiflexion:	"Flexing" the ankle so that the angle between the dorsal (top) part of the foot and anterior tibia decreases (lifting foot to point toes to head)
Plantar flexion:	"Extending" (planting) the ankle, increasing the angle between the dorsal (top) part of the foot and the anterior tibia (ballet dancer working on pointe)
Inversion:	Turning the ankle laterally inward so that the sole of the foot points toward the midline (soles of feet pointing toward each other)
Eversion:	Turning the ankle laterally outward so that the sole of the foot points away from the midline
Rotation:	Movement of a long bone clockwise or counterclockwise around its long axis—rotation toward midline is medial (internal) rotation and away from midline is lateral (external) rotation.
Circumduction:	The "swing" of a limb whose distal end forms a circle and whose proximal end forms the apex of the cone (combination of the movement of flexion, extension, abduction, and adduction, e.g., pitcher winding up to throw a ball, arm circles

* Pronation of the foot is a combination of the movements of eversion and abduction. Supination of the foot involves inversion and adduction.

Table 3–2. Types of Joints

Types	Movement	Example
Hinge	Flexion and extension one-axis	Knee, elbow, finger (between phalanges)
Ellipsiodal (condyloid)	Flexion, extension	Wrist (radius with carpals)
	Abduction, adduction biaxial	Knuckle (metacarpal with phalange of fingers)
Gliding (plane joints)	Slipping or gliding	Intercarpal (one carpal moving over another carpal bone) Intertarsal
Pivot	Rotation	Radius and distal end of humerus
Ball and socket	All movements (flexion, extension, abduction, adduction, and rotation)	Hip, shoulder
Saddle	All movements plus opposition	Carpal bone (trapezium and first metacarpal)

muscles, ligaments, and bones, and function as friction reducers between adjacent moving surfaces or structures.

The amount of movement within a specific joint, or range of motion (ROM), is limited by several factors:

1. Bony limitations: The structures of one or more of the two articulating bones may limit that joint's ROM (e.g., elbow extension is limited by the olecranon process of the ulna.)

2. Ligament limitations: For example, the ileofemoral ligament (connecting ilium of the pelvis to the femur) allows only a limited amount of trunk extension when the femur is fixed or stationary.

3. Muscular limitations: In addition to the proteins actin and myosin and the associated structures involved in the contractile process, skeletal muscle has connective tissue components with elastic properties that can limit

Table 3–3. Major Movement—Upper Extremity*

	Movement/Function	Prime Movers (Muscles Most Involved)
Scapula/thoracic	Fixation	Trapezius, serratus anterior, rhomboids, levator scapulae
	Adduction	Trapezius (middle fibers), rhomboids
	Abduction	Serratus anterior
Upper arm	Flexion	Anterior deltoid, pectoralis major (upper fibers)
	Extension	Latissimus dorsi, pectoralis major (lower fibers)
	Adduction	Latissimus dorsi, teres major, pectoralis major
	Abduction	Middle deltoid, supraspinatus
	Horizontal adduction	Pectoralis major, anterior deltoid
	Horizontal abduction	Posterior deltoid, intraspinatus, teres minor
	Internal (medial) rotation	Latissimus dorsi, teres major
	External (lateral) rotatation	Infraspinatus, teres minor
Forearm	Flexion	Biceps brachii, brachioradialis
	Extension	Triceps brachii
	Supination	Supinator, biceps brachii
	Pronation	Pronator teres

* Information for this table taken with permission from: Logan G. A. and Mckinney W. C. 1982. *Anatomic Kinesiology* Dubuque, Iowa: Wm. C. Brown.; Marieb E. N. 1992. *Human Anatomy and Physiology* Redwood City, CA: The Benjamin/Cummings Publishing Co.; Thompson C. W. 1989. *Manual of Structural Kinesiology* St. Louis, MO; Times Mirror/Mosby College Publishing.

ROM. Also, muscles that span across multiple joints may limit the ROM in other joints when they contract. For example, using the finger flexors to make a tight fist is close to impossible if the wrist is actively flexed.

In Tables 3–3 and 3–4, a summary is provided of the major joint movements, and the muscles producing these movements (i.e. prime movers). Figure 3–1 illustrates selected movements and the prime moves that produce them.

Table 3–4. Major Movements—Lower Extremity, Trunk*

	Movement/Function	Prime Mover (Muscles Most Involved)
Trunk	Flexion of the spine	Rectus abdominis, internal and external obliques (both sides of obliques contracting together)
	Extension of the spine	Erector spinae
	Rotation	Internal oblique (right side of muscle twists trunk to right)
		External oblique (right side of muscle twists trunk to left)
Upper leg	Flexion	Iliopsoas
	Extension	Gluteus maximus, hamstrings (semitendinosis, semimembranosis, long head biceps femoris)
	Adduction	Adductor group (magnus, longus, brevis), gracilis
	Abduction (or pelvis stabilization during one foot stance)	Gluteus medius
Lower leg	Flexion	Hamstrings
	Extension	Quadriceps femoris
Foot	Dorsiflexion	Anterior tibialis, extensor digitorium longus
	Plantar flexion	Gastrocnemius, soleus
	Inversion	Posterior tibialis, anterior tibialis
	Eversion	Peroneus group, extensor digitorium longus

* Information for this table from: Logan G. A. and Mckinney W. C. 1982. *Anatomic Kinesiology* Dubuque, Iowa: Wm. C. Brown.; Marieb E. N. 1992. *Human Anatomy and Physiology* Redwood City, CA: The Benjamin/Cummings Publishing Co.: Thompson C. W. 1989. *Manual of Structural Kinesiology* St. Louis, MO; Times Mirror/Mosby College Publishing.

Chapter 4

BIOMECHANICS OF FITNESS EXERCISES
Susan J. Hall and Stephen P. Messier

The biomechanics of human movements have implications not only for the relative skill and grace we attribute to those movements, but for efficacy and injury avoidance as well. When the purpose of human movement is exercise, movements are generally carried out with greater speed and/or greater force and any resulting impact forces are of greater magnitude than is normally the case during activities of daily living. As a result, the potential for injury is also heightened. This chapter begins with a review of selected basic mechanical concepts, then examines some biomechanic aspects of aerobic and muscular strength exercises.

BASIC MECHANICAL CONCEPTS

Center of Gravity and Balance

The ability to maintain the body's balance during many exercises is important for both proper exercise execution and injury prevention. From a mechanical perspective, maintaining balance involves controlling the position of the body's center of gravity (CG). The center of gravity is the point around which the body is balanced. In a symmetrically shaped object, the center of gravity is located at the object's geometric center. In a segmented body such as the human body, the position of the body segments determines the location of the center of gravity. Thus, each time a body segment is moved, there is a redistribution of body mass and a shift in the body's center-of-gravity location. The greater a given segment's mass, the greater that segment's location influences total body CG location. Because a given person's leg is typically more massive than his or her arm, the movement of a leg has a greater influence on the location of the center of gravity than does the movement of an arm.

To maintain balance, a line that passes vertically through the body's center of gravity must fall within the base of support. The base of support is the area of the body in contact with the ground, including the area between the points of body support when there is more than one support. For example, for a person in a standing position, the base of support consists of the area under the feet plus the area between the feet. When a person leans or topples far enough in any direction that the line of gravity falls outside of the base of support, balance is lost and a fall will result unless the line of gravity can be restored within the base of support.

There are several simple practical strategies for enhancing stability within the exercise setting. One is to keep the center of gravity in a comfortably low position, making it more difficult for the line of gravity to be forced outside of the base of support. Another is to manipulate the size of the base of support. Widening the stance, for example, makes it more difficult for the line of gravity to exceed the base of support in a lateral direction. It should be pointed out, however, that widening the stance side to side does not increase stability in the front-to-back direction. To increase stability in the front-to-back direction, stance should be widened by placing one foot in front of the other. A third strategy for enhancing stability is to choose footwear that is appropriately matched to the support surface so that the likelihood of foot slippage is reduced. The shoe should not slip or stick excessively to the surface.

Torque

From a mechanical perspective, the human body is composed of a series of semirigid links, or segments, connected at joints. Movement of the body segments can be initiated, decreased, or increased either internally by the muscles or externally by gravity or various other applied forces (e.g., contact with other objects, air resistance, friction).

When a force, either internal or external, acts on a body segment, the amount of movement that the force causes depends on several factors. One factor is the magnitude of the force. Equally as important as the force's magnitude, however, is the location at which it is applied. The amount of movement that a force produces depends on the perpendicular distance from the force's line of action to the axis of rotation of the body segment (Fig. 4–1). This distance is termed the moment arm of the force. The product of a force's magnitude and the length of the moment arm is called torque. It is torque that produces movement of a body or body segment about an axis of rotation. Torque is expressed in units called Newton-meters.

The direction and amount of body segment motion occurring at a given joint of the human body depend on the sum of all torques acting at that joint. For example, during the performance of a curl exercise, opposing torques act at the elbow joint. (Fig. 4–1). Torque in the direction of elbow extension (i.e., downward force) is created by the weight held in the hand. The magnitude of this torque is the product of the weight multiplied by the moment arm of the weight (perpendicular distance from the weight's line of action from the center of rotation at the elbow). Flexion torque (upward force) is created by the tension produced by the forearm flexor muscles. The magnitude of this torque is the product of the muscle force multiplied by the muscle force moment arm (perpendicular distance from the muscle force line of action to the center of rotation at the elbow). The *sum* of the opposing torques, flexion (muscle action) and extension (gravity acting on the weight), determines which way the forearm will move. When the torque produced by the elbow muscle flexors dominates, flexion occurs. When the elbow flexors relax sufficiently to allow the torque caused by the weight to dominate, extension occurs.

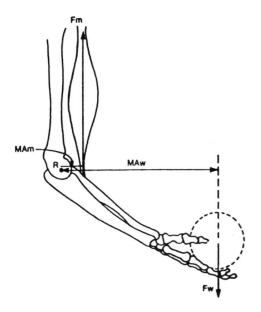

Fig. 4–1. Forces contributing to torque at the elbow. Muscle force (Fm) and the hand-held weight (Fw) are shown with their respective moment arms (MAm and MAw). (Adapted with permission from LeVeau B: *Biomechanics of Human Motion.* 2nd Ed. Philadelphia: W.B. Saunders, 1977.)

Sustaining Forces and Injury Potential

The human body is subjected to many forces on a daily basis. Forces are necessary for body movement and tissue maintenance. Without muscle forces, we could not move in opposition to gravity, and without gravitational and muscle forces, our bones would progressively lose mineral density and deteriorate. In addition, friction enables us to move about on a surface without slipping. Excessive forces sustained by the human body, however, result in injury.

Injury to biologic tissues can result from the application of a single traumatic force of relatively large magnitude (an acute injury), or from the prolonged application of forces of relatively small magnitude (a stress or overuse injury). Many biologic tissues, including muscle, tendon, ligament, and bone, tend to respond to appropriately applied increase in mechanical stress by becoming larger and stronger. When a runner's training protocol incorporates progressively increasing mileage, it is important that this occur in a sufficiently gradual fashion that the body can adapt to the increased mechanical stress without the occurrence of an overuse injury.

The direction in which forces are applied to the body may also influence the likelihood of injury. Bone, for example, is stronger in resisting forces applied along the long axis of the bone than forces applied perpendicular to the long axis of the bone. The anatomic arrangements of many of the joints of the human body also make them more susceptible to injury from a given direction. Lateral ankle sprains, for example, are much more common than medial ankle sprains because of the difference in the number and relative strength of the ligaments crossing the two sides of the joint.

AEROBIC EXERCISES

Walking

The most fundamental type of aerobic exercise is walking. Although walking may be the first step leading to a more strenuous exercise regimen, it has become increasingly popular as a primary exercise mode.

The gait cycle for both walking and running is divided into two phases, the stance and the swing (Fig. 4–2). At a normal walking speed of 1.56 m·sec^{-1} (3.5 mph), the stance phase comprises approximately 60% of the gait cycle. Three critical periods occur during the stance phase—heel strike, midstance, and push-off. The initial contact of the heel with the ground is termed heel strike, with the foot in a relatively flat position during midstance, and push-off then encompassing the time between midstance and toe-off.

Forward speed during walking and running is the product of stride length (SL) and stride frequency (SF). It has been shown that *self-selected* walking (or running) speed results in minimization of metabolic costs, and that at speeds greater than the preferred, increasing stride length produces a greater metabolic cost than increasing stride frequency.[1]

Impact forces sustained during walking and running are explained by Newton's third law of motion, which states that for every action there is an equal and opposite reaction. Each time the foot applies a force to the ground, an equal and opposite ground reaction force is generated on the foot. Because heavier and faster walkers tend to sustain larger ground reaction forces than their lighter and slower counterparts, footwear that provides adequate cushioning is particularly important for those who walk at a fast pace and/or for long distances, as well as for walkers who are overweight.

Running

Running is distinguished from walking by a period during which both legs are off the ground. Therefore, the swing phase of running is consequently sometimes referred to as the flight phase. Most runners initially land on the rear, lateral border of the shoe, with the subtalar joint in approximately 6° of supination (Fig. 4–3).[2] As the runner's center of gravity moves forward over the foot, pronation occurs. This pronation serves to reduce the magnitude of the ground reaction force by increasing the time interval over which the force is sustained.[3] Some runners tend to pronate more than others, however, and excessive pronation beyond the normal range of approximately 9.4° has been associated with

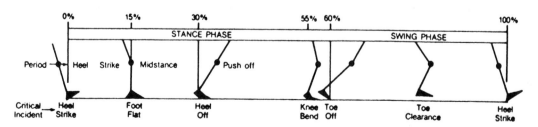

Fig. 4–2. Phases, periods, and critical incidents in the walking cycle. (Adapted with permission from Bowker JH, Hall CB: Normal walking gait. In *Atlas of Orthotics: Biomechanical Principles and Applications.* Edited by the American Academy of Orthopedic Surgeons. St. Louis: C.V. Mosby, 1975.)

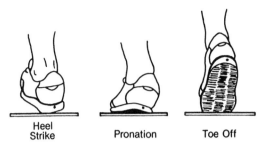

Heel
Strike   Pronation   Toe Off

Fig. 4–3. Rear-foot movement during running. (Adapted with permission from Nigg BM, et al.: Factors influencing kinetic and kinematic variables in running. In *Biomechanics of Running Shoes.* Edited by BM Nigg. Champaign: Human Kinetics Publishers, 1986.)

running injuries, including shin splints, chondromalacia, plantar fasciitis, and Achilles tendinitis. Many styles of running shoes are also designed to control pronation, and there is also some indication that increasing step width, or at least avoiding crossing over the body's midline, tends to reduce the amount of pronation that occurs.[4] It should be pointed out, however, that some runners who appear to pronate excessively are able to remain injury-free.[5] Several questions remain unanswered about the relationship between rearfoot motion and injury potential; analysis is complicated by complex interactions between the foot, the shoe, and the running surface.

Runners generally exhibit one of two types of foot strike patterns. The more common pattern, as described in the preceding paragraph, involves striking with the rear of the foot with the subtalar joint in supination, followed by pronation (Fig. 4–4A). Runners who exhibit this pattern are termed rearfoot strikers. The second, less common pattern is exhibited by the midfoot striker (Fig. 4–4B). The midfoot striker contacts the ground at midfoot and, after a brief backward movement, moves forward in preparation for toe-off.

The vertical force applied to the body during running displays a bimodal pattern that differs from that of walking gait in several important ways. First, the force peak associated with impact is constrained to a relatively short time interval of 50 ms following initial contact (Fig. 4–5). Second, almost immediately following impact, the

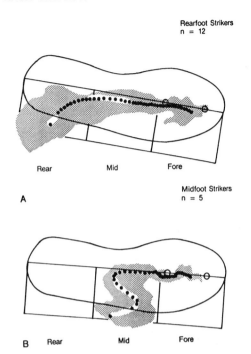

Rearfoot Strikers
n = 12

A   Rear   Mid   Fore

Midfoot Strikers
n = 5

B   Rear   Mid   Fore

Fig. 4–4. Center of pressure locations under the shoe at 2 msec intervals during surface contact in running. The shoe is divided into three equal regions. **A.** Rearfoot striker. **B.** Midfoot striker. (Courtesy of Cavanagh PR, LaFortune MA: Ground reaction forces in distance running. *J Biomech, 13:* 397, 1980.)

propulsive phase is initiated. Peak impact forces range from 1.6 to 2.3 times body weight as running speed increases from 3.0 $m \cdot s^{-1}$ (8:56 min mile^{-1}) to 5.0 $m \cdot s^{-1}$

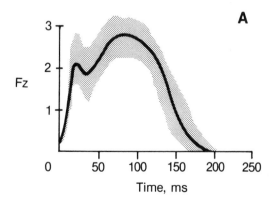

Fig. 4–5. Vertical force (in BW) versus time curve for a rearfoot striker, with range (shaded area) for the contact phase. (Courtesy of Cavanagh PR, LaFortune MA: Ground reaction forces in distance running. *J Biomech, 13:*397, 1980.)

(5:22 min·mile^{-1}). The propulsive peak ranges from 2.5 to 2.8 times body weight for this range of running speeds.[6] Hence, more force is exerted with each foot strike when one is running fast compared to running slow.

Because each foot strikes the ground approximately 1500 times per mile, many runners develop stress-related injuries, especially following an increase in training mileage. Because the musculoskeletal system requires time to adjust to increased levels of mechanical stress, it is essential that training increments take place in a gradual fashion if injury is to be avoided. The use of proper, correctly fitted footwear is also essential for minimizing the likelihood of injury during both running and walking. Although no one shoe can best meet the needs of every runner or of every walker, features to consider include good heel and forefoot cushioning, a stiff heel counter and a multidensity midsole to control rearfoot motion, a flexible forefoot, and an outsole that has good traction and will wear slowly.[7] Of special concern to the midfoot striker is the fact that the midfoot and forefoot must absorb the shock that occurs at touchdown and at toe-off. Therefore, the midfoot striker should select a running shoe that has excellent forefoot shock absorption.

As mentioned previously, running speed is the product of stride length and stride frequency. Several factors are believed to influence each runner's subconscious choice of SL and SF at a given running speed. These include anthropometric characteristics, developmental status, muscle fiber composition, footwear, grade, state of fatigue, and injury history.[8] At jogging and moderate running speeds, increases in running velocity are accomplished primarily by increasing SL. At speeds greater than approximately 5.5 m·sec^{-1} (12 mph), untrained runners rely on increasing SF to increase running velocity further.[9] Overstriding, or running with an excessively long stride length, should be avoided by untrained runners to reduce the likelihood of hamstring strains.

The reason that runners seem to prefer a given SF over a range of slow to moderate running speeds may be related to running economy. Economy is defined as the oxygen consumption ($\dot{V}O_{2submax}$) required for performance of a given task.[10] Most runners use a combination of SL and SF that minimizes metabolic cost during level running at a given speed.[11] It also appears likely that there is a most economical stride frequency for a given runner over the range of speeds used in distance running.[8] It should be noted that runners who appear to move efficiently, that is, without excessive range of motion and/or speed, are not necessarily more economical than runners who appear to move inefficiently.

Use of Hand and Ankle Weights

Some individuals who walk or run for exercise carry hand, wrist, or ankle weights to increase exercise intensity without necessitating an increase in walking or running speed. It has been shown that wearing light (0.45 kg) weight bands on the ankles does not appreciably alter lower extremity joint ranges of motion, but that carrying the same weights in the hands reduces the ranges of motion at the elbow and shoulder during running at a self-selected pace.[12] Modest increases in metabolic energy expenditure on the order of 8% accompany the use of such weights when carried both in the hand and on the ankles during a normal 30-minute workout.

The likelihood of increased injury incidence with the use of hand, wrist, or ankle weights is probably relatively small, so long as the added weights are light (0.45 kg, 1 lb, or less). However, adding weight to the hands imposes an additional stress at the elbow and shoulder joints, and adding weight to the ankles creates added stress at the knee and hip joints. As discussed previously, the heavier the weight and the greater the distance the weight is positioned from the joint center, the greater the increase in joint torque. Another factor that affects joint torque is the speed with which the body segments are moved, with joint torque proportional to the angular acceleration of the body segment. Thus, carrying hand or ankle weights during exercise places greater demand on the antagonist muscles that act as brakes at the end of the joint range of motion as the weight, the distance from the joint center, and the speed of motion are increased.

Therefore, weights should be used in a controlled manner, avoiding uncontrolled swinging at full ROM. Whereas only very light weights should be used during ballistic aerobic dance movements, somewhat heavier weights can be carried during walking at a slow pace with relatively low risk of joint injury. Use of hand and ankle weights is contraindicated for individuals with degenerative joint conditions.

Aerobic Dance

Aerobic dance has become an extremely popular form of exercise. Over the past decade, the nature of this activity has evolved in several directions. For example, a distinction is now made between "high-impact aerobics," involving repetitive jumping on one or both feet, and "low-impact aerobics," in which one foot remains on the ground at all times. Some aerobic dance activities incorporate the use of hand-held weights or weighted wrist and ankle bands to provide increased resistances. A relatively new approach within the realm of low impact aerobics involves the use of a low box or bench, with the participant stepping on and off the box, thus raising and lowering the body's center of gravity against the resistance of gravity (see Chap. 27).

Although it is not practical to address the biomechanical aspects of performance of the wide array of aerobic dance exercises presently used, it is important to mention the implications for aerobic dance injury prevention from a biomechanical perspective. A large percentage of aerobic dance class participants and an even larger percentage of instructors experience injuries.[13] Most of these are stress-related and occur to the lower extremity.

In many aerobic dance settings, especially those including a high-impact program component, the floor is probably the single most important factor relative to injury incidence.[14] It is critical that the floor have adequate cushioning properties to promote the dissipation of impact forces. A floor that is too soft, however, may provide an inadequate platform of support, thus promoting ankle sprains. The amount of friction between the floor and the shoe is also an important consideration, because the shoe should be able to slide without sticking, yet not slip unexpectedly. Floors that are extremely sticky or slick should be avoided.

Other factors related to injury potential include program design, footwear, and the use of hand and/or ankle weights. Just as with a running program, it is important that increments in the intensity and duration of an aerobic dance workout occur in a gradual fashion to allow the musculoskeletal system to adapt to increased levels of mechanical stress. Footwear should be selected in accordance with the nature of the aerobic dance program and the nature of the floor. It is important for participants in high impact programs to wear shoes with good forefoot cushioning. Shoe selection should also relate to whether the floor surface is wood or carpeted, because the soles should allow appropriate traction without slippage. As with walking or running, the addition of hand, wrist, or ankle weights adds to the torques imposed on the joints, but presents a low probability of increased injury incidence as long as light weights are used.

Cycling

Cycling is used as a means of exercise, recreation, and transportation, and stationary bicycles are used for exercise, therapy, and research. In recent years, a growing body of research has emerged on biomechanical factors related to cycling efficiency. A primary consideration is the ability of the cyclist to generate efficient force during pedalling. Only the component of force that is in the direction of the pedal movement generates torque that is transferred through the gears to the wheels to propel the bicycle. However, the cyclist's push on the pedals typically contains force components in other directions, so some amount of ineffective force is usually present.[15] Research has shown that as pedalling rate increases over a range from 40 to 120 rpm, the magnitude of the component of force in the pedal movement direction progressively decreases (Fig. 4–6).[16] The most economical pedalling rate, or the rate at which energy cost is minimal for a given power output, is therefore generally lower than the high pedalling rates used by competitive cyclists.

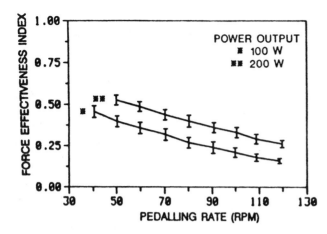

Fig. 4–6. Force effectiveness index (component perpendicular to pedal/total force) versus pedalling rate for 100 W and 200 W power outputs. With permission from Patterson RP, Moreno MI: Bicycle pedalling forces as a function of pedalling rate and power output. *Med Sci Sports Exerc*, 22:512, 1990.

When the cyclist's goal is exercise, rather than performance, other factors must be considered. If the exercise cyclist's intent is to develop leg strength, this goal is better achieved through a low pedalling rate at a high resistance. If improving aerobic endurance is the goal, a combination of pedalling rate and resistance should be selected that elevates the heart rate into the target zone, with the understanding that selection of a higher resistance is likely to result in reduced tolerance to exercise because of local fatigue in the leg muscles.

Another important consideration relative to both cycling efficiency and injury prevention is the "fit" of the cycle to the cyclist. Modern-day bicycles and ergometers have readily adjustable seat and handlebar heights. Seat height is a particularly important variable because it influences the ranges of motion of the hip, knee and ankle during pedalling as well as the lengths of many of the involved muscles. These factors, in turn, affect the lower extremity joint torques, and ultimately the energy of cycling. Optimal seat-to-pedal height is believed to be approximately 97 to 98% of leg length (measured standing from the floor to approximately the height of the crotch.)[17] The handlebar is generally positioned at the same height as the seat. Positioning the hands of the dropped portion of the bar as opposed to the top of the bar is advantageous in reducing the frontal, drag-producing area of the body. Body position is a critically important factor because aerodynamic drag is the major force opposing motion during cycling. Optimum

crank length has also been studied because a longer crank requires more leg movement but also requires less applied force for generation of a given torque. Optimum crank length has been reported to be 15.7% of leg length.[18]

The positioning of the foot on the pedal and the use of toe straps and cleats are other variables that have been studied. Foot position is important largely because of its influence on ankle torque. It has been reported that optimal foot position on the pedal for an individual of average anthropometry is at the middle of the foot.[17] Cleats are useful in that they prevent foot slippage and may enable faster effective pedalling rates. The use of toe straps or clips, however, is of more questionable value. Although some research has confirmed that cyclists using toe straps do pull upward on the pedal during the upstroke, other research has shown that even experienced cyclists fail to pull on the pedals during this phase.[19,20] There is evidence, however, that use of cleats or toe clips may alter load sharing among the muscles, ultimately reducing muscular fatigue.[15]

Serious cycling injuries may result from collision or loss of control of the bicycle. Injuries of a more chronic nature can also result from compression of the ulnar nerve or strains of the knee capsule.[21] Preventive measures for cycling injuries include wearing a helmet, avoiding strenuous cycling under conditions of high heat and/or humidity, avoiding cycling under prolonged fatigue, use of padded handlebars and frequent changing of the grip, and proper seat height adjustment and foot positioning on the pedal.

Swimming

Swimming is an important form of exercise in that it enables a strenuous non-weight-bearing cardiovascular workout. Because the resistance of the water tends to promote slow, controlled motions, exercise in the water enables reduced joint stresses, making swimming, water walking (on the bottom of the pool), and water running (with a buoyant support) excellent exercises for those with joint injuries or pathologies.

Although we know relatively little about what movements contribute effectively to propulsion in swimming, it appears that there are two general ways in which a swimmer can progress through the water. The first involves the application of a force against the water in the direction opposite the intended direction of propulsion. This occurs when a canoe paddle or a swimmer's hand is pushed vigorously backward through the water. The second approach to propulsion involves the generation of lift force. Lift is created by the motion of a foil shape (like the cross-section of an airplane wing) through a fluid. The term "lift" may be somewhat misleading, because the direction of lift force is always directed perpendicular to the foil, so that its direction varies with the orientation of the foil. (The lift force acting on a horizontal airplane wing is vertically upward). Because the human hand is shaped something like a foil, it is capable of generating a lift force when it is sliced through the water (Fig. 4–7). Propulsion in human swimming is believed to result from a complex combination of drag and lift forces.

Similar to the generation of velocity during walking and running, swimming velocity is the product of stroke length (SL) and stroke frequency (SF). A study of male and female competitors in the 100 m freestyle, butterfly, backstroke, and breaststroke races at the 1988 Olympic Games showed stroke length to be the most important contributor to swimming velocity. It was also shown that SL and SF were negatively correlated, with some swimmers using high SL and low SF, some using intermediate values

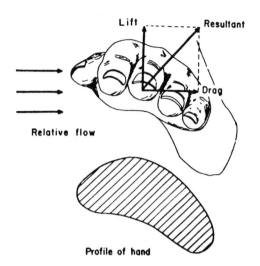

Fig. 4–7. The cross section of the human hand is sufficiently foil-shaped to enable the generation of lift force. With permission from Hay JG: *The Biomechanics of Sports Techniques* (2nd ed.). Englewood Cliffs: Prentice-Hall, 1978.

of both, and some using low SF and high SF.[22] The results of this study suggest that the recreational swimmer desiring to improve swimming performance should concentrate on applying more force to the water during each stroke to increase stroke length, as opposed to taking faster strokes.

RESISTANCE TRAINING EXERCISES

The number and variety of resistance-training regimens advocated today are enough to confuse even the most enthusiastic novice lifter, particularly since researchers do not concur as to the most effective method of increasing muscular strength. The intents of this section are to discuss the major approaches to resistance training and to describe two potentially dangerous weight-training exercises. See Chapter 26 for more specific information on strength training theory and methods.

Resistance Training Machines

A large assortment of resistance training machines is available—some elaborate, massive, perhaps computer-interfaced, and expensive, and some designed to be portable or readily storable for use in the home. The resistance itself may be provided by weights, hydraulic or air compression cylinders, springs, or even elastic cables.

The more basic among these machines provide an external resistance that can be changed, but remains constant throughout the user's range of motion. Proponents of resistance training machines cite increased exercise safety as an advantage to this approach because the resistance and the path of motion are controlled. Other advantages to constant resistance machines may include design simplicity, smaller size, and relatively low cost. The primary disadvantage of these machines relates to the fact that the amount of force a muscle can generate varies throughout the range of motion. This is because, as the joint angle changes, the moment arms of the muscles crossing the joint also change. Because of this, the extent to which the muscle is taxed by a constant external resistance varies, rather than being maximal, throughout the range of motion.

Variable resistance machines are designed to overcome this limitation, usually by incorporating variable radius pulley wheels or cams that function to provide changing levels of resistance through the user's range of motion. The more sophisticated machines enable specific designation of the resistance offered at any point in the range of motion through computer control. The concept is for the machine to accommodate the changing moment arms of the muscles by matching the maximal torque that the muscle group can generate throughout the range of motion. No research has conclusively demonstrated the superiority of variable resistance training over other methods, however.[23]

A third group of resistance training machines is termed isokinetic. These machines use hydraulic, electromechanical, or friction-based mechanisms that provide an adjustable, constant movement speed of the handle or arm upon which the user pulls, no matter how much force or torque the user applies. The intent is that a properly aligned joint will undergo rotation at a constant velocity, and that, if the user exerts maximal force or torque throughout the range of motion, that force or torque is matched by the machine. Disadvantages of this approach include velocity fluctuations that occur when force is initially applied to

this machine, and the fact that the user must be focused on exerting a maximal effort throughout the range of motion to derive the intended benefits. Although the versatility of isokinetic machines makes them ideal for use in rehabilitation settings, research has not generally supported the superiority of isokinetic training over other approaches for increasing strength or enhancing athletic performance.[23]

Free Weights

Manipulation of barbells and/or dumbbells is a popular form of resistance training. A major advantage attributed to training with free weights is the requirement that the user control the motion of the weight while at the same time controlling his or her own balance. Consequently, use of free weights is believed to be more commensurate with the demands of sport and ergonomic settings than the use of resistance training machines.[23] A disadvantage of free weights, however, is the fact that the user can accelerate the weight through part of the range of motion, thereby generating momentum of the weight that lessens the requirement on the muscle group(s) involved through the subsequent portion of the range of motion.

Because the user must control the path of motion of the weight during free weight exercises, use of proper lifting techniques is important for avoiding injuries. General safety tenets include avoiding arching of the back, avoiding full knee flexion, lifting in a relatively slow and controlled fashion, and working with a partner who can spot the weight. Use of a weight-belt has also been shown to provide some reduction of spinal compression and back muscle activity during the execution of heavy lifts.[24]

The Military Press and Squat Exercises

The military press and squat are two somewhat controversial free weight exercises.[25] Because a relatively heavy weight is lifted overhead during the military press, any anteroposterior or lateral sway lengthens the moment arm of the weight about the lumbar spine, thereby increasing the likelihood of low back injury. To avoid injury, the lifter should strive to keep his or her center of gravity directly over the center of the feet by executing the lift in a slow, controlled fashion.

Improper lifting mechanics during the execution of the squat exercise can increase the torques acting on both the trunk and the knees.[26,27] The mechanical flaws exhibited by less skilled lifters include increased forward trunk lean and greater speed during the downward squatting motion. Conversely, skilled lifters maintain a more vertical trunk position and lower the weight in a slow, controlled manner, thereby reducing stress on the trunk and knees. It has also been suggested that potentially damaging forces act upon the knees as the full squat position is approached. The half squat is therefore recommended as an alternate exercise to reduce knee strain.

REFERENCES

1. Holt KG, Hamill J, Andres RO: Predicting the minimal energy costs of human walking. *Med Sci Sports Exerc, 23:*491, 1991.
2. Nigg BM, et al.: Factors influencing kinetic and kinematic variables in running. In *Biomechanics of Running Shoes*. Edited by B. Nigg. Champaign: Human Kinetics, 1986.
3. Clarke TE, Frederick EC, Hamill C: The effects of shoe design parameters on rearfoot control in running. *Med Sci Sports Exerc, 15:*376, 1983.
4. Williams KR, Ziff JL: Changes in distance running mechanics due to systematic variations in running style. *Int J Sport Biomech, 7:*76, 1991.
5. Cavanagh PR: The shoe-ground interface in running. In *Symposium on the foot and leg in running sports*. Edited by RP Mack. St. Louis: CV Mosby, 1982.
6. Munro CF, Miller DI, Fuglevand AJ: Ground reaction forces in running: A reexamination. *J Biomech, 20:*147, 1987.
7. Ellis J: The Match Game. *Runner's World, October 20:*66, 1985.
8. Cavanagh PR, Kram R: Stride length in distance running: velocity, body dimensions, and added mass effects. In *Biomechanics of Distance Running*. Edited by P.R. Cavanagh. Champaign: Human Kinetics, 1990.
9. Saito M, Kobayashi K, Miyashita M, Hoshikawa T: Temporal patterns in running. In *Biomechanics IV*. Edited by RC Nelson and CA Morehouse. London: Macmillan, 1974.
10. Cavanagh PR, Kram R: The efficiency of human movement—a statement of the problem. *Med Sci Sports Exerc, 17:*304, 1985.
11. Cavanagh PR, Williams KR: The effect of stride length variation on oxygen uptake during distance running. *Med Sci Sports Exerc, 14:*30, 1982.
12. Claremont A, Hall SJ: Effects of extremity loading upon energy expenditure and running kinematics. *Med Sci Sports Exerc, 20:*167, 1988.
13. Francis LL, Francis PR, Welshons-Smith K: Aerobic dance injuries: A survey of instructors. *Phys Sports Med, 13:*105, 1985.
14. Francis PR, Leigh M, Berzins A: Shock absorbing characteristics of floors used for dance exercise. *Int J Sport Biomech, 3:*282, 1988.
15. Hull ML, Davis RR: Measurement of pedal loading in bicycling. I. Instrumentation. *J Biomech, 14:*843, 1981.
16. Patterson RP, Moreno MI: Bicycle pedalling forces as a function of pedalling rate and power output. *Med Sci Sports Exerc, 22:*512, 1990.
17. Gonzalez H, Hull ML: Multivariable optimization of cycling biomechanics. *J Biomech, 22:*1151, 1989.
18. Inbar O, Dotan R, Trousil T, Dvir Z: The effect of bicycle crank-length variation upon power performance. *Ergonomics, 26:*1139, 1983.
19. Faria I, Cavanagh PR: *The Physiology and Biomechanics of Cycling*. New York: John Wiley & Sons, 1978.
20. Ericson MO, Nisell R, Arbroelius UP, Ekholm J: Muscular activity during ergometer cycling. *Scand J Rehabil Med, 17,* 1985.
21. Pons DJ, Vaughan CL: Mechanics of cycling. In *Biomechanics of Sport*. Edited by C.L. Vaughan. Boca Raton, FL: CRC Press, 1989.
22. Kennedy P, Brown P, Chengalur SN, Nelson RC: Analysis of male and female Olympic swimmers in the 100-meter events. *Int J Sport Biomech, 6:*187, 1990.
23. Garhammer J: Weight lifting and training. In *Biomechanics of Sport*. Edited by C.L. Vaughan. Boca Raton, FL: CRC Press, 1989.
24. Lander JE, Simonton RL, Giacobbe JKF: The effectiveness of weight belts during the squat exercise. *Med Sci Sports Exerc, 22:*117, 1990.
25. Arnheim DD: *Modern Principles of Athletic Training*. St. Louis: Times Mirror/Mosby, 1989.
26. Ariel GB: Biomechanical analysis of the knee joint during deep knee bends with heavy load. In *Biomechanics IV*. Edited by RC Nelson and CA Morehouse. London: Macmillan, 1974.
27. McLaughlin TM, Lardner TJ, Dillman, CJ: Kinetics of the parallel squat. *Res Q, 49:*175, 1978.

Chapter 5

EXERCISE CONSIDERATIONS FOR THE BACK

Wendell Liemohn

LOW BACK PAIN SYNDROME

Low back pain (LBP) is one of the most common complaints among adults in the United States. Moreover, although it is not usually seen in youth it is not uncommon in this population.[1,2] LBP accounts for more lost person-hours than any other type of occupational injury and is the most frequent cause of activity limitation in individuals under age 45.[3] In the U.S., it costs at least $16 billion each year and disables 3.4 million individuals.[4] However, by exercising and being physically fit, one can decrease the likelihood of ever having this malady. Exercise and physical fitness are also important components of almost any rehabilitation program for individuals who have had LBP.[5]

Anatomy

The five lumbar vertebrae (L1 through L5) and the sacrum are presented in Figure 5–1. Although the ligaments of the spine are not depicted, the reader is reminded that the structural integrity of the spine is augmented by an extensive series of ligaments. A motion segment of the lumbar spine is shown in Figure 5–2. This segment consists of two adjacent vertebrae and their intervening disc. This joint complex is the smallest functional unit of the spine; it includes the anterior joint between the vertebral bodies and the disc and the posterior joints between the paired articular processes (i.e., facet or apophyseal joints). The intervertebral discs act as spacers and shock absorbers; they are also designed to resist rotational stresses (Fig. 5–3). If compressive forces are placed on the spine, the nucleus of the disc exerts pressure in all directions against its more rigid periphery (i.e., the annulus fibrosis and the vertebral endplates). The annulus fibrosis, in turn, distends to help dissipate the stress. If rota-

tional stresses are placed on the spine, the fibers of the disc are so oriented that some will always be in a position to resist this strain.

Etiology

Most low back problems occur in the lower motion segments of the spine (i.e., L4–L5 or L5–S1). LBP and/or symptoms result when there is chemical or mechanical stimulation of nociceptive (pain) nerve endings. The latter are located in liga-

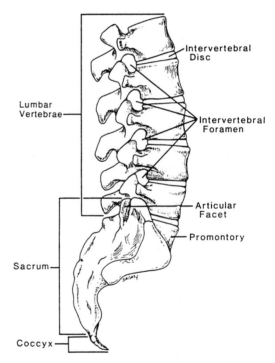

Fig. 5–1. Lumbar vertebrae and sacrum. The intervertebral foramen provide passageways for motor and sensory nerves of the lower extremities. Adapted with permission from Triano J, Cramer G. In *Conservative Care of Low Back Pain*. Edited by White AH and Anderson R. Baltimore: Williams & Wilkins, 1991.

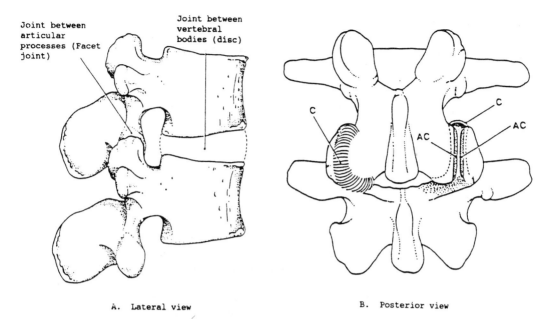

Joint between articular processes (Facet joint)

Joint between vertebral bodies (disc)

C   C

AC   AC

A. Lateral view   B. Posterior view

Fig. 5–2.   A. Lateral and **B.** Posterior view of a motion segment (i.e., two vertebra and the intervening disc) of the lumbar spine. The labels in the posterior view describe the junction of the superior and inferior articular process of the vertebra (facet joints). The ligamentous joint capsule is intact. Removing a portion of the ligamentous joint capsule reveals the articular cartilages in a facet joint. Adapted with permission from Bogduk N, Twomey LT: *Clinical Anatomy of the Lumbar Spine.* New York: Churchill Livingstone, 1987.

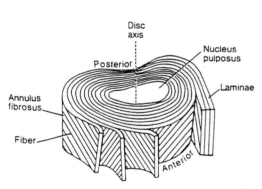

Disc axis

Nucleus pulposus

Posterior

Laminae

Annulus fibrosus

Fiber

Anterior

Fig. 5–3. Intervertebral disc. The outer portion, the annulus fibrosis, is composed of laminated collagen fibers oriented to resist rotational/torsional stress from either direction. The vertebral endplates (not depicted) provide top and bottom caps for the disc and blend with the fibers of the annulus and unite with the vertebra. Adapted with permission from Borenstein DG, Wiesel SW: *Low Back Pain—Medical Diagnosis and Comprehensive Management.* Philadelphia, W.B. Saunders, 1989.

ments, joint capsules, articular cartilage, the annulus portion of intervertebral discs, and tendinous material). Because the most common sources of acute LBP are "unvisualizable," they are unverifiable.[6] If collagen fibers in any of these structures are stressed, their deformation can place tension on nerve endings as well as nerve fibers, and pain results. It is important to understand that, regardless of the pain cause, LBP would not typically result from just *one* incorrect lift or from just *one* incorrect backhand stroke in tennis. Instead, LBP is more apt to result from cumulative microtrauma occurring over time, with the last one, so to speak, being "the straw that breaks the camel's back."[7] Thus there could be countless scenarios that could cause low back pain symptoms. An example of one scenario is presented.

Back Injury Scenario

In performing the backhand in tennis, a strong player can place an extreme amount of torsional (i.e., rotational) stress on the lower motion segments of the spine, particularly if the biomechanics of his or her movement are not good. The collagenous fibers of the annulus fibrosis (outer portion of the disc) could be strained. If this type of stress is repeated often enough, the annulus fibrosis gradually deforms in response to fatigue loading and protrudes into the spinal canal. This annulus deformation can place tension on its own pain receptors and potentially on nerve roots which innervate and receive sensation from the lower extremities (Fig. 5–4). In severe cases, the fibers of the annulus might become so severely damaged that part of the nucleus of the disc extrudes into the vertebral canal. Thus, what began as a herniation of a disc could lead to its rupture. Herniations are usually described as contained swellings or protrusions; extrusions or ruptures imply that nuclear material passes through the walls of the annulus fibrosis. This would only happen if the annulus were damaged because in a healthy disc the weakest link is the vertebral endplate. (In the popular literature, the term "slipped disc" is often used; it is a misnomer because discs are not likely to slip.) In

addition to upsetting homeostasis in the area, rupturing of a disc could lead to a progressive reduction in disc height. This would reduce the size of the adjacent intervertebral foramen (i.e., passageway for nerve roots) and also lead to an overriding of the facet joints. Because facet joints are synovial joints comparable to those seen in other articulations, any erosion or wearing away of their articular cartilage can lead to arthritis. If the afflicted individual limits movement at the injured motion segment, compensatory adaptations at adjacent motion segments can result in additional stress to tissue. Because the injury is usually not in the center of a disc or in only one of the paired facet joints, postural adjustments to the injury may be asymmetrical (e.g., a lateral shift of the spine), which can lead to additional compensatory adaptations and further problems.

SPINAL CURVATURES

The natural curvatures of the spine as viewed from the side include an anterior concavity in the cervical and lumbar regions and a convexity in the thoracic region. These curves are often described as lordotic and kyphotic, respectively. In some representations, the terms lordosis and kyphosis are used to infer abnormally increased curvatures, with lordosis meaning hollow back and kyphosis meaning hunched back. When viewed from the back, the spine is in a relatively straight vertical line. An appreciable lateral deviation is called scoliosis. Lordotic, kyphotic, and scoliotic deviations are functional if they can be removed voluntarily by modifying posture (Fig. 5–5); they are structural if postural adjustments do not affect the deviation.

Lordosis

A small lumbar lordotic curve is natural[8]; in fact, the lordotic curve assists the discs in cushioning compressive forces and shocks[9] (Fig. 5–6). Although there has been a common belief that an excessive lordosis is a risk factor for LBP, comparison studies have not shown a relationship between the shape of the lumbar lordosis and low back symptomatology.[10,11] Intrinsic features set the lumbar curve; extrinsic fac-

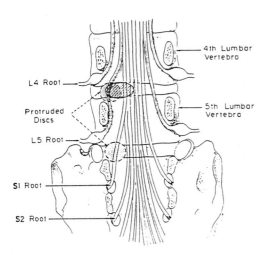

Fig. 5–4. Posterior view of the lumbosacral spine with the posterior elements removed. Because the spinal cord ends at the L1–L2 level, only nerve roots appear below this level. Although the herniated discs depicted in the figure protrude against nerve roots and could logically be expected to cause pain, the annulus also has its own pain receptors, which can also signal disc injury. Adapted with permission from Adams RD, Victor M: *Principles of Neurology, 4th Ed.* New York: McGraw-Hill, 1989.

In the figure labels:
- 4th Lumbar Vertebra
- L4 Root
- Protruded Discs
- 5th Lumbar Vertebra
- L5 Root
- S1 Root
- S2 Root

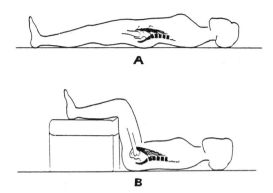

Fig. 5–5. A. If an individual assumes a supine position with the legs straight, the tension of the psoas muscle may lift the lumbar spine. **B.** When the lower extremities are supported, the tension diminishes and the lordotic curve is reduced. Adapted with permission from Lindh M. In *Basic Biomechanics of the Musculoskeletal System, 2nd Ed.* Edited by Nordin M, Frankel VH. Philadelphia: Lea & Febiger, 1989.

tors, such as being overweight, wearing of high heels, or muscle strength can also affect it. Even though strength training programs have not been shown to be effective in reducing the lordotic curve,[12] tightness in the hip flexors (e.g., psoas) could increase the curve, whereas tightness in the hamstrings could reduce it. There tends to

be a flattening of the lumbar lordosis with age.[13]

It is important to understand that, in performing the flexion movements seen in a sit-up, each lumbar vertebra rotates from its backward tilted position to a neutral or end-ROM position; flexion in the lumbar area beyond neutral (e.g., a reversal of the lordotic curve) is not expected.[14] However, an individual with structural lordosis will not even be able to reach the neutral position; thus he/she is apt to experience difficulty in performing many abdominal strengthening exercises because of this factor.

Kyphosis

In activities of daily living, spinal extension movements and postures are less often used than spinal flexion movements and postures. This would be one reason why greater losses are seen in spinal extension with age than in any other spinal ROM.[15] Habit could also be one of the causes of an increased dorsal kyphotic curve in the thoracic area. In Chapter 25, the importance of maintaining spinal ROM is stressed, it may also be a factor in counteracting a kyphosis.

A greater-than-average thoracic kypho-

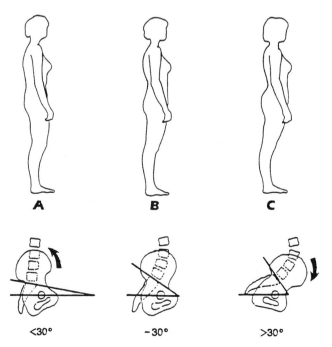

A   **B**   **C**

<30°   ~30°   >30°

Fig. 5–6. The sacral portion of the pelvis is the foundation for the spine; thus spinal integrity is dependent upon its positioning. In **A,** a backward or posterior rotation of the pelvis is depicted and there is little lumbar lordosis; a posture such as this could be caused by tight hamstrings. In **C,** there is excessive lumbar lordosis caused by an anterior tilting of the pelvis; this posture can also jeopardize low-back functioning. A more ideal posture is presented in **B.** Adapted with permission from Lindh M. In *Basic Biomechanics of the Musculoskeletal System, 2nd Ed.* Edited by Nordin M, Frankel VH. Philadelphia: Lea & Febiger, 1989.

sis is frequently associated with increased cervical and lumbar lordoses; however, it has not been shown that this will predispose one to LBP.[16] There are, however, two causes of kyphoses that warrant concern by exercise leaders: Scheuermann's disease and osteoporosis. In Scheuermann's disease, a somewhat rare condition also referred to as juvenile kyphosis, there may be a wedging of thoracic vertebrae. This condition is seen in youth and is caused by a disturbance of the normal pattern of vertebral ossification. A similar wedging may be seen in osteoporosis, wherein the vertebral deterioration is caused by bone demineralization. This condition, sometimes referred to as "dowager's hump," is seen mostly in women after menopause. It is important to obtain medical guidance before prescribing exercises to individuals with either condition.

Scoliosis

Although many causes of scoliosis have been suggested, in most cases the cause is unknown.[17] It is not surprising that leg-length discrepancy, leading to pelvic obliquity, is associated with scoliosis as well as LBP;[13] however, there is little hard evidence of scoliosis causing LBP.[16] Interestingly, asymmetric postures caused by sciatica (e.g., a type of LBP pain in which pain radiates from the back into one buttock and possibly the thigh) often present a scoliotic lateral shift as the afflicted individual tries to find the most comfortable position.

In young individuals with scoliosis, bracing is the mainstay of non-operative therapy. However, because bracing is rarely effective for adults, internal fixation devices such as Harrington rods are used.[17] The exercise program for the scoliotic patient with either external bracing or internal fixation must ascribe to the limitations that either device presents on mobility. Consultation with an orthopedist is particularly important before prescribing any fitness activity for the scoliotic individual with an internal fixation device.

EXERCISE AND THE BACK

Lack of strength and/or flexibility are often seen with the onset of LBP, and hence these variables are viewed as prog-

nostic indicators.[16,18] Although many of the musculoskeletal disorders that cause acute low back problems resolve themselves over time without treatment, rest alone is nothing more than a "Band-Aid" approach to solving the problem.

Flexibility and ROM Considerations

In Chapter 25, mention is made of the importance of ROM to low-back function. To reiterate, the muscles crossing the hip joint can be viewed as guy wires that support the pelvis. Because the sacral component of the pelvis is the foundation for the spine, tightness in these guy wires (e.g., psoas or hamstrings) can adversely affect spine biomechanics. The reader is referred to Chapter 25 for a discussion on hip-joint tightness and activities for the improvement of ROM. Because the biomechanics of the spine can also be adversely affected by structural lordosis or scoliosis, it is important that the exercise leader be aware of persons with such limitations before prescribing exercise for them.

Aerobic Exercise

It is accepted that aerobic exercise is important to cardiovascular condition and rehabilitation. A benchmark study by Cady et al. in 1979 presented a strong argument for the role of aerobic conditioning and general physical fitness in reducing the incidence of LBP.[19] More recently, aerobic exercise has been recognized as important not only in the prevention of LBP, but also in treatment of the condition.[20] Perhaps the following statement by Nutter[5] best summarizes its importance: "Though not a panacea, aerobic exercise should be a part of the treatment for virtually all causes of low back pain." The benefits of aerobic conditioning to low back function include (1) weight control, (2) increased muscle endurance, which facilitates better biomechanics in activities of daily living,[5] (3) higher endorphin levels and/or higher pain tolerance,[20] and (4) better nutritional maintenance of vascular articular cartilage and discs.[21]

Although aerobic activity can have a positive impact on spinal function, poor biomechanics can worsen existing problems as well as bring about new ones as compensatory adaptations are made. For example, poor running technique might include excessive forward lean; this must be counterbalanced by contraction of the back musculature, which may then become overly tired and/or result in stresses to the discs.[22] The biomechanics of running are also most important from the perspective of shock absorption. Factors to consider include cushioning with a heel-to-toe footstrike and by "giving" at the ankle, knee, and hip joints. To better understand the concept of cushioning footstrike, listen to the runners crossing the finish line at a road race. Typically, the faster runners are better at cushioning than many of the "plodding" slower runners.

Trunk Strength and Endurance

Research conducted since 1980 has permitted a better understanding of the unique intricacies of the functional anatomy of the lower back.[23–27] Figure 5–7 superficially covers some of these complexities; the reader may wish to refer to either the original research[23–28] or to a review article[29] for a more in-depth understanding. From the figure it can be seen that anteriorly and laterally the abdominal muscle group is uniquely arranged with stratified layers of muscle and aponeurosis (tendinous expansion/fascia). The fibers of the transversus abdominis run horizontally beneath the obliques and its thoracolumbar fibers are moored to the fascia that *envelops* the musculature of the spine. The internal and external obliques "criss-cross" the transversus and help it *envelop* the rectus abdominis with their aponeuroses. This engineering masterpiece has an amplifying effect because the lateral abdominal muscles exert tension on the fascia-*envelopes*, which house the rectus abdominis anteri-

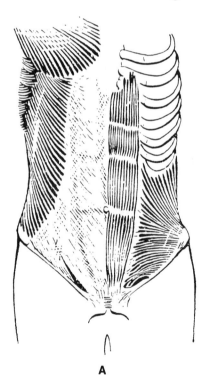
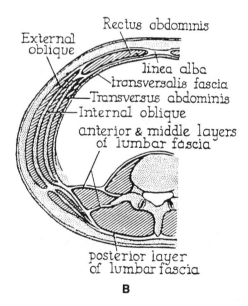

Fig. 5–7. **A.** The frontal figure demonstrates how the tendinous expansion (i.e., aponeurosis) of the lateral abdominal muscles (obliques) envelops the rectus abdominis muscle. In addition to noting this in the cross-sectional picture **(B)**, notice how the transversus abdominis attaches to the fascia of the low back, which envelops the musculature of the lumbar spine. The fascia of the low back is usually referred to as thoracolumbar or lumbodorsal fascia; the aponeurosis of the latissimus dorsi comprises its outer layer. Adapted with permission from Basmajian JV: *Primary Anatomy.* Baltimore: Williams & Wilkins, 1964.

orly and the muscles of the spine (erector spinae and multifidus) posteriorly. Its reinforcing nature is analogous to that presented by a Chinese finger trap. If nurtured and honed, these muscles can corset the trunk; however, if these muscles are not continually trained, the individual's chances of having LBP increase.

Abdominal Exercises

Because lumbar flexion is limited to removal of the lordotic curve (see Chap. 25), it is unnecessary and usually undesirable to raise the trunk more than 30 degrees in abdominal strengthening activities. In other words, raise one or both shoulder blades *but* keep the lumbar spine in contact with the floor or mat. It should be understood that, because the abdominal muscles do not cross the hip joint, any subsequent movement (e.g., full sit-up with or without the knees bent) is generated by the hip flexors as the abdominals contract isometrically. Although isometric exercises are often appropriate for the musculature of the trunk,[22] full sit-ups with the feet supported can place undue strain on the structures of the spine.[30] Crunch-type exercises, including those that emphasize use of the lateral abdominal muscles, are recommended. For variety, "isometric holds" of 5 to 30 seconds can be incorporated into these routines. Examples of abdominal strengthening exercises are presented in Figure 5–8.

Low-Back Exercises

Although abdominal strength is important to the integrity of the spine, the strength of the back musculature is often neglected even though it too is most important to spinal function.[18,31,32] This benign neglect appears to have been prompted by the concern that all hyperextension movements of the spine are contraindicated; such a belief is unfortunate. Active back extension movements can be most appropriate and are encouraged. However, the movement must *always* be under muscle control because ballistic hyperextension

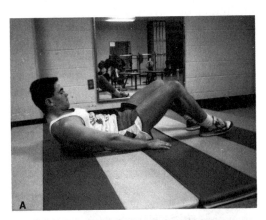

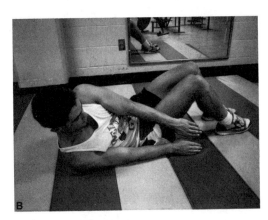

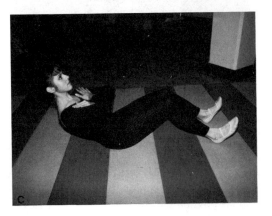

Fig. 5–8. The exercise demonstrated in **A** primarily involves the rectus abdominis; the one in **B** requires greater involvement of the obliques. The reverse curl with an isometric hold in **C** involves *all* abdominal muscles; the angle of inclination is commensurate with the strength of the exerciser. (Note that only the heels of the feet are touching the exercise surface in **C**.)

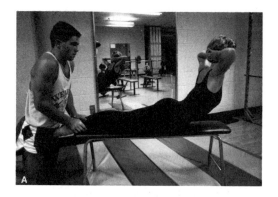
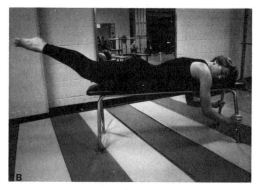

Fig. 5–9. In **A**, the movement is brought about by a slow and controlled contraction of the back musculature; it is stopped before end-ROM and held 5–30 seconds. In **B**, the gluteals and hamstrings are tightened unilaterally or bilaterally. (The lumbar lordosis on the individual shown is greater than is typically seen.)

movements are likely to result in tissue damage. *If* movement is carried into hyperextension, it should be stopped before reaching end-ROM. A guideline to follow is to limit extension to one's normal standing lumbar lordosis.[33] Examples of back-strengthening exercises are presented in Figure 5–9.

Trunk-Bracing Exercises

This type of exercise activity requires teamwork of all trunk muscles; it has been found most effective as part of an overall conservative treatment (i.e., nonsurgical) regimen for the individual suffering from disc disease.[33,34] This technique utilizes the trunk-corseting concept described earlier. Although designed specifically for back patients, some of these activities are appropriate for use in fitness programs as well. Examples of trunk-bracing exercises are presented in Figure 5–10.

SUMMARY

It is well established that having a high degree of physical fitness can decrease the likelihood of having LBP problems. The elements of physical fitness that are important include (1) flexibility/ROM, (2) aerobic condition, and (3) strength and endurance of the trunk musculature. Although the exercise leader is not apt to err if sound principles of biomechanics are followed in exercise selection for non-symptomatic individuals, care and counsel should be used before prescribing exercises for those who have had LBP because of the diversity and uncertainty of the specific causes of this malady.

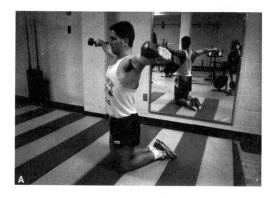
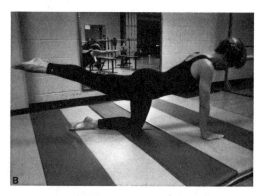

Fig. 5–10. **A** and **B**. To perform the spinal bracing exercises depicted, the exerciser must be able to "splint" the spine as the extremities are moved *slowly* to the position shown.

REFERENCES

1. Fairbank JCT, Pynsent PB, Van Poortvliet JA, Phillips H: Influence of anthropometric factors and joint laxity in the incidence of adolescent back pain. *Spine, 9:*461, 1984.
2. Harvey J, Tanner S: Low back pain in young athletes. *Sports Med, 12:*394, 1991.
3. Ashton-Miller JA, Schultz AB: Biomechanics of the human spine and trunk. In *Exercise and Science Reviews, Vol 16.* Edited by KB Pandolf. New York: Macmillan Publishing Co. 1988, p. 169.
4. Frymoyer JW: Back pain and sciatica. *N Engl J Med, 318:*291, 1988.
5. Nutter P: Aerobic exercise in the treatment and prevention of low back pain. *Occup Med: State Art Rev, 3:*137, 1988.
6. Adams RD, Victor M: *Principles of Neurology, 4th ed.* New York: McGraw-Hill, 1989, p. 155.
7. Triano J, Cramer G: Patient information: anatomy and biomechanics. In *Conservative Care of Low Back Pain.* AH White, R Anderson (eds). Baltimore: Williams & Wilkins, 1991, p. 46.
8. Bogduk N, Twomey LT: The lumbar muscles and their fascia. In *Clinical Anatomy of the Lumbar Spine.* New York: Churchill Livingstone, 1987.
9. Lindh M: Biomechanics of the lumbar spine. In *Basic Biomechanics of the Musculoskeletal System.* 2nd ed. Edited by M Nordin, VH Frankel. Philadelphia: Lea & Febiger, 1989.
10. Pope MH, Bevins T, Wilder DG, Frymoyer JW: The relationship between anthropometric, postural, muscular, and mobility characteristics of males ages 18–55. *Spine, 10:*644, 1985.
11. Hansson T, Bigos S, Beecher P, Wortley M: The lumbar lordosis in acute and chronic low-back pain. *Spine, 11:*154, 1986.
12. Suzuki N, Endo S: A quantitative study of trunk muscle strength and fatigability in the low-back-pain syndrome. *Spine, 8:*69, 1983.
13. Twomey LT, Taylor JR: Lumbar posture, movement, and mechanics. In *Physical Therapy of the Low Back.* Edited by LT Twomey, JR Taylor. New York: Churchill Livingstone, 1987, p. 51.
14. White AA, Panjabi MM: In *Clinical Biomechanics of the Spine.* Philadelphia: J.B. Lippincott Co., 1978.
15. Einkauf DK, Gohdes ML, Jensen GM, et al: Changes in spinal mobility with increasing age in women. *Phys Ther, 67:*370, 1987.
16. Pope MH: Risk indicators in low back pain. *Ann Med, 21:*387, 1989.

17. Borenstein DG, Wiesel SW: In *Low Back Pain—Medical Diagnosis and Comprehensive Management.* Philadelphia: W.B. Saunders, 1989, p. 3.
18. Biering-Sorensen F: Physical measurements as risk indicators for low back trouble over a one-year-period. *Spine, 9:*106, 1984.
19. Cady LD, Bischoff DP, O'Connell ER, et al: Strength and fitness and subsequent back injuries in firefighters. *J Occup Med, 21:*269, 1979.
20. McQuade PT, Turner JA, Buchner DM: Physical fitness and chronic low back pain. *Clin Orthop Rel Res, 233:*198, 1988.
21. Holm S, Nachemson A: Variations in the nutrition of the canine intervertebral disc induced by motion. *Spine, 8:*866, 1983.
22. Nachemson A: Towards a better understanding of low-back pain: a review of the mechanics of the lumbar disc. *Rheum Rehab, 14:*129, 1975.
23. Bogduk N: A reappraisal of the anatomy of the human erector spinae. *J Anat, 131:*525, 1980.
24. Bogduk N, Macintosh JE: The applied anatomy of the thoracolumbar fascia. *Spine, 9:*164, 1984.
25. Macintosh JE, Bogduk N: The biomechanics of the thoracolumbar fascia. *Clin Biomech, 2:*79, 1987.
26. Gracovetsky S, Farfan H, Helleur C: The abdominal mechanism. *Spine, 10:*317, 1985
27. Gracovetsky S, Farfan H: The optimum spine. *Spine, 11:*543, 1986.
28. Basmajian JV: *Primary Anatomy.* Williams & Wilkins, 1964.
29. Liemohn WP: Exercise and the back. Exercise and arthritis. *Rheum Dis Clin North Am, 16:*945–970, 1990.
30. Liemohn WP, Snodgrass LB, Sharpe GL: Unresolved controversies in back management—a review. *J Orthop Sports Phys Ther 9:*239, 1988.
31. Mayer TG, Smith SS, Keeley J, et al: Quantification of lumbar function Part II: Sagittal plane trunk strength in chronic low-back pain patients. *Spine, 10:*765, 1985.
32. Jorgenson K, Nicolaisen T: Trunk extensor endurance: determination and relation to low-back trouble. *Ergonomics, 30:*259, 1987.
33. Saal JS, Saal JA: Strength training and flexibility. In *Conservative Care of Low Back Pain.* Edited by AH White, R Anderson. Baltimore: Williams & Wilkins, 1991, p. 65.
34. Saal JA, Saal JS: Nonoperative treatment of herniated lumbar intervertebral disc with radiculopathy—an outcome study. *Spine, 14:*431, 1989.

Section II

EXERCISE PHYSIOLOGY

Chapter 6

FUNDAMENTALS OF EXERCISE METABOLISM

Scott K. Powers

Almost all changes occurring in the body during exercise are related to the increase in energy metabolism within the contracting skeletal muscle. For example, cardiac output and heart rate increase as a function of metabolic rate. At rest, a 70-kg human has an energy expenditure of about 1.2 kcal/min; less than 20% of this resting energy expenditure is estimated to be used by skeletal muscle, which is a surprisingly low value given that skeletal muscle constitutes almost 50% of total body weight.

During intense exercise, total energy expenditure may be increased 15 to 25 times above resting values, resulting in a caloric expenditure of approximately 18 to 30 kcal/min. Most of this increase is used to provide energy for the exercising muscles that may increase their energy utilization by a factor of 200 over resting levels.[1] The focus of this chapter in on muscle bioenergetics and exercise metabolism. By necessity, this section is concise, and the treatment of each topic is therefore brief. A detailed review of bioenergetics and exercise metabolism is provided in several sources.[2–6]

ENERGY FOR MUSCULAR CONTRACTION

Contraction of skeletal muscle is powered by the energy released through hydrolysis of the high-energy compound adenosine triphosphate (ATP) to form adenosine diphosphate (ADP) and inorganic phosphate (Pi). This reaction is catalyzed by the enzyme myosin ATPase:

$$ATP \xrightarrow{\text{myosin ATPase}} ADP + Pi + energy$$

The amount of ATP in muscle at any time is small, and thus it must be resynthesized continuously if exercise continues for more than a few seconds. Muscle fibers contain the metabolic machinery to produce ATP by three pathways: (1) creatine phosphate (CP) system; (2) glycolysis; and (3) aerobic oxidation of nutrients to produce CO_2 and H_2O.

The CP system involves the transfer of high-energy phosphate from CP to rephosphorylate ADP to ATP as follows:

$$ADP + CP \xrightarrow{\text{creatine kinase}} ATP + C$$

This reaction is rapid because it involves only one enzymatic step; however, CP exists in finite quantities in cells and thus the total amount of ATP that can be produced through this mechanism is limited. Note that oxygen (O_2) is not involved in the rephosphorylation of ADP to ATP in this reaction, and thus the CP system is considered anaerobic metabolism (without O_2).

A second metabolic pathway capable of producing ATP without the involvement of O_2 exists in the cytoplasm of the muscle cell; this is called glycolysis. Glycolysis is the degradation of carbohydrate (glycogen or glucose) to pyruvate or lactate and involves a series of enzymatically catalyzed steps (Fig. 6–1). The net energy yield of glycolysis is 2 or 3 ATP through substrate level phosphorylation. The net ATP production is 2 ATP when glucose is the substrate and 3 ATP when glycogen is the substrate. Although the process of glycolysis does not involve the use of O_2 and is thus considered an anaerobic pathway, pyruvate can participate in aerobic production of ATP when O_2 is available in the cell. Thus, in addition to being an anaerobic pathway capable of producing ATP without O_2, glycolysis can be considered the first step in the aerobic degradation of carbohydrate.

Historically, rising blood lactate levels during exercise have been considered

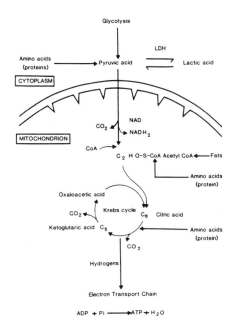

Glycolysis

Amino acids (proteins) → Pyruvic acid ⇌ Lactic acid

LDH

CYTOPLASM

MITOCHONDRION

CO_2

NAD

NADH$_2$

CoA

C_2 H O–S–CoA Acetyl CoA ← Fats

Amino acids (protein)

Oxaloacetic acid

CO_2 Krebs cycle C_8 Citric acid

Ketoglutaric acid C_5

Amino acids (protein)

CO_2

Hydrogens

Electron Transport Chain

ADP + Pi → ATP + H_2O

Fig. 6–1. Relationship between glycolysis, the Krebs cycle, and the electron transport chain.

an indication of increased anaerobic metabolism within the contracting muscle caused by a lack of oxygen.[7,8] However, whether the end product of glycolysis is pyruvate or lactate depends on several factors. First, if O_2 is not available in the mitochondria to accept the hydrogen released during glycolysis, pyruvate must accept the hydrogen and glycolysis will proceed. Second, if glycolytic flux is extremely rapid, hydrogen production may exceed the transport capability of the shuttle mechanisms required to move hydrogens from the cytoplasm (called sarcoplasm in muscle) into the mitochondria, where oxidative phosphorylation occurs. When glycolytic hydrogen production exceeds the mitochondria transport capability, pyruvate must again accept the hydrogen to form lactate so that glycolysis can continue. Finally, conversion of pyruvate to lactate (and vice versa) is catalyzed by the enzyme lactate dehydrogenase (LDH), which exists in several forms (isozymes). Fast-twitch muscle fibers contain an LDH isozyme that favors the formation of lactate, whereas slow-twitch fibers contain an LDH form that promotes the conversion of lactate to pyruvate. Therefore, lactate formation

might occur in fast-twitch fibers during exercise simply because of the type of LDH isozyme present, independent of O_2 availability in the muscle. In summary, debate continues over the mechanism(s) responsible for muscle lactate production during exercise. It seems possible that any one or a combination of the above possibilities (including lack of O_2) might provide an explanation for muscle lactate production during exercise. A detailed discussion of this topic is available from several sources.[3,7–9]

The final metabolic pathway found in cells to produce ATP is a combination of two complex metabolic processes (i.e., Krebs cycle and electron transport chain) and is located inside the mitochondria. As the name implies, oxidative phosphorylation involves the use of O_2 as the final hydrogen acceptor to form H_2O and ATP. Unlike glycolysis, aerobic metabolism can use fat, protein, and carbohydrate as substrate to produce ATP. The interaction of these nutrients is illustrated in Figure 6–1. Conceptually, a metabolic process called the Krebs cycle can be considered a "primer" for oxidative phosphorylation. Entry into the Krebs cycle begins with the combination of acetyl-CoA and oxaloacetic acid to form citric acid. In brief, the primary purpose of the Krebs cycle is to remove hydrogens from four of the reactants involved in the cycle. The electrons from these hydrogens then follow a chain of cytochromes (electron transport chain) in the mitochondria, and the energy released from this process is used to rephosphorylate ADP to form ATP. Oxygen is the final acceptor of hydrogens to form H_2O (Fig. 6–1). Note that glycolysis can interact with the Krebs cycle in the presence of O_2 by the conversion of pyruvate to form acetyl-CoA. For a detailed review of oxidative phosphorylation, see references 6 and 10.

REGULATION OF BIOENERGETIC PATHWAYS

The bioenergetic pathways that result in production of cellular ATP are under precise control. This control is achieved by regulation of one or more regulatory (allosteric) enzymes. A rate-limiting enzyme exists in each of the aforementioned bioenergetic pathways that can be "up-regulated" or "down-regulated," depending upon the cellular need for ATP. In other words, the catalytic activity of allosteric enzymes is regulated by cellular modulators. In general, important modulators of bioenergetic regulatory enzymes are cellular concentrations of ATP and ADP. For example, creatine phosphate breakdown is regulated by creatine kinase activity.[6] Creatine kinase activity is elevated when cytoplasmic concentrations of ADP increase and ATP levels decrease. Conversely, creatine kinase activity is inhibited by high cellular ATP levels. This type of negative feedback control is common among bioenergetic pathways in the muscle fiber.

The rate-limiting enzyme in glycolysis is phosphofructokinase (PFK). PFK is located early in the glycolytic pathway, and its regulation is similar to that of creatine kinase. PFK activity is increased by a rise in cellular ADP concentration and a decrease in ATP levels. PFK activity is inhibited by various factors, including high cellular concentrations of hydrogen ions, citrate, and ATP.

A detailed discussion of the regulation of mitochondrial respiration is beyond the scope of this chapter; therefore the following discussion is designed to provide a simple overview of the regulation of mitochondrial respiration. For a detailed discussion of the regulation of oxidative phosphorylation, see reference 10. Although oxidative phosphorylation is under complex control, it is clear that key allosteric enzymes in the Krebs cycle (i.e., isocitrate dehydrogenase) and electron transport chain (i.e., cytochrome oxidase) are regulated, in part, by cellular levels of ATP and ADP. Similar to the control schemes presented for the creatine phosphate system and glycolysis, an increase in cellular levels of ADP promotes oxidative phosphorylation and high concentrations of ATP inhibit this process.

METABOLIC RESPONSES TO EXERCISE

The importance of the interaction of the aforementioned metabolic pathways in the production of ATP during exercise should be emphasized. Although we often speak of aerobic versus anaerobic exercise, in reality, the energy necessary to perform most types of exercise comes from a combination of anaerobic/aerobic sources (see

Fig. 6–2). The contribution of anaerobic sources (PC system and glycolysis) to exercise energy metabolism is inversely related to the duration and intensity of the activity. That is, the shorter the activity, the greater the contribution of anaerobic energy production; the longer the activity, the greater the contribution of aerobic energy production. Although proteins can be used as a fuel for aerobic exercise, carbohydrates and fats are the primary energy substrates during exercise in a healthy, well-fed individual. In general, carbohydrates are used as the primary fuel at the onset of exercise and during high-intensity work.[3,11–13] During prolonged exercise (i.e., longer than 30 minutes), however, a gradual shift occurs from carbohydrate metabolism toward an increasing reliance on fat as a substrate (Fig. 6–3).[13–16] A detailed discussion outlining the interplay of substrates during exercise is available from several sources.[3,11–19] A brief discussion of the metabolic response to various types of exercise follows.

Short-term High-Intensity Exercise

The energy to perform short-term high intensity exercise (i.e., 5 to 60 seconds in duration) such as weight lifting or sprinting 400 meters comes primarily from anaero-

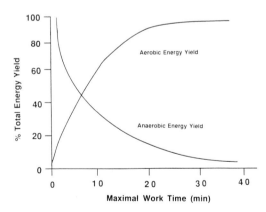

Fig. 6–2. Interaction between anaerobic and aerobic metabolism during exercise. Note that energy to perform short-term high intensity exercise comes primarily from anaerobic sources, whereas energy for muscular contraction during prolonged exercise comes from aerobic metabolism. Redrawn with permission from McArdle W, Katch F, Katch V: *Exercise Physiology*. Philadelphia: Lea & Febiger, 1991.

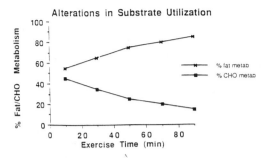

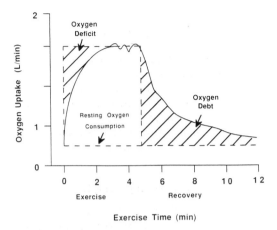

Fig. 6–3. Alterations in substrate utilization during prolonged submaximal exercise. CHO = carbohydrate. Data with permission from Powers S, Riley W, Howley E: Comparison of fat metabolism between trained men and women during prolonged aerobic work. *Res Q Exerc Sport, 51:*427, 1980.

Fig. 6–4. Oxygen uptake dynamics at onset and offset of exercise. See text for details.

bic pathways. Whether ATP production is dominated by the PC-ATP system or glycolysis depends on the duration of the muscular effort. In general, energy for all activities lasting less than 5 seconds comes from the CP system. In contrast, energy to perform a 200-meter sprint (i.e., 30 seconds) would come from a combination of the CP system and anaerobic glycolysis with glycolysis producing much of the required ATP. Note that the transition from the CP system to glycolysis is not an abrupt change but rather a gradual shift from one pathway to another as the duration of the exercise increases.

As illustrated in Figure 6–2, exercise bouts lasting longer than 45 seconds use a combination of the CP system, glycolysis, and oxidative phosphorylation. For example, the energy required to sprint 400 meters (i.e., 60 seconds) comes primarily from anaerobic pathways (~70%), whereas the remaining ATP production is provided by aerobic metabolism (~30%). The principal fuel used during this type of exercise is carbohydrates (glycogen) stored in muscle.[2-4,17]

Transition From Rest to Light Exercise

In the transition from rest to light exercise, oxygen uptake kinetics follow a monoexponential pattern, reaching a steady state generally within 1 to 4 minutes (Fig. 6–4).[20] The time required to reach a steady state increases at higher work rates and is longer in untrained subjects compared to

aerobically trained individuals. The fact that oxygen consumption ($\dot{V}O_2$) does not increase instantaneously to a steady state at the onset of exercise implies that anaerobic energy sources contribute to the required $\dot{V}O_2$ at the beginning of exercise. Indeed, evidence exists that both the CP system and glycolysis contribute to the overall production of ATP at the onset of muscular work.[21] Once a steady state is obtained, however, the body's ATP requirements are met by aerobic metabolism. The term O_2 deficit has been used to describe the inadequate O_2 consumption at the onset of exercise (Fig. 6–4). As in short term heavy exercise, the principal fuel used during the transition from rest to light exercise is muscle glycogen.[2-4,17]

Prolonged Submaximal Exercise

A steady-state $\dot{V}O_2$ can usually be maintained during 10 to 60 minutes of submaximal continuous exercise. Two exceptions to this rule exist. First, prolonged exercise in a hot and humid environment may result in a steady "drift upward" of $\dot{V}O_2$ during the course of exercise.[22] Second, continuous exercise at a high relative workload results in a slow rise in $\dot{V}O_2$ across time similar to that in observed during exercise in a hot environment. In both cases, this drift in $\dot{V}O_2$ probably occurs because of a variety of factors (i.e., rising body temperature and increasing blood catecholamines).[23,24]

As predicted from Figure 6–3, both carbohydrate and fats are used as substrates during prolonged exercise. As mentioned previously, during prolonged submaximal exercise, there is a gradual shift from carbohydrate metabolism toward the use of fat as a substrate. The percentage contribution fat versus carbohydrate as an energy substrate during prolonged exercise is determined by a complex interaction among exercise intensity, nutritional status of the individual, state of training, and duration of the activity.

Progressive Incremental Exercise

Figure 6–5 illustrates the oxygen uptake during a progressive-incremental exercise test. Note that oxygen uptake increases as a linear function to work rate until $\dot{V}O_{2max}$ is reached. After reaching a steady state, ATP used for muscular contraction during the early stages of an incremental exercise test comes primarily from aerobic metabolism. However, as the exercise intensity increases, the level of blood lactate rises (Fig. 6–6). Although much controversy surrounds this issue, many investigators believe that this lactate "inflection" point represents a point of increasing reliance on anaerobic metabolism. Although the precise terminology is controversial, this sudden increase in blood lactate levels—termed the "anaerobic threshold" or "lactate threshold"—has important implications for the prediction of performance and perhaps exercise prescription. For example, several investigators have shown that the anaerobic threshold used in combination with other physiologic variables (i.e., $\dot{V}O_{2max}$) is a useful predictor of success in distance running.[25,26] The anaerobic

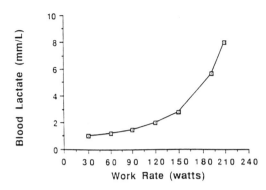

Fig. 6–6. Changes in blood lactate concentrations as a function of work rate during incremental exercise.

threshold might also prove to be a useful marker of the transition from moderate to heavy exercise for subjects, and thus could be useful in exercise prescription.

Recovery from Exercise

Oxygen uptake remains elevated above resting levels for several minutes during recovery from exercise (Fig. 6–4). This elevated postexercise O_2 consumption has traditionally been termed the "oxygen debt." The term "elevated post exercise oxygen consumption" has also been applied to describe this phenomenon.[2,23] In general, postexercise metabolism is higher after high-intensity exercise when compared to light and to moderate work. Furthermore, postexercise $\dot{V}O_2$ values remain elevated longer after prolonged exercise compared to values associated with short-term exertion. The mechanisms to explain these observations are probably linked to the fact that both high-intensity and prolonged exercise result in higher body temperatures, greater ionic disturbances, and higher plasma catecholamine levels than those values related to light or moderate short-term exercise.[23]

ENERGY COST OF ACTIVITIES

The energy cost of many types of physical activities has been established. Table 6–1 is a list of physical activities and their associated energy expenditures expressed in kilocalories per minute (kcal·min^{-1}). Activities that are vigorous and involve large muscle groups usually result in more

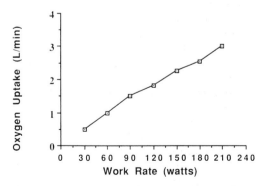

Fig. 6–5. Changes in oxygen uptake as a function of work rate during incremental exercise.

energy expended than activities that use small muscle mass or require limited exertion. The estimates of energy expenditure listed in Table 6–1 were obtained by measuring oxygen cost of these activities in an adult population. Although not precise, energy expenditure (kcal/min) can be estimated by multiplying the measured $\dot{V}O_2$ (L/min) and the coefficient 5 kcal/L (each liter of O_2 consumed represents an energy expenditure of 5 kcal). Clinicians often use the term "MET" to describe exercise intensity. One MET is equivalent to the amount of energy expended during 1 minute of rest. For example, an individual exercising at a metabolic rate that is five times his or her resting $\dot{V}O_2$ is working at a 5 MET work rate. In a strict sense, the absolute energy expenditure during exercise at a 5-MET intensity depends on the body size of the individual (i.e., a large individual is likely to have a larger resting $\dot{V}O_2$ when compared to a smaller individual). For simplic-

ity, individual differences in resting energy expenditures are often overlooked, and 1 MET is considered equivalent to a $\dot{V}O_2$ of 3.5 ml·kg^{-1}·min^{-1}. Hence, 1 MET represents an energy expenditure of approximately 1.5 kcal/min.

REFERENCES

1. Armstrong R: Biochemistry: Energy liberation and use. In *Sports Medicine and Physiology*. Edited by RS Strauss. Philadelphia: W.B. Saunders, 1979.
2. Brooks G, Fahey T: Exercise Physiology: Human Bioenergetics and its Applications. New York: John Wiley & Sons, 1984.
3. Powers S, Howley E: *Exercise Physiology: Theory and Application to Fitness and Performance.* Dubuque: William C. Brown, 1990.
4. McArdle W, Katch F, Katch V: Exercise Physiology. Philadelphia: Lea & Febiger, 1991.
5. Holloszy J: Muscle metabolism during exercise. *Arch Phys Med Rehabil, 63:*231, 1982.
6. Mathews C, van Holde K: *Biochemistry.* Redwood City: Benjamin Cummings, 1990.
7. Graham T: Mechanisms of blood lactate increase during exercise. *Physiologist, 27:*299, 1984.
8. Katz A, Sahlin K: Oxygen in regulation of glycolysis and lactate production in human skeletal muscle. In *Exercise and Sport Sciences Reviews.* Edited by Pandoff K, Holloszy J. Baltimore: Williams and Wilkins *18:*1, 1990.
9. Stainsby W, Brooks G: Control of lactic acid metabolism in contracting skeletal muscles during exercise. In *Exercise and Sport Sciences Reviews.* Edited by Pandoff K, Holloszy J. Baltimore: Williams and Wilkins *18:*29, 1990.
10. Senior, A: ATP synthesis by oxidative phosphorylation. *Physiological Reviews. 68:*177, 1988.
11. Gollnick P, Riedy M, Quintinskie J, Bertocci L: Differences in metabolic potential of skeletal muscle fibers and their significance for metabolic control. *J Exp Biol, 115:*191, 1985.
12. Gollnick P: Metabolism of substrates: Energy substrate metabolism during exercise and as modified by training. *Fed Proc, 44:*353, 1985.
13. Newsholme E: The control of fuel utilization by muscle during exercise and starvation. *Diabetes, 28(Suppl. 1):*1, 1979.
14. Powers S, Riley W, Howley E: Comparison of fat metabolism between trained men and women during prolonged aerobic work. *Res Q Exerc Sport, 51:*427, 1980.

Table 6–1. Energy Expenditure During Activities

Activity	Energy Expenditure (kcal/min/kg BW)
Badminton	0.06
Basketball	0.14
Boxing	0.22
Canoeing	
Leisure	0.04
Racing	0.10
Dancing	
Ballroom	0.05
Choreographed (vigorous)	0.17
Football	0.13
Golf (walking + carrying bag)	0.09
Running (horizontally)	
9 min/mile	0.19
8 min/mile	0.22
7 min/mile	0.24
6 min/mile	0.28
Swimming	
Backstroke	0.17
Breast stroke	0.16
Crawl, fast	0.16
Crawl, slow	0.13
Tennis (singles)	0.11
Volleyball	0.05
Walking (horizontal)	
16 min/mile	0.08
20 min/mile	0.07

15. Holloszy J, Coyle E: Adaptations of skeletal muscle to endurance exercise and their metabolic consequences. *J Appl Physiol, 56:* 831, 1984.

16. Holloszy, J. Utilization of fatty acids during exercise. In *Biochemistry of Exercise VII*. Edited by A Taylor et al. Champaign: Human Kinetics Publishers, 1990.

17. Stanley W, Connett R: Regulation of muscle carbohydrate metabolism during exercise. *FASEB J, 5:*2155, 1991.

18. Bonen A, McDermott J, Tan M: Glucose transport in muscle. *Biochemistry of Exercise VII*. Edited by A. Taylor et al. Champaign: Human Kinetics Publishers, 1990.

19. Powers S, Byrd R, Tulley R, Callender T: Effects of caffeine ingestion on metabolism and performance during graded exercise. *Eur J Appl Physiol, 50:*301, 1983.

20. Powers S, Dodd S, Beadle R: Oxygen uptake kinetics in trained athletes differing in VO_{2max}. *Eur J Appl Physiol, 54:*306, 1985.

21. diPrampero P, Boutellier U, Pietsch P: Oxygen deficit and stores at onset of muscular exercise in humans. *J Appl Physiol, 55:*146, 1983.

22. Powers S, Howley E, Cox R: Ventilatory and metabolic reactions to heat stress during prolonged exercise. *J Sports Med, 22:*32, 1982.

23. Gaesser G, Brooks G: Metabolic bases of excess post-exercise oxygen consumption: A review. *Med Sci Sports Exerc, 16:*29, 1984.

24. Powers S, Howley E, Cox R: A differential catecholamine response during prolonged exercise and passive heating. *Med Sci Sports Exerc, 14:*435, 1982.

25. Farrell PA, et al.: Plasma lactate accumulation and distance running performance. *Med Sci Sports Exerc, 11:*338, 1979.

26. Powers S, et al.: Ventilatory threshold, running economy and distance running performance of trained athletes. *Res Q Exerc Sport, 51:*179, 1983.

Chapter 7

CARDIORESPIRATORY RESPONSES TO ACUTE EXERCISE

J. Larry Durstine, Russell R. Pate, and J. David Branch

The cardiorespiratory system is the body's transportation network. The system functions by circulating blood through a closed network of blood vessels that infiltrate virtually all body tissues. The major components of the cardiorespiratory system (heart, blood vessels, and pulmonary tract) are subject to an integrated set of control processes that enable it to respond effectively to many physiologic perturbations.

A long-recognized fact is that the cardiorespiratory system plays a critical role in the physiologic responses to exercise. Vigorous exercise is associated with a marked increase in energy metabolism in active skeletal muscle. This increased metabolic activity can be sustained only if the muscles are provided with metabolic substrates (e.g., oxygen, glucose, and free fatty acids) and are cleared of metabolic end products (e.g., carbon dioxide and lactic acid) at rates that match their rates of utilization and production, respectively. Because the cardiorespiratory system is the only supply line for muscle tissue, sustained, vigorous exercise clearly necessitates marked alterations in cardiorespiratory function.

The major functions of the cardiorespiratory system during exercise are: (1) to deliver oxygen to the active muscles at a rate that matches the rate at which it is used in aerobic metabolism; (2) to clear carbon dioxide and other metabolic end-products from the active muscles at rates that match production; (3) to facilitate dissipation of metabolically produced heat to the environment by increasing blood flow to the skin; and (4) to support a properly integrated physiologic response to exercise by carrying regulatory substances such as hormones from sites of production to target tissues.

This chapter is a concise summary of the cardiorespiratory response to acute exercise. Major sections are dedicated to cardiovascular and respiratory responses. Within each of these major sections, the responses of key functional variables and their physiologic regulation are briefly discussed.

CARDIOVASCULAR RESPONSES

Absolute and Relative Rates of Energy Expenditure

Interpretations of the physiologic responses to acute exercise or exercise training and the comparison of physiologic information between individuals are influenced by how the physiologic data are referenced (i.e., the *absolute* energy expenditure or the *relative* energy expenditure). Although the absolute energy expenditure is the actual oxygen uptake (e.g., $300 \ mL \cdot min^{-1}$), relative energy expenditure is the percentage of maximal oxygen consumption ($\dot{V}_{O_{2max}}$) (e.g., 75% of $\dot{V}_{O_{2max}}$). Many physiologic variables such as blood flow distribution, ventilatory threshold, and blood and muscle concentrations of lactate depend on the *relative* intensity of exercise. The *relative* intensity of exercise also determines which energy system(s) supply ATP to exercising muscle. Comparison of physiologic variables at the same *absolute* exercise level is important when assessing changes in a given individual (i.e., submaximal changes resulting from training). However, interpretations may become confusing when comparing different individuals at the same *absolute* level of exercise. If two individuals have different $\dot{V}_{O_{2max}}$ values, the same *absolute* submaximal $\dot{V}_{O_{2max}}$ represents different *relative* percentages of $\dot{V}_{2max}$. For example, consider a trained subject and a sedentary subject with $\dot{V}_{O_{2max}}$ values of 60 and $40 \ mL \cdot kg^{-1} \cdot min^{-1}$, respectively. An *absolute* $\dot{V}_{O_{2max}}$ of $30 \ mL \cdot kg^{-1} \cdot min^{-1}$ represents *relative* rates of energy expenditure of

50% and 75%, respectively, for these subjects.

In this chapter, the phrase *work rate* defines an *absolute* power output (e.g., bicycle ergometry at 100 W). *Exercise intensity,* on the other hand, is the *relative* energy expenditure for a given *absolute* power output. Consider the two subjects described in the above paragraph. Bicycle ergometry at 100 W represents an approximate $\dot{V}O_2$ cost of 21 mL·kg^{-1}·min^{-1} for a 70 kg individual, an exercise intensity of 35% and 52.5% of the respective $\dot{V}O_{2max}$ for the trained subject and sedentary subject.

Orthostatic Hypotension

Orthostatic hypotension is a result of the body's inability to maintain arterial blood pressure against changes in posture because of decreased intravascular hydrostatic pressure, plasma volume, heart contractility, vasomotor tone, and venous return. As an individual moves from a supine to an upright position, there is a decrease in the intravascular hydrostatic pressure that must be compensated for by increased baroreceptor response. The result is an increase in heart rate to maintain arterial pressure. In hospitalized patients, orthostatic tolerance can be maintained by progressive exposure to an upright posture. Although supine exercise prevents deterioration in fitness, it is less effective in preventing orthostatic intolerance. At the same time, sitting is effective in preventing orthostatic hypotension, but will not prevent deterioration in fitness.[1]

A proper postexercise cool-down that involves low-intensity movement of the lower extremity musculature is an essential part of any workout. Failure to allow an adequate cool-down can result in pooling of blood in the lower extremities consequent to hypotension.

Cardiac Output

The primary function of the heart is to pump blood through the pulmonary and systemic arterial circulations of the body. Cardiac output ($\dot{Q}$), quantified as liters of blood pumped per minute, is a reflection of the overall functional activity of the heart and a principal determinant of the rate of oxygen delivery to peripheral tissues such as active skeletal muscle. Cardiac output is determined by heart rate, the frequency of the heart's contraction (contractions·min^{-1}), and stroke volume, the volume of blood pumped by the heart with each contraction (mL·contraction^{-1}). Thus, cardiac output is equal to the product of heart rate and stroke volume. At the onset of constant intensity exercise, $\dot{Q}$ increases rapidly at first and then more gradually until a plateau or "steady state" is attained. Subsequent increases in work rate and oxygen demand elicit similar responses in $\dot{Q}$ until a maximum is reached (Fig. 7–1). An average value for resting $\dot{Q}$ in normal healthy men is 5 liters·min^{-1}. During exercise, $\dot{Q}$ may increase to 4 to 5 times the resting level (20 to 25 liters·min^{-1}) in young, healthy men.[2] Somewhat lower maximal $\dot{Q}$ levels are observed in sedentary women (15 to 20 liters·min^{-1}).[3] Maximal $\dot{Q}$ values as high as 35 to 40 liters·min^{-1} have been observed in endurance athletes.[4]

Upright resting $\dot{Q}$ values are approximately 1 liter·min^{-1} less than those observed in a supine position.[5,6] The mechanism underlying this difference is not fully understood, but stroke volume values for supine subjects at rest are known to be higher than those reported for individuals while in the upright position.[5,6] In the upright position, gravity may impede venous return of blood to the heart and result in a diminished stroke volume and a lower $\dot{Q}$ value.

Heart Rate

Heart rate (HR), a major determinant of $\dot{Q}$, is controlled by factors intrinsic to the heart as well as by extrinsic neural and hormonal factors. The inherent rhythmicity of the heart, as established by its sinoatrial node, is regulated primarily by sympathetic and parasympathetic neurons emanating from the cardioregulatory center of the medulla. The sympathetic cardioaccelerator nerves release norepinephrine at their endings and cause HR to increase during exercise.[7] The parasympathetic vagus nerve releases acetylcholine, which tends to reduce HR. Under resting conditions, the vagal influences are dominant over sympathetic influences. During exercise, this rela-

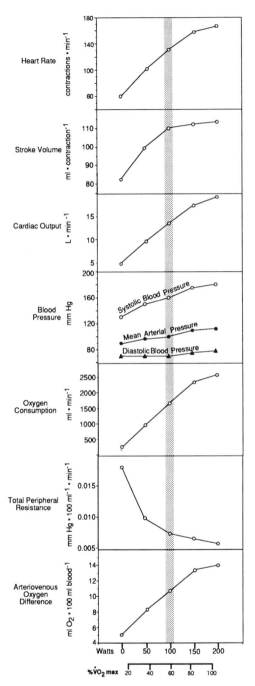

Fig. 7–1. Cardiovascular responses to graded exercise. Typical values for a sedentary individual are plotted against specific work rates and %V̇O$_{2max}$. The shaded area represents lactate threshold.

tionship is reversed, and HR consequently increases over its resting level. Also, circulating hormones such as epinephrine and norepinephrine, released by the adrenal glands into the blood, can increase the rate of contraction. In addition, factors such as increased temperature and stretch of the sinoatrial node (Bainbridge reflex) tend to increase HR.

The average resting HR for a sedentary individual is approximately 72 contractions·min^{-1}. The average resting HR for a trained person is somewhat lower, depending on the state of training. Maximal HR is relatively constant across various conditions, but tends to be slightly lower with the subject in the supine position than in the upright position.[6] Also, maximal HR decreases with aging.[8] A reasonably accurate estimate of average maximal HR for persons of a given age is obtained by using the equation:

$$\text{Average maximal HR} \\ (\text{contractions·min}^{-1}) = 220 - \text{age (years)}$$

This equation provides an indication of the age group average maximal HR; considerable variability in maximal HR exists among persons of a certain age (standard deviation of the mean is 10 to 12 contractions·min^{-1}).[9] Gender differences exist in the exercise heart rate response, with women generally having higher HR response to the same absolute work rate.[10] HR often rises in anticipation of exercise. This pre-exercise increase is controlled by the limbic system; a regulatory center situated in the basal area of the brain surrounding the hypothalamus. Nerve fibers originating from this center and ending in the medulla result in activation of the cardioaccelerator nerves and inhibition of the vagus nerve. At the beginning of exercise, HR increases almost instantaneously.[11] The mechanism for this rapid response is not well understood, but a neural reflex with origins in joint receptors and muscle spindles may be involved.[11,12]

A strong positive correlation exists between HR and oxygen consumption (Fig. 7-1).[9,13] Both parameters increase linearly with increasing intensity of exercise.[13] As shown in Figure 7–1, HR increases with increasing work rate until a maximal rate is reached. As a sedentary person experiences an improvement in aerobic fitness, the slope of the HR/$\dot{V}O_2$ relationship decreases (i.e., a lower post-training HR response results at the same pre-training work rate and $\dot{V}O_2$).

During sustained static exercise, HR is exaggerated because of the reduced venous return and activation of the baroreceptor reflex in response to decreased arterial pressure. Static exercise, especially involving the upper body, should be avoided by individuals with hypertension and/or coronary artery disease because of the associated increase in total peripheral resistance and myocardial oxygen demand.

Stroke Volume

Stroke volume (SV), the amount of blood pumped by the heart with each contraction, is regulated primarily by factors that are intrinsic to the heart. Principal among these factors is the Frank-Starling mechanism, which, stated simply, indicates that SV is determined by the rate at which blood is returned to the heart from the venous circulation (i.e., venous return). Increased venous return creates an increase in left ventricular end-diastolic volume, which increases the force of contraction of the myocardium through a mechanism that is similar to the length-tension relationship observed in skeletal muscle.[9] Factors extrinsic to the heart can also influence SV. Sympathetic neural stimulation of the myocardium, as well as epinephrine and norepinephrine released from the adrenal glands, can increase the contractile force of the heart.[9]

Stroke volume, unlike HR and $\dot{Q}$, does not increase linearly with work rate and oxygen consumption (see Fig. 7–1). During graded exercise, SV increases progressively only until a work rate that elicits 40 to 50% of the maximal rate of oxygen consumption is attained. After this intensity level is reached, only small increases in SV occur with increasing oxygen demand.[7] Stroke volume increases with both upright and supine exercise as a consequence of increased venous return and sympathetic stimulation.[6] Greater increases in SV during exercise are observed when the subject is in the upright position.[5,6] This greater SV is probably accomplished by a decrease in left ventricular end-systolic volume resulting in a greater ejection fraction. Ejection fraction is the ratio of the volume of blood ejected from the left ventricle with each contraction to the volume of blood in the left ventricle at the end of diastole.[6]

Normal resting values for SV approximate 70 mL of blood per contraction in sedentary individuals. Highly trained persons may have values as high as 100 mL per contraction.[4,14] During exercise, SV increases to approximately twice its resting value.[4] Women generally have a smaller stroke volume at rest and exercise than men because of smaller heart volume.[10]

Total Peripheral Resistance

Total peripheral resistance (TPR) is the sum of all forces that oppose blood flow in the systemic vascular bed. Factors that affect TPR include length of the arterial vasculature, blood viscosity, hydrostatic pressure, and vessel radius. Of these factors, vessel radius is the most important and, consequently, the balance between vasodilator and vasoconstrictor effects is a key determinant of TPR. Vessel radius is subject to neural control by the sympathetic nervous system; when the latter is activated, vasoconstriction results. Also, local control of vessels is exerted by chemical factors such as pH, P_{CO_2} and lactic acid concentration. Increased rates of muscle metabolism bring about local arterial vasodilation by decreasing pH and increasing P_{CO_2} and lactic acid concentration.

Total peripheral resistance decreases during exercise (Fig. 7–1).[15] This decrease occurs primarily through vasodilation of the arterial vascular beds in the active muscle tissues. The by-products from energy metabolism, released in the exercising tissue, override the sympathetic vasoconstrictor effect of the nervous system. The outcome is a diversion of blood flow to the working tissue and away from the inactive muscles and viscera.[15]

Mean Arterial Pressure

The cardiac cycle has two major phases: (1) diastole, during which the ventricles are at rest, and (2) systole, a contractile period during which blood is forced by the ventricles into the pulmonary and systemic arterial systems. Fluid pressure in the systemic arteries fluctuates between systolic (higher) and diastolic (lower) pressures. The average pressure exerted by the blood against the inner walls of the arteries is a function of systolic and diastolic pressures and is termed mean arterial pressure (MAP). The following equation includes the two major determinants of MAP, $\dot{Q}$ and TPR, and represents the mathematical model used to calculate MAP.

$$MAP = \dot{Q} \cdot TPR$$

An estimate of MAP is obtained easily by using the equation:

$$MAP = \text{Diastolic Pressure} + \frac{(\text{Systolic Pressure} - \text{Diastolic Pressure})}{3}$$

Normal resting MAP is in the range of 90 to 100 mm Hg. Exercise MAP rises steadily with increasing work rate (see Fig. 7–1). Maximal exercise MAP values approximate 130 mm Hg.[6] The systolic time interval (the period when the heart is in systole) represents approximately 33% of the resting cardiac cycle. Because the period of diastole is longer than the period of systole, MAP is less than the average of systolic and diastolic pressures. During exercise, the systolic time interval comprises a progressively larger proportion of the cardiac cycle. Thus, during exercising, this equation may provide a less accurate estimation of MAP. Some evidence indicates that resting and exercise MAP are not affected by body position.[6]

Systolic Blood Pressure

The pressure in the arterial vessels is highest during ventricular systole. Systolic blood pressure (SBP) is indicative of the force generated by the heart during ventricular contraction. Normal resting systolic pressure is about 120 mm Hg. Systolic blood pressure increases with exercise, but the magnitude of this response is specific to the type of exercise performed.

During dynamic, low-resistance exercise (e.g., jogging, swimming, and cycling), systolic blood pressure increases in proportion to exercise intensity (Fig. 7–1).[16] This overall response is the result of two countervailing effects of acute dynamic exercise. Dilation of arterial blood vessels in active muscles reduces peripheral resistance, and this response tends to decrease blood pressure.[15] This effect, however, is more than offset by increased $\dot{Q}$, which as previously discussed, increases linearly with work rate. Thus, the exercise-induced increase in SBP reflects an increase in $\dot{Q}$, the effect of which is partially offset by reduced peripheral resistance.

The magnitude of the response of SBP to dynamic exercise varies with body position and active muscle groups. Somewhat lower pressure values are recorded when the subject exercises while supine than when the erect position is maintained.[6] Researchers comparing leg and arm work have reported consistently higher SBP values (approximately 15%) associated with arm work.[16] This response is probably related to the smaller muscle mass of the arms, which offers greater resistance to blood flow than does the larger muscle mass of the legs.[16,17] In addition, a higher TPR could be expected from dynamic upper body exercise because of the relatively larger inactive muscle mass of the lower body.

Exercise activities that involve forceful isometric, isotonic, or isokinetic muscle contraction cause marked increases in SBP.[18,19] This is especially true for static exercise. In addition, the data presented by Seals et al. show that the SBP response to high-resistance exercise is directly related to the muscle mass activated.[20] These responses indicate that high-resistance dynamic or static exercise causes a substantial increase in myocardial work (and oxygen demand). As such, these activities should be used cautiously for persons with cardiovascular diseases.

Diastolic Blood Pressure

Diastolic blood pressure, the pressure in the arterial system during ventricular diastole, provides an indication of peripheral resistance. High diastolic pressure values indicate elevated peripheral resistance.

Normal resting diastolic blood pressure is approximately 80 mm Hg. Dynamic, low-resistance exercise usually causes little or no change in diastolic blood pressure (Fig. 7–1).[21–23] Investigators, comparing arm and leg work at the same relative percentage of Vo_{2max}, report somewhat higher diastolic blood pressures for arm work.[16] High-resistance static exercise may result in large elevations in diastolic pressure.[18,19]

Arteriovenous Oxygen Difference

The oxygen-carrying capacity of blood (C_aO_2) is approximately 20 mL of oxygen per 100 mL of arterial blood. Factors affecting C_aO_2 are hemoglobin concentration ([Hb]) and the percent of arterial oxyhemoglobin saturation (S_aO_2). Arteriovenous oxygen difference (a-$\bar{v}O_2$ diff) is the difference between the oxygen contents of the arterial blood and mixed venous blood. The a-$\bar{v}O_2$ diff is a reflection of the extraction of oxygen from the blood by the active muscle as well as the inactive muscle and tissue. Women generally have somewhat lower C_aO_2 and a-$\bar{v}O_2$ diff than males because of lower [Hb].[10] The average a-$\bar{v}O_2$ diff value at rest is 5 mL $O_2 \cdot 100$ mL^{-1} blood (i.e., 5 mL of oxygen are extracted from each 100 mL of blood circulated). During dynamic exercise, a-$\bar{v}O_2$ diff increases linearly with work rate to maximal values approximating 16 mL $O_2 \cdot 100$ mL^{-1} blood (Fig. 7–1).[14] Thus, about 85% of the oxygen in the blood is removed during maximal exercise. Capillary recruitment and vasodilation result in a longer blood transit time through active muscle and enhance O_2 diffusion from Hb to the mitochondria. The decreased blood flow to inactive tissues, caused by vasoconstriction, is offset to some extent by enhanced O_2 extraction to supply the necessary O_2 to these tissues. Even during maximal exercise, mixed venous blood returning to the heart contains some oxygen; some blood continues to flow through less active tissues and not all the oxygen is removed from the blood.

Blood Flow Redistribution

Acute exercise results not only in an increase in $\dot{Q}$, but also a redistribution of blood flow. As shown in Table 7–1, the general pattern of blood flow redistribution during exercise is away from the renal and splanchnic vascular beds and toward the metabolically active muscle tissue and skin. Increased muscle blood flow provides for increased O_2 delivery to these working tissues, and increased cutaneous flow is important in thermoregulation. Mechanisms responsible for this redistribution include sympathetic stimulation of the α-adrenergic receptors by norepinephrine resulting in vasoconstriction; stimulation of the β-adrenergic receptors by epinephrine resulting in vasodilation; the local increases in concentration of metabolites such as lactate, adenosine, H^+ and K^+, which stimu-

Table 7–1. Blood Flow Distribution to Various Tissues During Rest and Light, Moderate, and Strenuous Exercise*

| Tissue | Resting a-$\bar{v}O_2$ diff† | Resting Blood Flow‡ | Exercise Blood Flow‡ | | |
			Light	Moderate	Maximum
Splanchnic	4.1	1350 (27%)	1100 (12%)	600 (3%)	300 (1%)
Renal	1.3	1100 (22%)	900 (10%)	600 (3%)	250 (1%)
Cerebral	6.3	700 (14%)	750 (8%)	750 (4%)	750 (3%)
Coronary	14.0	200 (4%)	350 (4%)	750 (4%)	1000 (4%)
Muscle	8.4	1000 (20%)	4500 (47%)	12,500 (71%)	22,000 (88%)
Skin	1.0	300 (6%)	1500 (15%)	1900 (12%)	600 (2%)
Other		350 (7%)	400 (4%)	400 (3%)	100 (1%)
Total		5000 (100%)	9500 (100%)	17,500 (100%)	25,000 (100%)

* Modified from Anderson, K. L.: The cardiovascular system in exercise. In *Exercise Physiology*. Edited by H. B. Falls. New York: Academic Press, 1968.
† mL $O_2 \cdot 100$ mL^{-1} blood
‡ ml·min^{-1}

late local vascular receptors, resulting in vasodilation.

VENTILATORY RESPONSES

Minute Ventilation

Minute ventilation is the volume of air passing through the pulmonary system in one (1) minute. Minute volume is often measured as the volume of air expired and is expressed as liters of air expired per minute (liters·min^{-1}). Because the volume of a given amount of gas varies with environmental conditions, ventilatory volumes must be "corrected" to indicate the volume of the air under designated conditions. Ventilatory volumes are usually corrected to either BTPS (body temperature and pressure, saturated with water vapor) or STPD (standard temperature [0°C, 273°K] and pressure [760 mm Hg], for a dry gas). The latter convention is employed when minute ventilation is used with respiratory gas analysis in the measurement of oxygen consumption.

As shown in Figure 7–2, minute ventilation increases with increasing exercise intensity. Below approximately 50% $\dot{V}O_{2max}$, the relationship between ventilation and work rate is linear. At higher intensities, however, the relationship is curvilinear, with ventilation increasing at a rate greater than the rates of work output and oxygen consumption. Minute ventilation is equal to the product of tidal volume (volume expired per breath) and respiratory rate (breathing frequency). Across the lower range of exercise intensities, ventilation increases with increases in both tidal volume and breathing frequency.[24] At higher intensities, increases in ventilation are generated primarily by an increased respiratory respiratory rate.

The ventilatory response to exercise is controlled by a complex physiologic control process that is not fully understood.[9,25,26] The rate and depth of breathing are known to be controlled by nerve pathways that extend from the respiratory center in the medulla to the ventilatory musculature (i.e., diaphragm and intercostal and other muscles). Sensory input to the respiratory center comes from both neural and humoral sources. Central chemoreceptors, located on the ventral surface of the

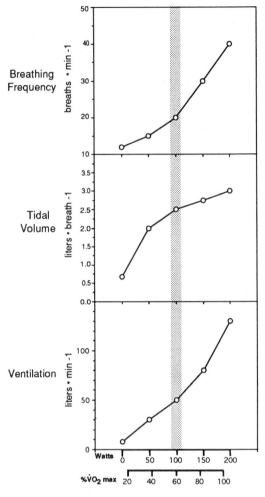

Fig. 7–2. Ventilatory responses to graded exercise. Typical values for a sedentary individual are plotted against specific work rates and %$\dot{V}O_{2max}$. The shaded area represents ventilatory threshold.

medulla, are sensitive to changes in the pH of cerebrospinal and medullary interstitial fluids, which are in turn affected by the pH and PCO_2 of arterial blood. Peripheral chemoreceptors, situated in the walls of the aorta and the carotid and brachycephalic arteries, are sensitive to fluctuation in partial pressure of PCO_2 in arterial blood. Both central and peripheral chemoreceptors function to alter ventilation in such a manner as to maintain normal pH, PCO_2, and PO_2 in arterial blood. For example, decreases in pH and PO_2 and increases in PCO_2 tend to cause increased ventilation.

Neural input to the respiratory center

comes from other sites in the brain. For example, nerve pathways from the motor cortex provide a "feed-forward" control in which ventilation increases as the skeletal muscles are activated in exercise. Also, afferent nerve pathways that arise from the skeletal muscles and joints likely play an important role in causing the rapid increase in ventilation that occurs at the onset of exercise.

Ventilatory Anaerobic Threshold (VANT)

As noted previously (also see Fig. 7–2), ventilation at higher intensities of exercise increases curvilinearly with increasing work rate. The work rate (or rate of oxygen consumption) at which the ventilatory response to graded exercise first departs from linearity is the ventilatory anaerobic threshold (VANT). Although the physiologic mechanism that underlies VANT is not fully understood, VANT usually occurs at a work rate that corresponds closely to that at which lactic acid begins to accumulate in the blood. The rapid increase in ventilation that occurs at exercise intensities above VANT may reflect activation of the bicarbonate buffer system that helps maintain blood pH by "blowing off" nonmetabolically produced carbon dioxide.

Most individuals who exercise regularly are able to perceive VANT as the exercise intensity at which breathing becomes somewhat labored and talking becomes difficult. Because VANT and blood lactic acid accumulation occur at similar exercise intensities in most persons, VANT provides a convenient marker for the upper end of the exercise intensity range usually applied in "aerobic" training programs. At exercise intensities above VANT, lactic acid accumulation in active muscle and blood may preclude prolonged activity. Thus, participants in aerobic exercise programs are often advised to maintain exercise intensities below VANT.

SUMMARY

The cardiorespiratory system responds to acute exercise in such a manner as to increase blood flow and oxygen delivery to the active skeletal muscles. Certain major functional adjustments contribute to this overall response: (1) increased cardiac output ($\dot{Q}$) owing to increased heart rate (HR) and stroke volume (SV); (2) increased arteriovenous oxygen difference (a-$\bar{v}O_2$ diff); (3) decreased total peripheral resistance (TPR) to blood flow owing to dilation of the arterial vasculature in active muscles; and (4) increased ventilation. The magnitude of these cardiorespiratory responses is graded to the intensity of the exercise. The responses are regulated by a complex and well integrated set of neural and humoral processes.

REFERENCES

1. Brooks GA, Fahey TD: *Exercise Physiology: Human Bioenergetics and Its Applications.* New York: John Wiley & Sons, Inc. 1984.
2. Hossack KF, et al.: Maximal cardiac output during upright exercise: approximate normal standards and variations with coronary artery disease. *Am J Cardiol 46:*204, 1980.
3. Hossack KF, Kusumi F, Bruce RA: Approximate normal standards of maximal cardiac output during upright exercise in women. *Am J Cardiol 47:*1080, 1981.
4. Ekblom B, Hermansen L: Cardiac output in athletes. *J Appl Physiol 25:*619, 1968.
5. Bevegard S, Holmgren A, Jonsson B: Circulatory studies in well trained athletes at rest and during heavy exercise with special reference to stroke volume and the influence of body position. *Acta Physiol Scand 57:* 26, 1963.
6. Poliner LR, et al.: Left ventricular performance in normal subjects: a comparison of the responses to exercise in the upright and supine positions. *Circulation 62:*528, 1980.
7. Astrand P-O, Cuddy TE, Saltin B, Stenberg J: Cardiac output during submaximal and maximal work. *J Appl Physiol 19:*268, 1964.
8. Londeree BR, Moeschberger ML: Effect of age and other factors on maximal heart rate. *Res Q Exerc Sports 53:*297, 1982.
9. Martin BJ, Sparks KE, Zwillich CW, Weil JV: Low exercise ventilation in endurance athletes. *Med Sci Sports Exerc 11:*181, 1979.
10. Pate RR, Kriska A: Physiological basis of the sex difference in cardiorespiratory endurance. *Sports Med 1:*87–98, 1984.
11. Petro JK, Hollandee AP, Bouman LN: Instantaneous cardiac acceleration in man induced by a voluntary contraction. *J Appl Physiol 29:*794, 1970.
12. Rowell LB: What signals govern the cardiovascular responses to exercise? *Med Sci Sports Exerc 12:*307, 1980.
13. Ekblom B, Goldberg AN, Kilbom A, Astrand P-O: Effects of atropine and pro-

pranolol on the oxygen transport system during exercise in man. *Scand J Clin Lab Invest 30:*35, 1972.

14. Saltin B: Physiological effects of physical conditioning. *Med Sci Sports Exerc 1:*50, 1969.

15. Clausen JP: Effect of physical training on cardiovascular adjustments to exercise in man. *Physiol Rev 57:*779, 1977.

16. Astrand P-O, et al.: Intra-arterial blood pressure during exercise with different muscle groups. *J Appl Physiol 20:*253, 1965.

17. Blomqvist CG, Lewis SF, Taylor WF, Graham RM: Similarity of the hemodynamic responses to static and dynamic exercise of small muscle groups. *Circ Res 48 (Suppl. 1):* 87, 1982.

18. Freedson PF, et al.: Intra-arterial blood pressure during free weight and hydraulic resistive exercise. *Med Sci Sports Exerc 16:* 131, 1984.

19. McArdle WP, Katch FI, Katch VL: *Exercise Physiology: Energy, Nutrition and Human Performance. 3rd Edition.* Philadelphia: Lea & Febiger, 1991.

20. Seals DR, et al.: Increased cardiovascular response to static contraction of larger muscle groups. *J Appl Physiol. 54:*434, 1983.

21. Ekelund LG, Holmgren A: Central hemodynamics during exercise. *Circ Res. 21 (Suppl. 1):*33, 1967.

22. Sheps DS: Exercise-induced increase in diastolic pressure: indicator of severe coronary artery disease. *Am J Cardiol 43:*708, 1979.

23. Hollman W, Hettinger T. *Sportmedizin-Arbeits-und-Trainingsgrundlagen. 2nd Ed.* Stuttgart: FK Schattauer, 1980.

24. Koyal SN, et al.: Ventilatory responses to the metabolic acidosis of treadmill and cycle ergometry. *J Appl Physiol 40:*864, 1976.

25. Grimby G: Respiration in exercise. *Med Sci Sports Exerc 1:*9, 1969.

26. Folinsbee LJ, et al.: Exercise respiratory pattern in elite cyclists and sedentary subjects. *Med Sci Sports Exerc 15:*503, 1983.

Chapter 8

CARDIORESPIRATORY ADAPTATIONS TO EXERCISE TRAINING

Michael L. Smith and Jere H. Mitchell

Endurance exercise training results in a general improvement in the ability to perform aerobic exercise. This chapter reviews the principal adaptations that facilitate this improvement associated with endurance exercise training (running, cycling, swimming, dance, etc.). Exercise training-induced improvement in fitness is achieved primarily by enhanced maximal exercise capacity and enhanced transport of oxygen to the working tissues. The most accepted index of work capacity is maximal oxygen consumption ($\dot{V}O_{2max}$), which represents the maximal rate of delivery of oxygen from the inspired air to the working tissues (skeletal muscle). Defined physiologically, $\dot{V}O_{2max}$ is the product of maximal cardiac output and maximal arteriovenous oxygen difference (amount of oxygen extracted from the blood). Exercise training can significantly improve the oxygen transport system and increase $\dot{V}O_{2max}$ by increasing both the maximal cardiac output and the maximal arteriovenous oxygen difference. These improvements are one or a combination of improvements in respiration, cardiac function, central circulation, peripheral circulation, and skeletal muscle metabolism. The extent of improvement is determined, in part, by the net training work rate performed, and thus depends on the frequency, intensity, and duration of each exercise session. In addition, the improvement depends on the initial level of fitness so that greater gains are achieved when the initial fitness is low.

RESPIRATION

Pulmonary function at rest is not changed after exercise training. However, some evidence suggests that exercise training may reduce ventilation at submaximal work rates and increase ventilation at maximal work rates.[1,2] These "adaptations" are at best modest and require months or years of training to be realized. If decreased submaximal exercise ventilation occurs, it is probably a secondary effect of reduced blood lactate at any given work rate that reduces ventilatory drive, and is mediated by reduced respiratory rate, whereas tidal volume is either slightly increased or not changed.[1-3] Increases in maximal ventilation appear to be the result of training effects on the respiratory muscle.

The importance of these adaptations in improving fitness is unclear because pulmonary factors do not limit oxygen transport during maximal exercise in healthy individuals. At sea level, arterial oxygen saturation is maintained at maximal work rates, demonstrating that pulmonary factors, ventilatory or diffusive, do not limit oxygen transport in healthy individuals. Thus, the limitation of oxygen transport appears to be imposed by maximal cardiac output or maximal oxygen extraction by the working tissues. In untrained individuals, the capacity for oxygen transport by respiration is greater than that for transport by the circulation. This mismatch is dramatically reduced as exercise training improves the cardiovascular capacity for oxygen transport.[4] Dempsey et al. demonstrated that oxygen saturation and content may begin to decrease near-maximal exercise in elite endurance athletes.[5] Therefore, in some elite athletes, the respiratory system may contribute to the limitation of $\dot{V}O_{2max}$ by reducing maximal arteriovenous oxygen difference because of a decreased arterial oxygen content.

As noted above, the respiratory system does not limit oxygen transport with the possible exception of that in elite endurance athletes. This is true for short-duration dynamic exercise to maximal work rates. However, respiratory muscle fatigue can occur after sustained (more than 1 hour) endurance exercise.[6] This post-exercise fatigue is not present in highly trained individuals[7]; therefore, training may improve endurance "performance" by minimizing respiratory fatigue during prolonged exercise.

CENTRAL CIRCULATION AND CARDIAC FUNCTION

Resting cardiac output is not remarkably altered by exercise training, whereas maximal cardiac output in a well-trained endurance athlete can be twice that of an untrained subject of similar body size (Fig. 8–1). The ability of an individual to have a high maximal cardiac output is probably related to both genetic factors and long-term participation in endurance training programs. By definition, maximal cardiac output is the product of maximal heart rate and maximal stroke volume. Maximal heart rate is not affected by endurance training; therefore, higher maximal cardiac outputs are attributed exclusively to lager stroke volumes (Fig. 8–1). Several factors are responsible for an increased maximal stroke volume. First, cardiac dimensions are increased. Left ventricular chamber size is greater in endurance-trained subjects, as evidenced by greater end-diastolic volumes at rest and during exercise.[8,9] Also, endurance-trained subjects have a significantly greater absolute left ventricular mass (eccentric hypertrophy) and left ventricular mass normalized to lean body mass than sedentary subjects.[10,11] This increased mass is proportional to both the $\dot{V}O_{2max}$ and the increase in end-diastolic volume.[12] Short-term endurance training (less than 20 weeks) results in very modest changes in wall thickness and chamber size[13]; therefore, the hypertrophy observed in trained individuals must develop gradually over months or years of training. The increased maximal stroke volume is attributable in part to the increases in chamber size, but is also improved by increased preload (venous return) and decreased afterload (vascular resistance) as discussed below.

An augmented preload produces an increase in stroke volume and cardiac output by the Frank-Starling mechanism. Preload appears to be significantly increased after endurance training. This effect of training

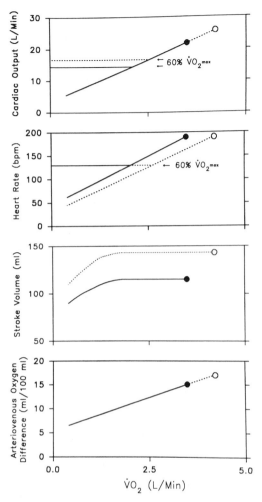

Fig. 8–1. Cardiovascular responses to increasing work rates to a maximum. Closed circles, untrained subject; open circles, trained subject. Solid line, submaximal responses in untrained subject; dashed line, submaximal responses in trained subject. Horizontal lines represent heart rates and cardiac outputs at 60% of $\dot{V}O_{2max}$ for untrained and trained subjects.

is related, in part, to an increase in total blood volume (specifically plasma volume).[14] In addition, the effective left ventricular diastolic compliance (ability of the chamber to accept blood) appears to be increased after endurance training, which can enhance preload at submaximal or maximal work rates.[15–17] Increased mechanical compression of the veins by the increased skeletal muscle mass probably also augments venous return.

Endurance training effects on autonomic function can contribute to alterations in cardiac output at submaximal and maximal work rates. Endurance-trained individuals often have a reduced heart rate at rest and at any level of submaximal exercise (Fig. 8–1). The resting bradycardia is attributable to a shift of autonomic balance in favor of the parasympathetic nervous system and a decrease in intrinsic heart rate, which is the rate obtained with complete ablation of the autonomic nervous system.[18,19] After training, heart rate is decreased at any absolute submaximal work rate, but is unchanged at submaximal work rates relative to maximum. This is illustrated in Figure 8–1. Heart rate at 60% of $\dot{V}o_{2max}$ is the same pre- and post-training, whereas cardiac output is greater at the same "relative" work rate. Cardiac output is not significantly changed at any absolute submaximal work rate[20]; hence, stroke volume is elevated at all levels of submaximal exercise after training (Fig. 8–1). The result is improved "efficiency" of the heart at rest and at submaximal work rates (i.e., the myocardium does not use as much oxygen at a given work rate) as illustrated by a decreased double product (heart rate times arterial pressure) at rest and submaximal work rates. Myocardial oxygen consumption is directly related to the double product; therefore, because blood pressure at submaximal work rates is either decreased or not changed after training, myocardial oxygen consumption is likely to be reduced at any submaximal work rate because of the lower heart rate and possible lower systolic blood pressure.

The effect of endurance training on ventricular performance or contractility is far less certain. Several authors suggest that contractility is enhanced by training (owing to increased sympathetic nervous system effects), whereas other investigators have found no training effect on contractility.[21] During maximal exercise, contractility is increased, resulting in a high ejection fraction and low end-systolic volume irrespective of training status.[9,17] Therefore, at maximal exercise, there is little to be gained from enhancing contractility further.

PERIPHERAL CIRCULATION

Endurance training is associated with a reduction in total peripheral vascular resistance, or afterload. This reduction in peripheral vascular resistance enables the endurance athlete to achieve levels of cardiac output at similar arterial pressures that are double that of a sedentary subject during maximal exercise. Although the mechanisms responsible for the augmented fall in peripheral vascular resistance are not fully understood, one factor is the increase in vasculature associated with endurance training.[21–23] The increased vascular space augments the fall in peripheral vascular resistance as maximal vasodilatation in skeletal muscle is approached during maximal exercise. Alterations in metabolic function at maximum exercise may also affect the maximal level of vasodilatation that is achieved. Together, these training effects reduce peripheral vascular resistance at maximal work rates, thereby augmenting maximal cardiac output. It is uncertain whether vascular resistance at submaximal work rates decreases more after training. Because vascular resistance is calculated from cardiac output and blood pressure, the occurrence of a training-induced decrease in vascular resistance at submaximal work rates would be associated with a decreased blood pressure. Most studies suggest that blood pressures taken at submaximal work rates are unchanged after training in normotensive subjects, whereas it may be decreased in hypertensive subjects, as discussed in Chapter 16.

The ability to vasodilate (and increase blood flow) in the active tissue does not reach a maximum even at maximal work rates. Stray-Gundersen et al.[24] found that removal of the pericardium in untrained dogs resulted in a greater rise in cardiac output and a greater fall in peripheral vascular resistance at maximal exercise. In fact, the vasculature of the contracting skeletal muscle appears to maintain some degree of tonic vasoconstriction such that if cardiac output is augmented further, the active muscle can receive a further increase in blood flow.[25] Saltin postulated that if most of the skeletal muscle of the body was engaged in maximal dynamic exercise, a cardiac output of more than 60 L/min would be required to prevent a measurable fall in blood pressure.[25] These findings support the hypothesis that the pump capacity of the heart is the primary limitation to $\dot{V}o_{2max}$ in man.

The maximal total body oxygen extraction (estimated from the arteriovenous oxygen difference) increases after endurance training (Fig. 8–1). This effect is brought about, in part, by an increase in the diffusion gradient for oxygen between the capillaries and the active skeletal muscle cells. The total myoglobin (the oxygen-carrying protein complex in skeletal muscle) content of trained muscle also increases.[26,27] These changes within the skeletal muscle tissue enhance the diffusion capacity of oxygen. Also, tissue oxygen extraction within the active muscle is enhanced by the increased capillary density that occurs with endurance training. The total number and the density (total number per gram of tissue) of capillaries increase.[22,23,28] The increased capillary density results in an increased capillary diffusion surface area, which is advantageous for nutrient and metabolite exchange. The arterial tree also may increase as a result of the opening of dormant collateral blood vessels. This change may contribute to improved extraction by improving blood flow to the working tissue. Musch et al. demonstrated that endurance training increases the degree of shunting of blood away from the splanchnic and renal circulations at maximal exercise.[29] This shift is associated with an increase in blood flow to the active skeletal muscle and acts in concert with the increased tissue extraction to augment total body arteriovenous oxygen difference. Hence, several training-induced adaptations within the skeletal muscle contribute to an augmented maximal arteriovenous oxygen difference.

MUSCLE METABOLISM

Although skeletal muscle metabolism is discussed in subsequent chapters, a few points are worth mentioning in this chapter. Endurance training increases the capacity for aerobic metabolism. This effect is accomplished by an increase in the total number of mitochondria and in mitochondrial enzyme activity.[26] These biochemical alterations result in an increase in the preferential use of free fatty acids released from adipose tissue as an energy substrate during sustained dynamic exercise. Skeletal muscle with an enhanced oxidative capacity is able to function at a lower oxygen tension, thereby delaying the onset of accelerated glycogenolysis and depletion of glycogen stores.[30] Therefore, trained individuals demonstrate enhanced endurance and are able to sustain longer periods of exercise at a given percentage of $\dot{V}_{O_{2}max}$.[31] This is also reflected in the balance of aerobic and anaerobic metabolism. Blood lactate levels serve as a marker for this balance and are decreased at submaximal work rates as training duration and intensity are increased (Figure 8–2). This metabolic balance is thought to influence the ventilation threshold (work rate at which ventilation increases sharply so that exercise cannot be sustained for long durations). The ventilation threshold has been related to anaerobic metabolism and the "anaerobic threshold," although the mechanisms of this relationship remain controversial. After training, ventilation threshold appears to be shifted to higher absolute and relative work

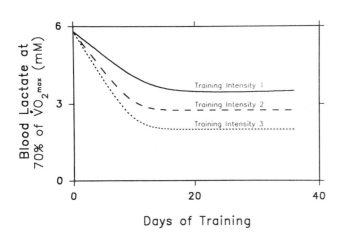

Fig. 8–2. Blood lactate levels at 70% of $\dot{V}_{O2max}$ during one month of training at three different hypothetical training intensities.

rates and has been used as an index for endurance exercise performance.[32–34]

GENDER DIFFERENCES

It is clear that endurance training elicits the same qualitative adaptations in women as in men.[35–37] Similar adaptations of the physiologic parameters discussed above are observed in both sexes. Importantly, when men and women were trained together with identical training regimens, the responses were the same.[38,39] The primary differences between men and women relate to body size. Generally, stroke volume, cardiac output and ventilation are larger at submaximal and maximal work rates in men; consequently, $\dot{V}O_{2max}$ also tends to be greater in men. In addition, arterial oxygen content and left ventricular mass per lean body mass tends to be lower in women.[36,37]

AGE EFFECTS

Training adaptations and improvements can be realized at any age. Adolescents can achieve improvements in fitness similar to those of adults, presumably by the same mechanisms described above.[40] Training effects also can be achieved in the elderly; however, the extent of improvement may be limited with age.[41,42] Figure 8–3 is a hypothetical illustration of the reduction of improvement that can be achieved with advancing age in a sedentary versus a previously trained individual. This age at which the inflection point occurs (i.e., when the decline in improvement begins) is un-

known and probably varies from person to person. Although this decline is well documented in the literature, it is difficult to distinguish effects attributable to age versus those attributable to life style, diet, and disease. The decline probably is related to several physiologic changes associated with advancing age. Maximal heart rate decreases from ~200 bpm at age 20 to ~160 bpm at age 60 to 65 by an unknown mechanism. Stroke volume at submaximal and maximal work rates is reduced significantly because of decreased heart chamber size and compliance (stiffness) and increased afterload caused by stiffness of the arterial tree.[42] Maximal ventilation is also reduced with advancing age, as much as 50%, because of increased stiffness of the respiratory muscles and chest wall and increased airway resistance.

A recent study suggests that a person's potential for benefitting from training may not decline with age. Makrides et al.[43] found that high-intensity endurance training can produce comparable increases in $\dot{V}O_{2max}$ in elderly and young subjects (38 and 29%, respectively). The pretraining values for $\dot{V}O_{2max}$ were very low in the elderly subjects and may reflect an underestimation of pre-training $\dot{V}O_{2max}$ that could have resulted in an overestimation of the training effect. Nevertheless, these data raise an important question of whether the reduced improvements documented in the literature may reflect an underestimation of the capacity for training in the elderly as a result of conservative training regimens employed in most studies with elderly subjects.

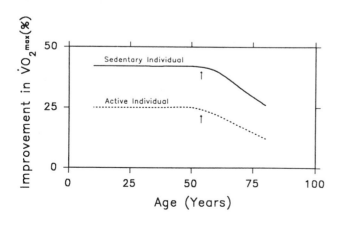

Fig. 8–3. Effect of age on maximal improvement in $\dot{V}O_{2max}$ that can be achieved in sedentary and active individuals. Arrows reflect hypothetical age at which decline in improvement begins. Age at which this occurs is dependent on life style, history of activity, and disease.

SUMMARY

Endurance training elicits several cardio-vascular adaptations evident both at rest and during exercise. These effects are summarized in Table 8–1. At rest, the only changes that occur are a decrease in heart rate and a concomitant increase in stroke volume. As a result, myocardial oxygen demand is moderately reduced at rest and at any given absolute work rate. When the work rate is considered as a percent of maximal capacity, the heart rate at any submaximal percent of capacity is the same, and stroke volume and cardiac output are greater. At maximal exercise, oxygen consumption, stroke volume, cardiac output, and the ability to extract oxygen increase significantly and result in enhanced exercise performance. Maximal heart rate is not changed, and maximal diffusion capacity is probably not increased significantly. Therefore, the oxygen delivery system is improved by augmentation of cardiac function, blood redistribution to the working tissue, and tissue extraction of oxygen. Cardiac pump function appears to be the primary limitation to maximal performance. Only in very elite athletes does respiratory function become a potential limitation. Improvements in aerobic metabolism in the skeletal muscle significantly improve the ability to sustain exercise at a given percent of $\dot{V}o_{2max}$. These training adaptations can be achieved regardless of gender or age.

Table 8–1. Endurance Training-Induced Changes in Some Cardiovascular Variables

Variable	Rest	Submaximal Exercise	Maximal Exercise
Oxygen consumption	NC	NC	↑
Heart rate	↓	↓	NC
Stroke volume	↑	↑	↑
Cardiac output	NC	NC	↑
Cardiac contractility	NC	NC	NC or ↑
Vascular resistance	NC	NC	↓
Muscle blood flow	NC	NC	↑
Splanchnic blood flow	NC	NC	↓
Oxygen extraction	NC	NC	↑
Ventilation	NC	NC	NC or ↑

NC = No change

REFERENCES

1. Ekblom B, Astrand PO, Saltin B, et al.: Effect of training on circulatory response to exercise. *J Appl Physiol, 24:*518, 1968.
2. Martin BJ, Sparks KE, Zwillich CW, Weil JV: Low exercise ventilation in endurance athletes. *Med Sci Sports Exerc, 11:*181, 1979.
3. Astrand PO: *Textbook of Work Physiology.* New York: McGraw-Hill Book Co., 1977.
4. Bender PR, Martin BJ: Maximal ventilation after exhausting exercise. *Med Sci Sports Exerc, 17:*164, 1985.
5. Anholm JD, Stray-Gundersen J, Ramanathan M, Johnson RL: Sustained maximal ventilation after endurance exercise in athletes. *J Appl Physiol, 67:*1759, 1989.
6. Johnson RL: Oxygen transport. In *Clinical Cardiology.* Edited by JT Willerson and CA Sanders. New York: Grune & Stratton, 1977.
7. Dempsey JA, Hanson P, Henderson K: Exercise-induced arterial hypoxemia in healthy humans at sea level. *J Physiol (Lond), 355:*161, 1984.
8. Morganroth J, Maron BJ, Henry WL, Epstein SE: Comparative left ventricular dimensions in trained athletes. *Ann Intern Med, 82:*521, 1975.
9. Rerych SK, Scholz PM, Sabiston DC, Jones RH: Effects of exercise training on left ventricular function in normal subjects: A longitudinal study by radionuclide angiography. *Am J Cardiol, 45:*244, 1980.
10. Keul J, Dickhuth HH, Simon G, Lehmann M: Effect of static and dynamic exercise on heart volume, contractility, and left ventricular dimensions. *Circ Res, 48:*1162, 1981.
11. Longhurst JC, Kelly AR, Gonyea WJ, Mitchell JH: Chronic training with static and dynamic exercise: Cardiovascular adaptation and response to exercise. *Circ Res, 48:*1171, 1981.
12. Milliken MC, Stray-Gundersen J, Peshock RM, et al.: Left ventricular mass as determined by magnetic resonance imaging in male endurance athletes. *Am J Cardiol, 62:* 301, 1988.
13. Peronnet F, et al.: Echocardiography and the athlete's heart. *Phys Sports Med, 9:*102, 1981.
14. Oscai LB, Williams BT, Hertig BA: Effect of exercise on blood volume. *J Appl Physiol, 26:*622, 1968.

15. LeWinter MM, Pavelec R: Influence of the pericardium on left ventricular end-diastolic pressure-segment relations during early and late stages of chronic volume overload in dogs. *Circ Res, 50:*501, 1982.

16. Levine BD, et al.: Left ventricular pressure-volume and Frank-Starling relations in endurance athletes: Implications for orthostatic tolerance and exercise performance. *Circulation, 84:*1016, 1991.

17. Poliner LR, et al.: Left ventricular performance in normal subjects. A comparison of the responses to exercise in the upright and supine position. *Circulation, 62:*528, 1980.

18. Smith ML, Hudson DL, Graitzer HM, Raven PB: Exercise bradycardia: Role of autonomic balance. *Med Sci Sports Exerc, 21:*40, 1988.

19. Lewis SF, Nylander E, Gad P, Areskog NH: Nonautonomic component in bradycardia of endurance trained men at rest and during exercise. *Acta Physiol Scand, 109:*297, 1979.

20. Rowell LB: Human cardiovascular adjustments to exercise and thermal stress. *Physiol Rev, 54:*75, 1974.

21. Blomqvist CG, Saltin B: Cardiovascular adaptations to physical training. *Ann Rev Physiol, 45:*169, 1983.

22. Hudlicka O: Growth of capillaries in skeletal and cardiac muscle. *Circ Res, 50:*451, 1982.

23. Ingjer F, Brodal P: Capillary supply of skeletal muscle fibers in untrained and endurance-trained women. *Eur J Appl Physiol, 38:*291, 1978.

24. Stray-Gundersen J, et al.: The effect of pericardiectomy on maximal oxygen consumption and maximal cardiac output in untrained dogs. *Circ Res, 58:*523, 1986.

25. Saltin B: Physiological adaptation to physical conditioning: Old problems revisited. *Acta Med Scand, 71:*11, 1986.

26. Holloszy JO: Adaptation of skeletal muscle to endurance exercise. *Med Sci Sports Exerc, 7:*155, 1975.

27. Meldon JH: Theoretical role of myoglobin in steady-state oxygen transport to tissue and its impact upon cardiac output requirements. *Acta Physiol Scand, 440:*S93, 1976.

28. Saltin B, Henrikson J, Nygaard E, Andersen P: Fiber types and metabolic potentials of skeletal muscles in sedentary man and endurance runners. *Ann NY Acad Sci, 3013:*3, 1977.

29. Musch TI, et al.: Training effects on regional blood flow response to maximal exercise in foxhounds. *J Appl Physiol, 62:*1724, 1987.

30. Gollnick PD, Saltin B: Significance of skeletal muscle oxidative enzyme enhancement with endurance training. *Clin Physiol, 2:*1, 1982.

31. Snell PG, Mitchell JH: The role of maximal oxygen uptake in exercise performance. In *Clinics in Chest Medicine.* Vol. 5. Edited by J. Loke. Philadelphia: WB Saunders, 1984.

32. Davis JA, Frank MH, Whipp BJ, Wasserman K: Anaerobic threshold alterations caused by endurance training in middle-aged men. *J Appl Physiol: Respirat Environ Exerc Physiol, 46:*1039, 1979.

33. Houmard JA, Costill DL, Mitchell JB, et al.: The role of anaerobic ability in middle distance running performance. *Eur J Appl Physiol, 62:*40, 1991.

34. McLellan TM, Jacobs I: Active recovery, endurance training, and the calculation of the individual anaerobic threshold. *Med Sci Sports Exerc, 21:*586, 1989.

35. Drinkwater BL: Women and exercise: Physiological aspects. *Exerc Sports Sci Rev, 12:*21, 1984.

36. Mitchell JH, et al.: Acute response and chronic adaptation to exercise in women. *Med Sci Sports Exerc, 24:*S258–S265, 1992.

37. Riley-Hagan M, et al.: Left ventricular dimensions and mass using magnetic resonance imaging in female endurance athletes. *Am J Cardiol, 69:*1067–1074, 1992.

38. Daniels WL, Kowal DM, Vogel JA, Stauffer RM: Physiological effects of a military training program on male and female cadets. *Aviat Space Environ Med, 50:*562, 1979.

39. Eddy DO, Sparks KL, Adelizi DA: The effects of continuous and interval training in women and men. *Eur J Appl Physiol, 37:*83, 1977.

40. Eisenman PA, Golding LA: Comparisons of effects of training on $\dot{V}O_{2max}$ in girls and young women. *Med Sci Sports Exerc, 7:*136, 1975.

41. Saltin B: Physiological effects of physical conditioning. *Med Sci Sports Exerc, 1:*50, 1969.

42. Raven PB, Smith ML: A guideline for cardiopulmonary conditioning in the middle-aged recreational athlete: A physiologic base. *Am J Sports Med, 12:*268, 1984.

43. Makrides L, Heigenhauser GJF, Jones NL: High-intensity endurance training in 20- to 30- and 60- to 70-yr-old healthy men. *J Appl Physiol, 69:*1792, 1990.

Chapter 9

SPECIFICITY OF EXERCISE, TRAINING, AND TESTING

Brian J. Sharkey and Daniel G. Graetzer

The responses and adaptations to exercise have been studied for more than a century. Not until 1967, however, when Holloszy reported the effect of endurance training on oxidative enzymes, did a theory of specificity begin to emerge.[1] Subsequent research has contributed to the principle that guides the development and conduct of exercise and training programs, the principle of specificity. This chapter focuses on the specificity of exercise and training, outlining responses and adaptations at the peripheral and central levels. Because exercise and training are specific, it follows that tests must be specific to the manner and mode of exercise if they are to reflect the effects of exercise and training.

SPECIFICITY OF EXERCISE

An exercise such as jogging recruits motor units and muscle fibers suited to the task. Slow oxidative fibers are recruited for slow contractions, with fast fibers becoming involved as the pace quickens. Both fiber types are recruited to lift heavy loads. The metabolic response within the individual fibers is also determined by the nature of the exercise. Anaerobic pathways provide energy for short-intense exertion, and aerobic pathways are utilized during extended contractions. Because the supply and support systems (respiratory, cardiovascular, and endocrine) are responsible for the support of these contracting muscle fibers, it follows that the systemic (central) response to a particular exercise is related to the fibers and energy systems employed, as well as the muscle mass involved.

Types of Contractions

Static versus Dynamic

Dynamic muscular contractions, such as in running, cycling, and swimming, are characterized by periods of relaxation between contractions, allowing blood flow in the working muscles during relaxation, and assisting venous return by means of the squeezing action of contractions (muscle pump). Static or isometric contractions, or contractions with a static component (shoveling snow), constrict blood vessels serving the muscles and prompt an exaggerated cardiovascular response relative to the level of oxygen uptake. When the contraction exceeds approximately 60% of the maximal voluntary contraction force, blood flow to the muscle is severely reduced. These differences are reflected in the heart rate and blood pressure responses during the two types of contractions.

Dynamic exercises are characterized by moderate increases in heart rate and systolic blood pressure. In contrast, static contractions provoke an exaggerated rise in heart rate, systolic, diastolic, and mean arterial pressures when compared with dynamic contractions at the same level of oxygen uptake (Figs. 9–1 and 9–2). Mean arterial blood pressure (MAP) is the product of cardiac output (CO) and total peripheral resistance (TPR).

$$MAP = CO \times TPR$$

When static contractions constrict arterioles, peripheral resistance rises, provoking an increase in heart rate and a dramatic rise in blood pressure. Thus static contractions elicit a dramatic rise in the rate-pressure product, the product of heart rate and systolic blood pressure, which is highly related to the oxygen needs of the myocardium.

A further complication of static effort is the possibility of a Valsalva maneuver, the forced expiratory effort against a closed glottis. Common in weightlifting and exercises with a pronounced static component,

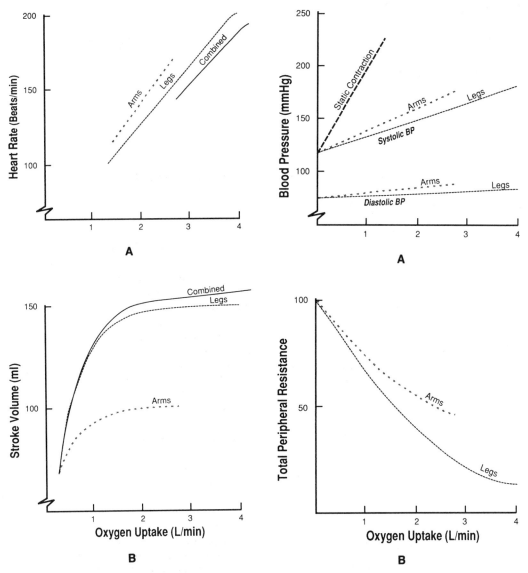

Fig. 9–1. Relationship of oxygen uptake to **A.** heart rate and **B.** stroke volume for arm, leg, and combined arm/leg exercise. Data for a cross-country skier with a leg $\dot{V}O_{2max}$ of 4 L, a peak arm value of 2.8 L (70% of leg max), and a combined max of 4.24 L (106% of leg value).

the increased thoracic pressure caused by the Valsalva can impede venous return, lower stroke volume, and interfere with blood flow in the coronary arteries. Proper breathing (exhaling during lifting phase) minimizes the problem. The exaggerated effects of static contractions, including in-tra-arterial pressures exceeding 300 mm Hg, call for care in the use of near maximal

Fig. 9–2. Relationship of oxygen uptake to **A.** blood pressure and **B.** total peripheral resistance for dynamic arm and leg exercise and static contractions with the arms (see **A**). Note the higher systolic blood pressure and peripheral resistance for a given level of oxygen uptake during exercise with the smaller muscle mass (arms), and the higher heart rate for arm versus leg exercise (Fig. 9–1A).

lifting or static exercises in untrained or coronary-prone populations.[2]

Concentric versus Eccentric

Dynamic contractions can be concentric or eccentric. In concentric contractions, the muscle shortens as it develops tension, while in eccentric contractions the muscle lengthens as it develops tension. Eccentric contractions occur during the pre-load or countermovement phase of the stretch-shortening cycle common in many forms of human movement. One example is in running, in which contracting thigh and calf muscles lengthen to absorb impact forces before the concentric contraction that propels the body forward. The stretch-shortening cycle makes the concentric contraction more powerful, or provides the same power with less expenditure of energy.[3] Ironically, this efficient method of force development has been called "cheating" in the weight room.

Unaccustomed eccentric contractions, as in weightlifting or downhill running, lead to delayed onset muscle soreness (DOMS). The soreness peaks 24 to 48 hours after the exercise, and declines slowly thereafter. Subsequent eccentric contractions are less likely to produce soreness. The DOMS is probably the result of structural damage in skeletal muscle, which could be caused by the relatively small number of contracting fibers relative to the load. The damage may take many weeks to repair, and performance is impaired during the recovery period. Eccentric training has been shown to prevent DOMS and the related muscle damage.[4]

Intensity and Duration of Contractions

The intensity and duration of contractions interact to influence the metabolic pathways and energy sources utilized during exercise. High intensity, short duration contractions are powered by anaerobic glycolysis, whereas low-intensity, long-duration contractions rely on aerobic pathways and the oxidation of carbohydrate and fat. The intensity of exercise also influences the type of muscle fiber recruited for the effort. Low intensity effort recruits slow oxidative fibers, medium intensity contractions recruit fast oxidative glycolytic fibers, and high intensity contractions recruit fast glycolytic fibers with limited oxidative capability. As increasing intensity causes a shift toward anaerobic glycolysis and recruitment of fast glycolytic fibers, blood lactate levels increase because of increased production and reduced removal of lactate.[5]

The lactate threshold (LT) or onset of blood lactate accumulation (OBLA) has been used to define exercise intensity, to determine training intensity, and to assess the effects of training. Lactate measurements are highly related to performance in endurance events ranging from 10 to 42 kilometers, probably because the measures reflect the oxidative capacity of the exercising muscles. More will be said about lactate measures in the sections on the specificity of training and testing.

Mode of Exercise

The mode of exercise refers to the activity or ergometer used to elicit a response. Walking, running, cycling, arm cranking, swimming, rowing, cross-country skiing, stair-stepping, and other aerobic exercises all elicit task specific responses. The responses are influenced by the muscle groups utilized (e.g., arm versus leg), the percent of total muscle mass involved (e.g., small versus large), the body position (e.g., upright versus recumbent), and whether the exercise involves full or partial weight bearing.

Arm versus Leg

At a given submaximal energy expenditure, arm work is performed at a greater physiologic cost than is leg work (see Figs. 9–1 and 9–2). Heart rate, systolic blood pressure, and blood lactate values are higher, whereas stroke volume is lower.[6] During arm exercise, heart rate is higher and stroke volume lower, partly because of pooling of blood in the legs. Furthermore, the involvement of a smaller muscle mass to accomplish the same task requires greater muscle tension and increased peripheral vascular resistance, which elicits an elevated heart rate and blood pressure in an effort to maintain blood flow.

Combined Arm/Leg Exercise

When upper and lower body musculature is involved in aerobic exercises such as swimming, rowing, or cross-country skiing, the heart rate is somewhat lower when compared to the same level of energy expenditure with legs alone (see Fig. 9–1A). Peak oxygen uptake scores for arm exercise range from 60 to 85% of leg values, depending on the amount of specific arm and leg training. Peak values seem limited by the smaller muscle mass in the arms and upper body. Maximal oxygen uptake levels in combined arm/leg exercise equal or slightly exceed values measured during legs-only exercise (e.g., 106% of legs alone). Athletes with highly trained arms can exceed legs-only values in a combined arm/leg test if the arm resistance is not excessive during the test.[7] Combined test values fall below legs-only scores when the arms are forced to contribute more than 40% of the total work. The combined demands of simultaneous arm and leg work limit blood flow to individual muscle groups, which adjust by increasing the amount of oxygen extracted from each unit of blood.

When a submaximal level of energy expenditure is shared in a combined arm/leg exercise, the effort is perceived as less strenuous than when it is performed with the arms or legs alone. Thus combined arm/leg exercises are well suited for caloric expenditure and weight control programs. Elite levels of performance in combined arm/leg sports require an elevated maximal oxygen uptake, which depends on the ability to serve both muscle groups with a high cardiac output.

Muscle Mass

As noted above, cardiovascular responses are exaggerated when work is performed with a smaller muscle mass. Resistance vessels (arterioles) dilate to allow blood flow in working muscles, thereby lowering total peripheral resistance. This effect is more pronounced during exercise with a large muscle mass such as the legs, in which relatively large energy expenditures can be accomplished with moderate increases in heart rate and blood pressure (see Figs. 9–1 and 9–2). When a small muscle mass is involved (e.g., arms), the peripheral resistance leads to a greater increase in heart rate and blood pressure. The increase in heart rate is especially pronounced in arm work that is performed

above the head, such as hammering nails or lifting hand weights.[8]

This exaggerated heart rate response has led some to believe that arm exercises (lifting hand weights, circuit weight training, or swinging arms above the head) could be used to increase aerobic fitness. Hempel and Wells have shown that the heart rate exaggerates the energy cost of circuit weight training.[9] Moreover, because each muscle is used only 20 to 30 seconds at a time, it is hard to imagine how circuit training could overload oxidative pathways and lead to improved aerobic fitness. This form of training may prompt some central circulatory changes, but it is not likely to bring about important peripheral adaptations in muscle. The exercise heart rate is a useful indicator of energy expenditure in a continuous dynamic activity utilizing a large muscle mass, but not in a discontinuous activity, one involving a small muscle mass, or arm work that is performed above the head.

Body Position

In the supine position (e.g., supine cycling), stroke volume and cardiac output are higher during moderate energy expenditure than during the same exercise performed in the upright position. The supine position allows a higher stroke volume at rest, and a near-maximal stroke volume during moderate exercise. As effort approaches maximal levels, the differences in supine versus upright stroke volume and cardiac output are diminished as upright values approach supine measurements. Arm tests in the upright position cause pooling of blood in the legs, lower stroke volumes, and higher heart rates. Body position is an important but often overlooked contributor to the specificity of exercise.

Weight Bearing

Physiologic responses differ in weight-bearing and nonweight-bearing exercises. Cyclists achieve higher maximal oxygen uptake scores when tested in the standing (weight-bearing) versus seated (nonweight-bearing) position.[10] The effort required to raise the center of gravity in weight-bearing exercise requires a larger muscle mass, hence a higher maximal oxygen uptake. In seated cycling, a smaller muscle mass is involved. Similarly, maximal oxygen uptake ($\dot{V}O_{2max}$) scores on the bicycle ergometer are typically lower than those measured on the treadmill. When subjects support a portion of their body weight by holding on to the support bar of a treadmill or stair climber, weight bearing is reduced. This practice may be acceptable for clinical testing or training programs, but it reduces caloric expenditure and invalidates the prediction of energy expenditure from treadmill rate and grade.

Summary

Exercise is specific to the type of contraction (static/dynamic, concentric/eccentric), the intensity and duration of contractions, the mode of exercise, the muscle mass involved, body position and the degree of weight bearing (on land, in water, or in space). The response to exercise is also influenced by environmental factors, including temperature, humidity, air movement, air quality, and altitude. And the emotional climate can exert an effect on the response to exercise.

SPECIFICITY OF TRAINING

Because exercise is specific, it follows that training must also be specific if performance goals are to be achieved. Training leads to improvements in neuromuscular skill and efficiency, to central changes in cardiovascular, respiratory and endocrine supply and support systems, and to peripheral adaptations in muscle fibers, energy sources, and metabolic pathways. The need for specificity increases with level of performance and competitive goals. Although a wide range of aerobic activities achieves the goal of energy expenditure in a weight-loss program, sport-specific training is necessary to improve performance in cross-country ski racing. As more is learned about the influence of exercise on clinical conditions (hypertension, diabetes, cancer, glaucoma), specific exercise prescriptions may emerge to aid in the achievement of therapeutic goals.

Peripheral Adaptations

When the tension-generating or metabolic properties of a skeletal muscle fiber are loaded or used beyond their usual range (overload), the fiber attempts to adapt to the new demand. Repeated and progressive overload of a fiber constitutes training, and the adaptations are specific to the manner and mode of exercise used in training. The overload of a training bout triggers a sequence of events including specific protein synthesis, probably involving messenger RNA to transmit a template from the nucleus, and transfer RNA to escort amino acids to the ribosome, where protein synthesis takes place.

These and other adaptations take place in the hours and days after a bout of training. Some adaptations occur in or around the muscle fiber (peripheral adaptations), and others occur in the cardiovascular, respiratory, and endocrine systems (central adaptations). Peripheral adaptations are usually specific to the manner and mode of exercise. Some central changes are specific and others are general, allowing some transfer of training. This discussion focuses on well-documented changes associated with aerobic (endurance) and strength training.

Aerobic Training

Initially called cardiovascular and later cardiorespiratory training, exercise programs that lead to improvements in endurance are now referred to as aerobic training. The change in terminology reflects changes of interpretation that began with the publication of Holloszy's landmark study of the effects of endurance training on oxidative (aerobic) enzymes. As research on the cellular effects of training began to accumulate, it became evident that peripheral effects are specific and that skeletal muscle (and not the heart) is the "target tissue" of training.

Aerobic or endurance training leads to increased concentrations of aerobic enzymes from the citric acid, electron transport and β-oxidation pathways. Aerobic training also increases the size and unit volume of mitochondria in which these pathways are housed. Pette has shown that prolonged exercise leads to increased oxidative capacity and eventual transformation of fast to slow twitch fiber characteristics in rat and rabbit muscle.[11] This shift of biochemical and contractile properties, which suggests the plasticity of skeletal muscle, has not been demonstrated in human muscle. Other peripheral adaptations to endurance training include increased concentrations of muscle myoglobin and triglyceride, and, when training is accompanied by a high carbohydrate diet, increased storage of muscle glycogen. All of these changes are specific to the fibers used in training. The capillary-to-fiber ratio is higher in endurance-trained muscle. These changes combine to enhance the endurance of trained fibers by improving adenosine triphosphate production by means of the efficient use of oxygen and fat, the conservation of muscle glycogen, and reduced blood lactate.

Strength Training

High-resistance strength training increases muscle size (hypertrophy) through the synthesis of contractile protein (actin and myosin) and thickening of connective tissue. The potential for creating additional fibers from fiber splitting or satellite cells in human muscle is still being investigated. The modest rise in creatine phosphate sometimes noted with strength training seems proportional to the increase in muscle mass. Strength training has been associated with loss of oxidative enzymes, and endurance training with the loss of contractile protein. Hickson has shown that simultaneous strength and endurance training can interfere with the development of strength in previously untrained subjects.[12] The effects of training occur within the muscle (myogenic) or the nervous system (neurogenic). Strength training elicits early neurogenic changes (decreased inhibitions, more effective application of force) followed by myogenic changes (increased contractile protein and myofibrils). Of course, significant changes only take place in the muscles directly involved in the training.

Central Changes

Aerobic Training

The peripheral adaptations to aerobic (endurance) training can occur in small or large muscle groups. When they occur in a small muscle group, such as those used by a barber to cut hair with scissors, they do not elicit adaptations in the cardiovascular, respiratory, or endocrine systems (central changes). But when a large muscle mass is involved, as in training for running, cycling, swimming, or cross-country skiing, supply and support systems also undergo adaptation.

Aerobic fitness is usually defined as the capacity to take in, transport, and utilize oxygen. Improved oxygen utilization, which takes place in the mitochondria of the muscle fiber, is a peripheral adaptation to training. The increased capacity to take in and transport oxygen depends on central adaptations. Although lung volumes are not highly related to performance, and the respiratory system is not viewed as a major limit to the maximal oxygen uptake, training can influence respiration by means of peripheral adaptations in previously untrained respiratory muscles. Respiration becomes more efficient with endurance training, leading to a larger tidal volume and slower respiration rate for a given level of oxygen uptake. Training also elevates the ventilatory threshold to a higher percentage of the $\dot{V}O_{2max}$.

Oxygen transport is accomplished by the heart, blood vessels, blood, red cells, and hemoglobin, as well as by redistribution of blood by means of vasomotor regulation. Endurance training leads to an improved stroke volume and lower heart rate at a given submaximal exercise level (Fig. 9–1), and increases the maximal stroke volume and cardiac output. The endurance-trained heart exhibits volume hypertrophy, an elevated left ventricular end-diastolic volume (LVEDV), which allows a greater stroke volume and slower heart rate for a given level of cardiac output. Although animal studies reveal minimal change in cardiac muscle enzymes with training, there is evidence of enlargement in the diameter of the coronary arteries.[13]

Other effects of training include an increase in blood volume and total hemoglobin, the ability to redistribute blood from inactive tissues to active muscles, decreased levels of some hormones (epinephrine), and increased sensitivity to others (insulin). Of course, training is also accompanied by improvements in skill and efficiency, leading to a lower energy cost for a given velocity. The importance of blood volume changes becomes evident during detraining, when important cardiovascular adaptations (increased stroke volume, decreased heart rate) regress to pretraining levels as blood volume declines.[14] It appears that some of the effects of training on the heart are secondary to other adaptations (increased blood volume, redistribution).

Strength Training

Strength, short-term endurance, and power training have minimal effects on the components of the oxygen transport system, including the heart and circulation. Echocardiographic studies of resistance athletes portray a cardiac hypertrophy characterized by increased left ventricular wall thickness, which could result from the afterload caused by vascular constriction and elevated blood pressure during lifting. This adaptation is the opposite of that found in endurance-trained athletes (greater left ventricular end-diastolic volume with normal wall thickness). However, when the wall thickness dimensions are adjusted for body size (surface area or lean body mass), the difference is reduced or nonexistent.[15] As previously noted, strength training and circuit weight training have little effect on the components of aerobic fitness. However, separate studies of strength training for the arms[16] and legs[17] have shown improvements in short-term endurance and total work output, even though there were no improvements in maximal oxygen uptake.

Implications

Transfer of Training

There is a temptation to speculate that the peripheral effects of training are specific, whereas the central effects are general, subject to transfer from one mode of exercise to another. But this is not always the case. Although blood volume and redistribution benefits should transfer to another endurance activity, heart rate changes may not. Saltin has shown that the cardiac responses to one-legged cycling are dependent on the level of training of the muscles used. Small nerve endings located in the muscle fibers sense the metabolic environment and influence the heart rate response by means of afferent nervous communication with the cardiac control center in the medulla. The slower heart rate during a given level of exercise with the trained leg allows more filling time and a greater end-diastolic and stroke volume.[18] Hence, some central responses to training are subject to peripheral influence and, therefore, unlikely to transfer to another mode of exercise (or the other leg, for that matter).

Mode of Training

Most peripheral and some central effects of training are task-specific, so a lack of transfer is not surprising. Training is even specific within one mode of exercise. For example, after 12 weeks of incline (uphill) training, the post-training $\dot{V}O_{2max}$ values on an inclined protocol were significantly greater than those measured on a horizontal test.[19] And when bicycle ergometer test values were correlated with flat and uphill bicycle race times, values for a seated protocol ($\dot{V}O_{2max}$, VT) predicted flat course results, while results from a standing protocol predicted hill climb performance.

The effects of cycle training do not transfer well to running, or vice versa. The same is true for swimming, cross-country skiing, rowing, or aerobic dance. When a cyclist shows improvement on a treadmill test, some of the increase can be attributed to generalizable central effects, such as increased blood volume, total hemoglobin, and redistribution. Related training is more likely to lead to improvements in $\dot{V}O_{2max}$ and performance. Arm training by means of swimming or on the swim bench improved $\dot{V}O_{2max}$ scores on tethered swim and swim bench tests, but not on a treadmill test.[20] There may be some transfer of training when the same muscles are used in similar ways; for example, standing cycling may improve performance in uphill running or cross-country skiing.

Arms and legs must both be trained to perform combined arm and leg activities, such as rowing, swimming, and cross-country skiing. Studies of arm training show that the initial limits to performance in previously untrained subjects are peripheral. As training progresses and peripheral adaptations take place, oxygen transport becomes the limiting factor.[21] In another study of moderately trained subjects, the addition of arm to leg work caused a decrease in blood flow to leg muscles.[22] The demands of combined arm and leg work limit blood flow to both muscle groups, which adjust by increasing oxygen extraction from each unit of blood. When the muscles are not sufficiently trained to utilize oxygen, or when blood flow (cardiac output) is inadequate, the muscles work anaerobically and become fatigued.

A possible peripheral effect with central implications is the hypothesized improvement in lactate utilization with training. Aerobically trained leg muscles could remove lactate produced during arm work, allowing improved arm performance after leg training.[23] However, in another study, arm training did not significantly affect the deterioration in the metabolic response to leg work that occurred with cessation of leg training.[24]

Cross-Training

A previous section has shown that training for one sport does little to improve performance in another. For a triathlete, swim training is unlikely to improve performance in running or cycling. But that does not imply that cross-training is without benefit. Cross-training provides a period of rest and recovery for overworked muscles and other tissues (connective tissue, tendons, bones), and could reduce the likelihood of overuse injury. Also, it serves to train and toughen accessory tissues and reduce the risk of injury associated with muscle imbalance. This concept has implications in occupational physiology, in which workers are being cross-trained in two or more jobs to reduce the risk of strains and overuse injuries.

Strength Training

The effects of strength training are specific to the muscles used, the mode of training (isometric, isotonic, or isokinetic), and the angle, range of motion, and speed of movement employed in training. Studies that demonstrate a cross-training effect (improvement in the untrained limb) probably involve neurogenic effects, such as learning, reduced inhibitions, and low levels of nervous stimulation in the control (untrained) limb. Because strength training is specific, strength tests must be spe-

cific if they are to reflect the effects of training.

Environment

Environmental factors such as heat, humidity, cold, altitude, and water immersion provoke specific responses and adaptations to exercise and training. Endurance performances are influenced more by the environment than are speed or resistance performances. Although training itself elicits some change in sweat rate, training in a hot environment is necessary to achieve full acclimatization and best possible endurance performances in the heat. Improvements in pulmonary ventilation and oxygen transport (red blood cells, hemoglobin) are part of the acclimatization process that occurs during training at moderate elevations (6000 to 9000 feet). Success in a particular environment requires training in that environment. And tests must be environmentally specific if they are to be used to predict performance in a particular environment.

SPECIFICITY OF TESTING

Because exercise and training are specific, the tests used to evaluate training should also be specific to the type of exercise and the method of training employed. Performance on a test is a function of neuromuscular skill, physiologic capacity, and motivation. Neuromuscular skill improves with practice and experience in the type or mode of exercise. The physiologic components include specific peripheral and more generalized central adaptations. Both the skill and physiology argue for specificity, and motivation should be higher when a test is similar to the manner of training. The best test is usually the activity itself. This section briefly reviews the need for specificity in testing, with examples from the literature on aerobic fitness or endurance.

Aerobic (Endurance) Tests
Mode

As previously noted, runners achieve best results when tested on a treadmill, cyclists on a cycle ergometer, swimmers in a swimming test, and rowers on a rowing ergometer. Unfortunately, no specific ergometers or protocols are available to assess the effects of aerobic dance or some other popular forms of training. Nonspecific testing can be counterproductive if participants become discouraged by an apparent lack of improvement. Arm tests cannot predict leg performance or vice versa. And arm movements for one sport cannot reflect improvements from another type of arm or upper body training. So specific arm tests must be developed to evaluate specific sports. Arm tests have been used to evaluate upper body endurance in rowers, swimmers, and cross-country skiers. Specific arm or upper body tests provide insights regarding performance in combined arm and leg sports. Low arm scores (peak $\dot{V}O_2$) relative to leg values correlate with poor combined (arm plus leg) test results and performances in cross-country skiing.[7] Peak values on arm tests depend on the ergometer used, the state of training, and specific test conditions, such as the degree of lower body immobilization. These factors and the state of leg training influence the percentage of arm to leg values.

Protocol

Because exercise and training are specific, test protocols should be adapted to the subject. In practice, however, most subjects are forced to adapt to the protocol. On the bicycle ergometer, the resistance and rate should be suitable for the subject.[25] Trained cyclists prefer 90 rpm, and untrained subjects do well with 60 to 70 rpm, but few have the leg strength to handle high resistances at 50 rpm, the rate of a popular bicycle protocol. When this rate is used with high resistance in a maximal test, subjects often experience leg fatigue before a true max is achieved. Similarly, speed and grade should be suited to the subject during a treadmill test. $\dot{V}O_{2max}$ tests yield best results when the test takes 8 to 12 minutes. Rate, grade, and workload increments should be adjusted to fit the training, experience, and preference of the subject. Hand signals allow the subject to select rate or grade increases in the final stages of the test, thereby avoiding early termination because of excess grade (leg cramps) or speed.

Of course, body position (upright versus recumbent), weight bearing (standing, seated, or weightless), and environmental conditions (temperature, humidity, altitude) should also be specific to those encountered in training. A nonacclimatized athlete does not do well on a test conducted in a hot environment, and testing in a cool environment does not reveal the effects of heat acclimatization.

Test Selection

Even the most specific tests may fail to account for all the peripheral and central effects of training. Davies, Packer, and Brooks studied the effects of treadmill training on the $\dot{V}O_{2max}$ and muscle enzyme levels of rats. They found that a maximal test on the treadmill was a relatively poor predictor of endurance, accounting for less than 50% of the variance in performance, whereas muscle oxidase levels accounted for 85%. Endurance improved five times and muscle oxidase increased four times (400%), and the $\dot{V}O_{2max}$ increased 14%. The $\dot{V}O_{2max}$ correlates with the maximum intensity of effort, while cellular oxidase capacity determines the duration of activity or endurance.[26] Similarly, in humans, tests other than the $\dot{V}O_{2max}$ (e.g., ventilatory and lactate thresholds) provide better relationships to endurance performance in running events ranging from 10 to 42 kilometers. The $\dot{V}O_{2max}$ may be the appropriate laboratory test for events up to 5 kilometers or 15 minutes, but for longer events or prolonged endurance, other measures are better correlated to performance.[27]

Purpose of Test

Tests that appear similar may have different purposes. For example, treadmill tests for aerobic fitness or $\dot{V}O_{2max}$ are used on asymptomatic subjects and athletes to assess fitness or the effects of training, and stress tests are used to screen clients, to search for hitherto undiagnosed disease, or to determine progress in rehabilitation. Max test protocols progress steadily to a plateau in oxygen intake, whereas stress test protocols designed for patients progress gradually to a percentage of the age-adjusted maximal heart rate, or until signs, symptoms, or fatigue necessitate a halt. Stress test protocols are often inappropriate for athletes because they take too long, involve nonspecific uphill walking (Balke), or slow running up steep grades (Bruce).

Job-Related Tests

Tests used to screen job applicants need to be valid indicators of work capacity. The principle of specificity suggests the use of actual job elements as tests of work capacity. However, such tests can be costly, time-consuming, and difficult to administer. When predictive tests must be used, they should be similar to the work tasks involved and significantly correlated to job performance. With legal tests of arbitrary age, sex, and work standards becoming more common, employers will place greater reliance on valid, reliable, objective tests that have been evaluated for fairness, adverse impact, and cultural bias.

SUMMARY

The responses to exercise and the adaptations to training are specific. Although some of the effects of training may be generalized to similar types of activity, all peripheral and some central effects are specific. It makes sense to concentrate training on the movements, muscle fibers, metabolic pathways, and supply and support systems that will be used in the activity or sport. This does not imply that athletes should ignore other exercises and muscle groups. Additional training is necessary to avoid injury, to achieve balance, and to provide backup for prime movers when they become fatigued.

Specificity applies to fitness as well. Fat metabolism and cardiovascular benefits are enhanced in regular moderate activity that employs major muscle groups for extended periods, but not when different muscle groups engage in a series of short lifting bouts. Bone mineral content is higher when bones are subjected to regular moderate stress, as in weight-bearing and resistance exercises. Endurance training does little for muscle strength and vice versa. The benefits of various activities are specific, and no single activity meets all fitness needs.

Finally, the capacity for performance or

the effects of training can be accurately assessed only when evaluated on tests specific to the activity. Failure to consider the principle of specificity will lead to improper conclusions and faulty program decisions.

REFERENCES

1. Holloszy J: Biochemical adaptations in muscle. *J Biol Chem, 242:*2278, 1967.
2. MacDougal J, et al.: Arterial blood pressure response to heavy resistance exercise. *J Appl Physiol, 58:*785, 1986.
3. Komi P: Stretch-shortening cycle. In *Strength and Power in Sport.* Edited by P. Komi, London: Blackwell Scientific Publishers, 1992.
4. Evans W: Exercise-induced skeletal muscle damage. *Phy Sports Med, 15:*89, 1987.
5. Brooks G: Anaerobic threshold: review of the concept and directions for future research. *Med Sci Sports Exerc, 17:*22, 1985.
6. Franklin B: Exercise testing, training and arm ergometry. *Sports Med, 2:*100, 1985.
7. Sharkey B, Heidel B: Physiological tests of cross-country skiers. *J Ski Coaches Assoc, 5:*5, 1981.
8. Carroll M, Otto R, Wygand J: The metabolic cost of two ranges of arm position height with and without hand weights during low impact aerobic dance. *Res Quart Exerc Sport, 62:*420, 1991.
9. Hempel L, Wells C: Cardiorespiratory cost of the Nautilus express circuit. *Phys Sports Med, 13:*82, 1985.
10. VanDorn K, Sharkey B: Unpublished data, 1986.
11. Pette D: Activity induced fast to slow transitions in mammalian muscle. *Med Sci Sports Exerc, 16:*517, 1984.
12. Hickson R: Interference of strength development by simultaneously training for strength and endurance. *Eur J Appl Physiol, 45:*255, 1980.
13. Kramsch D, et al.: Reduction of coronary atherosclerosis by moderate conditioning exercise in monkeys on an atherogenic diet. *N Engl J Med, 305:*1483, 1981.
14. Coyle E, Hemmert M, Coggan A: Effects of detraining on cardiovascular responses to exercise: Role of blood volume. *J Appl Physiol, 60:*95, 1986.
15. Fleck S: Cardiovascular response to strength training. In *Strength and Power in Sport.* Edited by P. Komi. London: Blackwell Scientific Publ, 1992, p. 305.
16. Washburn R, et al.: Dryland training for cross-country skiers. *Ski Coach, 6:*9, 1983.
17. Hickson R, et al.: Strength training effects

on aerobic power and short-term endurance. *Med Sci Sports Exerc, 12:*236, 1980.

18. Saltin B: The interplay between peripheral and central factors in the adaptive response to exercise and training. In *The Marathon.* Edited by P. Milvey. New York Acad Sci 1977, p. 224.

19. Freund B, Allen D, Wilmore J: Interaction of test protocol and inclined run training on maximal oxygen intake. *Med Sci Sports Exerc, 18:*588, 1986.

20. Gergley T, et al.: Specificity of arm training on aerobic power during swimming and running. *Med Sci Sports Exerc, 16:*349, 1984.

21. Boileau R, Mckeown B, Riner W: Cardiovascular and metabolic contributions to the maximal aerobic power of the arms and legs. *Int J Sports Cardiology, 1:*67, 1984.

22. Secher N, et al.: Maximal oxygen intake during arm cranking and combined arm plus leg exercise. *J Appl Physiol, 36:*515, 1974.

23. Rosler K, et al.: Transfer effects in endurance exercise. *Eur J Appl Physiol, 54:*355, 1985.

24. Pate R, et al.: Effects of arm training on retention of training effects derived from leg training. *Med Sci Sports Exerc, 10:*71, 1978.

25. Hagberg J, et al.: Effect of pedaling rate on submaximal exercise responses of competitive cyclists. *J Appl Physiol, 51:*447, 1981.

26. Davies K, Packer L, Brooks G: Biochemical adaptation of mitochondria, muscle and whole-animal respiration to endurance training. *Arch Biochem Biophys, 209:*539, 1981.

27. Sharkey B: New Dimensions in Aerobic Fitness. Champaign, IL: Human Kinetics Publishers, 1991.

Chapter 10

SKELETAL MUSCLE FUNCTION AND ADAPTATIONS TO TRAINING

Julia M. Lash and W. Michael Sherman

Skeletal muscle produces the force required for movement of the skeletal system during the performance of work and exercise. Therefore, an understanding of the structure, function, and adaptability of skeletal muscle is essential for individuals involved in fitness evaluation and exercise prescription.

SKELETAL MUSCLE STRUCTURE

Skeletal muscle is composed of parallel multinucleated cells attached to the skeletal system by three structured layers of connective tissue (Fig. 10–1). Skeletal muscle cells, or myofibers, are attached to adjacent fibers by a thin layer of connective tissue, the endomysium. Another connective tissue layer, the perimysium, encases and mechanically links groups of myofibers called fasciculi. The outermost surface of the muscle is covered by the epimysium. These three connective tissue sheaths fuse at the ends of the muscle to form tendinous attachments to the skeletal system.

As with all cells of the body, the contents of the myofiber are within the boundaries of a cell membrane, the sarcolemma. Invaginations of the sarcolemma, called T-tubules, occur at regularly spaced intervals along the surface of skeletal muscle cells (Fig. 10–2). The presence of the T-tubules allows the extracellular fluid to be in close proximity to the internal elements of the myofiber. The specialized endoplasmic reticulum of the myofiber, the sarcoplasmic reticulum (SR), consists of longitudinally oriented vesicles that store, release, and resequester calcium ions from the intracellular fluid. Enlargements of the SR, known as terminal cisternae, are closely associated with the T-tubules. A T-tubule and its two adjacent terminal cisternae form a structure called the triad. The anatomic relationship between the T-tubules and SR plays an important role in the series of events leading to muscle contraction.

The contractile capabilities of skeletal muscle are the result of interactions of the contractile proteins, myosin and actin (Figs. 10–2 and 10–3). The contractile proteins are arranged in parallel myofilaments within the cytoplasm of the myofiber. Myosin molecules attach to each other to form the thick filament, which is composed of long, light meromyosin strands and heavy, globular meromyosin heads, which project perpendicularly from the strands. The globular protein actin is arranged in a double helical pattern to form the basis of the thin filament. Actin-active sites, which are capable of binding to the heads of the myosin filament, are found at regular intervals along the thin filament. Strands of the protein tropomyosin lie in the grooves of the thin filament to cover the actin-active sites in relaxed skeletal muscle. Troponin, a three-subunit globular protein, is found at regular intervals along the thin filament. Each troponin subunit has unique binding characteristics: troponin-T attaches to tropomyosin, troponin-C binds calcium ions and is involved in the regulation of muscle contraction, and troponin-I is attached to actin.

Skeletal muscle is often referred to as striated because of the appearance of alternating dark and light bands along the length of the muscle (Fig. 10–1). The banded appearance is a result of partial overlap of the thick and thin filaments. The smallest subunit of skeletal muscle that is capable of contraction is known as a sarcomere. The sarcomere spans the region between two dark lines in the skeletal muscle, the Z-lines. The Z-lines are composed of Z-discs, to which parallel actin filaments are bilaterally attached. The wide, dark A-bands, which appear between Z-lines, are composed of both thin actin and thick

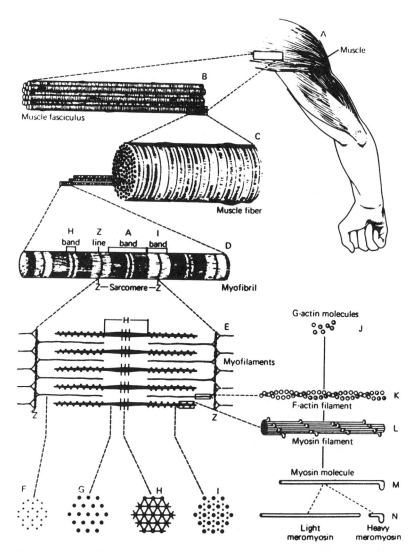

Fig. 10–1. Macroscopic and microscopic structure of human skeletal muscle. Individual muscle cells (myofibers) are mechanically linked through layers of connective tissue. The endomysium encompasses individual myofibers, the perimysium surrounds groups of myofibers called fasciculi, and the epimysium encapsulates the entire muscle. The striated appearance of skeletal muscle is caused by overlapping of actin and myosin myofilaments which form the basic contractile unit, the sarcomere. Drawing by Sylvia Colard Keene. From Bloom's *A Textbook of Histology.* Edited by DW Fawcett. Philadelphia: W.B. Saunders, 1975.

myosin filaments. The lighter H-bands, which appear in the middle of A-bands, contain only myosin filaments. The lightest bands of striations, the I-bands, are located adjacent to the Z-lines and contain only thin actin filaments. Of the protein in the contractile subunit, 84% is actin and myosin and 8% is tropomyosin. The remaining 6% includes alpha-actinin, a component of the Z-disc; beta-actinin, a compo-

nent of the thin filament; M-protein, which forms the M-line near the center of the A-band; and C-protein, which is a structural protein.[1]

EXCITATION AND MUSCLE CONTRACTION

As in most cells of the human body, there is a unequal distribution of ions across the sarcolemma of skeletal muscle cells. There

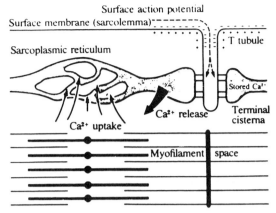

Fig. 10–2. Subcellular structure of skeletal muscle. The thin actin and thick myosin myofilaments overlap to form a striated appearance. The T-tubules, invaginations of the cell membrane, are closely associated with the terminal cisternae of the sarcoplasmic reticulum (SR) to form the triad. Graded depolarization of the T-tubule membrane results in calcium release from the SR, which initiates the sequence of events leading to muscle contraction. Calcium is resequestered by the SR during muscle relaxation. With permission from Selkurt EE: *Basic Physiology for the Health Sciences.* Boston: Little, Brown and Co., 1982.

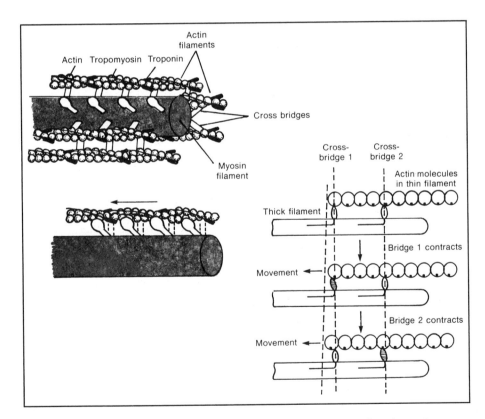

Fig. 10–3. Molecular components of skeletal muscle myofilaments. In relaxed muscle, tropomyosin covers the actin-active site, and there is no interaction between actin and myosin. In the presence of high calcium, tropomyosin is displaced, the actin-active site is exposed, and an actin-myosin cross-bridge is formed. A conformational change in the myosin head results in movement of the actin filament toward the center of the sarcomere, and muscle shortening occurs. Asynchronous cycling of cross-bridge attachment, movement, and detachment results in additional muscle shortening. With permission from McArdle WD, Katch F, Katch V: *Exercise Physiology.* Philadelphia: Lea & Febiger, 1985.

is a high concentration of potassium and low concentration of sodium inside the cells, and a high concentration of sodium and low concentration of potassium in the extracellular fluid. These concentration gradients are maintained by active electrogenic sodium-potassium pumps and the selective permeability characteristics of the sarcolemma. As a result of the unequal distribution of ions across the sarcolemma, there is a net electrical charge across the resting skeletal muscle cell membrane of approximately 90 mV, inside negative. The precise magnitude of the membrane potential varies with changes in the permeability of the sarcolemma or in response to alterations of the ionic composition of the extracellular fluid.[2]

The permeability characteristics of the muscle cell membrane may be altered by stimulation of the acetylcholine receptors located at the neuromuscular junction.[2] The neuromuscular junction is a specialized area along the sarcolemma of the skeletal muscle cell that is in close contact with a motor neuron. On stimulation, the motor neuron releases acetylcholine into the junctional region. The acetylcholine binds to the receptors on the skeletal muscle cell, and this binding produces local alterations in membrane permeability so that the membrane potential is decreased and endplate potentials (EPPs) develop. Individual EPPs sum together until a threshold level of depolarization occurs, at which point an action potential develops. The action potential is a progressive movement of membrane depolarization produced by changes in the sarcolemma permeability to sodium and potassium ions. Once initiated, the action potential propagates along the entire length of the cell membrane, and is therefore referred to as an all-or-none phenomenon.

The development of an action potential and membrane depolarization are linked to skeletal muscle contraction. As the action potential is propagated along the sarcolemma, it spreads into the T-tubules (Fig. 10–2). Graded depolarization of the T-tubule membrane causes release of calcium ions from the sarcoplasmic reticulum. As the cytosolic concentration of calcium increases, calcium ions bind to troponin C

and a conformational change in protein structure displaces troponin I, troponin T, and tropomyosin so that the actin-active sites along the thin filament are exposed and available for binding to the heads of the myosin filament (Fig. 10–3).

Skeletal muscle contraction, or muscle shortening, depends on the binding and interaction of the actin and myosin molecules and is described by the sliding filament and cross-bridge theories of muscle contraction.[3] Actin-myosin interaction is facilitated by two mechanisms. Increased cytosolic calcium results in exposure of the actin active sites, and the presence of ATP allows formation of the myosin-ADP-Pi complex, which has a high affinity for actin. Actin-myosin binding, or cross-bridge formation, results in conformational changes in the myosin molecule so that the myosin head rotates, pulling the actin filament toward the center of the sarcomere and reducing sarcomere length (Fig. 10–3). The energy required for the movement of the actin filaments is provided by completion of the hydrolysis of myosin-bound ADP-Pi. If sufficient ATP and calcium are available, the actin-myosin cross-bridge is broken and new attachments may be formed so that sequential cycles of cross-bridge formation, sliding of the filaments, and cross-bridge detachment result in increasing filament overlap and muscle shortening (Fig. 10–3). If ATP is not present, as in death, the actin-myosin complexes remain attached and the muscle remains in a state of rigor mortis. In contrast, when ATP is present but the myoneural stimulus for muscle contraction is removed, the actin-myosin complex detaches and calcium is resequestered into the sarcoplasmic reticulum by an ATP-dependent calcium pump. As a result, the number of calcium ions available for binding to troponin C decreases and tropomyosin returns to its original position, covering the actin active sites. Cross-bridge formation is inhibited and the muscle returns to its initial relaxed length. Single action potentials result in a consistent transient calcium release from the sarcoplasmic reticulum. Therefore, the mechanical response to a single action potential is also consistent and is referred to as a muscle twitch.

FUNCTIONAL PROPERTIES OF SKELETAL MUSCLE

Skeletal muscle performance, i.e., the force and velocity of contraction, can be voluntarily regulated by selective fiber recruitment, but is limited by the intrinsic properties of the muscle and the extrinsic properties of the load opposing muscle shortening.

Length-Tension Relationship

The ability of the individual myofiber to generate force depends on the number of actin-myosin cross-bridge interactions present at any single point in time.[4] The number of cross-bridge interactions is partially dependent on muscle length, as described by the length-tension relationship shown in Figure 10–4. When the myofiber is stretched beyond normal resting length, smaller portions of the myofilaments overlap within the sarcomere and the potential number of cross-bridge interactions is reduced, as is the capacity for force production (Fig. 10–4, point D). When the myofiber is excessively shortened, the opposing actin filaments overlap and interfere with cross-bridge formation near the center of the sarcomere, again reducing the potential for force generation (Fig. 10–4, point A). The sarcomere length required for optimal cross-bridge formation and force production is 2.0 to 2.2 μm.[2]

Under most in vivo conditions, the length-tension relationship is of little consequence in muscle force production because sarcomere length is maintained within the optimal range by the muscle attachments to the skeletal system.[5] However, the angle of muscle attachment (and joint angle) can significantly influence the fraction of total muscle force available for movement of the limb throughout its range of motion (Fig. 10–5). Muscle force generation is parallel to the long orientation of the myofibers. Therefore, the maximal amount of muscle force generation (nearly 100%) is available for limb movement when the long axis of the muscle is parallel to the direction of movement, e.g., when the long axis of the muscle is perpendicular to the attached bone. At all other joint angles, the muscle fibers are not parallel to the direction of movement and only a fraction of total muscle force generation is available to produce limb rotation. The remainder of the force generation acts to compress the joint. For example, during contraction of the biceps, the force available for lifting a weight held in the hand is maximal when the long axis of the biceps and the radius are at a 90° angle and the joint angle is approximately 60°.

Force-Velocity Relationship

The maximal shortening velocity of unloaded skeletal muscle is determined by the biochemical properties of the muscle. However, the maximal shortening velocity of loaded muscle is also dependent on the magnitude of the opposing load (Fig. 10–6). The greater the load, the slower muscle shortening occurs during maximal effort. For example, during a maximal isometric contraction, force production is maximal and the shortening velocity is zero. In contrast, unloaded muscles shorten very rapidly at near-maximal velocities.

Power output, or work per unit time, is equal to the product of force and velocity. As a consequence of the force-velocity relationship of skeletal muscle, there exists a

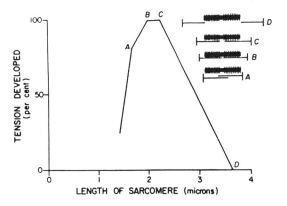

Fig. 10–4. Length-tension relationship of skeletal muscle. Excessive overlap (A) or extension (D) of the myofilaments decreases the number of potential effective cross-bridge interactions and the ability of the myofiber to generate force is inhibited. With permission from Guyton: *Textbook of Medical Physiology.* 6th Ed., Philadelphia: W.B. Saunders, 1981, p. 128.

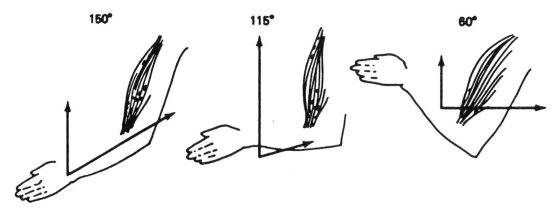

Fig. 10–5. Relationship between joint angle and portion of total muscle force mechanically available for limb movement. In this example, force is generated along the long axis of the biceps muscle. A major portion of this force is in the direction of limb movement when the joint angle is 115°. A smaller fraction of total muscle force is in the direction of limb movement at greater (150°) and lesser (60°) joint angles. With permission from Lamb DR: *Physiology of Exercise—Responses and Adaptations.* New York: Macmillan, 1978.

range of force production over which power output is optimized. Optimal power generation is achieved when force generation is equal to approximately 30% of maximal force production, corresponding to a

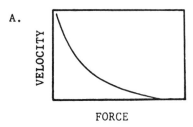

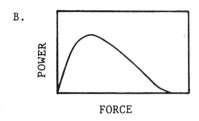

Fig. 10–6. **A.** Force-velocity and **B.** force-power relationships of skeletal muscle. Maximal shortening velocity is inversely related to the resisting force. Optimal power output (force·velocity) is achieved at about 30% of maximal force generation. With permission from Selkurt EE: *Basic Physiology for the Health Sciences.* Boston: Little, Brown and Co., 1982.

shortening velocity approximately 40% of maximal (Fig. 10–6).

Muscle Fiber Types

As previously mentioned, the maximal shortening velocity of unloaded skeletal muscle is determined by the biochemical properties of the muscle fibers. Distinct differences found in the shortening velocity of various muscle fibers have provided the basis for the primary classifications of slow-twitch and fast-twitch fiber types, and an additional subclassification of muscle fiber types is based on the principal metabolic pathway used for energy production.[4,6–8] As a result of these classification systems, human skeletal muscle is commonly divided into three basic fiber types: slow-twitch oxidative, fast-twitch oxidative, and fast-twitch glycolytic. However, the specific characteristics of an individual muscle fiber may lie anywhere along the continuum of fiber type characteristics so that a distinct classification of fiber type is often unclear.[4,9] Furthermore, the characteristics of a muscle fiber may change as the fiber adapts to the function for which it is most often recruited.

Slow-twitch fibers (also called Type I) have slow maximal shortening velocities and rely predominantly on oxidative metabolism, rather than anaerobic glycolysis, for metabolic energy. Type I fibers have a low activity of the enzyme myosin-ATPase. Myosin-ATPase is responsible for ATP hydrolysis, which provides the energy required for rotation of the myosin head and skeletal muscle contraction. As a consequence of the low myosin-ATPase activity, Type I (slow oxidative) fibers have slow contraction velocities and prolonged twitch durations (Fig. 10–7). Consistent with a high level of oxidative metabolism, Type I cells contain numerous and large mitochondria and high activity levels of mitochondrial enzymes such as succinate dehydrogenase and NAD dehydrogenase. In addition, Type I fibers have a rich capillary

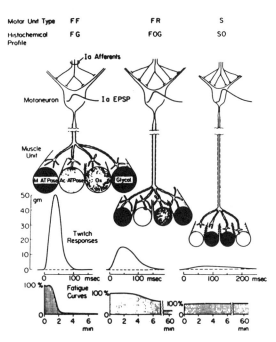

Fig. 10–7. Biochemical and functional characteristics of various motor unit types. Muscle fiber size and motor unit force generation and fatigue characteristics are scaled for comparison between motor unit types. Shading of fibers denotes the relative activities of various enzyme systems (identified in FF). Motor unit types are: FF-fast-twitch fatiguable or fast glycolytic; FR-fast-twitch fatigue resistant or fast oxidative/glycolytic; S-slow-twitch or slow oxidative. With permission from Saltin B, Gollnick PD: Skeletal muscle adaptability: Significance for metabolism and performance. In *Handbook of Physiology.* Edited by LD Peachy. Baltimore: Williams & Wilkins, 1983. Adapted from Burke RE, Edgerton VR: Motor unit properties and selective involvement in movement. *Exerc Sport Sci Rev,* 3:31, 1975.

supply, are small in diameter (25–40 μm), and have a high myoglobin content. These three characteristics facilitate the delivery of oxygen to the muscle cells, supporting oxidative metabolism. Because of the high capacities for oxidative metabolism, oxygen delivery, and preferential fat metabolism, Type I slow-twitch fibers are fatigue-resistant (Fig. 10–7) and are often found in continuously active postural muscles.

Fast-twitch, or Type II, fibers have relatively fast shortening velocities and short twitch durations because of their high myosin-ATPase activities (Fig. 10–7). Type II fibers are subdivided into Type IIa and IIb fibers on the basis of their metabolic oxidative capacities. Type IIa fibers, or fast oxidative fibers, have moderate capacities for both glycolytic and oxidative metabolism. The mitochondrial content and capillary supply of Type IIa fibers are relatively high and their diameters are relatively small (25–40 μm), favoring oxidative metabolism. Type IIa fibers are well suited for sustained phasic activities such as running and cycling. Type IIb fibers, or fast glycolytic fibers, have a high glycolytic metabolic capacity, as reflected by high activities of glycolytic enzymes such as phosphorylase. However, these muscle fibers have few mitochondria and a low oxidative capacity. Type IIb fibers are large in diameter (30 to 60 μm) and contain a larger number of actin and myosin filaments than their smaller counterparts. Therefore, Type IIb fibers can produce more force than Type I or Type IIa fibers, and are well suited for brief, powerful contractions that can be sustained by anaerobic metabolism, such as jumping and throwing.

Motor Unit Classifications

A myofiber is innervated by only one motor neuron, but a single motor neuron may innervate several muscle fibers. A motor unit is one motor neuron and all of the muscle fibers that it innervates.[4,6] A motor unit may be composed of few or many muscle fibers. For example, in the laryngeal and ocular muscles, there may be as few as two to three fibers per motor unit, whereas in the gastrocnemius muscle there may be thousands of fibers in a single motor unit. Motor units are composed of only one fiber type, and all myofibers within a single motor unit are stimulated to contract simultaneously (Fig. 10–7). Because skeletal muscle force production is proportional to the number of actin-myosin cross-bridge interactions, and is roughly proportional to the cross-sectional area of activated muscle, the force production of a single motor unit is determined by the size and number of muscle fibers comprising the unit. Motor units containing Type I (slow) or Type IIa (fast oxidative) fibers consist of relatively few muscle fibers and are recruited during sustained phasic contractions that require minimal to moderate force development, consistent with activities that can be sustained by oxidative metabolism. Motor units containing Type IIb (fast glycolytic) fibers are usually large, and simultaneous contraction of several large-diameter muscle fibers produces the high level of force required for powerful movements that must be supported by glycolytic metabolism (Fig. 10–7).

Graded Contractions

Contraction of a single muscle fiber is an all-or-none phenomenon. Therefore, the force produced by a myofiber in response to a single action potential results from the structural factors determining the number of actin-myosin cross-bridge interactions.[4] However, the force produced by an entire skeletal muscle can be regulated to meet the requirements of the movement. Graded force production is accomplished by varying the number and types of fibers contracting at any given time and by altering the frequency of muscle stimulation and contraction.

As previously noted, the number of muscle fibers contained in a single motor unit can range from few to many, and the force produced by a single motor unit depends on the size and number of muscle fibers activated (Fig. 10–7). The force production of an entire muscle depends on the number and type of motor units recruited during a given contraction. Muscle force production can be increased by recruitment of additional motor units. The additional force generation achieved by simultaneous contraction of multiple motor units is referred to as spatial summation. Motor unit recruitment occurs in a specific

sequential manner. During a muscle contraction, small motor units are recruited first, followed by recruitment of progressively larger motor units, until the desired force production is attained. The orderly progression of recruitment from small to large motor units is referred to as the size principle of motor unit recruitment.[10]

A single action potential produces a dis-

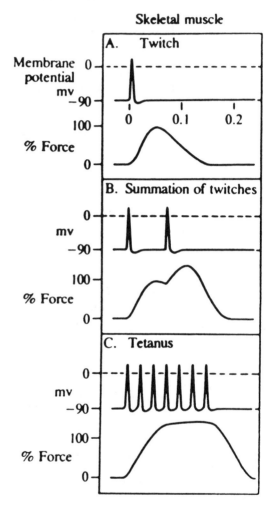

Fig. 10–8. Skeletal muscle force generation resulting from single and repetitive stimulation. A single action potential (panel **A**) results in a standard mechanical response. Initiation of a second contraction before complete relaxation is achieved results in enhanced force generation (panel **B**). This enhancement of force is referred to as temporal summation. When no relaxation or decrement in force is observed between sequential contractions, the maximal potential force production is attained and a tetanic contraction is observed (panel **C**).

tinct contraction and relaxation pattern known as a muscle twitch (Fig. 10–8A). A twitch is an all-or-none phenomenon that results in a specific magnitude of force generation roughly proportional to the cross-sectional area of muscle activated. Although the force produced by a single twitch is predetermined by the number of cross-bridge interactions, a graded increase in force production can be accomplished by a temporal summation (summation over time) of muscle twitches. Temporal summation occurs when a second action potential develops before the muscle completely relaxes from the previous twitch. In effect, the force and muscle shortening remaining because of incomplete relaxation are added to the standard twitch resulting from the second action potential. Therefore, total force production and muscle shortening are greater than would be expected from an isolated single twitch (Fig. 10–8B). As the frequency of stimulation (motor neuron firing) increases, the time available for relaxation decreases and additional force and shortening occur. When no relaxation or decrement in force is observed between sequential contractions, the maximal potential force production is attained and a tetanic contraction is observed (Fig. 10–8C). The stimulation frequency at which tetanus is observed is much lower in slow-twitch than fast-twitch fibers because

of the relatively long twitch duration of slow-twitch fibers (Fig. 10–7).

SKELETAL MUSCLE ADAPTATIONS TO EXERCISE TRAINING

As with most physiologic systems, skeletal muscle adapts to increased activity. The specific adaptations that occur depend on the frequency, duration, and intensity of the contractions. In general, the skeletal muscles used during the training activity become better equipped to perform the types of contractions encountered in training.[11] Skeletal muscle adaptations to endurance, sprint, and strength training are subsequently discussed and summarized in Table 10–1.

Endurance Training

The capacity of skeletal muscle to perform prolonged work of moderate intensity depends on its oxidative capacity. Endurance training regimens that produce an increase in aerobic capacity ($\dot{V}_{O_{2max}}$) also result in increased oxidative enzyme activities in muscles used in the training activity,[8,9,11] but the activity of the glycolytic enzymes remains relatively unchanged.[4] Mitochondrial size, number, and enzyme activities (e.g., cytochrome oxidase and succinate dehydrogenase) are increased in endurance-trained skeletal muscles.[7,8,12] Al-

Table 10–1. Skeletal Muscle Adaptations to Exercise Training

Properties of Muscle	Type of Training		
	Endurance	Sprint	Strength
Fibert type composition	+ ?	+ ?	0
Fiber size	0	+, −, 0	+
Metabolic enzyme activities			
carbohydrate oxidation	+ + +	+ +	+, −, 0
fatty acid oxidation	+ +	+	0
anaerobic glycolysis	0	+	+, 0
Myosin ATPase activity	+ ?	+ ?	0
Substrate storage			
ATP/CP	+	+	0, +
glycogen	+	+, 0	0
Myoglobin content	+ ?	+ ?	0
Mitochondria number	+ +	+	0
Capillary density	+	0?	0

Symbols indicate relative changes: +, + +, + + + = small, medium, and large increases; − = decrease; 0 = no change; ? = unknown or unconfirmed.

though the oxidative capacity is increased in all fiber types, the greatest training effects are observed in Type I fibers in response to continuous training, and in Type IIa fibers in response to interval training.[8,9,11,13]

The oxidative capacity for all fuel types (carbohydrates, fats, and proteins) appears to increase in parallel fashion.[4,8] Krebs cycle enzyme activities (e.g., succinate dehydrogenase), components of the electron transport chain (e.g., cytochrome oxidase and cytochrome c), and the capacity to transport and oxidize NADH (malate-aspartate shuttle) are all increased as a result of endurance training. In addition, the enzymatic capacities to phosphorylate and dispose of or metabolize glucose (e.g., hexokinase activity) and activate, transport, and oxidize fatty acids (e.g., carnitine palmitoyl transferase activity) are increased with endurance training.

The increases in oxidative enzyme activities most likely result from enhanced enzyme (protein) synthesis, stimulated by increased substrate flux through the oxidative pathways.[4,7] Physiologic conditions rarely elicit attainment of the maximal velocity of substrate utilization.[4] Therefore, the functional significance of the training-induced increase in oxidative potential cannot be fully appreciated. However, increased enzyme activities also enhance flux through the metabolic pathways at relatively low substrate concentrations, such as those that may occur during prolonged exercise. In addition, more precise control of oxidative metabolism may result from enhanced enzyme activities.[4,7,8,11]

In addition to the enhanced oxidative capacity, endurance training also results in an increase in substrate storage in active skeletal muscles. Although minor increases in the immediate stores of metabolic energy (ATP and creatine phosphate) have been reported in response to endurance training,[4] the small increases are most likely functionally insignificant during endurance activities because the total muscle phosphate stores can sustain only 10 to 15 seconds of muscle contraction. Therefore, the ability of the skeletal muscle metabolic machinery to replenish the high energy phosphates is of primary importance in endurance performance, rather than the actual size of the phosphate stores. Glycogen stores may increase as much as twofold in response to training, presumably because of increases in hexokinase and glycogen synthase activities.[4] However, dietary factors play the dominant role in determining skeletal muscle glycogen concentrations, and a combination of a high carbohydrate diet and endurance training can enhance muscle glycogen storage by as much as threefold.[4]

An additional biochemical alteration that occurs in response to endurance training is an increase in fatty acid utilization and a decrease in glycogen utilization during prolonged exercise.[7,8] This shift in fuel utilization appears to be a result of the increased oxidative capacity. For a given level of work, the training-induced increase in oxidative capacity minimizes the accumulation of ADP. Because ADP normally stimulates glycolysis, a decrease in ADP accumulation spares glycogen and enhances fat utilization. Furthermore, the enhanced oxidative capacity of Type I and Type IIa fibers allows more work to be done before anaerobic glycolysis and the recruitment of Type IIb fibers are required, which subsequently delays the onset of lactic acid accumulation.[13]

In addition to the enzymatic alterations that improve the ability of endurance-trained skeletal muscle to utilize oxygen, endurance training enhances the delivery of oxygen to muscle tissues by stimulating the growth of new capillaries. The number of capillaries per muscle fiber and per square millimeter of tissue is increased in the major muscle groups roughly in proportion to the total body aerobic capacity ($\dot{V}O_{2max}$).[4,11,14] Increases in both capillary number and diameter result in an increased capillary surface area for gas exchange and reduce the diffusion distances between blood and the core of the skeletal muscle tissue. These anatomic alterations facilitate the diffusion of oxygen and other metabolic substrates to the metabolic machinery of the active fibers. The myoglobin concentration of skeletal muscle may also increase as a result of endurance training, further facilitating the transport and storage of oxygen in the muscle tissue.[8,11]

Endurance training increases the oxidative capacity of all muscle fiber types. As a result, the oxidative capacities of Type I and Type IIa fibers become more similar after a period of endurance training. However, a true conversion of muscle fiber type or contractile properties has not been documented.[4] Although a few investigators have reported an increase in myosin ATPase activity with aerobic training, and chronic stimulation has been shown to prolong twitch duration in Type II fibers of the rat, a training-induced transformation of fast-twitch to slow-twitch fibers has not been clearly demonstrated in humans.[8,11] The fact that endurance athletes tend to have a relatively high proportion of Type I fibers is most likely the consequence of genetic predisposition rather than an adaptive response to endurance training.[4,7] Although Type I and Type II fiber conversion does not result from endurance training, the oxidative capacity of Type IIb fibers may increase to the point where they become histologically indistinguishable from Type IIa fibers.[7,14]

The performance effects of endurance training include the ability to perform a higher level of work for an extended period of time and a delay in the onset of fatigue during prolonged submaximal work. The increase in enzymatic oxidative capacity and capillary density support the increase in work capacity. The sparing of glycogen and decrease in lactic acid accumulation contribute to the delay in the onset of fatigue.

Sprint Training

The objective of sprint training is to recruit Type II muscle fibers to do aerobic work. This objective is met by performing an activity that requires a balance of power and endurance. Sprint training induces changes in skeletal muscle oxidative enzyme activities similar to those observed with endurance training: mitochondrial size and number and cytochrome oxidase activity increase, succinate dehydrogenase activity may increase or remain unchanged, and beta-oxidation of long-chain fatty acids increases in response to sprint training if the training regimen is of appropriate intensity and duration to elicit fatty acid mobilization.[4] The increase in oxida-

tive capacity resulting from sprint training is primarily evident in Type II fibers.[4] In addition to the enhancement of oxidative capacity, sprint training increased the activities of some glycolytic enzymes (e.g., phosphorylase and phosphofructokinase) in Type I muscle fibers.[8] Glycogen storage and glycogen synthase activity may also be enhanced in response to sprint training.[4,8] However, increased glycogen storage and substrate availability only enhance sprint performance during repeated bouts of intense exercise. Sprint training results in little or no change in the glycolytic capacity of Type II muscle fibers.[4]

A change in the contractile properties of muscle fibers can occur as a result of sprint training. Repeated bouts of exercise at 90 to 100% of Vo_{2max} can produce a shift in fiber type distribution from Type I to Type II fibers (slow-twitch to fast-twitch).[15] A decrease in Type I myofiber twitch time has also been reported as a result of placing endurance athletes on a high-intensity "anaerobic" training program.[16,17] Despite this evidence, there remains some doubt as to whether a true conversion of Type I to Type II fibers occurs as a result of sprint training.[4,11]

Strength Training

The objective of strength training is to increase the maximal force development capacity of a skeletal muscle. Increases in muscle size (hypertrophy) and muscle strength normally occur in response to strength training, and these two adaptations are physiologically related. The diameters of strength-trained muscle fibers (primarily Type IIa fibers) increase to accommodate new sarcomeres formed in parallel with the existing myofibrils.[4] This addition of parallel contractile units is directly related to an increase in muscle strength. The contractility of the muscle fibers (e.g., the maximal tension produced per square millimeter of cross-sectional area or the force produced per cross-bridge interaction) is not altered by strength training.[4] Therefore, the overall gain in strength is generally proportional to the increase in cross-sectional area of the muscle. However, in the early stages of strength training, muscle strength may increase more rapidly than muscle size. This early increase in functional muscle strength is a result of improved coordination and increased motor unit recruitment. In contrast, muscle size may increase more than functional strength if excessive hypertrophy alters the attachment angle to the bone in such a way that the biomechanical advantage is reduced. The cross-sectional area and strength of the connective tissue elements of skeletal muscle also increase in response to strength training to accommodate the increase in muscle strength.[4]

Traditional high-resistance isotonic strength training results in little or no enhancement of oxidative or glycolytic enzyme activities in skeletal muscle.[4] Mitochondrial enzyme activities may, in fact, be reduced because of the dilution effect of muscle hypertrophy in the absence of a compensatory increase in mitochondrial mass. In contrast, isometric training can result in increases in cytochrome oxidase and succinate dehydrogenase activities.[18] Isokinetic strength training may also alter enzyme activities. Isokinetic training consisting of 30-second bouts of maximal contractions has been shown to increase phosphorylase, phosphofructokinase, creatine kinase, malate dehydrogenase, and succinate dehydrogenase activities; conversely, 6-second bouts of isokinetic contractions resulting in similar strength gains produced only an increase in phosphofructokinase activity.[19] There is no evidence to support the idea that any method of strength training results in a conversion between muscle fiber types.[4]

Athletic performance and the ability to perform physical work are determined, at least partly, by the functional characteristics of skeletal muscle. Human skeletal muscle has the capacity to adapt to chronic use. These adaptations, which may include enhanced enzyme activities, protein synthesis, and capillary growth, enable the skeletal muscle and the overall human body to function more effectively in frequently encountered activities.[11]

REFERENCES

1. McArdle WD, Katch FU, Katch VL: *Exercise Physiology.* Philadelphia: Lea & Febiger, 1991.
2. Meiss RA: Muscle: Striated, smooth, cardiac. In *Basic Physiology for the Health Sciences.* Edited by EE Selkurt. Boston: Little, Brown, and Co., 1982.
3. Huxley, AF: Muscular contraction. *J Physiol (Lond), 243:*1, 1974.
4. Saltin B, Gollnick PD: Skeletal muscle adaptability: Significance for metabolism and performance. In *Handbook of Physiology.* Edited by LD Peachy. Baltimore: Williams & Wilkins, 1983.
5. Lamb DR: *Exercise Physiology—Responses and Adaptations.* New York: Macmillan, 1978.
6. Burke RE, Edgerton VR: Motor unit properties and selective involvement in movement. *Exerc Sport Sci Rev, 3:*31, 1975.
7. Holloszy JO, Coyle EF: Adaptations of skeletal muscle to endurance exercise and metabolic consequences. *J Appl Physiol, 56:*831, 1984.
8. Holloszy JO, Booth FW: Biochemical adaptations to endurance exercise in muscle. *Annu Rev Physiol, 38:*273, 1976.
9. Essen-Gustavsson B, Henriksson J: Enzyme levels in pools of microdissected human muscle fibers of identified type. *Acta Physiol Scand, 120:*505, 1984.
10. Henneman E, Clamann JD, Gillies JD, Skinner RD: Rank order of motorneurons within a pool: Law of combination. *J Neurophysiol, 37:*1338, 1974.
11. Salmons S, Henriksson J: The adaptive response of skeletal muscle to increased use. *Muscle Nerve, 4:*94, 1981.
12. Soar PK, Davies CTM, Fentem PH, Newsholme EA: The effect of endurance-training on the maximum activities of hexokinase, 6-phosphofructokinase, citrate synthase, and oxoglutarate dehydrogenase in red and white muscles of the rat. *Biosci Rep, 3:*831, 1983.
13. Baldwin KM, Winder WW: Adaptive responses in different types of muscle fibers to endurance exercise. *Ann NY Acad Sci, 301:*411, 1976.
14. Inger F: Effects of endurance training on fiber ATP-ase activity, capillary supply and mitochondrial content in man. *J Physiol (Lond), 294:*419, 1979.
15. Jansson E, Kaijser L: Muscle adaptation to extreme endurance training in man. *Acta Physiol Scand, 100:*315, 1977.
16. Henriksson J, Jansson E, Schantz P: Increase in myofibrillar ATPase intermediate skeletal muscle fibers with endurance training of extreme duration in man. *Muscle Nerve, 3:*274, 1980 (Abstract).
17. Staudte HW, Exner GU, Pette D: Effects of

short-term, high-intensity (sprint) training on some contractile and metabolic characteristics of fast and slow muscle of the rat. *Pflugers Arch, 344:*159, 1973.

18. Grimby G, et al.: Metabolic effects of iso-metric training. *Scand J Clin Lab Invest, 31:* 301, 1973.

19. Costill DL, et al.: Adaptations in skeletal muscle following strength training. *J Appl Physiol, 46:*96, 1979.

Chapter 11

MECHANISMS OF MUSCULAR FATIGUE

Robert H. Fitts

The etiology of muscle fatigue is an important question that has interested exercise scientists for more than a century. A definitive fatigue agent or agents have yet to be identified, although progress has been made and theories have been developed that, for the most part, explain the experimental findings. The problem is complex because muscle fatigue might result from deleterious alterations in the muscle itself (peripheral fatigue) and/or from changes in the neural input to the muscle. The latter factor could itself be mediated by changes of central and/or peripheral origin. Furthermore, the nature and extent of muscle fatigue clearly depend on the type, duration, and intensity of exercise, the fiber type composition of the muscle, individual level of fitness, and numerous environmental factors. For example, fatigue experienced in high-intensity, short-duration exercise is surely dependent on factors that differ from those precipitating fatigue in endurance activity. Similarly, fatigue during tasks involving heavily loaded contractions (e.g., weightlifting) are likely to differ from that produced during relatively unloaded movement (running and swimming).

In this review, we discuss muscle fatigue resulting from two general types of activity: short-duration, high-intensity, and endurance exercise. The current theories and important supportive experimental results are presented. Because of space limitations, this review cannot be complete. Detailed discussions are found in earlier reviews.[1-5]

SHORT-DURATION, HIGH-INTENSITY EXERCISE

Sites of Muscle Fatigue

Muscle fatigue is defined, for the purposes of this review, as a loss of force and power output leading to reduced performance of a given task. Fatigue during short-duration, high-intensity exercise could result from an impairment of the central nervous system (CNS), so that the optimal frequency of motor nerve activation is not maintained. Bigland-Ritchie and coworkers clearly showed that the frequency of motor nerve firing decreases during continuous contractile activity.[6] The question is whether this change precipitates muscle fatigue or results from neuronal feedback (muscle afferents) in an attempt to maintain an optimal activation frequency as fatigue develops. The preponderance of evidence suggests the latter. The fatiguing muscle generally shows a prolonged force transient (primarily because of a slower relaxation time) in response to a single stimulus. Consequently, a lower frequency of activation is required to elicit peak tension (force-frequency curve shifts to the left). The primary sites of fatigue are apparently located within the muscle, and do not generally involve the CNS, peripheral nerves, or neural-muscular (N-M) junction. The observation that fatigued muscles generate the same tension whether stimulated directly or by way of the motor nerve argues against N-M junction fatigue.

The major components of a muscle cell involved in excitation-contraction (E-C) coupling are shown in Figure 11–1. The numbers indicate possible sites within the cell where alteration during heavy exercise could induce fatigue. With fatigue, a 10 to 20 mv depolarization of the sarcolemma (muscle membrane) resting potential (V_m) is frequently observed, and the sarcolemma action potential (AP) amplitude and duration are depressed and prolonged, respectively.[7-10] It has been suggested that these changes in sarcolemma function induce fatigue by preventing cell activa-

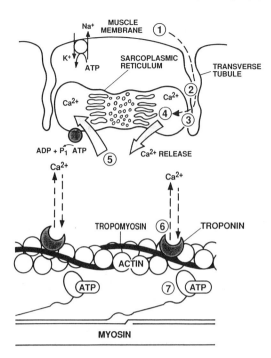

Fig. 11–1. A diagrammatic representation of the major components of a muscle cell involved in excitation-contraction (E-C) coupling. The numbers indicate possible sites of muscular fatigue during heavy exercise and include: one, surface membrane; two, T-tubular charge movement; three, unknown mechanism coupling T-tubular charge movement with SR Ca^{2+} release; four, SR Ca^{2+} release; five, SR Ca^{2+} reuptake; six, Ca^{2+} binding to troponin; and seven, actomyosin hydrolysis of ATP and crossbridge force development and cycling rate.

tion.[1,3-6] The general theory is that K^+ efflux and Na^+ influx and inhibition of the Na^+-K^+ pump cause cell depolarization, a reduced AP amplitude and, in some cells, complete inactivation. This hypothesis is known as the membrane mechanism of muscle fatigue.[1,3,4] Edwards[1] and Lindinger and Sjøgaard[4] speculate that the membrane mechanism of fatigue would allow contractions at reduced rates and forces while preventing catastrophic changes in cellular homeostasis that might lead to cell damage. It has been suggested, but not established, that cell depolarization and the reduced AP amplitude affect propagation of the sarcolemma AP into the T-tubules (No. 2, Fig. 11–1) and thus inhibit subsequent steps in E-C coupling.[3-5] In

support of this hypothesis, Lannergren and Westerblad[9] observed a steep decline in tension once V_m fell below -60 mv and, more recently, Westerblad et al.[11] found failure of Ca^{2+} release in the center of fatigued muscle fibers.

In nonfatigued muscle, the T-tubular AP produces a charge movement within the T-tubular membrane (see No. 3, Fig. 11–1) which subsequently, by an unknown process, leads to Ca^{2+} release from the sarcoplasmic reticulum (see No. 4, Fig. 11–1). In the past few years, considerable progress has been made in understanding the molecular mechanism of Ca^{2+} release.[12] The important proteins at the T-SR junction have been identified, and it is now clear that the T-tubular charge sensor (proteins responsible for the intramembranous charge movement) lies directly opposite and may contact the junctional foot protein (ryanodine receptor) which makes up the Ca^{2+} release channel of the SR.[12] The exact mechanism of transduction across the T-SR junction has not yet been established. The morphologic relationship between the SR Ca^{2+} release channel (ryanodine receptor) and the intramembranous T-tubular charge sensor [dihydropridine receptor (DHP)] supports the hypothesis that the main mechanism involves mechanical or allosteric coupling.[12] Two additional mechanisms, Ca^{2+}-induced Ca^{2+} release and activation by InsP3, are thought to play secondary or modulatory roles in regulating Ca^{2+} release in skeletal muscle.[12]

With activation, the T-tubular AP triggers a confirmational change in DHP receptor, which in turn opens the SR Ca^{2+} release channel. The elevated level of intracellular Ca^{2+} binds to troponin C (see No. 6, Fig. 11–1), a regulatory protein, producing a molecular change in the troponin-tropomyosin complex that in turn allows the contractile proteins actin and myosin to bind and to generate force.[13]

Fatigued muscle frequently shows prolonged twitch duration and reduced peak rate of tension development.[14] With activation, intracellular Ca^{2+} levels rise, triggering cross-bridge activation and force development. Prolonged twitch duration reflects a similar prolongation in the time course of the increase in intracellular levels of Ca^{2+}

(Ca^{2+} transient). The lengthened Ca^{2+} transient suggests either a reduced rate of release and/or reuptake of Ca^{2+} by the SR. Such changes could take place for any number of reasons, from alterations in T-tubular charge movement (see No. 3, Fig. 11-1) to changes in the intrinsic ability of the SR to release or remove Ca^{2+}. Blinks et al. and, more recently, Allen et al., Westerblad et al., and Westerblad and Allen have demonstrated that the amplitude of the Ca^{2+} transient decreases as fatigue develops.[11,15-17] The rate and extent of Ca^{2+} release from the SR could decline during contractile activity, even without an altered AP or intramembranous T-tubular charge movement, if either the coupling step between the T-tubular and SR membrane or the release process itself were inhibited. For example, low pH has been shown to decrease the open probability of the Ca^{2+} release channel.[18] Clearly, the exact role of alterations in E-C in the fatigue process awaits a better understanding of the basic steps in E-C coupling. Additionally, fatigue could result from a direct effect on the contractile proteins (see No. 7, Fig. 11-1).

Major Fatigue Agents

High-intensity exercise involves an energy demand that exceeds the individual's maximal aerobic power, and thus requires a high level of anaerobic metabolism. Consequently, the levels of high-energy phosphates, ATP, and phosphocreatine (PC) decrease, and levels of inorganic phosphate (P_i) ADP, lactate, and the H^+ ion increase as fatigue develops. All of these changes are possible fatigue-inducing agents, and since the development of the needle biopsy technique, each has been studied extensively.[2,19,20]

To avoid fatigue, adequate tissue ATP levels must be maintained, because this substrate supplies the immediate source of energy for force generation by the myosin cross-bridges. ATP is also needed in the functioning of the sodium-potassium pump, which is essential in the maintenance of a normal sarcolemma and T-tubular AP. Additionally, ATP is a substrate of the SR ATPase and thus is required in the process of Ca^{2+} reuptake by the SR. As discussed previously, a disturbance in any of these processes could lead to muscle fatigue. Although the tissue ATP concentration decreases during intense muscular contraction, this reduction does not appear to limit force output or cause muscle fatigue. The classic experiments of Karlsson and Saltin perhaps best illustrate the absence of correlated changes of ATP and performance.[21] In this work, the needle biopsy technique was used to evaluate substrate changes after exercise to exhaustion at three different workloads. After 2 minutes of work, ATP and PC were depleted to the same extent at all loads; however, fatigue occurred only with the highest workload. These results are equivocal, however, because the biopsy was acquired some seconds after work ceased, and the sample represented an average tissue ATP that might not reflect the concentration existing at the cross-bridges. We also observed, however, a lack of correlation between ATP and force in isolated muscles studied in vitro.[22,23] In these experiments, ATP showed complete recovery in the first 15 seconds after a fatiguing stimulation bout, whereas peak tetanic tension (P_o) remained depressed.

PC levels decline with contractile activity and some authors suggest that low muscle PC levels could induce fatigue.[19,24] The decline in PC level and in tension during contractile activity, however, follow different time courses, making a causal relationship unlikely.[23] PC participates in the movement of ATP from the mitochondria to the cross-bridges, a process called the PC-ATP shuttle.[25] The possibility exists that a critically low PC concentration may disrupt this shuttle system and slow the rate of ADP rephosphorylation to ATP. This interference could lead to a critically low ATP at the cross-bridges, thus producing muscle fatigue. This possibility seems unlikely in that varying degrees of fatigue have been associated with equal ATP and PC values, and the highest ATP utilization rate (and thus ATP synthesis) was observed in the exercise model giving the lowest force.[26] Furthermore, a recent single cell analysis found even the lowest postfatigue cell ATP concentration to be 100-fold higher than required for full cross-bridge activation.[27]

Muscular contraction involves the hydrolysis of ATP by the actomyosin ATPase-producing energy and yielding ADP, P_i, and the H^+ ion as end products. All three of these products increase during intense contractile activity and could cause fatigue by direct inhibition of hydrolysis.[28-31] Results that involved the use of the single-skinned fiber preparation have shown reduced peak tension in response to elevated values of H^+,[28,30] ADP,[31] and P_i.[29,30] The importance of ADP and P_i relative to other potential fatigue agents (particularly the H^+ ion) is unknown. The H^+ ion is a particularly interesting potential fatigue agent because it could produce fatigue at numerous sites. In addition to a direct inhibition of the cross-bridge actomyosin ATPase and ATP hydrolysis, a build-up in the intracellular H^+ ion (decreased intracellular pH, abbreviation pH_i) could induce fatigue by: (1) inhibiting phosphofructokinase and thus the glycolytic rate; (2) competitive inhibition of Ca^{2+} binding to troponin C-reducing crossbridge activation; and (3) inhibiting the SR-ATPase-reducing Ca^{2+} reuptake and subsequently Ca^{2+} release.[32-34]

A major source of H^+ ion production during intense muscular activity is the anaerobic production of lactic acid, the majority of which dissociates into lactate and H^+ ions. As early as 1907, lactic acid was implicated as a possible fatigue agent.[35] This hypothesis gained popularity after publication of the work of A.V. Hill in the late 1920s.[36] The general consensus now is that fatigue results from the elevated number of H^+ ions rather than lactate or the undissociated lactic acid. Resting skeletal muscle pH, determined by a variety of techniques, is approximately 7.00 and declines with intense muscular contraction to values below 6.5 (Table 11–1).

At least two observations lend support to the concept that an elevated H^+ ion concentration inhibits glycolysis. Hill found that lactate formation during muscle stimulation stopped when the intracellular pH dropped to 6.3.[36] Second, Hermansen and Osnes measured the pH of muscle homogenates and observed no change during a 60-second measurement period for the most acidic homogenates of fatigued muscle; the pH values of the homogenates from resting muscle fell markedly owing to significant glycolysis during the measurement period.[37] Sahlin et al.[38] suggest that this inhibition of glycolysis by the H^+ ion may be the limiting factor for performance of intense exercise, yet this conclusion is not supported by the aforementioned results in which the change in ATP and force were not significantly correlated.[22,23,26] If the inhibition of glycolysis was causative in fatigue, the decline in tissue ATP would be likely to reach limiting levels. Consequently, a significant correlation between force and ATP would exist during the development of, and recovery from, fatigue.

Results of studies on skinned fibers definitively showed that acidosis depressed the force output of skeletal as well as cardiac muscle.[28,30,43] Decreasing pH from 7.4 to 6.2 not only reduced the maximal tension generated in the presence of optimal free Ca^{2+}, but also increased the threshold of free Ca^{2+} required for contraction; the force-PCa curve shifted to the right so that higher free Ca^{2+} was required to reach a given tension.[28,43,44] Fast-twitch fibers were more sensitive to the acidotic depression of maximal tension than were the slow muscle fibers.[28,44] These effects may be mediated by a H^+ ion interference with Ca^{2+} binding to troponin.[33] The results reported by Bolitho-Donaldson and Hermansen as well as Fabiato and Fabiato

Table 11–1. Skeletal Muscle pH

Method	Rest Value*	Fatigue Value	Reference
Muscle Homogenate	6.92 ± 0.03	6.41 ± 0.04	Hermansen and Osnes[37]
Calculated from HCO_{3-} + PCO_2	7.04 ± 0.05	6.37 ± 0.11	Sahlin et al.[38]
Microelectrode	7.06 ± 0.04	6.33	Metzger and Fitts[39]
DMO method	7.06 ± 0.02		Roos and Boron[40]
NMR method	7.10 ± 0.02	6.40 ± 0.05	Miller et al.[41]
NMR method	6.99 ± 0.04	6.17 ± 0.33	Wilson et al.[42]

* Values are means $\pm$ SE except for findings of Sahlin et al., for which $\pm$ SD are listed.

indicate that the effect is not entirely a simple competitive inhibition of Ca^{2+} binding to troponin.[43,44] The observed depression of maximal tension was completely reversible when pH returned to a neutral value, but the depression could not be overcome by increasing free Ca^{2+}.[28,43,44] Fabiato and Fabiato suggest that the H^+ ion effect may act at some step in addition to the Ca^{2+} interaction with troponin, perhaps by directly affecting the myosin molecule (see No. 7, Fig. 11–1). A direct effect on myosin is supported by the observation that a 33% reduction in maximal rigor tension occurs when pH changes from 7.00 to 6.2. Recently, Metzger and Moss demonstrated low pH to reduce the force per cross-bridge in all fiber types, and the number of cross-bridges during maximal Ca^{2+} activation in the fast-twitch but not the slow-twitch fiber type.[45] These authors also reported low pH to depress the rate of myosin binding to actin during suboptimal, but not saturating, levels of Ca^{2+} activation.[46] They hypothesized that the fatigue-induced depression in the rate of tension development (dP/dt) could be partly caused by this pH effect on the kinetics of myosin and actin binding.[46]

The rate of ATP hydrolysis by actomyosin is thought to limit the maximal speed of muscle shortening (V_{max}). Consequently, an elevated H^+ ion concentration, which inhibits the ATPase, should decrease V_{max} as well as Po. Edman and Mattiazzi showed that V_{max} indeed decreases with fatigue, but not until peak tension falls by at least 10%.[47]

We observed a high negative correlation between free H^+ ion content and Po during recovery, a result fully consistent with the H^+ ion theory of muscular fatigue. This and previously published work, however, clearly show force to recover in two phases—a short (about 30-second), rapid phase followed by a slower, relatively prolonged (about 15-minute) phase of recovery.[22,39] The immediate, rapid phase of recovery cannot be explained by the H^+ ion theory because cell pH_i actually decreases during this time (probably because of the rapid resynthesis of PC, an H^+ ion-generating reaction). This rapid phase of force recovery is likely explained by the reversal of a non-H^+ ion-mediated alteration in E-

C coupling. The second, slower phase of recovery shows a high negative correlation with the H^+, which probably results partly from the removal of the excess intracellular H^+ ion.

Changes in pH may affect Ca^{2+} regulation by disturbing E-C coupling (see previous discussion) and/or Ca^{2+} reuptake. Nakamura and Schwartz noted decreased pH to increase the Ca^{2+}-binding capacity of isolated SR membranes, and suggested that a drop in pH might reduce the amount of Ca^{2+} released from the SR during excitation. Changes in free H^+ ion may also affect the Ca^{2+}-binding properties of the Ca^{2+} binding protein parvalbumin (a protein found in relatively high concentrations in fast-twitch fibers), which by itself would alter the Ca^{2+} transient and force output.

Nosek et al. and Wilkie suggested that an increased $H_2PO_4^-$ concentration induced fatigue by inhibiting the cross-bridge transition from the low to the high force state.[29,48] The primary support for this hypothesis comes from the observation in skinned fibers that high P_i (20 mM) reduced peak force.[29] Additionally, NMR studies show a close inverse relationship between P_i and force during the development of, and recovery from, fatigue.[27,42]

ENDURANCE EXERCISE

Numerous factors have been linked to fatigue resulting from prolonged endurance activity, including depletion of muscle and liver glycogen, decreases in blood glucose, dehydration, and increases in body temperature. Undoubtedly, each of these factors contributes to fatigue to a varying degree, their relative importance depending on the environmental conditions and the nature of the activity. This section is a review of some of these potential fatigue factors, particularly carbohydrate depletion, as well as of evidence linking an alteration in SR function to the development of fatigue during prolonged exercise.

Glycogen Depletion

In 1896, Chauveau suggested that the rate of carbohydrate utilization was dependent on the intensity of work. This belief was based on the observation that the respiratory exchange ratio (RQ) increased from

0.75 during rest to 0.95 during exercise. With the development of the needle biopsy technique, these early theories based on RQ were proven correct by direct measurements of glycogen utilization at different work intensities.[20,49] Glycogen utilization was found to increase from 0.3 to 3.4 glucose units $\times$ g^{-1} $\times$ min^{-1} as the relative workload increased from 25 to 100% of the maximal oxygen uptake ($\dot{V}O_{2max}$).[49] Muscle glycogen depletion coincided with exhaustion during prolonged work bouts that required approximately 75% of $\dot{V}O_{2max}$. With workloads below 50 or above 90% of $\dot{V}O_{2max}$, ample muscle glycogen remained at exhaustion.[49] The rate of body carbohydrate usage depends not only on the intensity of the work, but also on the state of the individual's fitness.[49] At a given workload, trained individuals have a lower RQ and deplete glycogen at a slower rate than untrained individuals.[49] The observation that the trained individual can work longer supports the hypothesis that depletion of body carbohydrate stores is not only correlated with, but causative of, muscular fatigue during endurance activity. The exact mechanism of this protective effect is unknown. Although muscle glycogen represents an important fuel source, adequate levels of free fatty acids (FFA) and, in most cases, blood glucose are available at exhaustion. One possibility is that a certain level of muscle glycogen metabolism is required for either the optimal production of NADH and electron transport or the maintenance of fat oxidation, perhaps intermediates of the Krebs cycle become limiting

without adequate glycogen metabolism. Alternatively, the translocation of FFA into mitochondria may be rate-limiting and/or a high concentration of long-chain FFA might inhibit ATP translocation across the mitochondria membrane. It seems apparent that future efforts should focus on the mechanisms by which glycogen depletion alters muscle function.

Other Factors

Glycogen depletion is probably not an exclusive fatigue factor during endurance exercise. Other potential candidates include disruption of important intracellular organelles, such as the mitochondria, the SR, or the myofilaments. Significant mitochondrial damage is an unlikely fatigue factor because the capacity of the mitochondria to oxidize substrate and generate ATP is unchanged by exercise to exhaustion.[2]

The contractile proteins and, in particular, the myofibril ATPase (turnover measured by V_{max}) appear relatively resistant to fatigue. After a prolonged swim, the myofibril Mg^{2+} ATPase of fast and slow rat hindlimb muscles was unaltered (Table 11–2). The V_{max} of the slow soleus muscle showed no significant change despite a 26% decline in peak tension. The fast-twitch extensor digitorum longus did undergo a significant 34% decline in V_{max}, but this muscle exhibited extreme fatigue, with a decrease in the Po of more than 70% (Table 11–2).[14] The fatigued (inactive) fibers might have provided a significant in-

Table 11–2. Effect of Endurance Swim to Exhaustion of Myofibril ATPase, V_{max}, and Po

Muscle	Myofibril ATPase (μmol/mg/min)	V_{max} (Fiber Lengths/Sec)	Po (g/cm²)
Slow Soleus			
Control	0.128 ± 0.008*	2.9 ± 0.2	2482 ± 208
Fatigued	0.104 ± 0.011	2.7 ± 0.2	1844 ± 203†
Fast Extensor Digitorum Longus			
Control	0.204 ± 0.031	7.6 ± 0.8	2397 ± 171
Fatigued	0.309 ± 0.030	5.2 ± 0.7†	633 ± 190†
Fast SVL			
Control	0.301 ± 0.021	9.5 ± 1.2	1757 ± 88
Fatigued	0.343 ± 0.021	9.8 ± 0.8	1713 ± 86

* Values represent means ± SE.
† Significantly different (< 0.05).

ternal drag during the unloaded and lightly loaded contractions. These results imply that the activity of the myofibril ATPase and its functional correlate V_{max} are relatively resistant to alteration during prolonged exercise.

In the same study, we evaluated the functional capacity of isolated SR membranes.[14] The SR is an intracellular membrane system primarily involved in the regulation of intracellular Ca^{2+}. Alteration in the force transient of contraction (a reflection of an altered Ca^{2+} transient) is a common observation with fatigue, and thus the SR may be involved in the etiology of muscular fatigue. Our results showed that the prolonged swim had no effect on the amount of SR isolated (mg/g time) from any of the fast muscles, but a significant decrease in SR protein isolated from the slow soleus did result (0.81 ± 0.05 versus 0.57 ± 0.05, mg/g, control versus fatigued). This decrease is unexplained, but it could reflect an elevated proteolytic enzyme activity shown to exist in fatigued muscle.[2] None of the muscles studied exhibited any change in the SR Ca^{2+}-stimulated ATPase activity. The uptake of Ca^{2+} by the SR vesicles (μmol mg SR), however, was depressed in the slow-soleus and fast-twitch red region of the vastus lateralis. A decreased degree of Ca^{2+} uptake with no change in the SR ATPase activity suggests either an uncoupling of the transport or a "leaky" membrane allowing Ca^{2+} flux back into the intracellular fluid. Although our results clearly show a major change in the SR, more experiments designed for studying the effects of prolonged activity on the kinetic properties of Ca^{2+} uptake and release during excitation are required before the exact nature of this change and its effect on muscle function can be elucidated.

The prolonged swim produced a significant decrease in glycogen concentration in muscles representative of the slow type I, fast type IIa, and fast type IIb fiber. Interestingly, the type IIb muscle showed no fatigue as reflected by an unaltered Po value. Furthermore, despite significant glycogen depletion, the fast type IIb muscle showed no change in any of the contractile or biochemical properties measured.[14] The apparent explanation is that the type IIb (fast white glycolytic) fiber was recruited less frequently during the endurance activity and that the heavy reliance of this fiber on glycolysis produced levels of muscle glycogen usage similar to those of other fiber types despite fewer total contractions. It is apparent from these results that muscle fatigue during endurance activity is related in some way to the degree of muscle usage, and is not entirely dependent on the extent of glycogen depletion. An important unanswered question is whether glycogen depletion somehow mediates (and hence is a prerequisite for) the disruption of intracellular organelles such as the SR.

The observed disruption in protein systems, such as the SR, coupled with an increased concentration of intracellular metabolites, is expected to increase the intracellular solute concentration and quantity of tissue water. An elevated level of tissue water produces swelling and thus could lead to muscle soreness. This possibility is supported by results of structural studies in which muscle soreness was related to changes in various intracellular organelles. The time course of recovery from muscle soreness (days) exceeds that observed with fatigue (minutes), and reflects the time required to synthesize new muscle protein.

The studies and findings described in this chapter illustrate the complex nature of muscle fatigue. After short duration, high-intensity exercise, recovery in force production usually shows two components that are probably caused by separate mechanisms: (1) a rapidly reversible non-H^+ ion-mediated perturbation likely related to changes in E-C coupling, and (2) a slower change that is likely mediated by the H^+ and P_i ions. The potential mechanisms of the deleterious effects of the H^+ and P_i are described.

In prolonged endurance exercise, the depletion of body carbohydrate stores frequently occurs, and muscle glycogen depletion is probably an important fatigue agent. Undoubtedly, other factors are involved, however, because muscle glycogen depletion can exist without fatigue. Muscle organelles, particularly the SR, are probably also involved in the fatigue process.

REFERENCES

1. Edwards RHT: Human muscle function and fatigue. In *Human Muscle Fatigue: Physi-*

ological Mechanisms. Edited by R Porter and J Whelan. London: Pitman Medical, 1981.

2. Fitts RH, Kim DH, Witzmann FA: The development of fatigue during high intensity and endurance exercise. In *Exercise in Health and Disease.* Edited by FJ Nagel and JH Montoye. Springfield: Charles C Thomas, 1981.

3. Sjøgaard G: Role of exercise-induced potassium fluxes underlying muscle fatigue: a brief review. *Can J Physiol Pharmacol, 69:* 238, 1990.

4. Lindinger MI, Sjøgaard G: Potassium regulation during exercise and recovery. *Sports Med, 11:*382, 1991.

5. Westerblad H, Lee JA, Lannergren J, Allen DG: Cellular mechanisms of fatigue in skeletal muscle. *Am J Physiol, 261 (Cell Physiol, 30):*C195, 1991.

6. Bigland-Ritchie B, Jones DA, Woods JJ: Excitation frequency and muscle fatigue: electrical responses during human voluntary and stimulated contractions. *Exp Neurol, 64:*414, 1979.

7. Hanson J, Persson A: Changes in the action potential and contraction of isolated frog muscle after repetitive stimulation. *Acta Physiol Scand, 81:*340, 1971.

8. Juel C: Potassium and sodium shifts during *in vitro* isometric muscle contraction, and the time course of the ion-gradient recovery. *Pflügers Arch, 406:*458, 1986.

9. Lännergren J, Westerblad H: Force and membrane potential during and after fatiguing, continuous high-frequency stimulation of single *Xenopus* muscle fibres. *Acta Physiol Scand, 128:*359, 1986.

10. Metzger JM, Fitts RH: Fatigue from high- and low-frequency muscle stimulation: role of sarcolemma action potentials. *Exp Neurol, 93:*320, 1986.

11. Westerblad H, Lee JA, Lamb AG, et al.: Spatial gradients of intracellular calcium in skeletal muscle during fatigue. *Pflügers Arch, 415:*734, 1990.

12. Rios E, Ma J, González A: The mechanical hypothesis of excitation-contraction (EC) coupling in skeletal muscle. *J Mus Res Cell Mot, 12:*127, 1991.

13. Vander AJ, Sherman JH, Luciano DS: Muscle (Ch. 10). In *Human Physiology: The Mechanisms of Body Function.* 3rd Ed. New York: McGraw-Hill, 1980.

14. Fitts RH, Courtright JB, Kim DH, Witzmann FA: Muscle fatigue with prolonged exercise: Contractile and biochemical alterations. *Am J Physiol, 242:*C65, 1982.

15. Allen DG, Lee JA, Westerblad H: Intracellular calcium and tension in isolated single muscle fibers from Xenopus. *J Physiol, 415:* 433, 1989.

16. Blinks JR, Rüdel R, Taylor SR: Calcium transients in isolated amphibian skeletal muscle fibers: detection with aequorin. *J Physiol, 277:*291, 1978.

17. Westerblad H, Allen DG: Changes of myoplasmic calcium concentration during fatigue in single mouse muscle fibers. *J Gen Physiol, 98:*615, 1991.

18. Ma J, Fill M, Knudson CM, Campbell KP, Coronado R: Ryanodine receptor of skeletal muscle is a gap junction-type channel. *Science, 242:*99, 1988.

19. Simonson E: Accumulation of metabolites. In *Physiology of Work Capacity and Fatigue.* Edited by E Simonson. Springfield: Charles C Thomas, 1971.

20. Bergstrom J: Muscle electrolytes in man. *Scand J Clin Lab Invest, 68:*1962.

21. Karlsson J, Saltin B: Lactate, ATP, and CP in working muscles during exhaustive exercise in man. *J Appl Physiol, 29:*598, 1970.

22. Fitts RH, Holloszy JO: Effects of fatigue and recovery on contractile properties of frog muscle. *J Appl Physiol, 45:*899, 1978.

23. Fitts RH, Holloszy JO: Lactate and contractile force in frog muscle during development of fatigue and recovery. *Am J Physiol, 231:*430, 1976.

24. Sahlin K, Edström L, Sjöholm H: Force, relaxation and energy metabolism of rat soleus muscle during anaerobic contraction. *Acta Physiol Scand, 129:*1, 1987.

25. Savabi F, Geiger FJ, Bessman SP: Myofibrillar end of the creatine phosphate energy shuttle. *Am J Physiol, 247:*424, 1984.

26. Bergström M, Hultman E: Energy cost and fatigue during intermittent electrical stimulation of human skeletal muscle. *J Appl Physiol, 65:*1500, 1988.

27. Thompson LV, Fitts RH: Muscle fatigue in the frog semitendinosus: the relationship of the high energy phosphates and inorganic phosphate. *Am J Physiol (Cell Physiol), 263:* C803, 1992.

28. Metzger JM, Moss RL: Greater hydrogen ion-induced depression of tension and velocity in skinned single fibres of rat fast rather than slow muscles. *J Physiol, 393:*727, 1987.

29. Nosek TM, Fender KY, Godt RE: It is diprotonated inorganic phosphate that depresses force in skinned skeletal muscle fibers. *Science, 236:*191, 1987.

30. Cooke R, Franko K, Luciana GB, Pate E: The inhibition of rabbit skeletal muscle contraction by hydrogen ions and phosphate. *J Physiol, 395:*77, 1988.

31. Godt RE, Nosek TM: Changes of intracellular milieu with fatigue or hypoxia depress contraction of skinned rabbit skeletal and cardiac muscle. *J Physiol, 412:*155, 1989.

32. Danforth WH: Activation of glycolytic pathway in muscle. In *Control of Energy Metabolites*. Edited by B Chance et al. New York: Academic Press, 1965.

33. Fuchs F, Reddy Y, Briggs FN: The interaction of cations with the calcium-binding site of troponin. *Biochim Biophys Acta, 221:*407, 1970.

34. Nakamura Y, Schwartz A: The influence of hydrogen ion concentration on calcium binding and release by skeletal muscle sarcoplasmic reticulum. *J Gen Physiol, 59:*22, 1972.

35. Fletcher WW, Hopkins FG: Lactic acid in mammalian muscle. *J Physiol, 35:*247, 1907.

36. Hill AV: The absolute value of the isometric heat coefficient T1/H in a muscle twitch, and the effect of stimulation and fatigue. *Proc R Soc Lond (Biol), 103:*163, 1928.

37. Hermansen L, Osnes J: Blood and muscle pH after maximal exercise in man. *J Appl Physiol, 32:*302, 1972.

38. Sahlin K, Harris RC, Nylind B, Hultman E: Lactate content and pH in muscle samples obtained after dynamic exercise. *Pflügers Arch, 367:*143, 1976.

39. Metzger JM, Fitts RH: Role of intracellular pH in muscle fatigue. *J Appl Physiol, 62:*1392, 1987.

40. Roos A, Boron WF: Intracellular pH transients in rat diaphragm and muscle measured with DMO. *Am J Physiol, 235:*C49, 1978.

41. Miller RG, Giannini D, Milner-Brown HS, et al.: Effects of fatiguing exercise on high energy phosphates, force, and EMG: Evidence for three phases of recovery. *Muscle and Nerve, 10:*810, 1987.

42. Wilson JR, McCully KK, Mancini DM, et al.: Relationship of muscular fatigue to pH and diprotonated P_i in humans: a ^{31}P-NMR study. *J Appl Physiol, 64:*2333, 1988.

43. Fabiato A, Fabiato F: Effects of pH on the myofilaments and the sarcoplasmic reticulum of skinned cells from cardiac and skeletal muscles. *J Physiol, 276:*233, 1978.

44. Donaldson SKB, Hermansen L: Differential, direct effects of H^+ on Ca^{2+}-activated force of skinned fibers from the soleus, cardiac and adductor magnus muscles of rabbits. *Pflügers Arch, 376:*55, 1978.

45. Metzger JM, Moss RL: Effect on tension and stiffness due to reduced pH in mammalian fast- and slow-twitch skinned skeletal muscle fibres. *J Physiol, 428:*737, 1990.

46. Metzger JM, Moss RL: pH modulation of the kinetics of a Ca^{2+}-sensitive crossbridge state transition in mammalian single skeletal muscle fibres. *J Physiol, 428:*751, 1990.

47. Edman KAP, Mattiazzi AR: Effects of fatigue and altered pH on isometric force and velocity of shortening at zero load in frog muscle fibers. *J Muscle Res Cell Motil, 2:*321, 1981.

48. Wilkie, DR: Muscular fatigue: effects of hydrogen ions and inorganic phosphate. *Fed. Proc. 45:*2921, 1986.

49. Saltin B, Karlsson J: Muscle glycogen utilization during work of different intensities. In *Muscle Metabolism During Exercise. Advances in Experimental Medicine and Biology, Vol. 11.* Edited by B Pernow and B Saltin. New York-London: Plenum Press, 1971.

Chapter 12

BED REST, DETRAINING, AND RETENTION OF TRAINING-INDUCED ADAPTATIONS

Susan A. Bloomfield and Edward F. Coyle

Physical training exposes the various systems of the body to potent physiologic stimuli. These stimuli induce specific adaptations that enhance an individual's tolerance for the type of exercise encountered in training. The level of adaptation and the magnitude of improvement in exercise tolerance are proportional to the potency of the physical training stimuli. Reduction of physical activity, on the other hand, also has physiologic consequences. The purpose of this chapter is to present the results of reducing physical activity through reduced levels of activity (detraining) and restricted activity (bed rest).

CONSEQUENCES OF BED REST

Enforced bed rest produces significant decrements in muscle mass, strength and cardiovascular function. Clinicians and exercise specialists working with any individual subjected to prolonged bed rest must be aware of the multiple deleterious effects of inactivity because decrements in strength and endurance may easily predispose the individual to injury if a full return to pre-bed rest activities is attempted too quickly.

To determine the effects of restricted activity alone (separate from whatever pathology may have necessitated a period of best rest or immobilization), most researchers have studied healthy young male volunteers subjected to prolonged bed rest or casting of limbs after extensive baseline testing. Valuable information has also been obtained from studies of clinical populations who represent the extreme of immobilization on a spectrum of disuse, e.g., spinal cord-injured patients with complete paralysis. Data from the latter group must be interpreted with caution, however, because coexisting pathologic sequelae may disallow exact comparisons with healthy individuals subjected to bed rest. Additional information has been obtained from the study of healthy individuals exposed to prolonged weightlessness.

This brief discussion focuses on available data from studies on the effect of immobilization on adult humans. The effects of disuse or inactivity in children or immature animals are not always equivalent to those in adults, particularly with reference to effects on normal bone growth and development, and are not considered here. "Immobilization" is used in a general sense to refer to the lack of weight bearing and reduced muscle contraction inherent in strict bed rest, casting of a limb(s), and exposure to weightlessness. It should be clearly noted that, in these conditions, muscle is still free to contract, at least isometrically, as opposed to the more complete immobilization of paralysis.

CARDIOVASCULAR CHANGES WITH BED REST

Cardiovascular changes occurring with bed rest are summarized in Table 12–1. The loss of cardiovascular function after bed rest results more from fluid shifts induced by a reclining posture than from inactivity. In addition to orthostatic intolerance, large reductions in maximal O_2 uptake and stroke volume result from bed rest.[1-3] Most investigators have reported decrements in $\dot{V}_{O_{2}max}$ of 17 to 28% following bed rest. The relative percentage change in $\dot{V}_{O_{2}max}$ may be related to the duration of confinement. A prediction from the body of data available suggests a rate change in $\dot{V}_{O_{2}max}$ of approximately 0.8% per day of bed rest.[4] However, longitudinal studies show that the rates of change may be more related to fluid/volume changes which occur within the first hours to days of confinement, than the actual duration

Table 12–1. Cardiovascular Changes with Bed Rest*

Plasma volume loss of 15–20%

Total blood volume loss of 5–10%

Decrease in heart volume of 11% after 20 days of bed rest

Decrease in left ventricular end diastolic volume of 6–11%

No change or an increase in basal heart rate

No change or decrease in supine cardiac output and stroke volume

Reduced orthostatic tolerance during standing, tilt, or lower body negative pressure

Reduced exercise tolerance; decreased $\dot{V}O_{2max}$

* With permission from Sandler H, et al.: Cardiovascular effects of inactivity. In *Inactivity: Physiological Effects.* Edited by H. Sandler and J Vernikos. Orlando: Academic Press, 1986.

of bed rest. The magnitude of decrease in $\dot{V}O_{2max}$ is also related to the pre-bed rest level of aerobic fitness. The decrements in $\dot{V}O_{2max}$ are associated with reductions in blood volume, stroke volume, cardiac output, skeletal muscle tone and strength, and aerobic enzyme capacities.

Several methods can be used as an attempt to counteract the deterioration of cardiovascular function. Blood volume expansion significantly improves cardiovascular status, but does not return normal function. Treatment designed to induce venous pooling (i.e., lower body negative pressure and reverse gradient garments) during bed rest to simulate conditions experienced in the upright position significantly reduce the deterioration in cardiovascular dysfunction.[1,5] Exercise in the supine position during bed rest, involving either dynamic or isometric contractions, tends to reduce cardiovascular deterioration, but is not capable of preventing dysfunction.[1,6] The effects of two types of exercise intervention during bed rest (isokinetic and isotonic) on $\dot{V}O_{2max}$ are shown in Figure 12–1.[7] This study showed that dynamic exercise can prevent deterioration of both muscle strength deterioration and dynamic exercise tolerance, and isokinetic training is best used to prevent deterioration of muscle strength, with minimal effect on dynamic exercise tolerance.[7]

MUSCLE AND BONE LOSS WITH IMMOBILIZATION

The magnitude of loss of muscle mass and strength, as well as the decrement in bone mineral density (BMD), is roughly proportional to the duration of the immobilization period. A summary of these changes is found in Figure 12–2. Cosmonauts returning from relatively brief mis-

Changes in $\dot{V}O_2$ during Control and Bed Rest Conditions

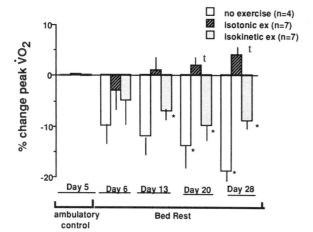

Fig. 12–1. Evidence that twice-daily, short-term, variable intensity isotonic leg exercise maintains peak $\dot{V}O_2$ during 30 days of bed rest while intermittent high-intensity isokinetic leg exercise reduces the decrement in peak $\dot{V}O_2$ but does not prevent it. Data with permission from Greenleaf JW, et al.: Work capacity during 30 days of bed rest with isotonic and isokinetic exercise training. *J Appl Physiol*, 67:1820–1826, 1989.

* p<.05 compared to control day zero

t p<.05 from no exercise group

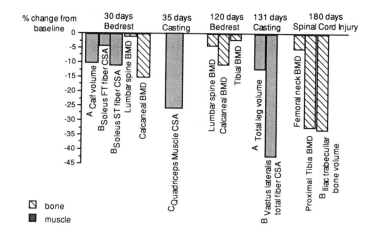

Fig. 12–2. Changes in lower limb volumes, fiber cross-sectional areas (CSA), muscle CSA and bone mineral density (BMD) at selected sites with various forms and durations of immobilization. Data taken from various cited references. FT = fast twitch; ST = slow twitch; [A] = anthropometric data; [B] = biopsy data; [C] = computed tomography data.

sions exhibited decrements in neuromuscular function leading to unstable gaits,[8] whereas those returning from flights of 185 to 237 days experienced such muscle weakness upon return to normal gravity that they had to be carried away from their return vehicles.[9] It is likely that the rate of loss of muscle mass and strength, as well as that for BMD, is at first rapid and then slows until a new steady-state is reached. For example, the rapid loss of cancellous bone mass during acute recovery from spinal cord injury plateaus after 6 months at 67% of pre-injury levels.[10]

The time course of changes in muscle is different from that observed in bone, no doubt because of the much slower turnover of bone tissue (3 to 4 months) versus that of muscle. One month of bed rest in healthy men resulted in a 10 to 20% decrease in muscle fiber cross-sectional area and a 21% decrease in peak isokinetic torque of knee extensors.[11] By contrast, decreases in BMD over a similar period of bed rest in healthy men ranged from 0.3 to 3.0% for the lumbar spine[12] and averaged 1.5% at the calcaneus.[13] These differences also reflect the causative role of muscle disuse atrophy in the bone loss of immobilization. The loss of normal mechanical strain patterns produced at origin and insertion sites during muscle contraction, particularly when weight bearing is removed, inevitably produces site-specific changes in bone morphology.

The muscle groups and bony sites most affected by prolonged immobilization are the antigravity postural muscles of the lower extremities and back and the corresponding limb and spinal bone. During prolonged weightlessness, greater loss of muscle strength has been observed in knee extensors than in elbow extensors; at both joints, extensors were significantly more affected than flexors.[8] The largest decrements in BMD following space flight or prolonged bed rest have consistently been in the calcaneus, with minimal to no change noted in the radius; significant losses of BMD also have been noted in the lumbar spine.[14]

CHANGES IN MUSCLE MORPHOLOGY AND FUNCTION WITH IMMOBILIZATION

Muscle Disuse Atrophy

The loss of muscle mass after a period of casting is a familiar observation. Indeed, the most comprehensive data on immobilization effects on muscle derive from experimental studies in which one or more limbs have been truly immobilized by a plaster cast for a period of 2 or more weeks. The first comprehensive "bed rest" studies actually involved casting of both legs up to waist level.[15,16]

Although isometric contraction of casted muscle is still feasible, the muscle atrophy noted after a period of casting is usually much more marked than that seen with simple bed rest or after prolonged weightlessness. With casting immobilization, the loss of limb volume frequently underestimates the degree of fiber shrinkage. Sargeant et al.,[17] for example, observed a

12% decrease in leg volume after 131 days of casting and a simultaneous 42% decrease in total fiber cross-sectional area.

By contrast, some portion of the decrease in leg volume seen after exposure to weightlessness or to bed rest is caused by the headward fluid shift that occurs within hours of take-off or the assumption of head-down tilt during ground-based bed rest studies; loss of muscle may therefore be over-estimated by anthropometric measurements. Decreases of 7 to 11% in leg volume have been noted after 28 to 84 days of weightlessness;[9] thigh cross-sectional area similarly decreased 8% after 30 days of head-down bed rest.[11] Computed tomography studies of erector spinae muscle volume[18] have documented a 5.5% decrease in the volume of erector spinae muscles in Soviet cosmonauts following missions of 150 to 180 days in duration.

That true muscle fiber shrinkage does occur with immobilization has been verified by muscle biopsy data from head-down tilt bed rest studies of 30 days duration; decreases in fiber cross-sectional area of the vastus lateralis have been documented for slow (Type I) (11% decrease) and fast (Type II) (18% decrease) fibers. In addition, histologic examination of these biopsies revealed necrotic changes in affected fibers, with evidence of cellular edema, disorganized myofibrils, and extracellular mitochondria.[19] Elevations in calcium-activated proteases, which preferentially affect myofibrillar proteins, may provide a mechanism for these ultrastructural changes.[20]

Capillary density (capillaries per muscle fiber) decreases significantly in the soleus (−38%) but not in the vastus lateralis after 30 days of bed rest in normal healthy men.[19] It may be that only very low levels of physical activity are required to maintain an elevated capillary density, as 84 days of detraining in highly conditioned athletes do not produce any decreases in capillary density.[21]

Changes in Muscle Strength and Neuromuscular Function

The most dramatic decrements in muscular strength are noted with casting of a limb. Casting of the leg for 27 to 43 days after knee surgery produces 40 to 80% decrements in quadriceps isometric strength; EMG measurements indicate a reduction in the number of motor units recruited at a given relative effort. After one week of remobilization, when half of the initial loss of muscle strength has been regained, EMG activity is back to normal (as measured in the contralateral leg).[22] This transient decrease in the ability to recruit motor units during voluntary contraction has been verified with EMG measures of decreased reflex potentiation following 35 days of casting immobilization of the thenar (thumb abductor) muscle.[23] These data argue for a neural component responsible for some portion of the strength decrements noted with disuse.

Ground-based bed rest studies confirm that the loss of muscle strength and impaired neuromuscular function noted after exposure to weightlessness affects the lower limbs more than the arms, and the postural, antigravity extensors more than the flexor muscle groups. With 30 days of 6° head-down tilt bed rest, which mimics the headward fluid shifts of weightlessness, Dudley et al.[11] documented a nonsignificant 6% decrease in peak torque output by knee flexors as opposed to a significant 19% decrease in knee extensor peak torque output. A 15% decrement in back extensor muscle strength was noted in Soviet cosmonauts after brief 2- to 5-day space flights; muscle tone was also reduced significantly in the tibialis anterior and quadriceps but not in the biceps brachii.[8] After an 18-day mission, significant postural instability and gait changes were noted in cosmonauts for up to 10 days on return to normal gravity.[8] A major concern for those returning to normal gravity after space flight or to normal activities in the upright position following bed rest, given these decrements in muscular strength and neuromuscular function, may be the increased risk for injury, particularly of the lower back.

Metabolic Alterations in Muscle

Oxidative metabolism of skeletal muscle is compromised with chronic inactivity. Significant declines in beta-hydroxyacyl-CoA dehydrogenase and citrate synthase are noted in the soleus and vastus lateralis following 30 days of bed rest; however, no changes are noted in glycolytic enzyme activities.[19] The more rigid immobilization of casting produces decreases in creatine phosphate and glycogen concentrations in skeletal muscle.[24] These biochemical adaptations clearly contribute to the increased fatigability of immobilized muscle.

Another often-overlooked metabolic consequence of prolonged bed rest in skeletal muscle is a rapid change in insulin receptor sensitivity. Glucose intolerance, with a marked hyperinsulinemic response to an oral glucose load, can be demonstrated after only 3 days of bed rest.[25] This alteration in glucose metabolism with even brief periods of bed rest has serious implications, particularly for adults at increased risk for development of adult-onset diabetes mellitus.

ALTERATIONS OF CALCIUM METABOLISM AND BONE MINERAL DENSITY WITH IMMOBILIZATION

Disuse atrophy of skeletal muscle contributes heavily to the loss of bone mass, or disuse osteopenia, noted after prolonged bed rest or exposure to zero gravity. Far less, however, is known about the cellular mechanisms contributing to the effects of immobilization on bone, partly because of its relative inaccessibility to sampling. Changes in bone mass are not reflected by alterations in external dimensions, but in a loss of bone mineral content and later a thinning of both cancellous and cortical bone detectable only by histomorphometric analysis of bone biopsies. Accurate methods for noninvasive measurement of bone mineral density (BMD) (e.g., computed tomography, x-ray absorptiometry) have only recently become available.

Changes in Calcium Balance With Immobilization

The maintenance of normal bone mass requires a balance between resorption of existing bone and formation of new bone. Prolonged bed rest or weightlessness appears to disrupt this balance, with either an absolute or relative increase in resorption as compared to formation.[26] The most obvious consequence of this increased bone resorption, with the attendant loss of bone calcium, is the negative calcium balance

that develops early during bed rest in healthy individuals and persists as long as 36 weeks.[27] There may also be decreased intestinal calcium absorption.[28] Elevations in urinary hydroxyproline (which derives in part from the collagenous organic matrix of bone) are routinely observed concurrent with hypercalciuria in immobilized subjects.[26]

Endocrine changes do not account for this loss of bone mineral with immobilization. Both parathyroid hormone and 1,25-dihydroxyvitamin D (the primary endocrine factors regulating bone metabolism) are typically suppressed in hypercalciuric spinal cord-injured patients;[29] no significant changes were noted in either hormone in astronauts flying the 8-day SpaceLab 2 mission.[30]

Decreases in Bone Mineral Density

Strict bed rest in scoliosis patients produces a mean BMD loss in the lumbar spine of 0.9% per week, as measured by photon absorptiometry.[31] However, normal healthy individuals experience much slower bone loss while on bed rest, at least in the spine. LeBlanc et al.[14] documented a total loss of 3.9% of lumbar spine BMD after 119 days of bed rest in adult men.

The bony sites most susceptible to decreases in BMD with immobilization are those in the normally weight-bearing lower limb. Dramatic losses with bed rest have consistently been documented in the calcaneus, ranging from −10.4%[14] to −49.5%[27] after 17 to 18 weeks in healthy male volunteers, and in the proximal tibia in monkeys immobilized in full-body casts (−27% over 180 days).[32] Increased porosity of cortical (compact) bone appears to develop much more slowly than does loss of cancellous (spongy) bone, consistent with the slower turnover of cortical bone. Cortical bone loss eventually, however, accounts for the major component of increased fragility of immobilized bone.[10]

Bone Biopsy Data

Histomorphometric measures on iliac crest biopsies taken from healthy men after 120 days of strict bed rest reveal no change in osteoblastic (bone-forming) activity, a decrease in mineralization rate, and an increase in bone resorption (osteoclastic) activity.[33] These changes in bone cell activities with bed rest do not result, however, in any decrease in cancellous bone volume (CBV), in contrast to the 33% decrement in CBV noted in the first 6 months after spinal cord injury.[10] Postmortem analysis of bone tissue from cosmonauts killed by accidental decompression of the Salyut-1 space station revealed increased resorption activity after 24 days of space flight similar to that observed during bed rest studies.[34] The primary effect, therefore, of immobilization on bone cell activity appears to be a disruption of the normal balance between bone formation and bone resorption. Whether this effect will produce bone volume loss of significant proportions in healthy individuals on bed rest or during space flight is as yet unknown.

REVERSIBILITY AND FUNCTIONAL CONSEQUENCES OF MUSCLE AND BONE LOSS WITH IMMOBILIZATION

Whether these decrements in musculoskeletal function with immobilization can be reversed is an issue of serious concern. Available evidence indicates fairly rapid reversal (within days to weeks) of muscle atrophy and loss of strength, particularly with aggressive rehabilitative exercise.[35] However, the time course of recovery of strength and mass is not yet documented; it is also unknown if the ultrastructural changes noted in muscle with bed rest deconditioning are completely reversed with remobilization.

The negative calcium balance observed during bed rest reverses within days of remobilization.[27] By contrast, reversal of decrements of bone mineral density appears to require weeks to months and may require 5 to 10 times longer than the period of immobilization.[36] Preliminary evidence suggests that bone loss in Skylab astronauts was not fully reversed 5 years later.[37] Many investigators believe that the potential for recovery is lost once disuse osteopenia is well established, after 3 to 6 months of immobilization.[28] Site-specific increases in bone mineral density in chronic spinal cord-injured patients can be produced, however, by electrical stimulation-induced muscle contraction of the paralyzed legs.[38]

Prevention of these decrements in muscle and bone during the period of immobilization or weightlessness is the focus of much current research activity. Vigorous exercise regimens of either isotonic or isokinetic nature appear to be effective in reducing losses of muscle strength with bed rest.[7,25] However, no effective exercise treatment has yet been defined to prevent losses of bone mineral during prolonged immobilization and is a clear research priority. In addition, there is a paucity of data on immobilization changes in muscle and bone, and the effectiveness of various countermeasures, in women and in elderly individuals.

Clinicians and exercise specialists working with any individual subjected to prolonged bed rest must be aware of the multiple deleterious effects of inactivity itself. Decreases in muscle strength and endurance may easily predispose the individual to injury if a full return to pre-bed rest activities is attempted too quickly. Special attention should be paid to strengthening the postural antigravity muscles of the lower limb and back. If the period of immobilization has been prolonged, significant decreases in bone mineral density increase the risk of fracture, particularly in the lower limb. Future research should help clarify the most effective countermeasures during bed rest, as well as the best rehabilitative approaches to achieve full recovery of function following immobilization.

REVERSIBILITY OF ADAPTATIONS INDUCED BY TRAINING

Inherent to the observations of training stimuli physiologic adaptation to training is the concept of the reversibility of the adaptations induced by training. The "reversibility concept" holds that when physical training is stopped (i.e., detraining) or reduced, the bodily systems readjust in accordance with the diminished physiologic stimuli. The focus of this chapter is on the time course of loss of the adaptations to endurance training as well as on the possibility that certain adaptations persist, to some extent, when training is stopped. Because endurance exercise training generally improves cardiovascular function and promotes metabolic adaptations within the exercising skeletal musculature, the reversibility of these specific adaptations is considered. Another approach to the study of the effects of reduced activity is to examine the exercise responses of people before and after prolonged bed rest. The idea that postural fluid shifts rather than inactivity account for the loss of cardiovascular function after bed rest is discussed.

CARDIOVASCULAR DETRAINING

Maximal Oxygen Uptake

Endurance training induces increases in maximal oxygen uptake (i.e., $\dot{V}O_{2max}$), cardiac output, and stroke volume.[39,40] When sedentary men participate in a 7-week, low-intensity training program (20 min/day; 3 days/week), $\dot{V}O_{2max}$ levels increase by 6%, with a return of $\dot{V}O_{2max}$ values to pretraining levels with 8 weeks of detraining.[41] Moderate endurance training increases $\dot{V}O_{2max}$ by 10 to 20%, yet again $\dot{V}O_{2max}$ may decline to pretraining levels when training is stopped.[42-44] Values of $\dot{V}O_{2max}$ decline rapidly during the first month of inactivity, whereas a slower decline to untrained levels occurs during the second and third months of detraining.[42-44] Therefore, the available evidence suggests that the increases in $\dot{V}O_{2max}$ produced by endurance training involving exercise of low to moderate intensities and durations are totally reversed after several months of detraining.

Investigators have not yet examined and then exposed untrained individuals to several years of intense endurance training and subsequent inactivity to determine if extreme training results in a persistent elevation of $\dot{V}O_{2max}$ above untrained levels. Our present knowledge is limited to findings of studies involving already trained endurance athletes who agreed to cease training so that reversibility of their physiologic adaptations could be studied periodically.[21] Figure 12–3 is a display of the time course of the decline in $\dot{V}O_{2max}$ (and its components of maximal stroke volume, cardiac output, and arteriovenous O_2 difference) when people become sedentary after training intensely for approximately 10 years.

The $\dot{V}O_{2max}$ value was relatively high in trained subjects (i.e., 62 ml/min^{-1} at 0 days

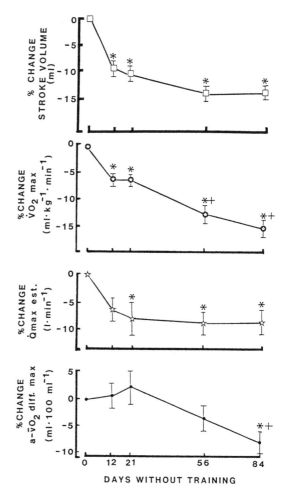

Fig. 12–3. Effects of detraining on percent changes in stroke volume during exercise, maximal O_2 uptake ($\dot{V}O_{2max}$), maximal cardiac output ($\dot{Q}_{max\ est}$), and maximal arteriovenous O_2 difference (a-$\bar{v}$ $O_{2diff.\ max}$). *, significantly lower than trained (day 0). +, significantly lower than 21 days. (Modified from Coyle EF, et al.: Time course of loss of adaptations after stopping prolonged intense endurance training. *J Appl Physiol*, 57: 1857–1864, 1984.)

without training) and it declined a total of 16% after 84 days of detraining. A rapid decline of 7% occurred in the first 12 to 21 days with a further decline of 9% during the period from 21 to 84 days.[21] The rapid, early decline in $\dot{V}O_{2max}$ was related to a reduction in maximal stroke volume measured during exercise in the upright position. Most of the decline in stroke volume occurred during the first 12 days of inactivity. Adaptive increases in maximal heart rate compensated somewhat for this loss of stroke volume. The decline in $\dot{V}O_{2max}$ during the 21- to 84-day period was associated with a decline in maximal arteriovenous O_2 difference.

The 84-day period of detraining resulted in a stabilization of $\dot{V}O_{2max}$ and maximal stroke volume. Thus, the subjects appeared to have detrained for a sufficient length of time to display a complete readjustment of cardiovascular response in accordance with their sedentary life-style. Note that maximal stroke volume during upright exercise in the detrained subjects was virtually the same as that observed in people who had never engaged in endurance training (Table 12–2). The idea that this finding does not necessarily imply a loss of heart function is subsequently discussed. Although maximal cardiac output and stroke volume declined to untrained levels, $\dot{V}O_{2max}$ levels in the detrained subjects remained 17% above that of untrained individuals, primarily because of an elevation of maximal arteriovenous O_2 difference. The persistent elevation of $\dot{V}O_{2max}$ values in the detrained subjects, the result of an augmented ability of the exercising musculature to extract oxygen, may be related to the observation that these subjects displayed no loss of the increased capillary density derived from the training and only a partial loss of the increase in muscle mitochondria (see *Detraining and Muscle Metabolism*).

Stroke Volume and Heart Size

Prolonged and intense endurance training is thought to promote an increase in heart mass, and researchers believe detraining results in a decline in heart mass.[39,45,46] What is not clear, however, is whether the training-induced increases in ventricular volume and myocardial wall thickness regress totally with inactivity. Athletes who become sedentary have enlarged hearts and an elevated $\dot{V}O_{2max}$ level in contrast to people who have never trained.[47]

One of the most striking effects of detraining in endurance-trained individuals is the rapid decline in stroke volume. To gain information regarding the cause of this large and rapid decline, Martin et al.[48] measured stroke volume during exercise in trained subjects in both the upright and supine positions and again after 21 and 56 days of inactivity (Fig. 12–4).

Simultaneous measurements of the diameter of the left ventricle were obtained echocardiographically. The large decline in stroke volume during upright cycling was associated with parallel reductions in the diameter of the left ventricle at end-diastole (i.e., LVEDD). When the subjects were evaluated during exercise in the supine position, a condition that usually augments ventricular filling because of the drainage of blood from the elevated legs, reduction in LVEDD was minimal. As a result, stroke volume during exercise in the supine position was maintained within a few percent of trained levels during the 56-day detraining period.

Role of Blood Volume

Along the same lines, results of recent studies indicate that the rapid reduction with detraining of stroke volume during exercise in the upright position is related to a decline in blood volume (Fig. 12–3).[49] Intense exercise training usually results in an increase in blood volume by approximately 500 mL through the expansion of

Table 12–2. Comparison of Untrained People and Detrained Subjects after 84 Days of Detraining

Population	$\dot{V}O_{2max}$ (ml·kg^{-1}·min^{-1})	SV$_{max}$ (ml)	HR$_{max}$ (beats·min^{-1})	a-$\bar{v}O_2$ Difference (ml·100 ml^{-1})
Untrained people	43.3	128	192	12.6
Detrained subjects	50.8*	129	197	14.1*
Percent difference from untrained	+17*	+1	+3	+12*

* Values for detrained subjects are significantly (p < 0.05) higher than untrained subjects. (Modified with permission from Coyle EF, et al.: Time course of loss of adaptations after stopping prolonged intense endurance training. *J Appl Physiol* 57:1857–1864, 1984.)

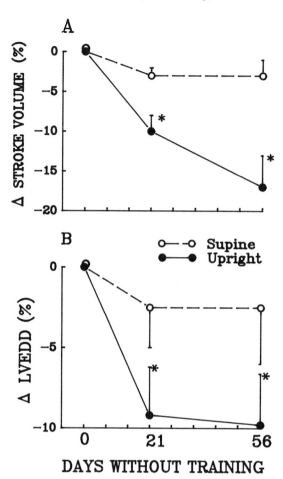

of detrained men expands to a level similar to that when the subjects were trained (Fig. 12–5).[49]

The observation that stroke volume during exercise is maintained at near trained levels when blood volume is high suggests that the ability of the heart to fill with blood is not significantly altered by detraining. If ventricular mass does indeed decline, a thinning of the ventricular walls and not a reduction in LVEDD is probably involved.[48] Thus, the reduction in intrinsic cardiovascular function is apparently mini-

Fig. 12–4. Percentage decline in exercise stroke volume (**A**) and left ventricular end diastolic diameter (LVEDD) (measured using echocardiography) (**B**) during exercise in upright and supine postures when trained and after 21 and 56 days of inactivity. *, responses in upright position are significantly (p < 0.05) lower than in supine position and lower than when trained (i.e., day 0). With permission from Martin WH, Coyle EF, Bloomfield SA, Ehsani AA: Effects of physical deconditioning after intense training on left ventricular dimensions and stroke volume. *J Am Coll Cardiol, 7*:982–989, 1986.

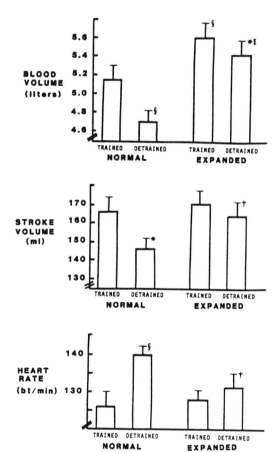

Fig. 12–5. Responses to upright exercise with normal and expanded blood volume when trained and detrained. Significantly different from trained normal (*, p < 0.05; §, p < 0.01). Detrained with expanded blood volume significantly different from detrained with normal blood volume (†, p < 0.05; ‡, p < 0.01). With permission from Coyle EF, Hemmert MK, Coggan AR: Effects of detraining on cardiovascular responses to exercise: Role of blood volume. *J Appl Physiol, 60*:95–99, 1986.

plasma volume.[50,51] This adaptation is gained after only a few bouts of exercise, and quickly reversed when training ceases.[50,51] The decline in stroke volume and the increase in heart rate during submaximal exercise, which normally accompanies several weeks of detraining, can be essentially reversed, and values return to near trained levels when the blood volume

mal after several weeks of inactivity in men who had been training intensely for several years.[49] The large reduction in stroke volume during exercise in the upright position is largely a result of reduced blood volume and not of a deterioration of heart function.[49]

DETRAINING AND MUSCLE METABOLISM

Enzymes of Energy Metabolism

Endurance exercise training induces enzymatic adaptations in the exercising musculature that result in slower rates of glycogen utilization and lactate production and improved endurance during submaximal exercise.[52] One of the more important alterations is an increase in the activity of mitochondrial enzymes, which results in an increased ability to metabolize fuels in the presence of oxygen. Moderate endurance training (2 to 4 months duration) increases

mitochondrial enzyme activity by 20 to 40% from untrained levels.[43,53] When moderate training ceases, however, and the stimuli for adaptation are removed, the increases in mitochondrial activity are quickly and totally reversed. Mitochondrial activity returns to pretraining levels within 28 to 56 days after the cessation of training.[43,53]

The pattern of change in enzyme activity observed when individuals who trained intensely for 10 years stopped training for 84 days is provided in Figure 12–6.[54] Mitochondrial enzyme activity in trained subjects (i.e., citrate synthase, succinate dehydrogenase, malate dehydrogenase, and β-hydroxyacyl-CoA dehydrogenase), which is initially twofold higher than those in untrained persons, declines progressively during the first 56 days of detraining and stabilizes at levels that are 50% higher than the values obtained from sedentary control subjects. The half-time of decline is approximately 12 days (i.e., declines one

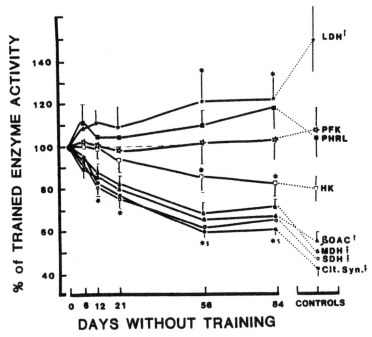

Fig. 12–6. Enzyme activity during detraining period and comparison to sedentary control subjects. Values expressed as percentage of trained values. Cit. Syn., citrate synthase. SDH, succinate dehydrogenase. MDH, malate dehydrogenase. BOAC, B–hydroxyacyl-CoA dehydrogenase. HK, hexokinase. LDH, total lactate dehydrogenase. PHRL, phosphorylase. PFK, phosphofructokinase. *, significantly different from trained ($p < 0.05$); significantly different from 21 days ($p < 0.01$); ‡, control significantly different from 84 days ($p < 0.05$); †, control significantly different from 84 days ($p < 0.001$). With permission from Coyle EF, et al.: Effects of detraining on responses to submaximal exercise. *J Appl Physiol, 59:* 853–859, 1985.

half the distance between trained and detrained in 12 days). Therefore, prolonged and intense training, in contrast to training programs that last only a few months, appears to result in only a partial loss of mitochondrial enzyme activity and thus a persistent elevation of activity above untrained levels. This elevation occurred almost entirely because of a persistent 80% elevation above untrained levels in the mitochondrial enzyme activity in fast-twitch muscle fibers.[55]

Muscle Capillarization

Endurance training promotes increased capillarization of the exercising musculature, which theoretically both prolongs the transit time of blood flow through the muscle and reduces diffusion distances, thus improving the availability of oxygen and nutrients to the muscle while also allowing better removal of metabolic waste products. Moderate endurance training of several months' duration increases muscle capillarization by 20 to 30% above pretraining levels.[43,56] Results of preliminary studies indicate that certain indices of muscle capillarization remain somewhat higher than pretraining levels 8 weeks after the cessation of moderate training.[43]

More prolonged and intense training increases muscle capillary density by 40 to 50% from untrained levels.[21,56] No indication exists that increases in muscle capillary density in highly trained people are reversed during 3 months of detraining.[21]

Muscular Adaptations That Persist With Detraining

The detraining responses in the skeletal musculature of highly trained people who regularly engaged in intense exercise for several years apparently differ from those in individuals who have trained for only a few months. No loss of the increase in muscle capillarization occurs with the cessation of prolonged intense training, although such a loss does occur when moderate training is stopped. The cessation of moderate training results in a complete reversal of the training-induced increases in mitochondrial enzyme activity, whereas only a partial decline and therefore a persistent elevation of mitochondrial activity above untrained levels occurs with the cessation of exercise after prolonged intense endurance training.[41,43,53,54]

EXERCISE RESPONSES OF DETRAINED SUBJECTS

Currently, scant evidence is available to imply that the cardiovascular or skeletal musculature adaptations derived from mild and moderate endurance training are maintained above pretraining levels with cessation of training for more than approximately 8 weeks. Therefore, a person should be stressed to the same degree during exercise of a given intensity whether untrained or after a prolonged detraining period. This hypothesis has yet to be fully evaluated, however, and one factor to consider is the possibility that people may perceive exercise to be more comfortable when they are in the detrained state having already experienced physical training, as compared to the untrained condition.

In agreement with the findings that individuals who exercised intensely on a regular basis for several years remain superior in the detrained state with respect to their muscle metabolism and intrinsic heart function (i.e., stroke volume when ventricular filling is high) compared with untrained people, it appears that these detrained people can exercise more intensely before becoming inordinately stressed. One indication of this ability is the observation that detrained persons not only possess a $\dot{V}O_{2max}$ level that is well above untrained values, but also maintain the ability to exercise at a high percentage of $\dot{V}O_{2max}$ before lactic acid begins to accumulate in the blood.[54]

SUMMARY

When physical training ceases (i.e., detraining), the bodily systems readjust in accordance with the diminished physiologic stimuli, and many training-induced adaptations are reversed to varying extents. The available evidence to date suggests that the increases in $\dot{V}O_{2max}$ produced by endurance training of low to moderate intensities and durations are totally reversed after several months of detraining. When people detrain after several years of intense training, they display large reductions (i.e., 5 to 15%) in stroke volume and $\dot{V}O_{2max}$ during the first 12 to 21 days of inactivity. These declines do not indicate a deterioration of heart function, but instead are largely a result of reduced blood volume and the ability to return venous blood to the heart. The $\dot{V}O_{2max}$ of endurance athletes continues to decline during the 21 to 56 days of detraining because of reductions in maximal arteriovenous O_2 difference. These reductions are associated with a loss of mitochondrial enzyme activity within the trained musculature, which declines with a halftime of approximately 12 days. Endurance athletes, however, do not regress to levels displayed by individuals who never participated in exercise training. Levels of mitochondrial enzyme activity remain 50% higher than those of sedentary subjects, skeletal muscle capillarization is maintained at high levels, and $\dot{V}O_{2max}$ and the maximal arteriovenous O_2 difference stabilize at a point that is 12 to 17% higher than untrained levels after 84 days of detraining. The aims of future studies should be to determine if these superior physiologic abilities of people who cease prolonged and intense training are maintained for longer than 84 days and if these abilities relate to persistent effects of physical training or to inherent genetic predispositions.

REFERENCES

1. Blomquist CG, Stone HL: Cardiovascular adjustments to gravitational stress. In *The Handbook of Physiology. The Cardiovascular System.* Edited by JT Shepherd, FM Abboud, SR Geiger. Bethesda, MD: Am Physiol Society, 1982.
2. Convertino VA, Hung J, Goldwater D, DeBusk R: Cardiovascular responses to exercise in middle-aged men after 10 days of bed rest. *Circulation, 65:*134, 1982.
3. Saltin B, et al.: Response to exercise after bed rest and after training: A longitudinal study of adaptive changes in oxygen transport and body composition. *Circulation, 7:*1, 1968.
4. Convertino VA: Exercise responses after inactivity. In *Inactivity: Physiological Effects.* Edited by H Sandler, J Vernikos. Orlando: Academic Press Inc., 1986.
5. Convertino VA, Sandler H, Weeb P, Annis JF: Induced venous pooling and the cardiorespiratory responses to exercise after bed rest. *J Appl Physiol, 52:*1343, 1982.
6. Stremel RW, Convertino VA, Bernauer

EM, Greenleaf JE: Cardiorespiratory deconditioning with static and dynamic leg exercise during bed rest. *J Appl Physiol 41:* 905–909, 1976.
7. Greenleaf JE, Bulbulian R, Bernauer EM, et al.: Exercise training protocols for astronauts in microgravity. *J Appl Physiol, 67:* 2191, 1989.
8. Convertino VA: Physiological adaptations to weightlessness: effects on exercise and work performance. *Exer Sport Science Rev, 18:*119, 1990.
9. Sandler H: Effects of inactivity on muscle. In *Inactivity: Physiological Effects.* Edited by H Sandler, J Vernikos. New York: Academic Press Inc., 1986.
10. Minaire P, Meunier P, Edouard C, et al.: Quantitative histological data on disuse osteoporosis: comparison with biological data. *Calcif Tiss Res, 17:*57, 1974.
11. Dudley GA, Duvoisin MR, Convertino VA, Buchanan P. Alterations of the *in vivo* torque-velocity relationship of human skeletal muscle following 30 days exposure to simulated microgravity. *Aviat Space Environ Med, 60:*659, 1989.
12. LeBlanc A, Schneider V, Krebs J, et al.: Spinal bone mineral after 5 weeks of bed rest. *Calcif Tissue Int, 41:*259, 1987.
13. Schneider VS, McDonald J: Skeletal calcium homeostasis and countermeasures to prevent disuse osteoporosis. *Calcif Tissue Int, 36:*S151, 1984.
14. LeBlanc AD, Schneider VS, Evans HJ, et al.: Bone mineral loss and recovery after 17 weeks of bed rest. *J Bone Min Res, 5(8):*843, 1990.
15. Cuthbertson DP: The influence of prolonged muscular rest on metabolism. *Biochem J, 23:*1328, 1929.
16. Deitrick JE, Whedon GD, Shorr E: Effects of immobilization upon various metabolic and physiologic functions of normal men. *Amer J Med, 4:*3, 1948.
17. Sargeant AJ, Davies CTM, Edwards RHT, et al.: Functional and structural changes after disuse of human muscle. *Clin Sci Molecular Med, 52:*337, 1977.
18. Cann CE, Oganov VS: Direct measurement of spinal muscle atrophy in long-term spaceflight. *Aviat Space Environ Med, 58(5):* 500, 1987.
19. Hikida RS, Gollnick PD, Dudley GA, et al.: Structural and metabolic characteristics of human skeletal muscle following 30 days of simulated microgravity. *Aviat Space Environ Med, 60:*664, 1989.
20. Riley DA, Ellis S, Slocum GR, et al.: Morphological and biochemical changes in soleus and extensor digitorum longus muscles

of rats orbited in Spacelab 3. *The Physiologist, 28(6 Suppl):*S207, 1985.

21. Coyle EF, et al.: Time course of loss of adaptations after stopping prolonged intense endurance training. *J Appl Physiol, 57:*1857, 1984.
22. Fuglsang-Frederiksen A, Scheel U: Transient decrease in number of motor units after immobilization in man. *J Neurol, 41:*924, 1978.
23. Sak DG, McComas AJ, MacDougall JD, Upton ARM: Neuromuscular adaptation in human thenar muscles following strength training and immobilization. *J Appl Physiol: Respirat Environ Exercise Physiol, 53:*419, 1982.
24. MacDougall JD, Ward GR, Sale DR, Sutton JR: Biochemical adaptation of human skeletal muscle to heavy resistance training and immobilization. *J Appl Physiol: Respirat Environ Exercise Physiol, 43:*700, 1977.
25. Greenleaf JE: Physiological consequences of reduced physical activity during bed rest. *Exerc Sport Sci Rev, 10:*84, 1982.
26. Arnaud SB, Schneider VS, Morey-Holton E: Effects of inactivity on bone and calcium metabolism. In *Inactivity: Physiological Effects.* Edited by H Sandler, J Vernikos. New York: Academic Press Inc., 1986.
27. Donaldson CL, Hulley SB, Vogel JM, et al.: Effect of prolonged bed rest on bone mineral. *Metabolism, 19(12):*1071, 1970.
28. Minaire, P: Immobilization osteoporosis: a review. *Clin Rheumatol, 8(suppl 2):* 95, 1989.
29. Stewart AF, Adler M, Byers CM, et al.: Calcium homeostasis in immobilization: an example of resorptive hypercalciuria. *N Engl J Med, 306:*1136, 1982.
30. Morey-Holton ER, Schnoes HK, DeLuca HF, et al.: Vitamin D metabolites and bioactive parathyroid hormone levels during Spacelab 2. *Aviat Space Environ Med, 59:*1038, 1988.
31. Krolner B, Toft B: Vertebral bone loss: an unheeded side effect of therapeutic bed rest. *Clin Sci, 64:*537, 1983.
32. Young DR, Niklowitz WJ, Steele CR: Tibial changes in experimental disuse osteoporosis in the monkey. *Calcif Tissue Int, 35:*304, 1983.
33. Vico L, Chappard D, Alexandre C, et al.: Effects of a 120 day period of bed-rest on bone mass and bone cell activities in man: attempts at countermeasure. *Bone Mineral, 2:*383, 1987.
34. Rambaut PC, Good AW: Skeletal changes during space flight. *Lancet, (Nov 9):*1050, 1985.
35. Herbison GJ, Talbot JM: Muscle atrophy during space flight: research needs and op-

portunities. *The Physiologist, 28(6):*520, 1985.
36. Mazess RB, Whedon GD: Immobilization and bone (editorial). *Calcif Tissue Int, 35:* 265, 1983.
37. Tilton FE, DeGioanni JJC, Schneider VS: Long-term follow-up of Skylab bone demineralization. *Aviat Space Environ Med, 51:* 1209, 1980.
38. Bloomfield SA, Mysiw WJ, Jackson RD: Change in bone mass and calcium metabolism in chronic spinal cord injury with functional electrical stimulation ergometry and calcium supplementation. *J Bone Min Res, 6(Suppl 1):*S128, 1991.
39. Blomqvist CG, Saltin B: Cardiovascular adaptations to physical training. *Annu Rev Physiol, 45:*169, 1983.
40. Rowell LB: Human cardiovascular adjustments to exercise and thermal stress. *Physiol Rev, 54:*75, 1974.
41. Orlander J, Kiessling KH, Karlsson J, Ekblom B: Low intensity training, inactivity and resumed training in sedentary men. *Acta Physiol Scand, 101:*351, 1977.
42. Fox EL, et al.: Frequency and duration of interval training programs and changes in aerobic power. *J Appl Physiol, 38:*481, 1975.
43. Klausen K, Andersen LB, Pelle I: Adaptive changes in work capacity, skeletal muscle capillarization and enzyme levels during training and detraining. *Acta Physiol Scand, 113:*9, 1981.
44. Drinkwater BL, Horvath SM: Detraining effects on young women. *Med Sci Sports Exerc, 4:*91, 1972.
45. Ehsani AA, Hagberg JM, Hickson RC: Rapid changes in left ventricular dimensions and mass in response to physical conditioning and deconditioning. *Am J Cardiol, 42:*52, 1978.
46. Hickson RC, Hammons GT, Holloszy JO: Development and regression of exercise-induced cardiac hypertrophy in rats. *Am J Physiol, 236:*H268, 1979.
47. Saltin B, Grimby GG: Physiological analysis of middle-aged and old former athletes: Comparison with still active athletes of the same ages. *Circulation, 38:*1104, 1968.
48. Martin WH, Coyle EF, Bloomfield SA, Ehsani AA: Effects of physical deconditioning after intense training on left ventricular dimensions and stroke volume. *J Am Coll Cardiol, 7:*982, 1986.
49. Coyle EF, Hemmert MK, Coggan AR: Effects of detraining on cardiovascular responses to exercise: Role of blood volume. *J Appl Physiol, 60:*95, 1986.
50. Convertino VA, et al.: Exercise training-induced hypervolemia: Role of plasma albu-

min, renin, and vasopressin. *J Appl Physiol, 48:*665, 1980.

51. Green HJ, et al.: Alterations in blood volume following short-term supramaximal exercise. *J Appl Physiol, 56:*145, 1984.

52. Holloszy JO, Coyle EF: Adaptations of skeletal muscle to endurance exercise and their metabolic consequences. *J Appl Physiol, 56:* 831, 1984.

53. Henriksson J, Reitman JS: Time course of changes in human skeletal muscle succinate dehydrogenase and cytochrome oxidase activities and maximal oxygen uptake with physical activity and inactivity. *Acta Physiol Scand, 99:*91, 1977.

54. Coyle EF, et al.: Effects of detraining on responses to submaximal exercise. *J Appl Physiol, 59:*853, 1985.

55. Chi MM-Y, et al.: Effects of detraining on enzymes of energy metabolism in individual human muscle fibers. *Am J Physiol, 244:* C276, 1983.

56. Ingjer F: Capillary supply and mitochondrial content of different skeletal muscle fiber types in untrained and endurance-trained men: A histochemical and ultrastructural study. *Eur J Appl Physiol, 40:*197, 1979.

57. Gaffney FA, et al.: Cardiovascular deconditioning produced by 20 hours of bed rest with head down tilt in middle-aged healthy men. *Am J Cardiol, 56:*634, 1985.

Chapter 13

ENVIRONMENTAL CONSIDERATIONS IN EXERCISE TESTING AND TRAINING

James A. Vogel, Paul B. Rock, Bruce H. Jones and George Havenith

When conducting exercise testing or prescribing exercise training regimens, health professionals must take into account the environment in which these activities are conducted, because hazards present in the environment may affect exercise performance or place an exercising individual at risk for injury or illness. Three prominent hazards—heat, cold, and low oxygen at high altitude—affect oxygen transport or thermoregulatory processes that are crucial to the ability to exercise. Atmospheric pollutants cause acute and chronic effects through a variety of pathophysiologic mechanisms. An understanding of the body's responses to these adverse environmental conditions provides a basis for adjusting exercise to minimize performance decrements and avoid injury in persons who may train, test, or compete in such adverse environmental conditions.

HIGH AMBIENT TEMPERATURE

Among the potential environmental hazards to exercising individuals, heat stress is the greatest concern. Heat stress is a common climatic condition that not only diminishes exercise capacity, but also poses the risk of potentially fatal consequences. Exercising in the cold can also have serious consequences if one is not aware of how the body can rapidly lose heat. Based on the physical capacities of the body and on how the body gains or loses heat, one can assess how thermally stressful the environment is and determine if exercise capacity or safety will be compromised.

Heat is a by-product of muscular activity. Even at moderate exercise intensities, uncompensated heat production is sufficient to raise the body's core temperature to lethal levels in 15 to 30 minutes. Physiologic mechanisms that dissipate heat maintain a near-constant internal temperature and prevent a lethal rise in body temperature.

Excess body heat is lost through radiation, convection, conduction from the skin surface (minor amounts) and, particularly during exercise, by production and evaporation of sweat.

Physiologic Responses to Heat Stress

Body temperature (i.e., core temperature of the deep tissues) is a result of factors that gain and lose core heat. This core or central temperature is regulated by mechanisms that occur at the surface (skin or periphery).[13]* Heat loss or gain by radiation occurs by electromagnetic heat waves. This is essentially how the sun's rays warm the earth. Usually our bodies are warmer than the environment, and radiant heat energy is lost through the air to the surrounding solid, cooler objects. When the temperature of surrounding objects in the environment exceeds skin temperature, radiant heat energy is absorbed from the surroundings. Dark-colored clothing absorbs light and adds to radiant heat gain, whereas light colors reflect heat rays.[13]

Heat exchange by conduction involves direct transfer of heat through liquid, solid, or gas. Heat loss by conduction involves transporting blood heated by the core to the shell (skin), where heat transfer occurs by warming air molecules and cooler surfaces in contact with the skin. The effectiveness of conduction depends also on convection or how rapidly the air (or water) next to the body is exchanged once it becomes warmed. If air movement is slow, air molecules next to the skin are warmed, act as insulation, and minimize further heat loss by conduction. On the other hand, if the warmer air surrounding the body is continually replaced by cooler air (on breezy days, by standing in front of

---

* 13 refers to No. 13 in Bibliography and Suggested Readings.

a fan, or while running), heat loss increases as convective currents carry away the heat.[1]

Heat loss by evaporation occurs when water is vaporized from the skin surface and respiratory passages. Heat is lost to the environment and a cooling effect occurs as sweat evaporates. In this way, the peripheral (skin) blood temperature is cooled and heat produced in the core is lost (dissipated). Sweating itself does not cool the skin; evaporation of the sweat cools the skin. "The total sweat vaporized from the skin depends on three factors: (1) the surface exposed to the environment, (2) temperature and humidity of the ambient air, and (3) convective air currents about the body. **By far, relative humidity is the most important factor that determines the effectiveness of the evaporative heat loss.**"[13] Relative humidity indicates how much moisture is in the air surrounding the body relative to how much moisture can be held by the air at that ambient temperature (e.g., at 60% relative humidity, the air is holding 60% of the air's moisture carrying capacity at that specific air temperature). When humidity increases, the ambient vapor pressure increases and reduces the ability of the body to lose heat by evaporation. Evaporation is limited by covering the skin areas where evaporation can take place and by constantly wiping sweat before it can evaporate. When evaporative cooling is combined with a large cutaneous (skin) blood flow, effective heat loss will occur.

When an individual is exercising in a thermally stressful environment, the circulatory system must try to meet two separate demands: (1) delivery of oxygen to the working muscles and (2) delivery of heated blood from the deep tissues to the periphery. Therefore, exercising in a thermally stressful environment results in a higher heart rate and lower stroke volume at a given intensity.

Metabolic heat is brought to the body surface for dissipation by increased skin blood flow. The body monitors both deep central and skin temperature through the thermoregulatory center in the hypothalamus, which, in turn, directs circulatory adjustments. During exercise, blood flow increases to the active muscle to support metabolic demands and also increases to the skin to dissipate the enhanced heat pro-

duction. The increased flow to muscle and skin is made possible by both increasing cardiac output (total blood flow) and redistributing regional blood flow, i.e., reducing flow to the visceral organs.

The body's ability to balance the competing demands for skin and muscle blood flow can be overwhelmed during exercise in high ambient temperatures and/or vapor pressures (high external heat load). High ambient temperature reduces the gradient between the skin temperature and the air temperature; reducing effective loss of heat by convection; a high ambient vapor pressure (relative humidity) reduces the vapor gradient from the skin to the environment, reducing sweat evaporation. The result of these compromised cooling mechanisms is increased heat storage in the body manifested by increasing core temperature. The body attempts to compensate by increasing the skin-to-air gradients through further enhanced skin blood flow. This peripheral shunting of blood causes a decline in central venous pressure, cardiac filling (end diastolic volume), and stroke volume. Heart rate then increases to maintain the cardiac output at a fixed exercise intensity. If the exercise and thermal load are sufficiently severe or prolonged, heart rate reaches its maximum and cardiac output is insufficient to meet the competing demands for blood flow to support both muscle metabolism and thermoregulation. The consequences are performance decrements, heat injury or both. These consequences can be avoided only by reduction of the exercise level and/or the thermal load.

Acclimatization

The ability to tolerate and exercise in the heat can be improved by repeated exposures to a hot environment. This adaptation is referred to as "heat acclimatization" (adaptation to natural climate change, i.e., seasonal or geographic) or "heat acclimation" (adaptation by deliberate controlled exposures/training). The primary physiologic mechanisms by which adaptation occurs include the following: (1) plasma volume increases, (2) sweating begins at a lower core and skin temperature, (3) sweat rates increase and can be sustained for longer periods of time, (4) sweat is more effectively distributed over the body, (5) sodium concentration in the sweat is reduced (i.e. sweat becomes more dilute), (6) cutaneous blood flow increases, and (7) cardiac output is more effectively distributed. These adaptations result in a reduced core temperature and heart rate response for a given heat exposure and exercise intensity. This process is achieved most effectively by moderate exercise during repeated heat exposures to produce elevated core and skin temperature, both of which are necessary stimuli for the acclima(tiza)tion. Moderate exercise (35 to 40% $\dot{V}o_{2max}$) in a warm to hot environment for approximately 1.5 to 2 hours a day during 8 or more consecutive days is usually sufficient. When body temperature measurements are available, the efficiency of the procedure can be increased by adjustment of the exercise intensity to produce a target core temperature of 38 to 38.5°C in the last half hour of the exercise bout. This regimen will result in a steady increase of the exercise intensity during the consecutive days as the subject's acclimation state steadily improves.

Acclimation is lost rapidly. After 2 days without heat exposure or training, a significant reduction in heat tolerance may be observed. As a general rule, one day of heat acclimation is lost during 2 to 3 days without heat exposure. Thus, after about 3 weeks, most of the beneficial effects of heat acclimation are lost.

Aerobically fit individuals can tolerate activity in heat stress better than individuals who are not aerobically conditioned. The aerobically fit individual who is acclimated is most efficient in coping with a heat load. Women and men who are aerobically trained and are exercising at similar relative work intensities can tolerate the thermal stress of exercise equally.[13] Because of differences in sweat rates and the differences in the ratio of surface area to volume, women probably rely more on circulatory mechanisms for heat dissipation, whereas men rely more on evaporative cooling.

Heat Stress Index

The environment must be evaluated in terms of its potential heat challenge. As-sessment of the hazards imposed by exercising in high-temperature environments necessitates using a heat stress index. Ambient temperature as measured by the ordinary dry-bulb thermometer (Tdb) is not an adequate index because it does not take into account the vapor pressure, which has a direct effect upon the ability to evaporate sweat. Wet-bulb temperature (Tnwb) is the temperature recorded by a thermometer with its mercury bulb surrounded by a wet wick. A sling psychgrometer measures the heat stress by exposing dry-bulb and wet-bulb thermometers to rapid air movements. If the relative humidity is high (and, therefore, evaporative cooling is compromised), the temperature of the dry and wet bulbs is similar. A large difference between the readings indicates little air moisture and a high rate of evaporation.[13] The conversion of dry-bulb and wet-bulb temperature to relative humidity can be completed using Table 13–1. One can then determine heat stress based on air temperature and relative humidity (Fig. 13–1). Table 13–1 and Figure 13–1 can be used to determine when dangerous heat stress conditions exist. The guidelines are recommendations. See Heat Stress Index in Figure 13–1 for other factors to consider when assessing heat stress for an individual.

Use of the natural wet-bulb thermometer, however, does not adequately incorporate the factor of solar radiant energy. Radiant energy can be quantified by the use of a black globe thermometer (Tg). To incorporate all these factors, the "wet-bulb globe temperature (WBGT) index" was developed to serve as a more accurate index of external heat load. WBGT is computed as: WBGT (outdoors) = (0.7 Tnwb) + (0.2 Tg) + 0.1 Tdb) or WBGT (indoors) = (0.7 Tnwb) + (0.3 Tg). See Figure 13–1 for interpretation of the WBGT.

The above indices are guidelines. Other factors should be considered when evaluating how successful an individual will be in coping with the heat load:

1. Body size and fat—individuals with a large surface area (see p. 161 in McArdle et al.[13] to calculate surface area) relative to body weight have a large area exposed to the environment and can cool at a faster rate.

Table 13–1. Determination of Relative Humidity Using Wet-Bulb (t° C) and Dry-Bulb (t° C) Temperature*

$t - t'$ / t	1.0	2.0	3.0	4.0	5.0	6.0	7.0	8.0	9.0	10.0	11.0	12.0	13.0	14.0	1⁻
16	90	81	71	63	54	46	38	30	23	15	8				
17	90	81	72	64	55	47	40	32	25	18	11				
18	91	82	73	65	57	49	41	34	27	20	14	7			
19	91	82	74	65	58	50	43	36	29	22	16	10			
20	91	83	74	66	59	51	44	37	31	24	18	12	6		
21	91	83	75	67	60	53	46	39	32	26	20	14	9		
22	92	83	76	68	61	54	47	40	34	28	22	17	11	6	
23	92	84	76	69	62	55	48	42	36	30	24	19	13	8	
24	92	84	77	69	62	56	49	43	37	31	26	20	15	10	
25	92	84	77	70	63	57	50	44	39	33	28	22	17	12	
26	92	85	78	71	64	58	51	46	40	34	29	24	19	14	
27	92	85	78	71	65	58	52	47	41	36	31	26	21	16	
28	93	85	78	72	65	59	53	48	42	37	32	27	22	18	
29	93	86	79	72	66	60	54	49	43	38	33	28	24	19	
30	93	86	79	73	67	61	55	50	44	39	35	30	25	21	
31	93	86	80	73	67	61	56	51	45	40	36	31	27	22	
32	93	86	80	74	68	62	57	51	46	41	37	32	28	24	
33	93	87	80	74	68	63	57	52	47	42	38	33	29	25	
34	93	87	81	75	69	63	58	53	48	43	39	35	30	26	
35	94	87	81	75	69	64	59	54	49	44	40	36	32	28	
36	94	87	81	75	70	64	59	54	50	45	41	37	33	29	
37	94	87	82	76	70	65	60	55	51	46	42	38	34	30	
38	94	88	82	76	71	66	61	56	51	47	43	39	35	31	
39	94	88	82	77	71	66	61	57	52	48	43	39	36	32	
40	94	88	82	77	72	67	62	57	53	48	44	40	36	33	

Example: (t) Dry Bulb = 27°
(t′) Wet Bulb = 20°
t − t′ = 7°
R.H. = 52%

* Adapted with permission from Sharkey BJ: *Physiology of Fitness.* Champaign, IL: Human Kinetics Books, 1990. Also from McArdle WD, Katch FI, and Katch VL: *Exercise Physiology: Energy, Nutrition, and Human Performance.* Philadelphia, Lea & Febiger, 1991.

Obesity is a liability when working in the heat. Obese individuals have lower conductive heat losses and have a relatively small body surface for evaporation. Larger-sized individuals with a relatively small surface area to mass ratio and higher percentage of body fat (e.g., football linemen) are less efficient in handling the heat load.[13]

2. State of aerobic training.
3. State of acclima(tiza)tion.
4. Intensity of exercise relative to one's maximal work capacity.
5. Clothing—heavy "sweatshirts" and clothing made of rubber or plastic produce high relative humidity close to the skin and inhibit or prevent evaporative cooling. Playing uniforms that cover most of the body and are heavy (i.e., football uniforms) can substantially add to the heat load.
6. Ground temperature—in certain situations, it is important to assess whether ground temperature is adding to the heat load. During later daylight hours of the summer, the ground is heated by solar radiation and is warmer than the air above. Ground temperature may even be higher if the surface is dark in color.

Testing and Training Adjustments

Depending on the state of acclima(tiza)tion, exercise capacity is adversely affected

HIGH HEAT STRESS: Extreme heat stress conditions exist; consider cancelling all exercise.

MODERATE HEAT STRESS: Heat-sensitive and nonacclimatized individuals may suffer; avoid strenuous activity in the sun; take adequate rest periods and replace fluids.

LOW HEAT STRESS: Use discretion, especially if unconditioned or unacclimatized; little danger of heat stress for acclimatized individuals who hydrate adequately.

Heat Stress Index Using Dry Bulb Temperature and Relative Humidity

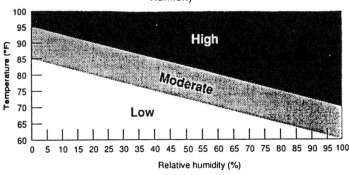

Fig. 13–1. Heat stress index. Adapted with permission from Sharkey BJ: *Physiology of Fitness.* Champaign, IL: Human Kinetics Books, 1990. Also from McArdle WD, Katch FI, and Katch VL: *Exercise Physiology: Energy, Nutrition, and Human Performance.* Philadelphia: Lea & Febiger, 1991.

WBGT HEAT STRESS INDEX

°F	°C	
80–84	26.5–28.2	Low Heat Stress
85–87	29.5–30.5	Moderate Heat Stress
88 or higher	31.2+	High Heat Stress

*F = (9/5 * °C) +32

if the heat index is sufficiently high and the exposure is prolonged enough to prevent the thermoregulatory system from adequately coping with the combined environmental and metabolic heat loads. Elevated heart rate (relative to the degree of activity) is a valid and useful indicator of the additional stress imposed by an environmental heat load. Thus, heart rate can be used both as an indicator of heat stress and as a guide for adjusting exercise training intensity to achieve a constant load on the cardiovascular system in a hot environment.

For laboratory exercise testing application, a cool or thermoneutral room temperature (22°C or less) is desirable, both for comfort and to prevent the adverse consequences of an exogenous heat load. If test periods are relatively brief, as maximal oxygen uptake determinations and clinical electrocardiographic "stress" testing are, room temperatures of as much as 26°C can be tolerated without adverse effects if air movement is increased by use of fans or other means.

Prolonged exercise for aerobic training or endurance testing is a different problem. Prolonged exercise causes the body heat load to increase when the heat-stress index is high. Training prescriptions or test protocols must be adjusted downward to maintain the same cardiovascular load as in a cooler environment. Heart rate can serve as a guide to cardiovascular load, as previously noted. Additional precautions are needed when assessing cardiac rehabilitation patients or others with compromised cardiovascular function who already have a narrowed heat tolerance because of impaired ability to increase cardiac output.

Heat Injury

Heat injury (or illness) is a category of pathologic conditions that occur when thermoregulatory mechanisms fail to cope effectively with the additive effects of external heat load and metabolically produced heat. Heat injuries exhibit a spectrum of clinical severity ranging from benign heat cramps to heat exhaustion and heat stroke; the latter two are potentially fatal. It is important that the individual conducting exercise training or testing be able to recognize heat injuries should they occur. Although the more benign conditions can be adequately treated following simple guidelines, definitive treatment of conditions such as heat stroke requires supervision of a physician.

Description and Treatment

Heat Cramp. Heat cramps involve benign, involuntary, sometimes painful cramping of muscles, usually in the calves or abdomen occurring as a result of exercise in a hot environment. These cramps probably result from an imbalance of sodium and potassium across muscle cell membranes as a result of salt loss through heavy sweating. Fluid and electrolyte (salt) replacement is the proper treatment. Salting of food and consumption of a balanced diet with adequate water intake is often adequate to restore appropriate electrolyte levels.

Heat Rash. Heat rash or "prickly heat" is a benign condition characterized by a prickling sensation in the skin during sweating. This skin condition is associated with prolonged wetting of the skin by sweat. The obvious but often impractical treatment is to limit exposure to high-temperature conditions that induce sweating.

Dehydration. Because it can occur in a number of conditions, dehydration is not considered exclusively a heat illness. In hot, humid environments, it occurs as a result of sweating, and invariably accompanies and complicates other heat injuries. For example, a 5% weight loss (3.5 kg), caused almost entirely by loss of water as sweat, is common for an average-sized man in the course of a 16-km (10-mile) run in 27 to 32°C (80 to 90°F) heat. This volume loss *must* be replaced, preferably by drinking water or dilute electrolyte solutions. Failure to adequately replace the volume loss predisposes the individual to heat injury if the exercise or heat exposure are continued.

Early signs of dehydration are decreased urine production, lethargy, anxiety, and irritability. Elevated heart rate and body temperature may also be present. Severe dehydration may be manifested by uncoordinated, spastic gait and altered consciousness. Untreated dehydration may lead to cardiovascular collapse and death. Individuals with symptoms of dehydration should be treated in the same manner as those with heat exhaustion and heat stroke (see below).

Salt Depletion. Like dehydration, salt depletion is exclusively the result of heat exposure. Salt depletion can occur in conditions of high sweat production over several hours or several days of repeated exposure, especially if the fluid loss is adequately replaced without replacing the electrolytes. Mild salt depletion causes symptoms similar to those of mild dehydration, including dizziness and fatigue; moderate to severe depletion leads to nausea, vomiting, and muscle cramps. Severe depletion can cause seizures, coma, and death. During heat exposure with exercise, daily salt loss in sweat can be 15 to 20 grams. Because salt uptake through the regular diet amounts to approximately 10 grams, it may take several days of heat exposure before significant depletion occurs. Prophylactic increased intake of salt by salting food or drinking dilute electrolyte solutions may be helpful in preventing and treating mild salt depletion. Moderate to severe depletion should be treated under the direction of a physician.

Heat Exhaustion. Heat exhaustion is a potentially serious condition, which occurs in the exercise setting as a result of increased metabolic heat load from physical activity and dehydration and/or salt depletion secondary to sweating. Although there is generally no evidence for significant tissue damage in heat exhaustion, it can progress to heat stroke, a potentially fatal condition with manifest tissue damage.

Common symptoms include "gooseflesh," headache, dizziness, shortness of breath, pallor, nausea, vomiting, and uncoordinated gait. Body temperature (rectal) is elevated but is usually less than 39.5°C (103°F), and subjects are usually normotensive. Treatment of heat exhaustion is similar to that for heat stroke (see below). The first treatment step is to eliminate sources of heat stress by stopping physical activity and removing the individual from the hot environment, if possible. Rehydration and replenishing of salt is essential. Active cooling measures may also be needed.

Heat Stroke. It is difficult to distinguish between heat stroke and heat exhaustion on the basis of symptoms alone because the initial manifestations are very similar. Heat stroke is notable for the loss of ability to thermoregulate, and affected individuals may have higher core temperatures (under 40°C, 104°F) if they are seen before cooling measures have been started. Contrary to popular belief, heat stroke victims may sweat profusely. Individuals with heat stroke may also be more likely to show symptoms of central nervous system dysfunction such as unsteady gait, disorientation, confusion, bizarre or combative behavior, and loss of consciousness. Heat stroke is ultimately diagnosed by detection of evidence of tissue damage using biochemical markers in the blood.

For purposes of the exercise professional who may be directing exercise training or testing, the distinction between heat stroke and heat exhaustion is not critical to initiate appropriate action. Symptoms of either type of heat injury require immediate action to discontinue the heat stress, institute cooling measures, and obtain appropriate medical attention promptly. If possible, affected individuals should be moved out of the hot environment, or to a cooler area (such as shade) within the environment. They should be laid down with their feet elevated above the level of the heart to help maintain blood pressure and circulation to the brain. Excess clothing should be opened or removed. Although people with heat exhaustion retain the ability to thermoregulate and may be able to cool with these measures alone, it is appropriate to institute active cooling measures on all those with symptoms. If core (usually rectal) temperatures are above 39.5°C (103° F), cooling should begin immediately. Sprinkling with water and fanning to increase evaporative cooling are effective

means of cooling, as is immersion in cool water. Although some controversy exists over the possibility of inducing vasoconstriction by rubbing ice over the large blood vessels in the groin, armpits and neck, ice can be used to wet large areas of the skin to increase evaporate cooling. Cooling by any means should continue until core temperature is 39°C (102°C). In addition to cooling, means of rehydration should be started. If the individual is conscious, alert, and not nauseated or likely to vomit, he or she should be given cool fluids to sip. If he or she cannot take fluids by mouth, intravenous fluids should be started under supervision of medical personnel. Definitive evaluation and treatment for heat stroke requires the attention of a physician, and appropriate medical care should be obtained as soon as possible.

Prevention

The key to the prevention of heat injuries associated with exercise is the avoidance of testing and training in hot ambient conditions that place the individual at increased risk. The WBGT index integrates the primary environmental risk factors into a practical index of the relative risk of injury. This risk indication has to be related to activity level and acclimation state. For the unacclimated, moderate risk exists at WBGT between 65°F and 73°F, high risk between 73°F and 82°F, and very high risk above 82°F. Figure 13–1 provides a means of translating known dry-bulb temperature and relative humidity into WBGT readings and risk levels. The ACSM Position Statement, "Prevention of Thermal Injuries During Distance Running," gives further information concerning these risk levels in runners. A summary of the strategies recommended in that document for minimizing the risks of running in the heat is presented below. The recommendations are appropriate for any exercise in the heat.

1. Allow time for acclimatization to the heat, usually 10 to 14 days.
2. Exercise during cooler parts of day.
3. Limit or defer exercise if heat stress indices are in high-risk zone (see Fig. 13–1).
4. The most effective defense against heat stress is adequate hydration.

Plan to drink before, during, and after exercise in the heat, even during training and acclima(tiza)tion (see ACSM guidelines). Recommended quantities are 400 to 500 mL (13 to 16 oz) of cold water about 20 minutes before exercising and 300 mL every 20 minutes during activity. Before and during exercise, fluid replacement should be either water or dilute commercially available fluid replacement drinks. After exercise, commercially available fluid replacement solutions should be ingested to ensure rehydration and to maintain a healthy thirst after exercise in the heat.[14]

5. Modulate training intensity by heart rate monitoring.
6. Monitor daily body weight closely. Acute weight losses are mostly water. If losses are greater than 3% of weight, they should be replaced by drinking before the next training session.
7. The electrolyte (sodium, potassium) requirements of most physically active individuals can be more than adequately met by consuming a balanced diet. Salt replacement becomes important:
   A. when exercising for more than 1 1/2 hours (especially in high humidity)
   B. if more than 2% of body weight has been lost by sweating
   C. during the initial stages of acclimatization to a hot environment
   D. during prolonged, repeated exposures to exercise and heat[6]
   In these cases, the salt loss can be accommodated by liberally salting food. Salt tablets are *not* recommended.
8. Clothing—loose fitting with a large area of skin exposed to the air to enhance evaporation. Clothing should be light in color to reduce radiant heat gain.

LOW AMBIENT TEMPERATURE

Physical performance decrements and injuries caused by exercise in cold environments are less frequent than those associated with exercise in heat. Part of the difference is because exercise itself generates heat to warm the body and clothing can be added to retain the heat produced. Nevertheless, cold weather can cause significant injury to the unprepared or inadequately equipped individual during exercise training or testing. The professional who may prescribe or supervise exercise in cold conditions should be familiar with health threats imposed by low temperature and take steps to avoid or prevent them.

Physiologic Responses

As described in the previous section, heat is lost from the body through radiation, conduction, and convection, or through evaporation of sweat. Although these processes are necessary to prevent overheating during activity in hot environments, they can cause excessive heat loss in cold conditions. Excessive heat loss is normally avoided by adding layers of clothing to reduce losses through radiation and convection and keeping the skin dry to reduce evaporative loss. If these measures are insufficient, and skin temperature falls, blood flow to the skin is reduced by cutaneous vasoconstriction, drawing blood away from the body surface and extremities to reduce heat loss and maintain core temperature. If the cold stress is severe enough that core temperature begins to fall, shivering occurs, resulting in the production of additional metabolic heat. Exercising can also produce additional heat in a cold environment. In general, however, the metabolic heat production capacity of an unprotected individual through increased activity is insufficient to compensate for prolonged exposure to severe cold.

Body heat is lost about two to four times faster in water than at the same temperature in air. This is because water can absorb several thousand times more heat than air, therefore heat is more rapidly lost by conduction.[13]

Acclimatization

Humans apparently do not exhibit the pronounced physiologic acclima(tiza)tion response to cold that they do to the heat. Some evidence exists, however, that people who are habitually active in cold temperatures develop the ability to burn more calories per unit of exercise than others. The best protection against the cold is to dress appropriately and to maintain a high level of aerobic fitness.

Training Adjustments

Acute cold exposure, at least down to −20°C, does not significantly affect maximal oxygen uptake, probably because the oxygen transport system to active muscles is not compromised. Cold exposure can reduce submaximal endurance performance, although the mechanism(s) are not understood. The reduction is not large and should not be a major concern in training prescription during cold periods. The most important concern for an exercise program in the cold is prevention of cold injuries.

Cold Exposure Index

The effect of cold exposure on the body depends on the rate of heat loss, which, as in heat exposure, depends on air movement, humidity, and precipitation in addition to absolute temperature. Quantification of cold stress must account for all of these factors. Humidity is less of a factor at temperatures below freezing. Wind velocity, however, is a major factor in the severity of cold stress on unclothed skin or skin covered by wet clothing because it markedly increases heat loss by convection, and evaporation. The extent of the air velocity factor (or wind-chill effect) is shown in Table 13–2. Protective clothing that prevents air movement across the skin eliminates the wind-chill effect for the areas that are covered. For the clothed person, other "cold" indices are available that account for the insulating effects of clothes.

Cold Injury

Description and Treatment

Although many cold-induced injuries are known to occur, those of primary concern to the exercise professional are hypothermia and frostbite. These conditions can range in severity from mild to life-threatening or causing extensive tissue damage and loss of appendages. In addition to ensuring that exercise regimens are designed to avoid these injuries, the exercise professional must be able to recognize them when they occur to obtain appropriate medical treatment. Two additional cold-related conditions of which an exercise professional should be aware when prescribing or supervising exercise in cold conditions are the effects of breathing cold air on the reactivity of the airways and cold-induced urticaria.

Hypothermia. Hypothermia is a potentially fatal condition characterized by a sufficient lowering of the body core temperature to affect normal body function. Lowering of core temperature occurs when metabolic heat production is insufficient to match the rate of heat loss. In the setting of exercise activity, insufficient heat production can result from relative inactivity, a decrease of energy substrate in very prolonged exercise, or metabolic compromise caused by medication or underlying illness. Increased heat loss during exercise can re-

Table 13–2. Wind-Chill Index

Wind Speed (mph)	Thermometer Reading (°F)										
	50	40	30	20	10	0	−10	−20	−30	−40	−50
	(Equivalent temperature [°F])										
5	48	37	27	16	6	−5	−15	−26	−36	−47	−57
10	40	28	16	4	−9	−24	−33	−46	−58	−70	−83
15	36	22	9	−5	−18	−32	−45	−58	−72	−85	−99
20	32	18	4	−10	−25	−39	−53	−67	−82	−96	−110
25	30	16	0	−15	−29	−44	−59	−74	−88	−104	−118
30	28	13	−2	−18	−33	−48	−63	−79	−94	−109	−125
35	27	11	−4	−20	−35	−51	−67	−82	−98	−113	−129
40	26	10	−6	−21	−37	−53	−69	−85	−100	−115	−132
	Minimal Risk			*Increasing Risk*				*Great Risk*			

sult from an excessive work rate (fatigue), insufficient insulating clothing, clothing becoming wet, or consumption of drugs and alcohol that impair normal thermoregulatory mechanisms.

When the body begins to lose heat faster than it can be produced, an individual is at risk for hypothermia. Early signs of hypothermia are the result of the physiologic responses to decreasing core temperature and include shivering and cold extremities caused by shunting of blood to the body core to conserve heat. As the core temperature continues to drop, all body functions are progressively depressed, including heart rate, respiration, and reflexes. As exposure continues and mild hypothermia develops, judgment and ability to reason are lost. The person may complain of being cold and focuses all activity on getting warm. As hypothermia progresses, speech may become slurred; the person has trouble with precise hand movements, and then begins to stumble. As severe hypothermia develops, the person may appear agitated and show bizarre or inappropriate behavior and wants to lie down and rest. Hypothermia frequently occurs in air temperatures above 30°F because of the wind-chill factor, fatigue, and the person's becoming wet.

Mild hypothermia can be managed by removing the affected individual from the cold to a warm environment, increasing the person's insulation against further heat loss with dry clothes or blankets, and allowing him or her to consume warm beverages if he or she is sufficiently alert. Moderate to severe cases require treatment under the direction of a physician in a hospital setting. Gentle handling during transportation to medical care is crucial to avoid precipitating dangerous cardiac arrhythmias. The individuals should be kept still to prevent recirculation, and transportation should take place with the individual lying down to avoid shock.

Frostbite. Frostbite is the consequence of water crystallization within tissues, causing subsequent cellular dehydration and tissue destruction. In the setting of exercise, it is most likely to occur on exposed or insufficiently insulated skin. High windchill factor creates a significant risk for frostbite injury. Exercise that involves speed, such as running, skiing, and cycling, can create wind-chill conditions by increasing air movement over exposed skin.

Frostbite injuries can be serious, resulting in extensive tissue loss and the necessity of amputation of the affected body part. Even when no detectable tissue damage occurs (a condition often referred to as "frost nip"), the affected area may be more prone to cold injury on subsequent exposures. Early signs and symptoms of frostbite include numbness and white or yellowish color in the affected area. Clear or blood-containing blisters occur with more severe injury. Although numb when frozen, the affected tissue may be very painful when rewarmed.

The key to early management of significant frostbite is to ensure that the affected tissue does not refreeze after it has been rewarmed, because that cycle leads to more extensive tissue damage. When there is no risk of refreezing, frostbitten tissue can be rapidly rewarmed in water within the temperature range of 40 to 42°C (104 to 108° F which is warm but not hot water). Do **not** massage the affected area. Rewarming is best accomplished in a medical care setting when possible. Definitive treatment of significant frostbite should be under the direction of a physician.

Cold-Air inhalation. Inhalation of cold air does not usually cause tissue damage in the respiratory tract, although it may be uncomfortable. This is because the respiratory system is efficient in warming and humidifying air, and even in very cold weather inhaled air is warmed to about 75 to 80°F by the time it reaches the bronchi.[13] Cold air can cause constriction of the bronchi in patients with exercise-induced asthma, inhalation of very cold air can also cause angina in persons with coronary artery disease. Precautions should be taken to avoid unnecessary exposure to inhalation of cold air when prescribing exercise training or rehabilitation programs for these individuals.

Cold Urticaria. Cold urticaria is the development of redness, itching, and large blister-like wheals on skin that is cold-exposed. Although these skin manifestations usually resolve after the cold exposure is terminated, they can be accompanied by life-threatening anaphylaxis on rare occasions. Individuals with cold urticaria should be evaluated by medical personnel, and probably should not exercise in cold conditions.

Prevention

Because the harmful effects of cold exposure are a function of the balance between heat production and heat loss, any factor that either compromises metabolic heat production or accelerates the loss of body heat to the environment can be considered "risk factors." Prevention of cold injuries is accomplished by recognizing specific risk factors and taking steps to modify or avoid them. In the setting of exercise, metabolic heat production is largely a function of work intensity and heat loss a function of protective clothing. Prevention of cold injuries in this setting is primarily a function of balancing work rate and the insulative effect of protective clothing to match the specific environmental conditions.

Adequate protective clothing is very important in preventing cold injuries during exercise. Windproof and water-repellent (not watertight) outer garments are necessary when wind and precipitation are present. If wind-chill temperatures are $-15°F$ or less, extra care should be taken to protect areas of skin such as the face, nose, ears, and hands, which are often left exposed under less harsh conditions. Increased insulation under the protective outer garments is best achieved with layers of loose-fitting clothing. Layered clothing is more efficient in insulating than bulkier single garments and has the advantage that partial layers can be removed as temperature and sweating increase and put back on as the person becomes cold. If possible, the garment closest to the skin should be of a material that will "wick" moisture away from the skin and prevent excessive accumulation of sweat and minimizes evaporative cooling. Several newer synthetic materials (e.g., polypropylene) have been specifically designed for this purpose.

The key consideration in adjusting exercise intensity for training in the cold is to avoid periods in which there is a decrease in metabolic heat production that is not compensated by either leaving the cold environment or adding clothing for extra insulation. Cool-down periods after stopping exercise or a reduced pace at the end of extended training periods are important to consider in this regard. Individuals who are fatigued and depleted of energy should avoid extended periods of activity. Running a series of loops rather than a long run out and back should be considered. If a wind is present, it is best to run first into the wind and return with the wind at the back.

HIGH TERRESTRIAL ALTITUDE

Exercise testing and training at high altitude are unavoidable for those who reside there normally, but others choose to train at altitude in the belief that training in conditions of reduced oxygen partial pressure will improve their performance at lower altitudes. Although the question of whether training at altitude enhances sea-level performance is somewhat controversial, the reduced oxygen availability at high altitude has profound effects on physical performance and can cause serious illness in unacclimatized individuals. Awareness of these hazards is necessary to plan a safe and effective exercise program in a high-altitude environment.

Physiologic Responses

The amount of hemoglobin saturated with oxygen depends on the partial pressure of oxygen in the inspired air. The partial pressure of any gas is a product of the barometric pressure and the percentage of concentration of the gas in the ambient air. The partial pressure of oxygen in the air decreases with the decline in barometric pressure that occurs with increasing altitude (% concentration of oxygen in the air is the same at various altitudes). For example, the ambient oxygen pressure declines from 159 mm Hg at sea level to 132 mm Hg in Denver, Colorado (5280 feet) and to as low as 94 mm Hg on the top of Pike's Peak (14,110 feet). With a decline in inspired oxygen pressure, there is a concomitant fall in arterial oxygen saturation and a decrease in the maximal amount of oxygen available to the cells. This decrease in arterial oxygen saturation triggers compensatory mechanisms that function to increase oxygen transport to body tissues.

The immediate physiologic response to increases in altitude above 1500 to 2000 meters (5000 to 6500 feet) is an increase in pulmonary ventilation. This hyperventilation is an attempt to increase the arterial saturation of oxygen by increasing inspired air volume. On the other hand, the increased volume of expired air tends to "wash" out the carbon dioxide in the blood. Therefore, respiratory alkalosis develops and the acid-base balance of the body is affected. The alkalosis, in turn, causes a "left shift" in the oxygen-hemoglobin dissociation curve, which allows oxygen to be more available to the tissue at a given oxygen pressure.

In the early stages of altitude adaptation, submaximal heart rate and cardiac output increase, while stroke volume remains essentially unchanged. The increase in submaximal blood flow is the body's compensatory mechanism to try to keep oxygen available to the cells with the decrease in oxygen in the arterial blood. The major affect of altitude is observed during maximal exercise. The maximal oxygen uptake ($\dot{V}_{O_{2}max}$) is decreased approximately 10% for every 1000 meters (3300 feet) gain in altitude above 2000 meters (6500 feet). There is little or no change in maximal cardiac output; however, maximal cardiac output occurs at a lower exercise intensity than that at sea level. Because of the increased cardiac output at submaximal workloads, there is no change in oxygen uptake for any of those exercise intensities. However, because of the decreased $\dot{V}_{O_{2}max}$, the absolute submaximal uptake represents a higher relative value expressed as percent of the $\dot{V}_{O_{2}max}$. Simply stated, the body can achieve the same submaximal performance, but requires relatively more physiologic work to do so.

Acclimatization

With prolonged (days to weeks) residence at high altitude, acclimatization occurs. Resting ventilatory rate remains elevated, but the initial respiratory alkalosis is moderated through bicarbonate excretion by the kidneys. Cardiac output for a given submaximal exercise intensity decreases, largely because of a decrease in stroke volume (submaximal HR remains elevated). Red cell production increases (polycythemia), leading to a sustained increase in hemoglobin, hematocrit and arterial oxygen content. Additionally, prolonged (months to years) residence at high altitude may lead to adaptation at the tissue level with increased mitochondria, increased aerobic enzymes, increased 2,3 DPG, and tissue capillary density. The changes that occur with acclimatization result in improved exercise performance *at altitude,* as evidenced by increased in $\dot{V}_{O_{2}max}$ and submaximal exercise endurance from the initial days of altitude exposure. The changes are sufficient to completely offset the decrements caused by lowered ambient availability at submaximal exercise. Maximal performance never fully recovers to sea-level values, even in well acclimatized individuals. As a general guideline, about 2 weeks are needed to adapt to altitudes up to 2300 meters (7500 feet). For each 610 meters (2000 feet) increase, an additional week is required for full adaptation.[13]

Testing and Training Adjustments

Because of the reduced oxygen intake ability above 1500 meters (5000 feet), usual exercise intensity has a larger anaerobic component than at sea level. Upon arriving at altitude, an individual has a choice of exercise at the usual intensity for short distances, exercise at lower intensity for longer duration, or taking a few days off as the body adjusts physiologically to the reduced arterial oxygen saturation. For athletes wishing to compete at altitude, intense training should begin as soon as possible. Remember that it will be difficult to engage in intense training in the early days of altitude exposure. It is important to allow enough time to acclimatize fully before the event (see section on Acclimatization).

Aerobic events are affected greatly at altitude, whereas anaerobic events are affected little if at all. Activities with a large anaerobic component which also involve rapid movement through air, such as sprinting, may actually be improved because of decreased air resistance.

Professionals who supervise or prescribe

exercise training in high-altitude environments should be aware of the controversy regarding the benefits of that training. Although it is well documented that training at high altitude will improve performance *in that setting,* too few well-controlled studies have been done to show any significant effect of altitude training on sea-level performance. Despite this, there is currently a great deal of enthusiasm for using altitude training in an attempt to enhance sea-level performance based largely on anecdotal reports and theoretical arguments. When $\dot{V}O_{2max}$ is the criterion, sea-level maximal aerobic capacity is about the same as pre-altitude measures.[13] Physiologic changes that occur at altitude return to pre-altitude values within 2 to 3 weeks of sea-level living.

High-Altitude Illness

High-altitude exposure, with or without exercise, can cause numerous illnesses ranging in seriousness from mild symptoms that resolve with acclimatization to potentially fatal edema of the brain and lungs. The incidence of these conditions is directly related to the speed of ascent and the elevation achieved. Because altitude illness can affect performance, anyone supervising exercise in mountainous environments should be aware of the potential of these illnesses to occur. Additionally, exercise professionals should recognize serious altitude illness so that they can arrange appropriate medical care for the affected individual.

Description and Treatment

Acute Mountain Sickness. Acute mountain sickness (AMS) is characterized by the presence of a severe headache often accompanied by nausea, vomiting, decreased appetite, weariness, and sleep disturbances. It is very common in people who make rapid ascents, such as those afforded by airplanes and automobiles, to altitudes over 2500 meters (8000 feet). The symptoms begin 4 to 6 hours after ascent and may last 48 to 72 hours before resolving on their own. In very few individuals, the symptoms of AMS can be early indications of a condition of fluid leakage into

the brain called "high-altitude cerebral edema." These individuals often have behavioral changes and ultimately lapse into unconsciousness and die if they do not get proper medical attention.

The only effective treatment for AMS that is not resolved within 2 to 3 days is descent. Recently, some success has been reported in treating AMS using a portable hyperbaric chamber called the "Ganow Bag." Supplemental oxygen is also useful, but rarely available in sufficient quantity to be useful for treating AMS. Individuals with signs and symptoms of cerebral edema should be evacuated to low altitude *immediately,* with supplemental oxygen if it is available. A physician should direct the medical care of these seriously ill individuals.

High Altitude Pulmonary Edema. High altitude exposure can cause fluid leakage into the lung, termed "high altitude pulmonary edema" or HAPE. The fluid causes shortness of breath, a cough, and cyanosis or purple color of the lips and extremities. Affected individuals can cough up frothy or blood-tinged sputum. The difficulty in breathing can rapidly progress to coma and death if these people are not appropriately treated. Of special interest to the person directing or supervising exercise training at high altitude is that exercise by unacclimatized individuals, especially the young, seems to confer a greatly increased risk of developing HAPE.

Treatment of this often rapidly fatal condition should be under the direction of a physician. Afflicted individuals should be evacuated to lower altitude *immediately.* If oxygen is available, it can be administered during the evacuation, but one should not wait for oxygen to start descent. If evacuated to lower altitude promptly, individuals with HAPE tend to recover swiftly with few complications. Individuals who have had a previous episode of HAPE appear to have an increased risk of developing it again during subsequent trips to high altitude. These individuals should probably be discouraged from participating in vigorous exercise testing or training at high altitude.

Prevention

Most severe altitude illness occurs in unacclimatized individuals who ascend too high and/or too rapidly, and therefore it can be prevented by adjusting the extent and speed of ascent. This can be achieved by an interrupted ascent with several days to acclimatize at lower altitudes before reaching the final elevation, or by limiting the daily gain in altitude to 300 meters (1000 feet) or less per day. Vigorous exercise should be avoided during the initial acclimatization period. Other actions that may help prevent altitude illness are attention to adequate hydration and eating a high carbohydrate diet. Although many drugs have been suggested to prevent altitude illness in persons who cannot or do not wish to take time to acclimatize properly, acetazolamide is the only one approved by the FDA for that purpose. This drug can affect exercise performance, however, and probably has little role in exercise training or testing at high altitude.

AIR POLLUTION

Organizers of sports events and those participating in exercise activities are increasingly confronted with problems related to air pollution. Sporting events or exercise training sessions are often performed within large cities, which are sites of high pollution levels produced by traffic and industry. Acute exposure to air pollution can affect exercise performance and affect an individual's health and well-being. Chronic exposure can also have significant adverse health effects. Although this discussion concentrates on effects of short-term exposure, it should be remembered that regular exercise in a polluted atmosphere may contribute significantly to the effects of chronic exposure.

Two general classes of air pollutants exist. "Primary" pollutants are those that remain unchanged after their introduction to the atmosphere and include carbon monoxide, sulfur and nitrogen oxides, and particulate matter (soot, smoke, and dusts). "Secondary" pollutants are formed within the atmosphere by interaction of primary pollutants with each other, sunlight, and moisture. Common secondary pollutants include ozone, peroxyacetyl nitrate (PAN), and various aerosols.

Biologic Effects

The effects of atmospheric pollutants are partly related to their penetration in the body. The major route of penetration is through the respiratory tract, which functions to limit the entry of many pollutants. The mucous membranes in the nose remove large particles and highly soluble gases very effectively (e.g., 99.19% of inhaled sulfur dioxide is removed in the nose), but smaller particles and agents with low solubility pass to the lower tract. During exercise, when mouth breathing must play an important role, this air filtration process is less efficient and more pollutants reach the lungs. Within the lungs, pollutants contact respiratory surfaces through deposition or diffusion and may be removed by the mucous layer and white blood cells in the tissue, or taken into the blood stream and circulated through the body. Because the respiratory tract is the largest surface of the body to come in contact with atmospheric pollution, many of the adverse effects occur there. The biologic effects of air pollution include:

- Irritation of conducting airways (specifically vasoconstriction of bronchial tubes causing increased airway resistance)
- Effect on diffusing surface (alveolar breakdown or increased mucus secretion affecting diffusion capacity)
- Reduction in oxygen transport capacity.[20]

Description

Carbon Monoxide (CO). Carbon monoxide emissions in urban areas are greater than emissions of all other pollutants combined. Although usually associated with motor vehicle exhaust gasses outdoors, it can also play a role in indoor events where emissions from gas-powered equipment are the primary source. CO is also a component of cigarette smoke (primary or secondary). Carbon monoxide strongly binds to hemoglobin in the blood creating carboxyhemoglobin (COHb), which reduces ability of hemoglobin to combine with oxygen and diminishes oxygen transport from the lungs to the tissues. Although COHb saturations greater than 30% cause headache and fatigue, and saturations greater than 50% are fatal, the concentration of carbon monoxide in outdoor air is virtually never high enough to cause those levels of saturation.

The effect of CO on exercise depends on the saturation of COHb induced and the intensity of exercise. For submaximal exercise, COHb levels above 20% are needed to produce effects, but these levels are much higher than those found in typical air pollution, and little effect is observed. For maximal exercise, the critical level is approximately 4.3% COHb. Above this level, both exercise time and $\dot{V}O_{2max}$ are inversely related to CO concentration. Considering that the COHb saturation during prolonged exposure to heavy traffic can reach 5%, the 4.3% critical level is of practical importance. Additionally, cigarette smokers may have baseline COHb saturations in the 4 to 8% range.

In contrast to healthy subjects, individuals with ischemic heart disease are affected by CO even during submaximal exercise. Levels as low as 2.5 to 3% COHb have been found to decrease the exercise time before onset of angina and prolong the duration of the ischemia.

Sulfur Oxides (SO$_2$). Sulfur oxide pollutants, mainly in the form of sulfur dioxide, quickly dissolve in the moisture coating the mucous membranes and cause irritation of the upper respiratory tract. This irritation can cause reflex bronchoconstriction and increased airway resistance. Nose breathing, compared to mouth breathing, strongly reduces this effect by absorbing more sulfur oxides before they get to the bronchi. The threshold level before pulmonary function effects are observed during submaximal exercise lies between 1 and 3 ppm. Threshold levels for maximal exercise have not been reported. For individuals with asthma, the threshold values are much lower for elicitation of the bronchoconstrictor response during submaximal exercise (0.2–0.5 ppm of SO$_2$).

Nitrogen Oxides (NO$_2$). Of the several nitrogen oxides, only nitrogen dioxide (NO$_2$) has been studied during exercise in humans. Although exposure to high concentrations of NO$_2$ (200 to 400 ppm) can cause lung damage and fatalities, the levels usually present in the atmosphere are not high enough to induce those effects. No significant effect of NO$_2$ levels up to 1 to 2 ppm has been observed during submaximal exercise. Effects of higher concentrations during maximal exercise have not been reported.

Particulate Matter (Soot, Dust, and Smoke). Although particulate pollutants are often encountered during outdoor (and sometimes indoor) exercise, the physiologic effect of minute particles on exercise performance has not been evaluated directly. The penetration of particles in the respiratory system is related to their size. Sizes below 3 microns may reach the alveoli; sizes between 3 and 5 microns usually settle in the upper respiratory tract, and those above 5 microns are filtered in the nose. As previously noted, mouth breathing during exercise allows larger particles to penetrate farther into the respiratory tract. Generally, a bronchoconstrictive response is associated with particulate inhalation. Particles smaller than 5 microns can cause inflammation, congestion, or ulceration in the lower respiratory tract.

Ozone (O$_3$). In contrast to the ozone in the upper atmosphere, high levels of ozone at ground level create a health risk. Ozone is a secondary pollutant generated by the action of sunlight on hydrocarbon and nitrogen dioxide pollutants in the air. Because they depend on sunlight, ozone levels are highest, and exert their greatest effect on exercise, from mid-day to afternoon. Like the effect of sulfur and nitrogen oxides, the primary effect of ozone in concentrations normally encountered during exercise outdoors in polluted areas is inanition of the respiratory tract, often causing constriction of the airways. The magnitude of exposure is determined by both the ozone concentration and the length of exposure. Exercise effectively increases exposure by increasing ventilation and shifting to more mouth breathing.

During light to moderate submaximal exercise of several hours duration, exposures to 0.3 to 0.45 ppm O$_3$ cause decrements in pulmonary function and increased subjective discomfort. Limitations of exercise time appear to be secondary to the symptoms of respiratory discomfort, and little effect in terms of cardiorespiratory system limitations has been observed. For heavy submaximal, and probably also for maximal, exercise levels, performance can be significantly limited because of severe respiratory discomfort and greater changes in pulmonary function. The effect of ozone exposure on maximal exercise performance has not been well studied, however.

Organic Nitrogen Oxide. The organic nitrogen oxides, of which peroxyacetyl nitrate (PAN) is the most common, are secondary pollutants formed in the atmosphere from nitrate oxides and organic compounds. In their usual concentrations in polluted air, their main effects are eye irritation and minor changes in pulmonary function, presumably from airway constriction caused by irritation of the respiratory tract. PAN is the only one of this class of compounds for which the results of exposure on exercise have been reported. No significant decrement in submaximal or maximal exercise performance was noted at PAN levels approximately twice as high as those normally found in polluted air. Thus, the main impact of PAN and the other organic nitrate oxides may be eye irritation.

Aerosols. Aerosols are fine suspensions of liquid or solid particles in a gas or mixture of gases. The particulate matter discussed earlier in this chapter can be a form of aerosol. Numerous liquid aerosols can also be air pollutants. Most of these are secondary pollutants formed by dissolution of pollutants in water vapor. Commonly encountered aerosol pollutants include sulfur and nitrogen salts and acids, and aldehydes.

Similar to primary particulate matter, liquid aerosols are filtered out of inhaled air in relation to the size of the droplet particles, and only those smaller than 3 microns reach the alveoli of the lungs. The main adverse effect of acute exposure to the common aerosol pollutants is airway irritation, which can cause airway constriction. As is the case with particulate matter, exercise increases the severity of exposure to aerosols by increasing ventilation and promoting mouth breathing, thereby negating the filter function of the upper respiratory tract. When studied, however, the common aerosol pollutants seem to have minimal effects on exercise performance.

Interactions

Given the many sources of atmospheric pollution and the fact that sources involving combustion produce multiple different pollutants, an exercising individual is much more likely to be exposed to combinations of pollutants than to a single pollutant. These combinations can have interactive effects. When studied, several combinations have been shown to have either additive or synergistic effects on parameters of exercise performance, whereas other combinations do not appear to have interactive effects. An additive interaction implies that the total effect is equal to the sum of the individual pollutants (e.g., O_3 and NO_2). Synergistic effect is that in which the combined effect of pollutants is *greater* than the sum of the individual pollutants (e.g., O_3 and PAN).[18] Considering the range of combinations, concentrations of pollutants, and intensity and duration of exercise that can exist, more study is needed to adequately define the extent of the problem.

Just as combinations of atmospheric pollutants can induce responses that are different from those of the individual pollutants alone, exposure to the combination of atmospheric pollutants and environmental factors such as thermal stress or high altitude might affect exercise performance. Little information is available on this subject, however, because relatively few studies have been reported.

Heat, high humidity, and air pollution often occur together. The few studies that have been reported suggest that low levels of CO or PAN combined with a warm environmental temperature do not significantly affect maximal or submaximal exercise, but that pulmonary function and submaximal exercise are affected by the combination of ozone and warm temperature. No information is available on the effects of other pollutants or humidity in warm environments.

Cold air and exercise are known to stimulate airway constriction in many individuals, especially those with asthma. It has been suggested, therefore, that the combination of cold air, exercise, and airborne pollutants that irritate the respiratory tract may cause increased airway constriction, but no information is available.

Carbon monoxide is a common pollutant at high altitudes because of poor combustion of fuels. Because CO interferes with oxygen delivery from lungs to tissue by creating COHb, it could be expected to worsen the altitude-induced hypoxia and decrease exercise performance. The few studies reported confirm this effect for altitudes above 2000 meters (approximately 6500 feet). No information is available on other atmospheric pollutants and altitude exposure.

Table 13–3 summarizes the effects on exercise performance factors that enhance the various pollutants.

Prevention

Because air pollution can affect an individual's health and exercise performance, consideration of pollution levels can be relevant when planning an athletic event or prescribing an exercise training regimen. Such consideration is essential when prescribing exercise programs for individuals with health conditions such as asthma or coronary artery disease, which make these individuals particularly sensitive to the effects of specific pollutants.

The fundamental strategy for dealing with air pollution in the exercise setting is to prevent the effects of pollution by avoid-

Table 13–3. Primary and Secondary Pollutants: Mechanism of Effect, Effect on Exercise Performance, and Factors that Enhance the Effect*

Pollutant	Mechanism of Effect	Submaximal Exercise	Maximal Exercise (VO_{2max})	Factors Enhancing the Effect	
				Environmental Conditions	Conditions and/or Disease
PRIMARY POLLUTANTS:					
Carbon Monoxide (CO)	Decreased H6 saturation with oxygen Decreased ability to deliver O_2 to cells	Little impairment unless levels of COHb greater than 20%	Inversely related to concentration of CO Significant effect when levels >4.3%	Altitude Cigarette smokers Time of day with heaviest traffic patterns Midwinter (peak values)	Impaired exercise tolerance with CV disease People with CV may have effect at submaximal exercise with levels as low as 2.5–3%)
Sulfur Oxides (SO₂, sulfuric acid, sulfate)	Upper respiratory irritant Bronchoconstriction Increased air-way resistance	Threshold level of effect: 1.0 to 3.0 ppm in healthy individuals	Unknown	Burning of fossil fuels High humidity Oral breathing	Asthmatics (threshold levels between 0.2 and 0.5 pm) Respiratory illness Elderly
Nitrogen Oxides (Primarily NO₂)	Constriction of small airways and alveoli Increased airway resistance	Does not appear to have adverse effects in healthy people	Unknown	Peak values with heavy motor vehicle traffic Increase with smoke (cigarette or fire) Oral breathing Midwinter (peak values)	Possibly those with chronic bronchitis, COPD, and other respiratory disorders
Primary Particles [TSP] (dust, soot, smoke)	Bronchoconstriction Increased airway resistance Possible inflammation, congestion	Unknown	Unknown	Soot: incomplete combustion of fossil fuels Dust storms, forest fires, wind storms Volcanoes	Asthma Chronic lung disease Aggravation of CR disease symptoms
SECONDARY POLLUTANTS:					
Ozone (O₃)	Bronchoconstriction of small airways and proximal alveoli	No effect at light to moderate exercise (increased respiratory discomfort)	Unknown (Performance potentially limited at high levels of O₃)	Peak values in afternoon (related to hours of sunlight) Early autumn/summer Heat stress	Asthma Respiratory diseases
Peroxyacetyl Nitrate (PAN)	Minor pulmonary function alterations Eye irritant	No effect	No effect	Ozone	
Aerosols, sulfate, nitrate, sulfuric acid	Particles <3 microns reach alveoli Airway irritation with possible airway constriction	Minimal	Minimal		

* Adapted with permission from Pandolf KB: Air quality and human performance. In *Human Performance Physiology and Environmental Medicine at Terrestrial Extremes.* Edited by Pandolf KB, Sawka MN, Gonzalez RR. Indianapolis: Benchmark Press, 1988.

Table 13–4.   Comparison of the Pollution Standard Index Values with Pollutant Concentrations and Descriptor Words

Index Value	Air Quality Level	TSP (24-hr) $\mu g/m^3$	SO$_2$ (24-hr) $\mu g/m^3$	CO (8-hr) $\mu g/m^3$	O$_3$ (1-hr) $\mu g/m^3$	NO$_2$ (1-hr) $\mu g/m^3$	Health Effect Descriptor
500	Significant harm	600	2620	57.5	1200	3750	
400	Emergency	500	2100	46.0	1000	3000	Hazardous
300	Warning	420	1600	34.0	800	2260	Very unhealthful
200	Alert	350	800	17.0	400	1130	Very unhealthful
100	NAAQS†	150	365	10.0	235	*	Moderate
50	50% of NAAQS	50	80	5.0	118	*	Good
0		0	0	0.0	0	*	

TSP = total suspended particulates, SO$_2$ = sulfur dioxide, CO = carbon monoxide, O$_3$ = ozone, NO$_2$ = nitrogen dioxide

$\mu g/m^3$ = ppm × molecular weight/0.024

* No index values reported at concentration levels below those specified by "alert level" criteria.

† NAAQS = National Average Air Quality Standards

Data with permission from Pandolf KB: Air quality and human performance. In *Human Performance Physiology and Environmental Medicine at Terrestrial Extremes*. Edited by Pandolf KB, Sawka MN, Gonzalez RR. Indianapolis: Benchmark Press, 1988.

ing exercise activity in locations or at times when pollution levels are elevated. Information on air pollution levels can usually be acquired from local meteorologic authorities. Table 13–4 is included to aid in interpreting that information. Further, daily and seasonal fluctuations in air pollution levels should be taken into account. For example, the CO level in cities peaks during the rush hours, and the ozone levels are usually low all winter and increase during daylight hours in the summer with a daily peak around 3 pm. Maximal peak values for ozone are seen in early autumn.

As a guideline for health risks, Table 13–4 presents values for the pollution standards index (PSI), the pollutant concentration, and the associated health effects descriptor.

BIBLIOGRAPHY AND SUGGESTED READINGS

1. ACSM Position Statement: Prevention of thermal injuries during distance running. *Med Sci Sports Exerc, 16:*ii, 1984.
2. Armstrong LE, Dziados JE: Effects of heat exposure on the exercising adult. In *Sports Physical Therapy*. Edited by DB Bernhardt. New York: Churchill Livingstone, 1986.
3. Armstrong LE, Hubbard RW: High and dry. *Runners World*, June: 38, 1985.
4. Brown CF, Oldridge NB: Exercise-induced angina in the cold. *Med Sci Sports Exerc, 17:* 607, 1985.
5. Burton AC, Edholm OG: *Man in a Cold Environment*. London: Arnold, 1955.
6. Coleman E: Sports drink update. *Sport Science Exchange (Gatorade Sports Science Institute)*, *1:*5, August, 1989.
7. Hackett P: *Mountain Sickness: Prevention, Recognition and Treatment*. New York: American Alpine Club, 1980.
8. Hartley LH: Effects of high-altitude environment on the cardiovascular system of man: *JAMA, 215:*241, 1971.
9. Heath D, Williams D: *Man at High Altitude*. Edinburgh: Churchill Livingstone, 1977.
10. Horvath SM: Exercise in a cold environment. In *Exercise and Sport Sciences Reviews*. Vol. 9. Edited by DI Miller; Philadelphia: Franklin Institute, 1981.
11. Houston C: *Going High*. New York: American Alpine Club, 1980.
12. Khogali M, Hales JRS: *Heat Stroke and Temperature Regulation*. Sydney: Academic Press, 1983.
13. McArdle WD, Katch FI, Katch VL: *Exercise Physiology: Energy, Nutrition, and Human Performance*. Philadelphia; Lea & Febiger, 1991.
14. Nadel ER (ed): *Problems with Temperature Regulation during Exercise*. New York: Academic Press, 1977.
15. Nadel ER: New ideas for rehydration during and after exercise in hot weather. *Sports Science Exchange (Gatorade Sports Science Institute)*. *1:*3, June, 1988.
16. Pandolf KB: Effects of physical training

and cardiorespiratory physical fitness on exercise-heat tolerance: Recent observations. *Med Sci Sports Exerc, 11:*60, 1979.

17. Pandolf KB, Sawka MN, Gonzalez RR (eds): *Human Performance and Physiology and Environmental Medicine at Terrestrial Extremes.* Indianapolis: Benchmark Press, 1988.

18. Pandolf KB: Air quality and human performance. In *Human Performance Physiology and Environmental Medicine at Terrestrial Extremes.* Edited by KB Pandolf, MN Sawka, RR Gonzalez. Indianapolis: Benchmark Press, 1988, pp. 591–629.

19. Patton JF, Vogel JA: Effects of acute cold exposure on submaximal endurance performance. *Med Sci Sports Exerc, 16:*494, 1984.

20. Sharkey BJ: *Physiology of Fitness.* Champaign, IL: Human Kinetics Books, 1990.

Section III

PATHOPHYSIOLOGY

Chapter 14

THE RISK FACTOR CONCEPT OF CORONARY HEART DISEASE

Carl J. Caspersen and Gregory W. Heath

Beginning in the middle to the late 1960s, the number of deaths related to coronary heart disease (CHD), stroke, and associated cardiovascular problems has continuously declined.[1] Still, the overall economic impact and the number of people afflicted with these three disease entities make cardiovascular disease (CVD) a major national health problem. Educating both health professionals and lay persons about how to reduce this problem is of paramount importance. Hence, identifying and implementing effective ways to reduce risk factors associated with the development of CHD are necessary.

Epidemiologic research seeks to identify the distribution and determinants of disease. Specifically, the risk factor concept has emerged from the identification of disease determinants. A risk factor may be defined as "an aspect of personal behavior or lifestyle, an environmental exposure, or inherited characteristic, which on the basis of epidemiologic evidence is known to be associated with health-related condition(s) considered to be important to prevent."[2] The risk factor concept is well evolved for coronary heart disease.

Multiple factors are responsible for the development of CHD in an individual. Therefore, estimating risk and managing intervention measures are important in controlling CHD. The optimal time to begin preventive steps to combat CHD is not firmly established. However, evidence suggests that the longer potentially reversible risk factors are allowed to operate in a person, the greater is the impact on the individual. The impact is especially pronounced when multiple risk factors coexist. The rises in serum lipid levels, blood pressure, weight, and blood glucose concentration often seen in the transition from childhood to adulthood are not necessarily inevitable, desirable, or part of normal physiologic growth. There is no absolute proof that all recommended interventions will fully eliminate CHD risk. The size of the CHD burden, however, mitigates against delaying the application of interventions until definitive proof becomes available. Similarly, the logic for secondary prevention in patients with documented CHD is also reasonable; secondary prevention corresponds with knowledge of the natural history of the disease and the control of risk factors. The following hygienic proposals should therefore be appropriate components of a total cardiovascular health program:

1. Identify and control blood lipid levels
2. Promote cessation and prevention of cigarette smoking
3. Enhance hypertension control (drug and nondrug)
4. Encourage (prescribe) regular physical activity and exercise training
5. Facilitate weight control
6. Identify and control diabetes
7. Identify and modify type A behavior.

Our discussion of these proposals follows the same order.

RISK FACTORS

Blood Lipids

Cholesterol is the predominant lipid constituent of the atherosclerotic lesion. Retrospective comparisons of populations with large differences in CHD mortality reveal consistent correlations between serum cholesterol levels and CHD. For example, the Seven Countries Study revealed very low serum cholesterol levels and very low CHD in Japan. Conversely, both serum cholesterol and CHD were very high in Finland (Fig. 14–1).[3,4] A contrasting view of those two vastly different cultures reveals the differences in the range of serum cholesterol

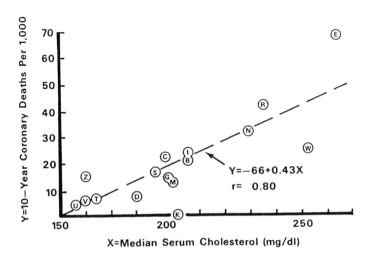

X=Median Serum Cholesterol (mg/dl)

$$Y = -66 + 0.43X$$

$$r = 0.80$$

Fig. 14–1. Coronary heart disease age-standardized 10-year death rates versus the median serum cholesterol levels (mg/dL) for 16 cohorts. All men judged free of coronary heart disease at entry. Correlation coefficient is r = 0.80. B = Belgrade, C = Crevalcore, D = Dalmatia, E = East Finland, G = Corfu, I = Italian railroad, K = Crete, M = Montegiorgio, N = Zutphen, R = American railroad, S = Slavonia, T = Tanushimaru, U = Ushibuka, V = Velika Krsna, W = West Finland, Z = Zrenianin. With permission from Keys A: *Seven Countries: A Multivariate Analysis of Death and Coronary Heart Disease.* Cambridge: Harvard University Press, 1980.

(Fig. 14–2). In the American population under age 50 years, the difference in risk that is related to the differences in serum cholesterol levels is more than fivefold. Further, this risk is magnified in the presence of other risk factors (Fig. 14–3).[5] Hypercholesterolemia is sometimes a familial trait, but rarely results from a demonstrable monogenetic disorder. A recent study revealed that even persons possessing specific lethal genes for hypercholesterolemia

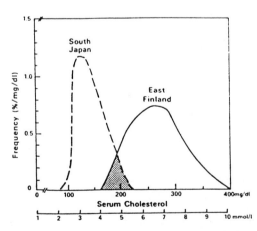

Fig. 14–2. Cultural differences in serum cholesterol levels. With permission from Blackburn H: Diet and mass hyperlipidemia: A public health view. In *Nutrition, Lipids, and Coronary Heart Disease.* Edited by RI Levy, et al. New York: Raven Press, 1976.

can reduce their risk of CHD through lifestyle alterations.[6] Genetic factors influence the broad range of cholesterol levels in the general population. However, the high average level is thought to result from dietary factors. Dietary studies show that the serum cholesterol level rises predictably by increasing saturated fat and cholesterol in the diet. Conversely, serum cholesterol levels decrease substantially by reducing the dietary intake of these nutrients.[7]

The association between elevated serum total cholesterol levels and an increased risk of CHD arises principally from the low-density lipoprotein (LDL) cholesterol fraction. LDL cholesterol is the principal carrier of cholesterol in the serum. An elevated LDL cholesterol level consistently correlates with a higher incidence of CHD.[8] One experiment reduced LDL cholesterol levels with the drug cholestyramine, which resulted in a convincing decrease in the incidence of CHD.[9] Another important study is the National Heart, Lung, and Blood Institute Type II Study[10,11] in which lowering LDL and raising high-density lipoprotein (HDL) cholesterol levels in persons with documented CHD impeded the progression of atherosclerosis.

Other studies show an inverse relationship between an elevated HDL cholesterol fraction and CHD.[12] In some persons who

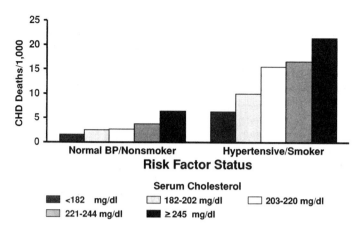

Fig. 14–3. CHD deaths per 1000 in men aged 35–57 with an average follow-up of 6 years according to serum cholesterol quintile and presence or absence of other risk factors. With permission from Kannel WB, et al.: Overall and CHD mortality rates in relation to major risk factors in 325,348 men screened for MRFIT. *Am Heart J, 112*:825, 1986.

undertake weight reduction, physical exercise, avoidance of cigarettes, and moderate ingestion of alcohol, there is an increase in HDL cholesterol blood levels.[13–15] However, the relationship among alcohol, HDL, and CHD is as yet imperfectly defined. Because HDL cholesterol transports cholesterol out of the system, higher levels are desirable to reduce the risk of CHD. Therefore, the partitioning of the serum total cholesterol value into the LDL and HDL fractions helps to clarify the risk, particularly in persons aged 50 years and older.[16,17]

The National Institutes of Health (NIH) convened a consensus development conference that concluded that lowering blood cholesterol levels reduces the incidence of CHD.[18] The National Cholesterol Education Program (NCEP) arose from the results of the consensus conference. The NCEP convened an Expert Panel on Detection, Evaluation, and Treatment of High Blood Cholesterol in Adults to determine cholesterol levels that would aid in identifying individuals at risk of developing CHD and in need of treatment.[19] Table 14–1 provides the values set forth by the panel for adults aged 18 years and older.[19] The panel also made recommendations for follow-up of persons with elevated levels of total cholesterol (Table 14–2). The NCEP also convened an Expert Panel on Population Strategies for Blood Cholesterol Reduction[20] whose recommendations are designed to help healthy Americans lower their blood cholesterol levels through changes in eating patterns to reduce their likelihood of developing CHD. The treat-

ment panel and the population panel also recommended dietary and drug therapy to reduce cholesterol in persons determined to be at moderate or high risk.

Results of international dietary comparisons, human metabolic studies, and feeding experiments in animals each clearly implicate the dietary intake of large amounts of saturated fat and cholesterol in the hypercholesterolemia found in populations where CHD is highly prevalent.[3] A diet that also includes an intake of calories in excess of need worsens hypercholesterolemia. However, the conclusive demonstration of this relationship is difficult in populations (e.g., the United States) because of a high consumption of foods considered to be atherogenic. Similarly, persons following a vegetarian diet have lower-than-average levels of blood lipids and also have a lower incidence of CHD.[7,21]

Table 14–1. Classification of Risk Based on Total Blood Cholesterol*

Blood Cholesterol Level	Initial Classification
<200 mg/dL	Desirable blood cholesterol
200–239 mg/dL	Borderline-high blood cholesterol
≥240 mg/dL	High blood cholesterol

* With permission from National Cholesterol Education Program. Report of the Expert Panel on Detection, Evaluation, and Treatment of High Blood Cholesterol in Adults. Bethesda, U.S. Department of Health and Human Services, Public Health Service, National Institutes of Health, National Heart, Lung, and Blood Institute, January 1988, *NIH Publication 88-2925.*

Table 14–2.　Recommended Follow-up for Blood Cholesterol Management Based on Total Cholesterol*

Blood Cholesterol Level	Recommended Follow-up
Total cholesterol < 200 mg/dL	Repeat within 5 years
Total cholesterol 200–239 mg/dL without definite CHD or two other CHD risk factors	Dietary information and recheck annually
Total cholesterol 200–239 mg/dL with definite CHD or two other CHD risk factors (one of which can be male sex) Total cholesterol ≥ 240 mg/dL	Lipoprotein analysis: further action based on LDL-cholesterol level

* With permission from National Cholesterol Education Program. Report of the Expert Panel on Detection, Evaluation, and Treatment of High Blood Cholesterol in Adults. Bethesda, U.S. Department of Health and Human Services, Public Health Service, National Institutes of Health, National Heart, Lung, and Blood Institute, January, 1988, *NIH publication 88-2925.*

Dietary modification can alter serum lipid values in humans and animals.[22] A high intake of complex carbohydrate is generally associated with low CHD mortality rates, particularly when complex carbohydrate replaces saturated fat in the diet. Several recent reports are designed to assist health professionals who provide dietary therapy. The U.S. Department of Health and Human Services recently presented a synopsis of effective methods of dietary counseling.[23] In addition, the NCEP recommends a two-step approach of dietary therapy to reduce high levels of serum cholesterol (Table 14–3).[20] Each step emphasizes weight control. Step 1 is a moderately low-fat, low-cholesterol plan for persons with desirable cholesterol levels; it is offered as a "prudent diet." Step 1, however, is also the starting point in attempting to modify the diet of persons with moderate or high-risk cholesterol levels. Step 2, which further restricts dietary cholesterol, is for persons who fail to respond to step 1 efforts. Drug therapy is reserved for individuals who fail to respond to rigorous dietary modification, weight control, and exercise. A recent multicenter, double-blind, placebo-controlled study examined the utility of Lovastatin, a 3-hydroxy-3-methylglutaryl coenzyme A reductase inhibitor, as a form of drug therapy.[24] That study showed effective lowering of total and low-density lipoprotein cholesterol levels of about 33% in patients with diagnosed type IIa or IIb hypercholesterolemia. Lovastatin is an important pharmacologic agent for persons unable to respond to nonpharmacologic approaches to lowering cholesterol levels.[24]

Smoking

Substantial evidence incriminates cigarette smoking in CHD. Overall, smokers have a 70% greater level of CHD risk than nonsmokers. Persons who smoke two or more packs of cigarettes per day have a two- to threefold greater risk of CHD (Table 14–4 and Fig. 14–4).[25] The CHD

Table 14–3.　Dietary Therapy of High Blood Cholesterol, a Two-Step Approach*

Nutrient	Step One-Diet Intake	Step Two-Diet Intake
Total fat	<30% of total Kcal	<30% of total Kcal
Saturated fat	<10% of total Kcal	<10% of total Kcal
Polyunsaturated fat	≤10% of total Kcal	≤10% of total Kcal
Monounsaturated fat	10–15% of total Kcal	10–15% of total Kcal
Carbohydrates	50–60% of total Kcal	50–60% of total Kcal
Protein	10–20% of total Kcal	10–20% of total Kcal
Cholesterol	<300 mg/day	<200 mg/day
Total Kcal carbohydrates	Achieve and maintain desirable weight	Achieve and maintain desirable weight

* With permission from the National Cholesterol Education Program. Report of the Expert Panel on Population Strategies for Blood Cholesterol Reduction: Executive Summary. *Arch Intern Med, 151:*1071, 1991.

Table 14–4. Standardized CHD Incidence Ratio and Risk Ratios by Smoking Behavior in Five Cohort Studies (Individual and Pooled Results)*

Smoking Behavior	Standardized Incidence Ratio by Study Group					
	Pooling Project Research Group	Albany Cardiovascular Health Study	Chicago Peoples Gas Company Study	Chicago Western Electric Company Study	Framingham Heart Disease Epidemiology Study	Tecumseh Health Study
All	100	100	100	100	100	100
Nonsmokers	58	55	48	59	67	53†
Never smoked	54	45	53†	44	77†	60†
Past smoker	63	67	56	89	46†	50†
<½ pack/day	55	67†	43†	78	43†	†
Cigar and pipe only	71	78	58†	98	57	61†
Cigarette smokers						
About ½ pack/day	104	52†	64†	139	106	151†
About 1 pack/day	120	108	125	128	119	117
>1 pack/day	183	200	190	162	174	151
Risk ratio						
≥1 pack/ day:Nonsmokers	2.5	2.7	3.3	2.4	2.2	†
95% confidence interval	(2.1, 3.1)	(1.8, 4.3)	(2.1, 6.2)	(1.6, 3.7)	(1.5, 3.4)	
Risk ratio						
>1 pack/ day:Nonsmokers	3.2	3.7	4.0	2.8	2.6	†
95% confidence interval	(2.6, 4.2)	(2.4, 6.1)	(2.5, 8.4)	(1.2, 5.5)	(1.8, 4.5)	
Number of men at risk	8,282	1,796	1,258	1,926	2,162	1,140
Person-years of experience	70,970	17,240	11,017	16,072	19,756	6,885
Number of first events	644	154	123	140	178	49

* With permission from the Pooling Project Research Group. Relationship of blood pressure, serum cholesterol, smoking habit, relative weight, and ECG abnormalities to incidence of major coronary events: Final report of the Pooling Project. *J Chron Dis, 31*:202, 1978.
† Based on fewer than 10 first events

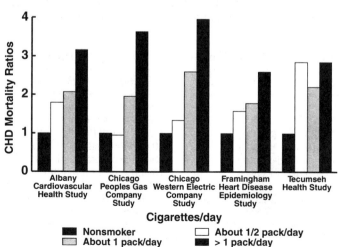

Fig. 14–4. Coronary heart disease mortality ratios according to the amount of cigarettes smoked in five populations. With permission from The Pooling Project Research Group: Relationship of blood pressure, serum cholesterol, smoking habit, relative weight, and ECG abnormalities to incidence of major coronary events: Final report of the Pooling Project. *J Chron Dis, 31:* 202, 1978.

risk also increases with depth of inhalation and with the total number of years as a smoker. However, persons who give up the smoking habit reduce their risk level to one that is close to that of nonsmokers.[25,26] Findings of laboratory studies suggest that smoking can accelerate atherogenesis and provoke myocardial infarction. Smoking increases platelet adhesiveness, damage to arterial endothelium, susceptibility to ventricular dysrhythmia, oxygen transport and utilization, heart rate, and blood pressure.[27,28] Cigarette smoking has an independent effect on CHD risk and acts synergistically with other well-established CHD risk factors. A variety of behavioral approaches can successfully promote smoking cessation.[29] Nicotine gum has also been proposed as a pharmacologic measure to assist smoking cessation efforts.[30]

Hypertension

The role of high blood pressure as a major risk factor for CHD and stroke is beyond serious doubt.[31-33] Blood pressure-related risk for CHD appears to increase continuously from lowest to highest values (Fig. 14–5).[34] No "ideal" blood pressure value truly exists; however, evidence suggests that with each increment in both systolic and diastolic pressure, the risk for adverse cardiovascular effects increases with time. Elevated blood pressure seldom works alone; it tends to work in concert with other well-identified risk factors including dietary intake, elevated lipids, obesity, smoking, diabetes mellitus, and lack of exercise.

The appropriate treatment of the pa-

Table 14–5. Classification of Blood Pressure in Adults Aged 18 Years and Older*

Range, mm Hg	Category
Diastolic	
< 85	Normal blood pressure
85–89	High normal blood pressure
90–104	Mild hypertension
105–114	Moderate hypertension
≥115	Severe hypertension
Systolic, when diastolic is < 90	
< 140	Normal blood pressure
140–159	Borderline isolated systolic hypertension
≥ 160	Isolated systolic hypertension

(With permission from National High Blood Pressure Education Program. The 1988 Report of the Joint National Committee on Detection, Evaluation, and Treatment of High Blood Pressure. *Arch Intern Med, 148*: 1023, 1988.)

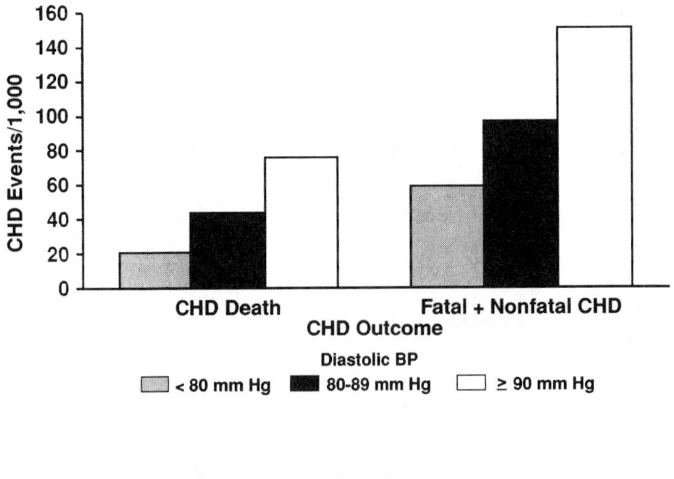

tient with elevated blood pressure begins with adequate documentation that the blood pressure values are elevated and the degree of elevation when discovered. Table 14–5 outlines the appropriate classifications of persons according to their measured levels of diastolic and systolic blood pressure.[35] After confirming hypertension, one must undertake an appropriate history, a physical examination, and an assessment of pathology. The primary goal of treating hypertensive patients is to prevent premature morbidity and mortality; therefore, successful treatment must reduce elevated blood pressure to a level that

Fig. 14–5. Rates of major coronary events in 12 years in relation to baseline diastolic blood pressure: Framingham Study, men aged 40 to 54 years at entry. With permission from The Framingham Study: An Epidemiological Investigation of Cardiovascular Disease. Section 31. The results of the Framingham Study applied to four other U.S.-based epidemiological studies of cardiovascular disease. Bethesda: National Heart, Lung, and Blood Institute, *DHEW Publication 76-1083*, 1976.

eliminates excessive cardiovascular risks. Table 14–6 outlines the recommended follow-up criteria for blood pressure measurement and steps towards effective therapeutic intervention of high blood pressure.

Therapeutic approaches include non-pharmacologic therapy, particularly weight reduction and reduced dietary sodium intake. Other ions including potassium, calcium, and magnesium, are suspected of influencing blood pressure, but the limited data for those ions do not warrant specific therapeutic recommendations.[36] Exercise is a recommended form of therapy. Recent reports suggest that regular physical activity that emphasizes rhythmic, sustained, and regular, moderate, muscular movement substantially lowers elevated blood pressure.[37] Epidemiologists, too, have identified a lower prevalence of hypertension in individuals who are more physically active.[38] Other therapeutic approaches include assessing alcohol consumption. Heavy consumption of alcohol (five drinks or more per day) is often associated with elevated blood pressure and cardiovascular damage. A dietary history of fat consumption, particularly the polyunsaturated to saturated ratio, appears critical. Appropriate intervention for tobacco use is also an integral part of a complete therapeutic process.[39,40]

Pharmacologic intervention to treat hypertension revolves around several available drugs. The choice of drug clearly relates to the level of blood pressure, and to the presence of target organ damage, diabetes mellitus, or other major risk factors for CHD and stroke. An ultimate goal of drug therapy is to maximize blood pressure control to achieve a normal or near normal level with a minimum of side effects. The 1988 Report of the Joint National Committee on Detection, Evaluation, and Treatment of High Blood Pressure offered guidelines for the stepped-care approach to treatment of hypertension.[35] One unresolved issue relates to the wisdom in treating patients with "mild" hypertension with drugs. Another unresolved issue is the "best" form of therapy for the elderly patient with so-called isolated systolic hypertension.[41–43]

Physical Inactivity

Powell and co-workers undertook an extensive review of 43 epidemiologic studies and concluded that physical activity has a protective effect on CHD.[44] Figure 14–6 represents the type of decline often noted in CHD risk with increasing physical activity.[45] Two thirds of the 43 studies showed

Table 14–6. Follow-up Criteria for Initial Blood Pressure Measurement for Adults Aged 18 Years or Older*

Range, mm Hg	Recommended Follow-up
Diastolic	
<85	Recheck within 2 years
85–89	Recheck within 1 year
90–104	Confirm within 2 months
105–114	Evaluate or refer promptly to source of care within 2 weeks
≥115	Evaluate or refer immediately to source of care
Systolic, when diastolic is <90	
<140	Recheck within 2 years
140–199	Confirm within 2 months
≥200	Evaluate or refer promptly to source of care within 2 weeks

* With permission from National High Blood Pressure Education Program. The 1988 Report of the Joint National Committee on Detection, Evaluation, and Treatment of High Blood Pressure. *Arch Intern Med, 148:* 1023, 1988.)

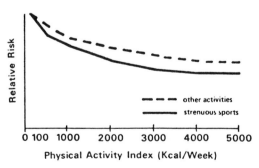

Fig. 14–6. Relative risks of first heart attack by physical activity index for strenuous sports and other activities in 6- to 10-year follow-up study of Harvard male alumni (first-order multiple logistic model). With permission from Paffenbarger RS Jr, Wing AL, Hyde RT: Physical activity as an index of heart attack risk in college alumni. *Am J Epidemiol, 108:*161, 1978.

a significant inverse relationship. However, an important additional finding was that the methodologically superior studies were more likely to report a significant inverse association. As the quality of the measure of physical activity, the measure of CHD outcome, and the epidemiologic methods improved, the results were more pronounced. Additional evidence reveals that physical activity may improve the likelihood of survival from a myocardial infarction.[46] Several studies of patients with documented CHD reveal that endurance exercise training may reduce morbidity and mortality.[47-51]

A variety of mechanisms may account for the protective effect of physical activity in reducing the risk of CHD and its progression. For example, physical activity may be a useful adjunct in eliminating or controlling other risk factors such as obesity, glucose intolerance, insulin insensitivity, and mild hypertension.[52,53] Exercise training can even lower blood lipid levels in normolipemic men.[54] In addition, studies show higher levels of HDL cholesterol in cross-sections of populations ranging from low to high on the physical activity continuum, in men who simply report some regular strenuous activity, and in endurance-trained athletes.[55-57] One study revealed higher HDL cholesterol level in previously inactive men after physical training.[58] Vigorous physical activity also reduces fasting triglyceride concentrations and enhances intravenous fat clearance. The net effect of these two alterations is to reduce the number of potentially atherogenic, triglyceride-rich lipoproteins.[59,60]

Studies of physical activity in animals have produced encouraging results regarding the reduction of CHD factors. However, these studies have not been successfully applied to humans. A physical training program applied to monkeys resulted in higher HDL and lower LDL and very low-density lipoprotein (VLDL) cholesterol and triglyceride levels with a concomitant lower incidence of coronary atherosclerosis.[61] Similar studies of coronary atherosclerosis in humans are not conclusive.[62] Also, studies of physical training in animals have shown an increase in the diameter of coronary arteries and proliferation of coronary collateral develop-

ment.[61,63,64] Angiographic investigations have failed to demonstrate collateral development in CHD patients after an extended period of physical training.[65,66]

Other effects of physical activity are acute increases in fibrinolysis and enhanced fibrinolytic capacity in response to venous occlusion, which may combat coronary thrombosis.[67,68] Physical activity can enhance myocardial electrical stability and decrease coronary vasospasm in response to adrenergic stimulation.[66,70] Physical training in humans increases cardiac parasympathetic tone, reducing the risk of ventricular fibrillation during cardiac ischemia.[71-73] These sources of experimental evidence show that physical activity may reduce the risk of CHD through risk factor modification, enhancement of myocardial perfusion, or offsetting the likelihood of acute coronary events.

No randomized, controlled clinical trials demonstrating the role of physical activity in CHD prevention exist or are currently under way. Such trials will not likely be forthcoming because of the expense, the required sample size to show a statistically significant effect, and problems with adherence to physical activity.[74,75] An analogous situation exists with conducting definitive dietary studies designed to lower CHD risk.

The review by Powell and co-workers also revealed that the calculated relative risk for CHD with reduced physical activity was about 1.9. This value was essentially similar to the relative risks associated with increased systolic blood pressure (2.1), cigarette smoking (2.5), and serum cholesterol (2.4) as found in the Pooling Project.[25] The number of individuals who are inactive is substantially greater than the number of persons who smoke cigarettes, have high levels of serum cholesterol, or have hypertension. Hence, the overall impact of stimulating Americans to be more physically active could effectively lower the country's CHD rates even more than by reducing any single one of the other three CHD risk factors.

Obesity

With rare exceptions, obesity evolves from eating too much and exercising too

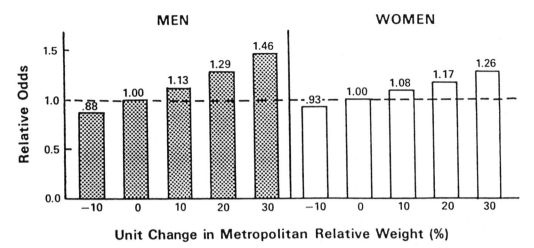

Fig. 14–7. The relative odds of developing cardiovascular disease corresponding to degrees of change in metropolitan relative weight between age 25 years and entry into the Framingham Study. The odds ratios reflect adjustments for the effects of relative weight at age 25 years and risk factor levels at exam 1. With permission from Hubert HB, et al.: Obesity as an independent risk factor for cardiovascular disease: A 26-year follow-up of participants in the Framingham Heart Study. *Circulation, 67*:968, 1983.

little. Obesity is associated with an excessive number of CHD deaths, especially sudden death in men and congestive heart failure in women. This high death rate appears to result largely from the influence of obesity on blood pressure, blood lipid levels, and the risk of precipitating the onset of diabetes. Recent reports from the Framingham Study, however, indicate the independence of obesity as a risk factor for CHD (Figs. 14–7 and 14–8).[76–78] An eating pattern low in saturated fat and cholesterol often leads to weight reduction. The weight reduction will, in time, improve the level of all major atherogenic risk factors with the exception of cigarette smoking.[79] Obesity is also associated with depressed HDL cholesterol levels. Weight control is a logical first step in the control of mild hypertension, hyperlipidemia, and impaired glucose tolerance. Further, weight control may eliminate the necessity of lifelong drug therapy for those conditions. Therapeutic efforts for weight control have been disappointing. Nonetheless, researchers have shown the effectiveness of combined programs of behavior modification and exercise.[52] Therapeutic approaches emphasizing increased levels of physical activity enhance caloric expenditure, and also draw on the beneficial effects of exercise in influencing blood lipids, blood pressure, mood, and attitude.[80–82] A public health approach entails a more comprehensive intervention strategy; the individual approach integrates itself within a stepped-care approach to weight reduction (Table 14–7).[52]

Table 14–7. Stepped-care Model for the Management of Obesity*

	Step			
	1	2	3	4
Action	Media programs Competitions Popular books Brochures Self-diet	Commercial programs Self-help groups	Clinical groups Aggressive diets	Individual programs Residential programs Surgery

* With permission from Brownell, K.D.: Public health approaches to obesity and its management. *Annu Rev Public Health, 7*:521, 1986.

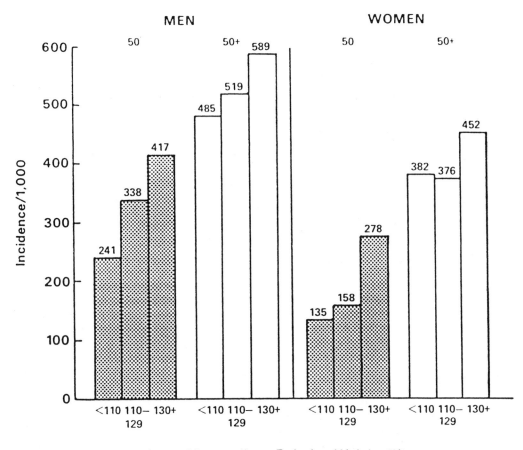

Fig. 14–8. Twenty-six year incidence of cardiovascular disease by metropolitan relative weight at entry among Framingham men and women aged < 50 years and ≥ 50 years. Numbers above the bars give the incidence rate per 1000. With permission from Hubert HB: The importance of obesity in the development of coronary risk factors and disease: The epidemiological evidence. *Annu Rev Public Health, 7:* 493, 1986.

Diabetes and Glucose Intolerance

Glucose intolerance, a direct effect of obesity, is often associated with hypertriglyceridemia, hypertension, elevated LDL cholesterol values, and depressed HDL values. Each of these factors may result in increased risk of CHD. Diabetes mellitus appears to have a vasculotoxic effect, which is greatest for occlusive peripheral vascular disease. However, the most common macrovascular manifestation of diabetes is CHD (Fig. 14–9).[83] The risk of CHD is twofold greater for diabetic men and threefold greater for diabetic women than for persons free of clinical diabetes.

The mortality rate from CHD for diabetic women appears to be similar to the rate for nondiabetic men of the same age. The control of hyperglycemia alone does not appear to reduce the risk of the macrovascular sequelae of diabetes mellitus. The excess risk is also not clearly related to the duration of diabetes. Clearly, individuals with diabetes are more likely than those without diabetes to have characteristics associated with an increased risk of CHD. Hence, it is critical to apply direct, aggressive attention toward the management of these risk factors. Special attention must center on effective weight control, adequate treatment of hypertension, smoking cessation, and increased levels of physical activity. A diet high in fiber, rich in com-

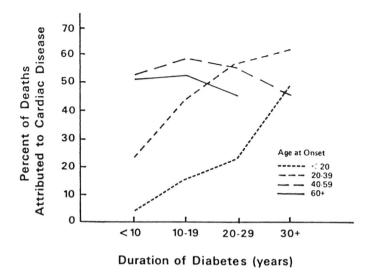

Fig. 14–9. Percent of deaths during 1956–68 attributed to cardiac disease among diabetic patients, by age at onset and duration of diabetes, Joslin Clinic. With permission from Barrett-Connor E, Orchard T: Diabetes and heart disease: In *Diabetes in America*. Edited by MI Harris and RF Hamman. Bethesda: *NIH Publication 85-1468*, 1985.

plex carbohydrate, and low in fat may be helpful. However, definitive evidence of the effectiveness of such dietary alterations is not yet available.

Psychosocial Stress

According to several prospective studies, persons with an overdeveloped sense of time-urgency, drive, and competitiveness (type A behavior) develop an excess of CHD (Fig. 14–10).[84–86] The mechanism is obscure but appears to be associated with the sympathetic nervous system and the se-

cretion of catecholamines.[87] The established major CHD risk factors seem to have a greater impact among type A persons. These relationships have been described primarily in white middle-aged men. Few studies exist implicating type A behavior as a CHD risk factor among women, blacks, Hispanics, and young adults. In addition, one study reveals that hostile type A persons are more likely to develop CHD than are nonhostile type A persons;[88] hostility may be the more explanatory factor.

Difficulty in assessing the behavior pattern has contributed to the discrepancies

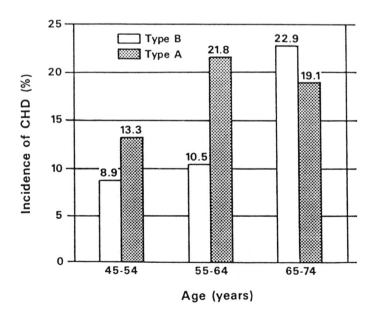

Fig. 14–10. Eight-year incidence of coronary heart disease among men by the Framingham Type A and B behavior patterns. With permission from Haynes SG, Feinleib M, Kannel WB: The relationship of psychosocial factors to coronary heart disease in the Framingham Study. III. Eight-year incidence of coronary heart disease. *Am J Epidemiol, 111:37,* 1980.

noted in studies investigating type A persons and CHD. Structured interviews tend to be the most reliable and valid forms of assessing the behavior pattern; pencil-and-paper methods are less effective.[89] Because authors of current reports emphasize results from studies employing various assessment tools, a consensus regarding the role of type A behavior and CHD is difficult to develop. Matthews and Haynes tried to evaluate these discrepancies.[89]

Various intervention methods can be effective in controlling the physiologic variables of type A behavior (e.g., heart rate, blood pressure, and catecholamine response). These methods include biofeedback, behavior modification, meditation, and exercise.[90] Currently, no researchers of intervention measures have documented a reduction in morbidity and mortality. Nonetheless, such intervention measures may enhance the quality of one's life.

Family History

A history of premature fatal or nonfatal stroke, fatal or nonfatal myocardial infarction, or sudden coronary death in siblings or parents suggest increased risk of CHD. A family history of diabetes, hypertension, or hyperlipidemia also increases the risk of CHD. The familial aggregation of CHD risk factors may often account for this familial aggregation of diseases. Authors have shown that, when considering the effects of CHD risk factors, the effect of family history on CHD risk appears to be minimal.[91] This finding was most recently shown in persons having a true family history of heart attack.[92] Therefore, the most prudent approach to CHD prevention and control is to direct efforts toward control of hyperlipidemia and hypertension, prevention and cessation of smoking, weight control, and increased physical activity. Researchers place special emphasis on interventions among persons possessing a familial tendency toward these modifiable risk factors and their premature disease outcomes.

CLUSTERING OF CHD RISK FACTORS

Many CHD risk factors aggregate with one another as well as with CHD (Fig. 14–11).[76,93,94] Therefore, individuals with

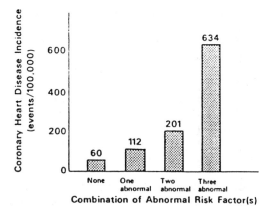

Fig. 14–11. Relationship between a combination of abnormal risk factors (cholesterol $\geq$ 250 mg/dL; systolic blood pressure $\geq$ 160 mm Hg; smoking $\geq$ 1 pack of cigarettes/day) and incidence of coronary heart disease. With permission from Kannel WB, Gordon T: The Framingham Study: An epidemiological investigation of cardiovascular disease. Section 30. Washington, Public Health Service, NIH, DHEW Publication (NIH) 74-599, 1974.

combinations of risk factors are at an increased risk for CHD. Obesity is an example of a risk factor for CHD that influences other potent risk factors, including hyperlipidemia, hypertension, and diabetes mellitus. Physical inactivity is associated with obesity, lipid abnormalities, hypertension, and diabetes mellitus.

Many risk factors evolve from similar health behavior patterns, and can be influenced by similar, and in some cases identical, intervention approaches. Thus, one must carefully evaluate any individual having one risk factor for CHD for the presence of other risk factors. Intervention strategies should focus on the specific health behavior patterns known to influence the greatest number of risk factors, then pay careful attention to these particular health behaviors in hope of simultaneously lowering the levels of multiple risk factors. The result could be a substantial reduction in overall risk for CHD.

INTERVENTION MEASURES

High-Risk Versus Population-Based Interventions

Substantially different rates of reduction in cardiovascular disease (including CHD) deaths may result when interventions target only persons with the highest risk factor levels rather than the entire population. Using data from the North Karelia Study, Kottke and coworkers applied a logistic risk function to a group at the top 10% of serum cholesterol and diastolic blood pressure risk distributions, as well the general North Karelia population.[95] They examined three types of intervention results and formulated specific criteria for attaining "achieved," "goal," and "ideal" intervention results for both approaches (Fig. 14–12). Achieved, goal, and ideal results in the high-risk approach would decrease individual serum cholesterol levels (only for persons with levels higher than 325 mg/dL) by 10%, by 20%, and to 190 mg/dL. Further, the achieved, goal, and ideal results would decrease individual diastolic blood pressure (only for people with levels higher than 105 mm Hg) to 95, 90, and 85 mm Hg, respectively. Achieved, goal, and ideal results in the population-based approach would decrease the population mean of serum cholesterol levels by 10%, by 20%, and to 190 mg/dl. Also, the achieved, goal, and ideal results would decrease the population mean diastolic blood pressure by 5%, by 10%, and to 80 mm Hg, respectively. As shown in Figure 14–12, the population-based intervention strategy would yield a cardiovascular disease death rate in the entire population that was nearly two times lower for each of the three intervention results. In fact, lowering the risk factor levels to the ideal level for the high-risk group would not yield death rates that were substantially lower than the achieved results of the population based approach. The findings support the use of the population-based intervention approach because so many persons should lower their levels of CHD risk factors. In addition, an approach that includes a focused strategy for persons known to be at high risk appears warranted.

Many practical problems arise when treating a patient with several risk factors. The critical issue becomes which intervention measures to use and in what order to use them. Because of the many ways in which cigarette smoking can affect the cardiorespiratory system, smoking is probably the most important risk factor to attack. A group of researchers in Oslo demonstrated the utility of both smoking cessation and dietary intervention among high-risk patients.[96] Hypertension control can also bring about immediate reductions in risk. Although it is not empirically established, patients may find that changing their physical activity pattern is less imposing and more enjoyable than giving up cigarettes and high-fat foods. After the patient establishes a stable physical activity pattern, it may be feasible to integrate steps to promote smoking cessation and dietary modification. Changes in physical activity should not be used as an excuse to avoid making changes in the other high-risk factors for CHD. Use of health education techniques is also important to provide information on all the risk factors and to es-

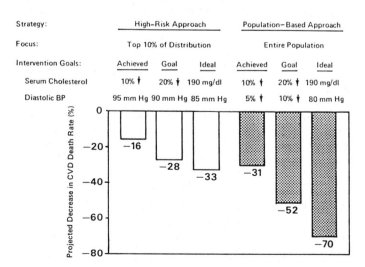

Fig. 14–12. Projected decrease in cardiovascular disease death rates using high-risk versus population-based approaches for three types of intervention goals. With permission from Kottke TE, et al.: Projected effects of high-risk versus population-based prevention strategies in coronary heart disease. *Am J Epidemiol, 121:*697, 1985.

tablish the patient's perceived ability and willingness to make changes.

REFERENCES

1. Goldman L, Cook EF: The decline in ischemic heart disease mortality rates. *Ann Intern Med, 101:*825, 1984.
2. Last JM: *A Dictionary of Epidemiology.* 2nd Edition. New York: Oxford University Press, 1988.
3. Keys A: *Seven Countries: A Multivariate Analysis of Death and Coronary Heart Disease.* Cambridge, Harvard University Press, 1980.
4. Blackburn H: Diet and mass hyperlipidemia: A public health view. In *Nutrition, Lipids, and Coronary Heart Disease.* Edited by RI Levy, et al. New York: Raven Press, 1976.
5. Kannel WB, et al.: Overall and CHD mortality rates in relation to major risk factors in 325,348 men screened for MRFIT. *Am Heart J, 112:*825, 1986.
6. Williams RR, et al.: Evidence that men with familial hypercholesterolemia can avoid early coronary death. *JAMA, 255:*219, 1986.
7. Glueck CJ, Connor WE: Diet-coronary heart disease relationships reconnoitered. *Am J Clin Nutr, 31:*727, 1978.
8. Tyroler HA: Total serum cholesterol and ischemic heart disease in clinical and observational studies. *Am J Prev Med, 1:*18, 1984.
9. Lipid Research Clinics Program: The Lipid Research Clinics Coronary Primary Prevention Trial results. I & II. *JAMA, 251:*351, 1984.
10. Brensike JF, et al.: Effects of therapy with cholestyramine on progression of coronary arteriosclerosis: Results of the NHLBI Type II Coronary Intervention Study. *Circulation, 69:*313, 1984.
11. Levy RI, et al.: The influence of changes in lipid values induced by cholestyramine and diet on progression of coronary artery disease: Results of the NHLBI Type II Coronary Intervention Study. *Circulation, 69:*325, 1984.
12. Castelli WP, et al.: HDL cholesterol and other lipids in coronary heart disease. The cooperative lipoprotein phenotyping study. *Circulation, 55:*767, 1977.
13. Olefsky JM, Reaven GM, Farquhar JW: Effects of weight reduction on obesity: Studies of lipid and carbohydrate metabolism in normal and hyperlipoproteinemic subjects. *J Clin Invest, 53:*64, 1974.
14. Wood PD, et al.: Increased exercise level and plasma lipoprotein concentrations: A one year randomized, controlled study in sedentary middle aged men. *Metabolism, 32:*31, 1983.
15. Hartung GH, et al.: Effect of alcohol intake and exercise on plasma high-density lipoprotein cholesterol subfractions and apolipoprotein A-1 in women. *Am J Cardiol, 58:*148, 1986.
16. Miller GJ, Miller NE: Plasma HDL concentration and development of ischemic heart disease. *Lancet, 1:*16, 1975.
17. Gordon T, et al.: The prediction of coronary heart disease by high-density and other lipoproteins: An historical perspective. In *Hyperlipidemia: Diagnosis and Therapy.* Edited by B.M. Rifkind and R.I. Levy. New York: Grune and Stratton, 1977.
18. Consensus Conference: Lowering blood cholesterol to prevent heart disease. *JAMA, 251:*365, 1984.
19. National Cholesterol Education Program. Report of the Expert Panel on Detection, Evaluation, and Treatment of High Blood Cholesterol in Adults. Bethesda, U.S. Department of Health and Human Services, Public Health Service, National Institutes of Health, National Heart, Lung, and Blood Institute; *NIH publication 88-2925,* 1988.
20. National Cholesterol Education Program. Report of the expert panel on population strategies for blood cholesterol reduction: Executive summary. *Arch Intern Med, 151:*1071, 1991.
21. Sacks FM, et al.: Plasma lipids and lipoproteins in vegetarians and controls. *N Engl J Med, 292:*1148, 1975.
22. Vesselinovitch D, et al.: Reversal of advanced atherosclerosis in rhesus monkeys. I. Light microscopic studies. *Atherosclerosis, 23:*155, 1976.
23. Heart to Heart: A Manual on Nutrition Counseling for the Reduction of Cardiovascular Disease Risk Factors. Bethesda, U.S. Department of Health and Human Services, Public Health Service, *NIH publication 83-1528,* 1983.
24. The Lovastatin Study Group II: Therapeutic response to Lovastatin (mevinolin) in nonfamilial hypercholesterolemia. A multicenter study. *JAMA, 265:*2829, 1986.
25. Pooling Project Research Group. Relationship of blood pressure, serum cholesterol, smoking habit, relative weight, and ECG abnormalities to incidence of major coronary events: Final report of the Pooling Project. *J Chronic Dis, 31:*202, 1978.
26. Gordon T, Kannel WB, McGee D: Death and coronary attacks in men after giving up cigarette smoking. *Lancet, 2:*1348, 1974.
27. Kannel WB, Castelli WP, McNamara PM: Cigarette smoking and risk of CHD: Epidemiologic clues to pathogenesis. The Framingham Study: *NCI Monograph, 28:*9, 1968.

28. U.S. Department of Health and Human Services: Smoking and Health: A report of the Surgeon General. Washington, *DHHS Publication (PHS) 79-50066, 1979.*

29. Health and Public Policy Committee, American College of Physicians: Methods for stopping cigarette smoking. *Ann Intern Med, 105:*281, 1986.

30. Hughes JR, Miller SA: Nicotine gum to help stop smoking. *JAMA, 252:*2855, 1984.

31. Gordon T, Sorlie P, Kannel WB: Problems in the assessment of blood pressure. The Framingham Study. *Int J Epidemiol, 5:*327, 1976.

32. Freis E: Salt volume and the prevention of hypertension. *Circulation, 53:*589, 1976.

33. Berglund G, et al.: Coronary heart disease after treatment of hypertension. *Lancet, 1:* 1, 1978.

34. The Framingham Study: An epidemiological investigation of cardiovascular disease. Section 31. The results of the Framingham Study applied to four other U.S.-based epidemiological studies of cardiovascular disease. Bethesda, National Heart, Lung, and Blood Institute, *DHEW publication (NIH) 76-1083, 1976.*

35. National High Blood Pressure Education Program. The 1988 Report of the Joint National Committee on Detection, Evaluation, and Treatment of High Blood Pressure. *Arch Intern Med, 148:*1023, 1988.

36. An epidemiological approach to describing risk associated with blood pressure levels: Final report of the Working Group on Risk and High Blood Pressure. *Hypertension, 7:* 641, 1985.

37. Levine DM, et al.: Health education for hypertensive patients. *JAMA, 241:*1700, 1979.

38. Paffenbarger RS Jr, et al.: Physical activity and incidence of hypertension. *Am J Epidemiol, 117:*245, 1983.

39. Stamler R, et al.: Primary prevention of hypertension. *Circulation, 68:*362, 1983.

40. Boyer JL, Kasch FW: Exercise therapy in hypertensive men. *JAMA, 211:*1668, 1970.

41. Toth PJ, Horwitz RI: Conflicting clinical trials and the uncertainty of treating mild hypertension. *Am J Med, 75:*482, 1983.

42. Hypertension Detection and Follow-up Program Cooperative Group: Results of the Hypertension Detection and Follow-up Program. *N Engl J Med, 307:*976, 1982.

43. Working Group on Hypertension in the Elderly, National High Blood Pressure Education Program: Statement on hypertension in the elderly. JAMA, *256:*70, 1986.

44. Powell KE, Thompson PD, Caspersen CJ, Kendrick JS: Physical activity and the incidence of coronary heart disease. *Annu Rev Public Health, 8:*253, 1987.

45. Paffenbarger RS Jr, Wing AL, Hyde RT: Physical activity as an index of heart attack risk in college alumni. *Am J Epidemiol, 108:* 161, 1978.

46. Morris JN, et al.: Coronary heart disease and physical activity of work. *Lancet, 2:* 1053, 1953.

47. May GS, et al.: Secondary prevention after myocardial infarction: A review of long term trials. *Prog Cardiovasc Dis, 24:*331, 1982.

48. Barnard RJ: Effects of an intensive exercise and nutrition program in patients with coronary artery disease: Five year follow-up. *J Cardiac Rehab, 3:*183, 1983.

49. Kavanagh T, et al.: Prognostic indexes for patients with ischemic heart disease enrolled in an exercise-centered rehabilitation program. *Am J Cardiol, 44:*1230, 1979.

50. Oldridge NB, Guyatt GH, Fisher ME, Rimm AA: Cardiac rehabilitation after myocardial infarction. Combined experience of randomized controlled trials. *JAMA, 260:*945, 1988.

51. O'Connor GT, et al.: An overview of randomized trials of rehabilitation with exercise after myocardial infarction. *Circulation, 80:*234, 1989.

52. Brownell KD: Public health approaches to obesity and its management. *Annu Rev Public Health, 7:*521, 1986.

53. Kemmer FW, Berger M: Exercise and diabetes mellitus: Physical activity as part of daily life and its role in the treatment of diabetic patients. *Int J Sports Med, 4:*77, 1983.

54. Farrell PA, Barboriak J: Time course in alterations in plasma lipid and lipoprotein concentrations during eight weeks of endurance training. *Atherosclerosis, 27:*231, 1980.

55. LaPorte RE, et al.: The spectrum of physical activity, cardiovascular disease and health: An epidemiologic perspective. *Am J Epidemiol, 120:*507, 1984.

56. Haskell WL, et al: Strenuous physical activity, treadmill exercise test performance and plasma high-density lipoprotein cholesterol. The Lipid Research Clinics Program Prevalence Study, *Circulation, 62:*53, 1980.

57. Wood PD, et al.: The distribution of plasma lipoproteins in middle aged male runners. *Metabolism, 25:*1249, 1976.

58. Kiens B, et al.: Increased plasma HDL-cholesterol and apo A-1 in sedentary middle age men after physical conditioning. *Eur J Clin Invest, 10:*203, 1980.

59. Sady SP, et al.: Prolonged exercise augments plasma triglyceride clearance. *JAMA, 256:*2552, 1986.

60. Zilversmit, DB: Atherogenesis: A postpran-

dial phenomenon. *Circulation, 60:*473, 1979.

61. Kramsch DM, et al.: Reduction of coronary atherosclerosis by moderate conditioning exercise in monkeys on an atherogenic diet. *N Engl J Med, 305:*1483, 1981.

62. Stamler J, et al.: Prevalence and incidence of coronary heart disease in strata of the labor force of a Chicago industrial corporation. *J Chronic Dis, 11:*405, 1960.

63. Wyatt HL, Mitchell J: Influences of physical conditioning and deconditioning on coronary vasculature of dogs. *J Appl Physiol, 45:*619, 1978.

64. Neill WA, Oxendine JM: Exercise can promote coronary collateral development without improving perfusion of ischemic myocardium. *Circulation, 60:*1513, 1979.

65. Nolewajka AJ, et al.: Exercise and human collateralization: An angiographic and scintigraphic assessment. *Circulation, 60:*114, 1979.

66. Kennedy CC, et al.: One-year graduated exercise program for men with angina pectoris. Evaluation by physiologic studies and coronary arteriography. *Mayo Clin Proc, 51:*231, 1976.

67. Rosing DR, et al.: Blood fibrinolytic activity in man. Diurnal variation and in response to varying intensities of exercise. *Circ Res, 27:*171, 1970.

68. Williams RS, et al.: Physical conditioning augments the fibrinolytic response to venous occlusion in healthy adults. *N Engl J Med, 302:*987, 1980.

69. Bove AA, Dewey JD: Proximal coronary vasomotor reactivity after exercise training in dogs. *Circulation, 71:*620, 1985.

70. Maseri A, et al.: Coronary vasospasm as a possible cause of myocardial infarction. A conclusion derived from the study of "preinfarction" angina. *N Engl J Med, 299:*1271, 1978.

71. Kenney WL: Parasympathetic control of resting heart rate: Relationship to aerobic power. *Med Sci Sports Exerc, 17:*451, 1985.

72. Billman GE, Schwartz PJ, Stone HL: The effects of daily exercise on susceptibility to sudden cardiac death. *Circulation, 69:*1182, 1984.

73. Noakes TD, Higginson L, Opie LH: Physical training increases ventricular fibrillation thresholds of isolated rat hearts during normoxia, hypoxia, and regional ischemia. *Circulation, 67:*24, 1983.

74. Friedewald WT: Physical activity research and coronary heart disease. *Public Health Rep, 100:*115, 1985.

75. Taylor HL, Buskirk ER, Remington RD: Exercise in controlled trials of the prevention of coronary heart disease. *Fed Proc, 32:*1623, 1973.

76. Kannel WB, Gordon T: The Framingham Study: An epidemiological investigation of cardiovascular disease. Section 30. Washington, Public Health Service, *NIH, DHEW Publication (NIH) 74-599,* 1974.

77. Hubert HB, et al.: Obesity as an independent risk factor for cardiovascular disease: A 26-year follow-up of participants in the Framingham Heart Study. *Circulation, 67:*968, 1983.

78. Hubert HB: The importance of obesity in the development of coronary risk factors and disease: The epidemiological evidence. *Annu Rev Public Health, 7:*493, 1986.

79. Ashley FW Jr, Kannel WB: Relation of weight change to changes in atherogenic traits. The Framingham Study. *J Chronic Dis, 27:*103, 1974.

80. Seals DR, Hagberg JM: The effect of exercise training on human hypertension: A review. *Med Sci Sports Exerc, 16:*207, 1984.

81. Blair SN, Jacobs DR Jr, Powell KE: Relationships between exercise or physical activity and other health behaviors. *Public Health Rep, 100:*172, 1985.

82. Taylor CB, Sallis JF, Needle R: The relation of physical activity and exercise to mental health. *Public Health Rep, 100:*195, 1985.

83. Barrett-Connor E, Orchard T: Diabetes and heart disease. In *Diabetes in America.* Edited by MI Harris and RF Hamman. Bethesda, *NIH Publication 85-1468,* 1985.

84. Jenkins CD, Rosenman RH, Zyzanski SJ: Prediction of clinical coronary heart disease by a test for coronary-prone behavior pattern. *N Engl J Med 290:*1271, 1974.

85. Haynes SG, Feinleib M, Kannel WB: The relationship of psychosocial factors to coronary heart disease in the Framingham Study. III. Eight-year incidence of coronary heart disease. *Am J Epidemiol, 111:*37, 1980.

86. Jenkins CD: Psychological and social precursors of coronary disease. *N Engl J Med, 244:*207, 1971.

87. von Eulen US: Quantitation of stress by catecholamine analysis. *Clin Pharmacol Ther, 5:*398, 1964.

88. Shekelle RB, et al.: The MRFIT Behavior Pattern Study II: Type A behavior and the incidence of coronary heart disease. *Am J Epidemiol, 122:*559, 1985.

89. Matthews KA, Haynes SG: Type A behavior pattern and coronary disease risk: Update and critical evaluation. *Am J Epidemiol, 123:*923, 1986.

90. Elliot RS, Forker AD, Robertson RJ: Aero-

bic exercise as a therapeutic modality in the relief of stress. *Adv Cardiol, 18:*231, 1976.

91. Perkins KA: Family history of coronary heart disease: Is it still an independent risk factor? *Am J Epidemiol, 124:*182, 1986.

92. Khaw KT, Barrett-Connor E: Family history of heart attack: A modifiable risk factor? *Circulation, 74:*239, 1986.

93. Criqui MH, et al.: Clustering of cardiovascular disease risk factors. *Prev Med, 9:*525, 1980.

94. Gotto A: Interactions of the major risk factors for coronary heart disease. *Am J Med, 80(Suppl):*48, 1986.

95. Kottke TE, et al.: Projected effects of high-risk versus population-based prevention strategies in coronary heart disease. *Am J Epidemiol, 121:*697, 1985.

96. Hjermann I, et al.: Effect of diet and smoking intervention on the incidence of coronary heart disease: Report of the Oslo Study Group of a randomized trial in healthy men. *Lancet, 2:*1303, 1981.

Chapter 15

CORONARY ATHEROSCLEROSIS AND ACUTE MYOCARDIAL INFARCTION

Ray W. Squires and William L. Williams

Atherosclerosis is the leading cause of death in industrialized countries, and although the disease was recognized in the 19th century, it has become more prevalent and appreciated in the 20th century.[1] Atherosclerosis involving the coronary arteries (coronary artery disease, ischemic heart disease) may result in the clinical problems of angina pectoris, myocardial infarction, sudden cardiac death, and congestive heart failure. Annually, in the United States, approximately 1,500,000 persons suffer myocardial infarction (MI), and one quarter of all deaths in the United States result from MI.[2] Coronary artery disease is not necessarily an inevitable consequence of a genetic predisposition and the aging process. Multiple environmental risk factors are suggested by the variation in incidence of coronary artery disease around the world.[3] This is powerfully illustrated by the observation that migrants, on leaving an area of lower incidence of cardiovascular mortality, assume the higher incidence in their new country.[4]

Arteries undergo changes associated with the aging process such as thickening of the intima, loss of elastic connective tissue, an increase in calcium content, and an increase in diameter.[5] These natural changes occur throughout the arterial tree and are referred to as *arteriosclerosis*.[5] In contrast, *atherosclerosis* is a pathologic phenomenon resulting in obstructive lesions primarily in the aorta, coronary, carotid, iliac, and femoral arteries.[6] The disease is a multifactorial process, and many risk factors (characteristics associated with an increased probability of developing the disease) have been identified, such as cigarette smoking, a blood lipid profile including elevated low-density lipoprotein cholesterol (LDL-C) and depressed high-density lipoprotein cholesterol (HDL-C) concentrations, hypertension, genetic factors, dia-

betes mellitus, sedentary lifestyle, psychosocial disturbances, male gender, and obesity.[3,4] Risk factors may be causally related to the disease or merely associated with an increased chance of developing the disorder. This chapter reviews the process of coronary atherosclerosis, the clinical syndromes resulting from the disease, and the medical therapies used in the management of the disease.

THE NORMAL CORONARY ARTERY

Arteries are lined by a single layer of metabolically active cells, the *endothelium,* which serves as a barrier between the blood and the artery wall (Fig. 15–1). The channel for blood flow within the artery is the *lumen.* The endothelial cells are connected to each other at their borders and rest on a basement membrane.[7] The endothelium is selectively permeable and controls the passage of molecules from the blood into the arterial wall. Various receptors (for example, low-density lipoprotein and growth factors) are located on the endothelium, and endothelial cells are capable of producing several vasoactive substances, such as prostacyclin (a vasodilator and inhibitor of platelet aggregation) angiotensin-converting enzyme (important in vasoconstriction), and connective tissue molecules.[7,8] The endothelium can produce substances capable of dissolving blood clots, such as plasminogen, or molecules which promote clotting (von Willebrand factor).[6] Endothelium can synthesize a form of platelet-derived growth factor that stimulates growth of connective tissue and smooth muscle. When activated to produce growth factors, the endothelium plays a role in atherosclerosis.[6,7,9]

Underneath the endothelial basement membrane is the *intima,* a thin layer of connective tissue with an occasional smooth muscle cell (Fig. 15–1). The intima is the

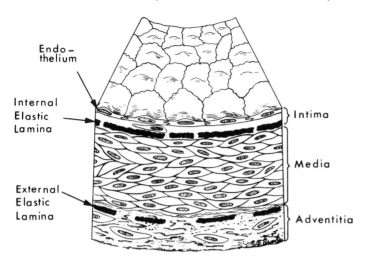

Endo-thelium

Internal Elastic Lamina

External Elastic Lamina

Intima

Media

Adventitia

Fig. 15-1. The normal coronary artery wall. With permission from Ross R, Glomset J: The pathogenesis of atherosclerosis. *N Engl J Med*, 295:369, 1976.

area of the arterial wall in which the obstructive lesions of atherosclerosis form.[7]

The *media* contains most of the smooth muscle cells of the arterial wall in addition to elastic connective tissue, and is located between the internal and external elastic laminae just under the intima (Fig. 15-1). The laminae consist of elastic connective tissue with pores to allow passage of cells and other substances in either direction.[7] Advanced atherosclerosis is characterized by proliferation of smooth muscle cells derived from the media. Smooth muscle cells maintain arterial tone by their characteristic prolonged contractions. The smooth muscle responds to various vasoactive stimuli, such as epinephrine and angiotensin which cause vasoconstriction, and vasodilators like prostacyclin. Smooth muscle cells possess receptors for numerous particles, which include low-density lipoprotein, insulin, and platelet-derived growth factor.[10,11] Smooth muscle cells in the artery are capable of either functioning as contractile cells (as in maintenance of arterial wall tension) or, when properly stimulated, as synthetic cells.[12] When in the synthetic mode of action, these cells are sensitive to growth factors and become involved in the formation of connective tissue and are directly implicated in the atherosclerotic process.

The *adventitia* is the outermost layer of the artery and consists of collagen, elastin, fibroblasts (another cell capable of forming connective tissue), and some smooth muscle cells (Fig. 15-1). This layer is highly vascular (its blood supply from small vessels is called the vasa vasorum) and provides the media with oxygen and nutrients.[7]

ATHEROGENESIS: RESPONSE TO INJURY

Research performed over the past several decades has revealed much about the development and progression of atherosclerosis (*atherogenesis*), although our understanding of the disease is incomplete. The initial event is injury to the arterial wall with a subsequent inflammatory response leading to a proliferation (growth) of tissue in the arterial wall, which may result in obstruction of blood flow.[6,7] The process may begin in childhood and progress over many years before symptoms occur.

Injury to endothelial cells may result from the following factors: tobacco smoke or other tobacco substances, hypercholesterolemia, hypertension, turbulent blood flow, immune complexes, vasoconstrictor substances, and viral infections.[6,13-15] Injury may result in *endothelial dysfunction*, leading to increased permeability to substances in the blood, an increased tendency to form small blood clots (increased *thrombogenesis*), and greater tendency for adherence of substances to the endothelial cells.[7,16] LDL-C may alter the surface characteristics of the endothelial cells, thus potentiating the adherence of cells and other substances to the arterial wall.

Platelets adhere to the injured endothelium (*platelet aggregation*), form small blood clots (*mural thrombi*), and release growth factors and vasoactive agents. Atherosclerosis appears to thrive in a hyperthrombotic state. Platelets, after adhering to the endothelium, release thromboxane A_2, a potent vasoconstrictor, and may cause additional vascular injury.[6,7] A hyperthrombotic state may result from excessive catecholamine levels or may represent a genetic trait.[17,18] An impaired ability to dissolve intra-arterial thrombi (*fibrinolysis*) may result from higher than normal levels of lipoprotein (a) [Lp(a)], a potentially atherogenic lipoprotein distinct from LDL.[19] Platelet-derived growth factor (PDGF) binds to specific receptors on the endothelium and causes growth of certain tissues (*mitogenic* effect) and the migration of specific types of cells into the area of injury (*chemotactic* effect).[6,20]

Monocytes, from the blood, also adhere to the endothelium, accumulate cholesterol from the blood and are transformed into a different type of cell, the *macrophage*.[7] Growth factors, such as PDGF, are believed to enhance monocyte binding to endothelial cells; and to increase the number of LDL receptors on the endothelium, thus inducing greater LDL binding, increased deposition of cholesterol into the arterial wall, and increased cholesterol synthesis within the macrophage.[7,10]

In response to growth factors, *smooth muscle cells* and *fibroblasts* (a type of relatively nondifferentiated connective tissue cell that can form fibrous tissue) migrate from the media to the intima.[7,20] These cells then accumulate cholesterol (cholesterol is also deposited extracellularly), forming *foam cells*, which give rise to *fatty streaks*, the earliest visually detectable (yellow macroscopic appearance) lesion of atherosclerosis (Fig. 15–2).[21] *T-lymphocytes* (immune cells) are present in early fatty streaks, and are associated with monocytes and macrophages.[22] Their place in atherogenesis is unknown, but may indicate a role for the immune system in the process.[23]

Additional production of growth factors from several different cell types (platelets, injured endothelial cells, monocytes, smooth muscle cells) results in continued *proliferation* (increased cell numbers and cell size) of smooth muscle cells as well as the formation of *fibrous connective tissue* by fibroblasts and smooth muscle cells.[7,24] With continued accumulation of connective tissue, smooth muscle, other cellular debris, and cholesterol, the lesion progresses in size and appearance to a *fibromuscular plaque* (Fig. 15–2). The plaque is firm in texture and pale gray in color, and often contains a yellow cholesterol core called the *atheroma*. As the plaque increases in size and reduces the vessel internal diameter, obstruction of blood flow may begin.[6,7] Progression in size of the lesion occurs at

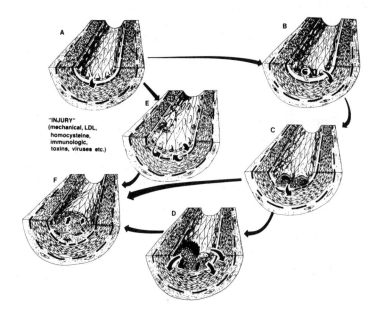

Fig. 15–2. The atherosclerotic process—response to injury. **A.** Injury to endothelium with release of growth factors (small arrow). **B.** Monocytes attach to endothelium. **C.** Monocytes migrate to intima, take up cholesterol, form fatty streaks. **D.** Platelets adhere to the endothelium and release growth factors. **F.** The result is a fibromuscular plaque. An alternative pathway is shown with arrows from A to E to F, with growth factor-initiated migration of smooth muscle cells from the media to the intima (**E**). With permission from Ross R: The pathogenesis of atherosclerosis—An update. *N Engl J Med, 314*:496, 1986.

extremely variable rates. Some lesions appear stable over many years; other lesions progress wildly in a matter of months. A plausible explanation for the varying rates of progression is not currently available.

As a result of local stress on the atherosclerotic lesion (for example, turbulent blood flow or vasoconstriction), *fissuring* or *rupture* of the plaque may occur, exposing the contents of the inside of the lesion to the blood.[25] These sites may form thrombi of varying sizes. Over time, fibrous organization of the thrombi occurs and the tissue is incorporated into the plaque. These thrombi may form repeatedly, giving a layered appearance to the lesion and resulting in progression of the size of the lesion. These complicated lesions, which include organized thrombus, are called *advanced atherosclerotic plaques* (Fig. 15–2).[6,7]

Coronary atherosclerosis tends to affect vessels in a diffuse manner with occasional discrete, localized areas of more pronounced narrowing that produce obstruction of blood flow.[26] Selective coronary angiography is used to diagnose the extent and severity of disease and is considered the gold standard (best available technique). However, based on comparisons of angiography and autopsy findings, other than in instances of complete blockage, the degree of stenosis (obstruction) tends to be underestimated by angiography because of the diffuse characteristic of the disease.[27] Obstructive coronary atherosclerosis tends to occur more frequently in the first 4 to 5 centimeters of the epicardial coronary arteries, although lesions can occur anywhere in the coronary tree (Fig. 15–3).[26] Ostial lesions (at the origin of the left main and main right coronary arteries) may occur. Women tend to lag 5 to 20 years behind men in the extent and severity of coronary atherosclerosis.[28] The precise reasons for the gender differences remain to be determined.

Coronary risk factors are associated with the development of atherosclerosis on the basis of epidemiologic studies evaluating factors common to persons with the disease.[3,4] (See Chap. 14.) Possible mechanisms of the effect of some risk factors on atherogenesis have been investigated, although a clear understanding of all actions of risk factors is not presently available.

It is known that tobacco smoke increases platelet activity and hence the tendency for thrombi to form on the endothelial cells.[29] Smoking also reduces HDL-C, which is involved in reverse cholesterol transport (described in more detail below) and increases blood catecholamine levels, which may injure the endothelium directly. The carbon monoxide in smoke results in arterial wall hypoxia.[30–32]

Much investigation into the roles of plasma lipoproteins in the atherosclerotic process has occurred over the past several decades. Data from epidemiologic and experimental studies have strengthened the cholesterol-atherosclerosis hypothesis, although a complete understanding of the precise mechanisms is not yet available. The plasma lipoproteins are water-soluble

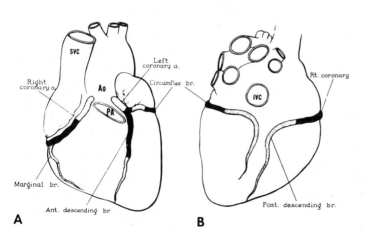

Fig. 15–3. The epicardial coronary arteries. **A.** Anterior view. **B.** Posterior view. Black segments are prime sites for the development of high grade stenoses. Ao = aorta, IVC = inferior vena cava, SVC = superior vena cava, PA = pulmonary artery. With permission from Lie JT: Atherosclerosis B. Pathology of coronary artery disease. In *Cardiology: Fundamentals and Practice.* Second Edition. Edited by ER Giuliani, V Fuster, BJ Gersh, MD McGoon, DC McGoon. Chicago: Mosby Yearbook, 1991, pp. 1211–1231.

complexes of lipids (cholesterol, triglycerides, phospholipids) and specific proteins (apolipoproteins).[33] They originate in the liver and/or intestine. Five classes have been described as follows.

1. *Chylomicrons*—triglyceride-rich particles produced in the intestine after a fatty meal, which enter the circulation through the thoracic duct. After a half-life of a few minutes, they are degraded to remnant particles by the enzyme lipoprotein lipase and are taken up by the liver. They are probably not atherogenic.

2. *Very Low Density Lipoprotein* (VLDL)—secreted by the liver into the circulation and transport mostly triglyceride and a small amount of cholesterol (10 to 15% of the total cholesterol). VLDL undergoes degradation in the blood by lipoprotein lipase to intermediate density lipoprotein. Some epidemiologic data suggest that elevated VLDL (increased triglycerides) may be a risk factor for atherosclerosis.

3. *Intermediate Density Lipoprotein* (IDL)—converted to low density lipoprotein by the liver.

4. *Low Density Lipoprotein* (LDL)—transports 60 to 70% of the total cholesterol. The major apolipoprotein is apo B, and this lipoprotein is felt to be the most atherogenic particle. In the disorder called familial hypercholesterolemia, a genetic LDL receptor defect is present, which dramatically affects total cholesterol concentrations and coronary risk.[34] In heterozygous familial hypercholesterolemia, one defective and one normal LDL receptor gene are present (this occurs in 1 in 500 persons); total cholesterol is 350 to 400 mg/dL; and coronary atherosclerosis often becomes symptomatic in the fourth or fifth decade of life. The homozygous form of the disease is very rare (1 in 1,000,000 persons) and results in total cholesterol concentrations of over 600 mg/dL with myocardial infarction often in childhood or adolescence. Polygenic hypercholesterolemia is a much more common abnormality that involves a relative deficiency of functioning LDL receptors with elevated total cholesterol concentrations in the setting of a high fat/cholesterol diet.[35]

5. *High Density Lipoprotein* (HDL)—transports 20–30% of the total cholesterol. Apo A_1 is the major apolipoprotein and is inversely related to the risk of developing coronary artery disease. HDL probably mediates reverse cholesterol transport, the process by which cholesterol is removed from sites of deposit and transported to the liver for excretion. Extremely low HDL-C levels are seen in familial hypoalphalipoproteinemia caused by a reduced synthesis of apo A-I.[36] Individuals with this condition develop premature coronary artery disease. With ultracentrifugation, HDL subfractions (HDL_2, HDL_3) may be identified, although these subfractions do not predict coronary atherosclerosis risk any better than HDL-C.

Hypercholesterolemia is a potent risk factor, as illustrated by the very early atherosclerosis in patients with a familial LDL receptor abnormality and extremely high levels of LDL-C.[34] Elevated cholesterol concentrations in the blood may directly injure the endothelium, increase platelet activity, accumulate in the intimal plaque, and promote the proliferation of smooth muscle cells. The lipoprotein Lp(a) may impair natural fibrinolysis.[19]

The blood lipid profile may be influenced by genetics as well as by the shared environment of family life. Familial hypercholesterolemia and hypoalphalipoproteinemia are examples of genetic traits that result in the development of atherosclerosis at a young age.[34,36,37] Hyperhomocyst(e)inemia, a rare genetic abnormality, is also associated with a high incidence of coronary artery disease.[38] There is evidence that genetic differences exist in the amount and rate of proliferation of smooth muscle cells and fibroblasts in the intima.[6]

Hypertension worsens the prognosis of patients with documented coronary artery disease and probably directly impacts atherogenesis.[39] Elevated blood pressure may enhance smooth muscle proliferation, cause plaque rupture, increase endothelial cell permeability, and increase platelet and monocyte interaction with the vessel wall.[6,39,40]

Coronary artery disease is a major complication of diabetes mellitus.[41] Inadequately controlled diabetes worsens the blood lipid profile and activates platelets.[42]

The vast majority of obstructive coronary disease is atherosclerosis. Nonatherosclerotic coronary obstruction, although relatively rare, may result from the following: vasospasm (primary or cocaine-induced), embolism (thrombi from cardiac valves or chambers, calcium, tissue from tumors), primary thrombus, arteritis, spontaneous and traumatic coronary dissection, coronary artery aneurysm, and congenital abnormalities of the coronary arteries (for example, anomalous origin of the right or left main stem).[26]

ACCELERATED ATHEROSCLEROSIS AFTER CARDIAC INTERVENTIONS

Accelerated atherosclerosis is a major obstacle for cardiac interventions such as saphenous vein bypass graft surgery, percutaneous transluminal coronary angioplasty (PTCA) (either balloon or laser), coronary atherectomy, coronary stent placement, and cardiac transplantation. Platelet activation and the proliferative response of smooth muscle cells and connective tissue play a more prominent role in this process than does cholesterol deposition.[6]

Injury to saphenous vein grafts may occur at the time of harvesting, during operative handling, with the high pressure and flow characteristics of their new location in the circulation (arterialization of the vein), or from other factors. At 5 years after the operation, up to 35% of vein grafts are occluded.[43]

Restenosis rates of approximately 35% at 6 months after coronary angioplasty have been reported.[44] Mechanical disruption of the endothelial surface appears to be the stimulus (vascular injury) for the process to begin.

After cardiac transplantation, *accelerated graft atherosclerosis* may lead to significant blood flow reduction in less than 1 year, and affects approximately 40% of patients at 5 years after surgery.[45] The initiating injury to the coronary vessels probably results from the immune system, viruses, and the denervated state of the heart. The result is usually diffuse, longitudinal intimal thickening of the affected arteries.

IS CORONARY ATHEROSCLEROSIS REVERSIBLE?

In human studies of established coronary atherosclerosis involving very aggressive improvement of blood lipids (marked lowering of LDL-C and increasing of HDL-C), with coronary angiography performed before and after lipid treatment, there is evidence that some degree of *regression of obstructive lesions may occur in a minority of patients.*[46-49] Most investigations used one or more lipid-improving medications, and some used very-low fat and cholesterol diets with other lifestyle factors such as aerobic exercise, avoidance of tobacco, and stress reduction activities. One study used intestinal bypass surgery to markedly reduce LDL-C.[50] Among investigators, there is a consensus that early, less complicated lesions that are lipid-rich are more likely to show improvement than advanced plaques with incorporation of thrombus and fibromuscular tissue, although a systematic evaluation of this concept has not been performed. It should be pointed out that regression of coronary atherosclerosis has been documented in control subjects, whose blood lipids were not modified, in some of the investigations.

It is clear that, because coronary atherosclerosis begins in early life and requires decades to progress to symptomatic levels, prevention of lesion development is of paramount importance.[6,7] Risk factor identification and modification in children, grandchildren, and siblings of patients with established symptomatic coronary artery disease should become a high priority.

MYOCARDIAL BLOOD FLOW AND ISCHEMIA

Normal cardiac function depends on adequate levels of high energy phosphate (ATP) supplies in the myocardium. The heart produces ATP with the aerobic metabolic pathway under normal conditions (the heart has a poor anaerobic metabolic capability), consuming 8 to 10 mL O_2 per 100 g of myocardium at rest. During exercise, the oxygen requirement may increase 200 to 300%.[51] Because the myocardium extracts nearly all of the oxygen from the arterial blood, which flows through its capillary beds (70% extraction), coronary blood flow must be closely regulated to the needs of the myocardium for oxygen.[52] With an increase in myocardial work, which increases oxygen demand (myocardial oxygen demand is determined by the heart rate, the contractile state of the left ventricle, the end-diastolic pressure, and the aortic pressure), coronary blood flow is augmented to adequately provide the required amount of oxygen.[53]

Blood flow is determined by the arterial blood pressure and the resistance to the flow of blood offered by the vasculature, primarily the arterioles, which may change caliber and dramatically alter the resistance to flow in a given portion of the circulation.[52] Because of the high intramyocardial pressure generated during systole, which compresses the coronary arteries and inhibits forward flow, coronary blood flow to the left ventricle occurs primarily during diastole (Fig. 15–4). Control of coronary blood flow comes primarily from metabolic factors produced locally in the myocardium, such as the vasodilators adenosine and prostacyclin.[54,55] These substances are released during myocardial contraction. Mechanical forces that increase intramyocardial pressure during systole, as mentioned previously, may inhibit blood flow by increasing vascular resistance. The autonomic nervous system exerts some effect over myocardial blood flow as well.[56]

A substantial reduction in vessel internal diameter may occur before a decrease in blood flow can be measured distal to a narrowed coronary artery segment. When the stenosis reduces the luminal cross-sectional area by 75% or more, blood flow through the artery will be reduced under resting conditions (termed a hemodynamically significant lesion).[43] Beyond this level of *critical stenosis*, further small decreases in cross-sectional area of the vessel will result in abrupt reductions in flow.

The reduction in the cross-sectional area of the coronary artery may be caused by atherosclerosis, *vasospasm* of an otherwise normal artery, or vasospasm superimposed over an atherosclerotic plaque.[57] Coronary vasospasm is defined as a temporary increase in epicardial coronary artery smooth muscle contraction, which leads to a reduced luminal cross-sectional area.[58] Coronary vasospasm may result from a variety of factors: local arterial wall abnormalities which result in an exaggerated response to vasoconstrictor agents such as thromboxane A_2 and serotonin released from platelets adhering to the artery wall, neurogenic stimulation resulting in activation of alpha adrenergic receptors in the artery which lead to vasoconstriction (for example, coronary vasoconstriction resulting from cold pressor stimulation), and blood-borne factors such as epinephrine, which also stimulates alpha receptors. There is evidence that atherosclerotic arteries are deficient in the production or release of endothelium-derived relaxing factor and may exhibit an exaggerated vasoconstrictor response to blood-borne agents.[59]

Myocardial ischemia is a pathophysiologic state in which blood flow to the myocardium is reduced below the level needed to provide adequate amounts of oxygen to

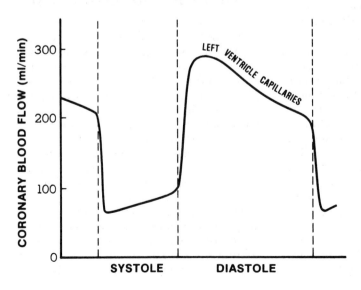

Fig. 15–4. Coronary blood flow during systole and diastole. With permission from Guyton AC: *Textbook of Medical Physiology.* Seventh Edition. Philadelphia: WB Saunders, 1986, pp. 295–304.

match the needs of the organ for APT production (oxygen supply less than demand).[51,53] Ischemia may result in tissue hypoxia (insufficient oxygen for aerobic metabolism), accumulation of toxic metabolic substances, and the development of acidosis. Ischemia requires the heart to shift from aerobic to anaerobic ATP production, and the myocardium produces lactic acid rather than extracting it from the arterial blood as it does under nonischemic conditions.

Ischemia may result in progressive abnormalities in cardiac function referred to as the *ischemic cascade*.[60] The first abnormality is a stiffening of the left ventricle, which decreases the ability of the chamber to fill with blood during diastole (diastolic dysfunction). Second, systolic emptying of the left ventricle becomes impaired, as demonstrated by the development of segmental wall motion abnormalities, and a reduction of left ventricular ejection fraction and stroke volume. Third, electrocardiographic changes associated with altered repolarization, ST-segient depression or elevation and T wave inversion or pseudonormalization, occur as a result of nonuniformity of repolarization through the ischemic and surrounding tissue. Ischemia may initiate life-threatening ventricular arrhythmias. Finally, the patient may develop symptoms of *angina pectoris*.

Angina pectoris is transient, referred cardiac pain resulting from myocardial ischemia.[61] Some patients with severe ischemia do not develop pain (*silent ischemia*), but most do have symptoms if the ischemia is moderate to severe. The locations and sensations of angina pectoris are diverse. The pain is usually located in the substernal region, jaw, neck, or left arm, although the sensation may occur in the epigastrium and interscapular regions. The characteristic pain is usually described as a feeling of pressure, heaviness, fullness, squeezing, burning, aching, choking, or boring. The pain may vary in intensity and may radiate. If the myocardial ischemia leads to an increase in left ventricular end-diastolic pressure and increased pulmonary pressure, the patient may experience dyspnea (*anginal equivalent*). *Typical angina* is usually provoked by exertion, emotions, cold or heat exposure, meals, and sexual intercourse,

and relieved by rest or nitroglycerin. *Atypical angina* refers to similar symptoms, but with some characteristic that is apart from typical angina, such as no relationship with exertion. *Unstable angina* is described as new onset of exertional angina, increasing frequency or intensity or duration of previously stable angina, or angina that occurs at rest.[61] Unstable angina is believed to result from dynamic myocardial ischemia because of the development of partially occlusive transient platelet thrombi (thrombi that form and then dissolve) or periodic coronary vasospasm (*variant or Prinzmetal's angina*) mediated by local vasoconstrictors such as endothelin, which is produced by the injured endothelium.[25]

If the episode of myocardial ischemia is brief, the abnormalities in cardiac function described above are reversible. With prolonged ischemia, myocyte necrosis (irreversible damage) may occur.[60] If ischemia is prolonged but not severe enough to result in myocyte necrosis, chronic but reversible left ventricular contraction abnormalities may result (*hybernating myocardium*).[51] This phenomenon appears to be a protective mechanism whereby myocytes reduce their oxygen demand when the oxygen supply is inadequate for normal function. In the case of hybernating myocardium, medical therapy or revascularization that eliminates the ischemia restores cardiac contraction to normal.

ACUTE MYOCARDIAL INFARCTION

Acute myocardial infarction is the necrosis of myocytes resulting from prolonged myocardial ischemia caused by complete occlusion of a coronary artery.[62] Precipitating factors include none in most cases, physical exertion, emotional stress, and surgery with associated blood loss. Slightly more myocardial infarctions occur in the morning hours than at other times.[62,63] The current concepts regarding the transition from coronary atherosclerosis to complete vessel occlusion are provided in the following section.

The initiating factor in complete coronary artery occlusion appears to be *rupture (or fissuring) of an atherosclerotic plaque* with subsequent thrombus development, which completely blocks the forward flow of blood.[25,64] The forces leading to plaque rupture may be hemodynamic stress on the plaque, increased blood pressure and/or heart rate, local vasoconstriction, hyperlipidemia, or circulating nicotine or immune complexes. In addition, macrophages located within the plaque may release proteases and tumor necrosis factor, which may erode the plaque from within. Rupture is more common in cholesterol-rich plaques.

After plaque rupture, circulating platelets come in direct contact with the internal environment of the plaque which provides an excellent setting for the development of thrombus.[25,64] Thrombus formation may follow, and if the thrombus superimposed on the atherosclerotic plaque becomes completely occlusive, a myocardial infarction results. Unstable angina may occur if the thrombus is partially occlusive or if the total occlusion lasts only a short period of time.[25] A few hours of severe ischemia produce a myocardial infarction.[62] A key event in differentiating reversible from irreversible (infarction) cell damage is the disruption of the myocyte membrane. This appears to be the lethal event, and the myocyte cannot recover if membrane disruption occurs that spills cytoplasmic contents (such as enzymes) into the circulation.[62]

It is extremely important to note that plaque rupture with thrombus formation leading to myocardial infarction commonly occurs in patients with noncritical lesions, some less than 50% occlusive before rupture.[65] A severe stenosis is not a necessary requirement for the development of acute myocardial infarction. This may explain the finding that many patients who experience acute myocardial ischemia do not possess a prolonged history of myocardial ischemia or angina pectoris before their myocardial infarction.

Current medical care of patients with acute myocardial infarction includes prompt reperfusion of the occluded artery by the use of thrombolytic agents and/or PTCA, if possible. These procedures do salvage myocardium and may reduce the size of the infarct, but the reperfusion of an ischemic area may cause accelerated myocyte necrosis (*reperfusion injury*) or a pro-

longed postischemic contraction abnormality (*stunned myocardium*).[51,62,63]

The diagnosis of acute myocardial infarction is based on symptoms of myocardial ischemia, electrocardiographic (ECG) hallmarks, and evaluation of the presence of cardiac enzymes in the blood (evidence of myocyte necrosis).[62,63]

The most common symptom of myocardial infarction is chest pain or discomfort, although some patients experience painless infarctions (*silent myocardial infarction*). The pain is usually severe, but all intensities of discomfort may be experienced.[63] Common additional symptoms are gastrointestinal upset and diaphoresis.

Myocardial infarctions may involve the entire thickness of the ventricle (*transmural infarction*) or only a portion of the wall of the ventricle (*subendocardial infarction*). Transmural infarction can be diagnosed from the ECG in the vast majority of cases, but subendocardial infarction cannot be reliably diagnosed from the ECG.[63] The most common ECG findings in subendocardial infarction are ST segment depression and T-wave inversion. Transmural myocardial injury resulting from ischemia produces ST segment elevation. During the acute phase of a transmural myocardial infarction, three zones of affected myocardium may be distinguished: a central core of necrosis, a surrounding zone of ischemic injury, and a peripheral area of ischemia. The necrotic core produces a *pathologic Q wave,* the zone of ischemic injury results in *ST segment elevation* in the leads facing the infarct, and the peripheral ischemic zone produces an *inverted T wave*.[66] Figure 15–5 shows the evolution of the ECG changes in transmural myocardial infarction with hyperacute ST segment elevation as the most recognizable abnormality in the early hours of the infarction, the development of Q waves and T wave inversion, and the return of the ST segment to baseline. Over time, the scar tissue of the infarct tends to shrink and the Q-wave becomes smaller. Categorization of infarcts into transmural and subendocardial has been replaced by the designation of *Q-wave* and *non-Q-wave* based on the ECG. This reflects the fact that there is no clear relationship between the level of necrosis into the ventricular wall and the presence or absence of a Q-wave. Also, a pathologic Q-wave may be absent when a transmural infarction is present.[66]

Criteria for Q-wave infarct localization are as follows:

1. Inferior myocardial infarction (usually right coronary artery occlusion)
   Q-wave (over 40 msec duration, amplitude over 25% of R wave) in leads II, III, aV_f
   QS pattern in leads II, III, aV_f

2. Anterior myocardial infarction (usually left anterior descending coronary artery occlusion)
   Q-wave in leads V_1-V_3 (anteroseptal)
   QS pattern in leads V_1-V_3 (anteroseptal)
   Q-wave in leads V_2-V_4 (anterior)
   QS pattern in leads V_2-V_4 (anterior)

3. Lateral wall myocardial infarction (usually circumflex coronary artery occlusion)
   Q-wave in leads V_4-V_6
   QS pattern in leads V_4-V_6

4. Posterior wall myocardial infarction (usually right coronary artery occlusion)
   Prominent R-wave in leads V_1-V_2 with positive T-wave

5. High lateral wall myocardial infarction (usually circumflex artery occlusion)
   Q-wave in leads I and aV_L
   QS pattern in leads I and aV_L

Myocardial infarction may involve more than one area simultaneously. Two or more infarcts, some acute and some chronic, may coexist.[66] Diagnosis of a transmural myocardial infarction from the ECG is difficult or impossible in patients with the electrocardiographic abnormalities of left bundle branch block, left ventricular hypertrophy, and Wolff-Parkinson-White syndrome.

Myocardial infarction results in the disruption of the myocyte membrane and the release of cytoplasmic contents into the blood. Cardiac enzymes released by the necrotic areas of the myocardium are useful in the diagnosis of acute infarction.[63] Lactate dehydrogenase (*LDH*) catalyzes the conversion of pyruvic acid to lactic acid in anaerobic glycolysis. The enzyme is found in most tissues and investigation into the five isoenzymes (different molecular forms of an enzyme) of LDH is necessary to evaluate myocardial necrosis. More than 50% of the total LDH is in the form of isoenzymes *LDH-I* and *LDH-II*. Under normal conditions, the blood level of LDH-II is greater than that of LDH-I. Within 12 to 24 hours after myocardial infarction, the level of LDH-I increases dramatically, becoming greater in serum concentration than LDH-II.[63,67]

Creatine phosphokinase (*CK*) catalyzes the hydrolysis of creatine phosphate resulting in the release of energy for the resynthesis of ATP. The enzyme exists in three isoenzymes: BB, found primarily in the brain and kidney; MM, located in skeletal

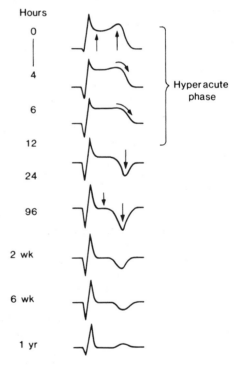

Fig. 15–5. The evolution of electrocardiographic changes in Q-wave myocardial infarction. With permission from Gau GT: Standard electrocardiography, vectorcardiography and signal-averaged electrocardiography. In *Cardiology: Fundamentals and Practice*. Second Edition. Edited by ER Giuliani, V Fuster, BJ Gersh, MD McGoon, DC McGoon. Chicago: Mosby Yearbook, 1991, pp. 273–317.

muscle; and MB, found in the heart and skeletal muscle (small amounts). An increase in *CK-MB* is the most specific enzyme marker for myocardial necrosis.[68] CK-MB appears in the blood as early as 3 hours after the onset of myocardial infarction and peaks at 12 to 24 hours. If a patient is seen within the first 24 hours after the onset of myocardial infarction, only total CK and CK-MB need to be measured. If the patient presents more than 24 hours after the beginning of suspicious symptoms, the peak level of CK may be missed and the additional measurement of LDH isoenzymes is generally performed.[63]

Serious complications often arise from acute myocardial infarction and may result in early or late mortality.[62,63] The most common complications are significant ventricular arrhythmias (*ventricular tachycardia* and *ventricular fibrillation*). Additional serious situations include *rupture of the ventricular free wall* (most commonly during the first week after infarction, 1 to 3% of all infarcts), development of a *left ventricular aneurysm, interventricular septal rupture, myocardial infarction extension or recurrence,* and severe congestive heart failure leading to *cardiogenic shock* with its characteristic downward cascade of pump failure resulting in further reduction in coronary blood flow (caused by hypotension and inadequate cardiac output), which leads to a further worsening of heart failure with almost certain death as the endpoint,[62] and *papillary muscle rupture* leading to severe mitral valve regurgitation. The pathophysiologic sequelae of acute myocardial infarction include changes in left ventricular pump function, the healing process within the infarcted myocardium, and a process termed ventricular remodeling.

Contraction abnormalities affecting the ventricle(s) are almost universal after myocardial infarction.[62] Diastolic abnormalities (a reduced ability to accept venous blood) are common and represent a stiff, noncompliant ventricle. Systolic contraction abnormalities are defined as follows: *hypokinesis*—a decrease in the extent of myocyte shortening, *akinesis*—a complete cessation of shortening, and *dyskinesis*—systolic bulging or expansion (the opposite of the normal behavior of the myocardium).

Myocardial infarction, particularly in situations of extensive myocardial necrosis (anterior location of infarction, for example), may produce changes over time in the geometry and contractile function of the ventricle (*ventricular remodeling*).[69] Left ventricular dilation involving the infarcted myocardium (*infarct expansion*), as well as dilation of the adjacent noninfarcted tissue, may occur. This dilation, which can continue for months to years after infarction, may result in progressive thinning of the ventricular wall and worsening contractile performance, culminating in congestive heart failure.

After myocardial infarction, patients may be risk stratified for reinfarction and sudden cardiac death, based on selected clinical criteria.[70,71] The state of left ventricular systolic function is of paramount prognostic importance. Patients who experienced congestive heart failure during hospitalization or who have left ventricular ejection fractions of less than 40% are at higher risk of sudden death and reinfarction. Patients who suffer non-Q-wave myocardial infarction experience only 50% of the hospital mortality as patients with Q-wave infarctions, but 20% of these patients develop Q-wave infarctions within 3 months of the initial event, and should be classified at high risk for recurrent myocardial infarction. Psychologic factors also play an important role in survival after myocardial infarction. Patients with a non-Q-wave myocardial infarction who have an elevated stress score while hospitalized experience a much higher 1-year cardiac mortality than patients with a similar cardiac history who do not appear to be under high stress.[72] Further, living alone and not having adequate social support is an independent risk factor for a recurrent cardiac event.[73] A history of a prior infarction is an independent risk predictor of a future cardiac event. Patients with unstable angina pectoris are at high risk for infarction or sudden death. Exercise-testing variables are helpful in risk prediction with a poor exercise capacity (less than 4 METs), the presence of myocardial ischemia (especially at low work levels), and systolic hypotension portending a poor survival. Some studies have demonstrated that complex ventricular arrhythmias are a risk factor for sudden cardiac death. Finally, ad-

vanced heart block (Mobitz type II, or 3°
AV block) and a new interventricular conduction delay are predictive of future cardiac events.[70,71]

TREATMENT OF CORONARY ARTERY DISEASE

Coronary Angioplasty

The introduction of percutaneous transluminal coronary angioplasty (PTCA)
by Dr. Andreas Gruntzig in 1979 has revo-
lutionized our approach to the symptomatic control of ischemic heart disease.[74]
PTCA has become a practical, safe, and effective means of nonsurgically augmenting
coronary flow for the prolonged palliation
of angina and improvement in left ventricular function. Improvements in equipment
design, imaging technology, operator experience, and patient selection have
yielded a procedural success rate approaching 90%, with PTCA accounting for
half of all coronary revascularization procedures in most institutions.

Technique of PTCA

PTCA has evolved as an elegant technique to guide an inflatable balloon
through the labyrinth of the coronary tree,
to straddle an offending coronary stenosis and squash it flat with the simple
application of compressive pressure. A
PTCA system is comprised of the following elements:[75] (1) a guiding catheter
shaped like a coronary diagnostic catheter
but strengthened for support, (2) a slender
double-lumen dilatation balloon catheter
that can be inflated to a specified pressure with a solution of contrast media,
and (3) a flexible nontraumatic guide wire
that can be guided past the lesion under
fl009scopic control. (Fig. 15–6)

Once the PTCA catheter has been advanced to the middle of the stenosis, the
balloon is inflated to the minimally effective pressure, usually 5 to 7 Atm. Reduction
of the coronary constriction is achieved by
physically splitting the offending atheromatous plaque and stretching the arterial
wall (Fig. 15–7). Usually, a variable degree
of localized longitudinal intimal and medial tearing occurs that heals with subse-

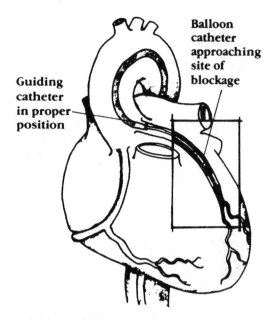

Fig. 15–6. Guiding catheter directs balloon catheter used for percutaneous transluminal coronary
angioplasty (PTCA). Balloon catheter ultimately
advanced to middle of coronary artery stenosis.
With permission from Department of Professional
Clinical Education Services, USCI Division: *A Patient's Guide to PTCA.* Billerica, MA: CR Bard,
1985.

quent vascular remodeling. In about 5% of
cases, arterial delamination is more extensive, resulting in a dissection that abruptly
occludes. This is the most common serious
PTCA complication. After successful
PTCA, in approximately 30% of patients,
overexuberant healing with proliferation
and migration of smooth muscle cells into
the arterial lumen culminates in symptomatic restenosis within the first 3 to 6
months.[76] This is the most frustrating
shortcoming of PTCA.

Indications and Patient Selection for PTCA

The overwhelming indication for PTCA
is the symptomatic control of disabling angina, to improve the quality of life among
patients with ischemic heart disease. Most
patients have chronic stable angina, but
PTCA can also be effective in those with
uncontrollable symptoms of unstable angina. Safe and effective acute coronary reperfusion has been achieved by PTCA dur-

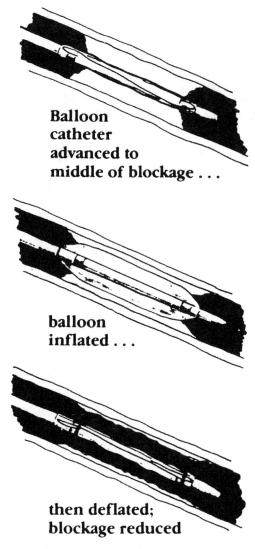

Balloon catheter advanced to middle of blockage . . .

balloon inflated . . .

then deflated; blockage reduced

Fig. 15–7. Events leading to successful percutaneous transluminal coronary angioplasty (PTCA). With permission from Department of Professional Clinical Education Services, USCI Division: *A Patient's Guide to PTCA.* Billerica, MA: CR Bard, 1985.

ing evolving acute myocardial infarction, with postinfarction angina. Among patients who have received thrombolytic therapy, PTCA is safer when it can be postponed several weeks.[77] Balloon angioplasty is usually limited to patients who would otherwise be considered appropriate candidates for bypass surgery. Access to this contingency must be available.

The anatomic criteria for PTCA have been considerably expanded over the last decade, but certain prerequisites prevail. The ideal short, proximal, concentric, discrete, noncalcified Type A lesion on a straight segment of vessel now comprises the minority of dilated arteries. With improved experience and catheter design, longer and more distal lesions, multiple stenosis, eccentric, irregular, calcified lesions, and recent total occlusion can now be dilated with a good measure of safety and success. Coronary angioplasty can be performed on saphenous vein bypass and internal mammary artery grafts with equivalent initial results. These broadened indications for PTCA have resulted in approximately 200,000 procedures per year in the United States. Guidelines for indications and selection of patients for PTCA have been set out by the American Heart Association and the American College of Cardiology.[78]

Results and Outstanding Problems with PTCA

Initial success rates greater than 95% can be achieved in proximal lesions with an emergency surgery risk of 1%.[79] Overall complication-free success is achieved in 90% of lesions attempted, with success defined as less than 50% residual stenosis (Table 15–1). Success rates fall to 75% when considering total occlusions or calcified eccentric lesions distally situated in a tortuous vessel.

Uncontrolled coronary dissection resulting in early abrupt occlusion remains the most feared PTCA complication. Occurring in 5% of cases, it can be controlled without bypass 70% of the time with an infarction rate of 10 to 15% and a mortality of 3 to 5%.[80] Abrupt occlusion is more likely to occur in association with the following factors: long or calcified stenosis, lesions on a bend or branch point, in situ

Table 15–1. Results of PTCA

Initial success per lesion	90%
5-year event-free survival	80%
Complication rate:	
Emergency bypass	2%
Q-wave infarction	1%
In-hospital death	0.3%
Symptomatic restenosis	30%

thrombus, multiple lesions, and female gender.[79]

The Persistent Problem of Restenosis

Since the inception of PTCA, restenosis still constitutes its "soft underbelly," occurring in about 30% of patients within 4 to 6 months. Redilation is usually feasible and effective and remains the most practical tactic. To date, all mechanical strategems to curb restenosis have been disappointing. A tremendous research effort continues to target this problem. Restenosis is more frequent with ostial and proximal left anterior descending artery stenosis, in midvein graft lesions, and in total occlusions. Recurrence after a second angioplasty remains at 30%, but is somewhat less for those that occur late (more than 5 months after PTCA).

Newer Devices and Future Directions

Recent innovations have included an array of intracoronary cutters, gougers, drills, scaffolding, stents, laser vaporizers, and extractors. Despite the excellent initial cosmetic results achieved with extraction atherectomy, high-speed rotational atherectomy and intravascular stents, the long-term efficacy of these expensive technologies remains to be established.

Summary

Balloon angioplasty, when used with skill and discretion, has become well established as an effective tool for the symptomatic control of ischemia. The quality of life of anginal patients can be immeasurably improved, with acceptable cost and minimal morbidity, by this invaluable technique.

Coronary Artery Bypass Grafts

Coronary atherosclerosis involves a localized accumulation of lipid and fibrous tissue within the coronary artery, causing progressive narrowing of the vessel lumen. Fatty streaks progress to fibrous plaques, which usually develop in the proximal, epicardial segments of the coronary artery at sites of abrupt curvature or branching. Clinically significant lesions, producing either or both angina pectoris and ischemic ST segment depression usually exceed

75% of the vessel lumen (Fig. 15–8).[81] Atheroma or complex atherosclerotic plaques may then become complicated by hemorrhage, ulceration, calcification, or thrombosis, producing myocardial infarction with accompanying tissue necrosis.[82]

The objective of coronary artery bypass graft surgery (CABGS) is to increase blood flow and oxygen delivery to ischemic myocardium beyond an obstructive arterial lesion. The surgical technique involves bypassing the critically obstructed coronary artery with either a saphenous vein, removed from the patient's legs, or an internal mammary artery, one of the major arteries carrying blood to the chest wall (Fig. 15–9).[83] The internal mammary artery is not as versatile a conduit, however, and is technically more difficult to construct.

Indications

Recommendations for CABGS may include: (1) disabling or unstable angina that is refractory to pharmacologic treatment; (2) lesions threatening major portions of viable myocardium (i.e., left main coronary artery obstructions); (3) multivessel disease; (4) severe proximal left anterior de-

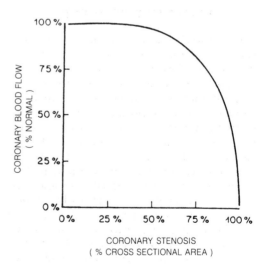

Fig. 15–8. Relationship between myocardial perfusion and coronary artery stenosis. Coronary blood flow not significantly impaired until stenosis exceeds 75% of cross-sectional area of vessel. With permission from Dehn M, et al.: Clinical exercise performance. In *Clinics in Sports Medicine.* Edited by B Franklin and M Rubenfire. Philadelphia: WB Saunders, 1984.

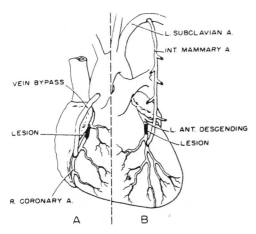

Fig. 15–9. Coronary artery bypass graft procedures. **A.** Saphenous vein bypass graft. Leg vein is sutured to ascending aorta and to right coronary artery beyond critical stenosis, creating vascular conduit to shunt blood around blockage to ischemic myocardium. **B.** Mammary artery graft procedure. Mammary artery is anastomosed to anterior descending branch of left coronary artery distal to blockage so blood flow is re-established. With permission from Price SA, Wilson LM: *Pathophysiology: Clinical Concepts of Disease Processes.* New York: McGraw-Hill, 1978.

scending coronary artery disease; and (5) ongoing ischemia after myocardial infarction.[83]

Complications

Major complications associated with CABGS occur in about 13% of revascularization patients.[84] Complications, including perioperative infarction in 2 to 8% of cases, occur more frequently in women, obese patients, patients with impaired left ventricular function (ejection fraction of less than 30%), and persons undergoing emergency bypass surgery.[85] Overall operative mortality rate is currently 1 to 2% in many institutions; however, this figure varies somewhat depending on the patient's age, extent of disease, and degree of left ventricular dysfunction. Sex is another determinant of risk in that the operative mortality rate is slightly higher in women, probably because of greater severity of angina and smaller coronary arteries. Finally, for patients who require repeat bypass, the mortality rate is twice that for the initial procedure.

Graft Patency

Current patency rates for saphenous vein grafts are 90% after 1 year and 80% after 5 years.[83] A marked attrition of vein grafts occurs between postoperative years 6 and 11, however, which is related to the development of atherosclerosis. After 11 years, only 60% of vein grafts are patent and nearly one half of these grafts are severely atherosclerotic.[83] In contrast, internal mammary grafts have a 93% 10-year graft patency and appear to be resistant to atherosclerosis.[86] This fact may partially explain the impressive 10-year actuarial survival advantage in patients undergoing CABGS who received internal mammary grafts when compared to patients who received saphenous vein grafts.[87]

Relief of Angina

Total relief of angina typically occurs in 60 to 75% of patients during the first 5 postoperative years; an additional 20 to 25% of patients report a significant reduction in symptoms.[85] Angina recurs in about 15% of CABGS patients over this same time period; however, primarily because of incomplete bypass grafting, progression of disease in native vessels, or graft occlusion.

Prolongation of Life

A recent review of three major randomized trials, in which researchers compared surgical intervention with medical management, concluded that: (1) CABGS improved survival in patients with left main disease; (2) CABGS improved survival in patients with three-vessel disease and impaired ventricular function; and (3) CABGS offered no survival advantage to mildly symptomatic or asymptomatic patients.[88]

Thrombolytic Therapy

Thrombolytic therapy for acute myocardial infarction is a promising new therapeutic approach that can re-establish vessel patency and achieve reperfusion in a high percentage of patients. Consideration of this strategy emerged when investigators showed the acute transmural myocardial infarction was associated with a high incidence of coronary thrombosis. Such findings rekindled interest in using thrombolytic enzymes to limit infarct size and to preserve ventricular function.

Agents and Mechanism of Action

Streptokinase, urokinase, and tissue-plasminogen activator (tPA) are specific thrombolytic agents that may be used to activate the fibrinolytic process. Activation results in the conversion of plasminogen, the inactive enzyme precursor, to plasmin, the active fibrinolytic enzyme, which is then able to lyse (dissolve) the clot. Plasminogen activation with either streptokinase or urokinase, however, results in the production of circulating plasmins, sytemic lysis, and frequent bleeding complications, regardless of the method of infusion (intravenous or intracoronary). In contrast, tPA dissolves thrombi but does not produce serious generalized bleeding.

Effectiveness

Reperfusion was achieved in about 75% of patients when streptokinase was infused directly into a thrombosed coronary artery within the first 6 hours after the onset of infarction. Intravenous infusion of streptokinase, which can be done more simply and more rapidly than intracoronary infusion, can restore perfusion in about 50% of patients with acute myocardial infarction.[89] In addition, successful thrombolytic therapy may provide sudden relief of angina and rapid resolution of ST-segment elevation. High-grade stenoses usually remain, however, with an attendant risk of reinfarction.

Several clot-selective plasminogen activators that do not induce systemic fibrinolysis are currently under investigation. Of these activators, tPA appears to have the greatest potential in that it produces in vivo clot dissolution without systemic effects. In the European Cooperative tPA Trial, patients treated with tPA demonstrated a 70% reperfusion rate as compared with a 55% rate in patients treated with intravenous streptokinase.[90] Successful thrombolysis was also accompanied by a lower incidence of systemic bleeding in the tPA-treated patients. In the Thrombolysis in Myocardial

Infarction (TIMI) trial, reperfusion was achieved in 60 and 35% of the tPA and streptokinase-treated patients, respectively.[91] Results of these prospective clinical trials showed that tPA is significantly more effective in achieving coronary reperfusion and may be associated with fewer bleeding complications.

REFERENCES

1. Report of the Working Group on Arteriosclerosis of the National Heart, Lung, and Blood Institute, Vol 2. DHEW Publication No. (NIH) 82-2035, Washington, D.C., US Government Printing Office, 1981.
2. American Heart Association: 1987 Heart Facts. Dallas, American Heart Association National Center.
3. Marmot MG: Epidemiological basis for the prevention of coronary heart disease. *Bull WHO, 57:*331, 1979.
4. Kannel WB: Cardiovascular disease: A multifactorial problem (insights from the Framingham study). In *Heart Disease and Rehabilitation.* Edited by ML Pollock, DH Schmidt. Boston: Houghton Mifflin Professional Publishers, 1979, pp 15–31.
5. Lobstein JF: Cited in Li P-L: Adaptation of veins to increased intravenous pressure, with special reference to the portal system and inferior vena cava. *J Pathol Bacteriol, 50:* 121, 1940.
6. Fuster V: Atherosclerosis, A. Pathogenesis, pathology, and presentation of atherosclerosis. In *Cardiology: Fundamentals and Practice.* Second Edition. Edited by ER Giuliani, V Fuster, BJ Gersh, MD McGoon, DC McGoon. Chicago, Mosby Yearbook, 1991, pp 1172–1210.
7. Ross R: The pathogenesis of atherosclerosis. In *Heart Disease: A Textbook of Cardiovascular Medicine.* Third Edition. Edited by E Braunwald. Philadelphia: WB Saunders Company, 1988, pp. 1135–1152.
8. Renkin EM: Multiple pathways of capillary permeability. *Circ Res, 41:*735, 1977.
9. Gajdusek CM, DiCorleto PE, Ross R, et al.: An endothelial cell-derived growth factor. *J Cell Biol, 85:*467, 1980.
10. Chait A, Ross R, Albers JJ, et al.: Platelet-derived growth factor stimulates activity of low density lipoprotein receptors. *Proc Natl Acad Sci USA, 77:*4084, 1980.
11. Bowen-Pope DF, Seiffert RA, Ross R: The platelet-derived growth factor receptor. In *Control of Animal Cell Proliferation: Recent Advances.* Vol 1. Edited by AL Boynton, HL

Leffert. New York: Academic Press, 1985, p 281.

12. Campbell GR, Campbell JH: Smooth muscle phenotypic changes in arterial wall homeostasis: Implications for the pathogenesis of atherosclerosis. *Exp Mol Pathol, 42:* 139, 1985.

13. Ross R, Glomset J: Atherosclerosis and the arterial smooth muscle cell. *Science, 180:* 1332, 1973.

14. Clowers AW, Reidy MA, Clowers MM: Kinetics of cellular proliferation after arterial injury. I. Smooth muscle growth in the absence of endothelium. *Lab Invest, 49:*327, 1983.

15. Faggiotto A, Ross R, Harker L: Studies of hypercholesterolemia in the nonhuman primate. I. Changes that lead to fatty streak formation. *Arteriosclerosis, 4:*323, 1984.

16. Leary T: The genesis of atherosclerosis. *Arch Pathol, 32:*507, 1941.

17. Rowsell HC, Hegardt B, Downie HB, et al.: Adrenaline and experimental thrombosis. *Br J Haematol, 12:*465, 1972.

18. Hampton JR, Gorlin R: Platelet studies in patients with coronary artery disease and in their relatives. *Br Heart J, 34:*465, 1972.

19. Scott J: Thrombogenesis linked to atherogenesis at last? *Nature, 341:*22, 1989.

20. Ross R, Glomset J, Karija B, et al.: A platelet-dependent serum factor stimulates the proliferation of arterial smooth muscle cells in vitro. *Proc Natl Acad Sci USA, 71:*1207, 1974.

21. Stary HC: Evaluation of atherosclerotic plaques in the coronary arteries of young adults. *Arteriosclerosis, 3:*471a, 1983.

22. Van Furth R: Current view on the mononuclear phagocyte system. *Immunobiology, 161:* 178, 1982.

23. Hansson GK, Jonasson L, Seifert PS, et al.: Immune mechanisms in atherosclerosis. *Arteriosclerosis, 9:*567, 1989.

24. Assoian RK, Grotendorst GR, Miller DM, et al.: Cellular transformation by coordinated action of three peptide growth factors from human platelets. *Nature, 309:*804, 1984.

25. Chesebro JH, Zoldelyi P, Fuster V: Plaque disruption and thrombosis in unstable angina pectoris. *Am J Cardiol, 68:*9c, 1991.

26. Lie JT: Atherosclerosis B. Pathology of coronary artery disease. In *Cardiology: Fundamentals and Practice.* Second Edition. Edited by ER Giuliani, V Fuster, BJ Gersh, MD McGoon, DC McGoon. Chicago: Mosby Yearbook, 1991, pp. 1211–1231.

27. Arnett EN, Isner JM, Redwood DR, et al.: Coronary artery narrowing in coronary heart disease: comparison of cineangiographic and necropsy findings. *Ann Intern Med, 91:*350, 1979.

28. Strong JP, McGill HC Jr: The natural history of coronary atherosclerosis. *Ann J Pathol, 40:*37, 1962.

29. Brinson K: Effect of nicotine on human platelet aggregation. *Atherosclerosis, 20:*137, 1974.

30. Astrup P: Some physiological and pathological effects of moderate carbon dioxide exposure. *Br Med J, 4:*447, 1972.

31. Mustard JF, Murphy EA: Effect of smoking on blood coagulation and platelet survival in man. *Br Med J, 1:*846, 1963.

32. Haft JI: Cardiovascular injury induced by sympathetic catecholamines. *Prog Cardiovasc Dis, 17:*73, 1974.

33. Lavie CJ, Gau GT, Squires RW, et al.: Management of lipids in primary and secondary prevention of cardiovascular diseases. *Mayo Clin Proc, 63:*605, 1988.

34. Goldstein JL, Brown MS: Regulation of low-density lipoprotein receptors: implications for pathogenesis and therapy of hypercholesterolemia and atherosclerosis. *Circulation, 76:*504, 1987.

35. Brown MS, Goldstein JL: How LDL receptors influence cholesterol and atherosclerosis. *Sci Am, 251:*58, November 1984.

36. Scheidt S: Lipid regulation: A clinician's view of patient management. *Am Heart J, 112:*437, 1986.

37. Kottke BA: Lipid markers for atherosclerosis. *Am J Cardiol, 57:*11C, 1986.

38. Malinow MR: Hyperhomocyst(e)inemia: A common and easily reversible risk factor for occlusive atherosclerosis. *Circulation, 81:* 2004, 1990.

39. Kannel WB, Cuppler LA, D'Agostino RB, et al.: Hypertension, antihypertensive treatment, and sudden coronary death: The Framingham study. *Hypertension, 11(Suppl 2):*45, 1988.

40. Leung DYM, Glagov S, Mathews MB: Cyclic stretching stimulates synthesis of matrix components by arterial smooth muscle cells in vitro. *Science, 191:*475, 1976.

41. United States Department of Health, Education, and Welfare: Report of the National Commission on Diabetes to the Congress of the United States (DHEW Publication No [NIH] 76-1022). Vol 3, Pt, 2, Washington, DC, Government Printing Office, 1976.

42. Sagel J, Colwell, Crook L, et al.: Increased platelet aggregation in early diabetes mellitus. *Ann Intern Med, 82:*733, 1975.

43. Lie JT, Lawrie GM, Morris GC Jr: Aortocoronary bypass saphenous vein graft atherosclerosis: anatomic study of 99 vein grafts from normal and hyperlipoproteine-

mic patients up to 75 months postoperatively. *Am J Cardiol, 40:*906, 1977.

44. McBride W, Lange RA, Hillis DL: Restenosis after successful coronary angioplasty: pathophysiology and prevention. *N Engl J Med, 318:*1734, 1988.
45. Billingham ME: Pathology of the transplanted heart and lung. *Cardiovasc Clin, 20:* 71, 1990.
46. Blankenhorn DH, Nessim SA, Johnson RL, et al.: Beneficial effects of combined colestipol-niacin therapy on coronary atherosclerosis and coronary venous bypass grafts. *JAMA, 257:*3233, 1987.
47. Brown G, Albers JJ, Fisher LD, et al.: Regression of coronary artery disease as a result of intense lipid-lowering therapy in men with high levels of apolipoprotein B. *N Engl J Med, 323:*1289, 1990.
48. Ornish D, Brown SE, Scherwitz LW, et al.: Can lifestyle changes reverse coronary heart disease? *Lancet, 336:*129, 1990.
49. Kane JP, Malloy MJ, Ports TA, et al.: Regression of coronary atherosclerosis during treatment of familial hypercholesterolemia with combined drug regimens. *JAMA, 264:*3007, 1990.
50. Buchwald H, Moore RB, Varco RL: Surgical treatment of hyperlipidemia. *Circulation, 4(Suppl I):*I1, 1974.
51. Garratt KN, Morgan JP: Coronary circulation B. Pathophysiology of myocardial ischemia and reperfusion. In *Cardiology: Fundamentals and Practice*. Second Edition. Edited by ER Giuliani, V Fuster, BJ Gersh, MD McGoon, DC McGoon. Chicago: Mosby Yearbook, 1991, pp. 1150–1158.
52. Guyton AC: *Textbook of Medical Physiology*. Seventh Edition. Philadelphia: WB Saunders, 1986, pp. 295–304.
53. Braunwald E, Sobel BE: Coronary blood flow and ischemia. In *Heart Disease: A Textbook of Cardiovascular Medicine*. Third Edition. Edited by E Braunwald. Philadelphia: WB Saunders, 1988, pp. 1191–1221.
54. Rubio R, Wiedimeier VT, Berne RM: Relationship between coronary flow and adenosine production and release. *J Mol Cell Cardiol, 6:*561, 1974.
55. Schor K: Possible role of prostaglandins in the regulation of coronary blood flow. *Basic Res Cardiol, 76:*239, 1981.
56. Bove AA, Santamore WP: Coronary circulation A. physiology of the coronary circulation. In *Cardiology: Fundamentals and Practice*. Second Edition. Edited by ER Giuliani, V Fuster, BJ Gersh, MD McGoon, DC McGoon. Chicago: Mosby Yearbook, 1991, pp. 1131–1149.
57. Maseri A: Myocardial ischemia in man: Current concepts, changing views and future investigation: *Can J Cardiol, Suppl A:* 225A, 1986.
58. McGoon MD, Fuster V: Myocardial ischemia syndromes B. coronary artery spasm and vasotonicity. In *Cardiology: Fundamentals and Practice*. Second Edition. Edited by ER Giuliani, V Fuster, BJ Gersh, MD McGoon, DC McGoon. Chicago: Mosby Yearbook, 1991, pp. 1307–1317.
59. Griffith TM, Lewis MJ, Newby AC, et al.: Endothelium-derived relaxing factor. *J Am Coll Cardiol, 12:*797, 1988.
60. Hurst JW: Coronary heart disease: the overview of a clinician. In *Rehabilitation of the Coronary Patient*. Third Edition. Edited by NK Wenger, HK Hellerstein. New York: Churchill Livingstone, 1992, pp. 3–18.
61. Shub C: Myocardial ischemia syndromes A. angina pectoris and coronary heart disease. In *Cardiology: Fundamentals and Practice*. Second Edition. Edited by ER Giuliani, V Fuster, BJ Gersh, MD McGoon, DC McGoon. Chicago: Mosby Yearbook, 1991, pp. 1276–1306.
62. Pasternak RC, Braunwald E, Sobel B: Acute myocardial infarction. In *Heart Disease: A Textbook of Cardiovascular Medicine*. Third Edition. Edited by E Braunwald. Philadelphia: WB Saunders, 1988, pp. 1222–1313.
63. Gersh BJ, Clements IP, Chesebro JH: Acute myocardial infarction A. diagnosis and prognosis. In *Cardiology: Fundamentals and Practice*. Second Edition. Edited by ER Giuliani, V Fuster, BJ Gersh, MD McGoon, DC McGoon. Chicago: Mosby Yearbook, 1991, pp. 1318–1361.
64. Frick RJ, Ostrach LH, Rooney PA, et al.: Coronary thrombosis, ulcerated plaques and platelet/fibrin microemboli in patients dying with acute coronary disease. A large autopsy study. *J Inv Cardiol, 2:*199, 1990.
65. Shah PK, Forrester JJ: Pathophysiology of acute coronary syndromes. *Am J Cardiol, 68:* 16C, 1991.
66. Gau GT: Standard electrocardiography, vectorcardiography and signal-averaged electrocardiography. In *Cardiology: Fundamentals and Practice*. Second Edition. Edited by ER Giuliani, V Fuster, BJ Gersh, MD McGoon, DC McGoon. Chicago: Mosby Yearbook, 1991, pp. 273–317.
67. Agress CM, Kim JHC: Evaluation of enzyme tests in the diagnosis of heart disease. *Am J Cardiol, 6:*641, 1960.
68. Sobel BE, Shell WE: Serum enzyme determinations in the diagnosis and assessment of myocardial infarction. *Circulation, 45:* 471, 1972.

69. Pfeffer MA, Braunwald E: Ventricular remodeling after myocardial infarction: Experimental observations and clinical implications. *Circulation, 81:*1161, 1990.

70. Krone RJ: The role of risk stratification in the early management of a myocardial infarction. *Ann Intern Med 116:*223, 1992.

71. American College of Sports Medicine. *Guidelines for Exercise Testing and Prescription.* Fourth Edition. Philadelphia: Lea & Febiger, 1991, pp. 122–125.

72. Frasure-Smith N, Lesperance F, Juneau M: Differentiated long-term impact of in-hospital symptoms of psychological stress after non-q-wave and q-wave acute myocardial infarction. *Am J Cardiol, 69:*1128, 1992.

73. Case RB, Moss AJ, Case N, et al.: Living alone after myocardial infarction: Impact on prognosis. *JAMA 267:*515, 1992.

74. Gruentzig AR, Senning A, Segenthaler WE: Non-operative dilatation of coronary artery stenosis: Percutaneous transluminal coronary angioplasty. *N Engl J Med, 301:* 61–68, 1979.

75. Block PC: Mechanism of transluminal angioplasty. *Am J Cardiol 53:*69C, 1984.

76. Califf RM, Fortin DF, Frid DJ, et al.: Restenosis after coronary angioplasty: An overview. *J Am Coll Cardiol, 17:*2B–13B, 1991.

77. Topol EJ, Califf M, George BS, et al.: Thrombolysis and angioplasty in myocardial infarction study group. A randomized trial of immediate versus delayed elective angioplasty after intravenous tissue plasminogen activator in acute myocardial infarction. *N Engl J Med, 317:*581–87, 1987.

78. Ryan TJ, Faxen DP, Gunnar RM, et al.: Guidelines for percutaneous transluminal angioplasty. *J Am Coll Cardiol, 12:*529–545, 1988.

79. Linkoff AM, Popma JJ, Ellis SG, et al.: Abrupt vessel closure complicating the coronary angioplasty: Clinical, angiographic and therapeutic profile. *Am J Cardiol, 19:* 926–935, 1992.

80. Topol EJ, Faxen DP, (Editors): Symposium on restenosis: From basic studies to clinical trials. *Am J Cardiol, 19:*Supplement B, 1991.

81. Dehn M, et al.: Clinical exercise performance. In *Clinics in Sports Medicine.* Edited by B Franklin and M Rubenfire. Philadelphia: WB Saunders, 1984.

82. Price SA, Wilson LM: *Pathophysiology: Clinical Concepts of Disease Processes.* New York: McGraw-Hill, 1978.

83. Timmis GC, et al.: *Cardiovascular Review.* 8th Ed. New York: Pergamon Press, 1987.

84. Kuan P, Bernstein SB, Ellestad MH: Coronary artery bypass surgery morbidity. *J Am Coll Cardiol, 3:*1391, 1984.

85. Loop FD: Coronary artery surgery—1982. *Coronary Club Bulletin, 11:*1, 1982.

86. Lytle BW, et al.: Young adults with coronary atherosclerosis: 10 year results of surgical myocardial revascularization. *J Am Coll Cardiol, 4:*445, 1984.

87. Loop FD, et al.: Influence of the internal-mammary-artery graft on 10-year survival and other cardiac events. *N Engl J Med, 314:* 1, 1986.

88. Killip T, Ryan TJ: Randomized trials in coronary bypass surgery. *Circulation, 71:*418, 1985.

89. Laffel GL, Braunwald E: Thrombolytic therapy: A new strategy for the treatment of acute myocardial infarction. *N Engl J Med, 311:*770, 1984.

90. European Cooperative Study Group: Randomised trial of intravenous recombinant tissue-type plasminogen activator versus intravenous streptokinase in acute myocardial infarction. *Lancet, 1:*842, 1985.

91. TIMI Study Group: The thrombolysis in myocardial infarction (TIMI) trial: Phase I findings. *N Engl J Med, 312:*932, 1984.

Chapter 16

PATHOPHYSIOLOGY OF CHRONIC DISEASES AND EXERCISE TRAINING

Peter Hanson

HYPERTENSION

Hypertension is the most common cardiovascular disease in human populations. The prevalence of hypertension in most Western industrialized countries is 15 to 20%. The prevalence of hypertension in the black population is substantially higher (25 to 30%).

Blood pressure values are deemed "hypertensive" on the basis of epidemiologic criteria that show an exponential rise of cardiovascular morbidity and mortality with increasing systolic and diastolic pressures. The World Health Organization defines normal resting blood pressure as less than 140/90 and hypertension as greater than 160/95. Intermediate blood pressure values are defined as borderline or mild hypertension. However, many authorities have emphasized that risk from hypertension may begin at values of 135/85.

Hypertension is a major risk factor for coronary artery disease, stroke, and congestive heart failure and chronic renal failure. Hypertension may contribute to 2,000,000 excess deaths every 10 years. In several blood pressure intervention trials, however, mortality and morbidity, particularly from stroke, were substantially reduced when adequate antihypertensive treatment was maintained.

Pathophysiology

For clinical purposes, hypertension is divided into two subgroups: *primary hypertension* and *secondary hypertension*. Primary hypertension (essential hypertension) accounts for sustained high blood pressure in over 95% of patients. Multiple regulatory mechanisms contribute to the evolution of primary hypertension, including abnormal central (sympathetic) mediation of increased peripheral resistance; renal and metabolic control of vascular volume; decreased vascular compliance, and possibly impairment of endothelial-mediated vasodilation. In various studies of primary hypertension, authors reported variable increases in circulating catecholamines; increased, normal, and low renin levels; hyperinsulinemia; and evidence of abnormally high calcium content within vascular smooth muscle cell in hypertensive patients.

These neurohumoral and metabolic disturbances all contribute to the gradual increase in systemic vascular resistance that is characteristic of primary hypertension. In addition, an alteration of arterial baroreceptor function occurs, leading to a "resetting" of baroreflexes to accommodate higher systemic pressure levels. In hemodynamic studies involving subjects with primary hypertension, systemic vascular resistance was increased at rest and throughout exercise. During the early phases of primary hypertension, cardiac output may be increased, whereas in the later stages, cardiac output is normal or reduced as systemic vascular resistance continues to increase.

Secondary hypertension is caused by specific endocrine or renal abnormalities. Examples include tumors of the adrenal medulla, which release catecholamines (epinephrine and norepinephrine), and tumors of the adrenal cortex, which release hypertension-mediating steroid hormones (cortisol and aldosterone). Renal vascular disease causes increased production of renin, which stimulates the conversion of plasma angiotensin and the release of aldosterone. Angiotensin is a potent mediator of peripheral vasoconstriction, and aldosterone stimulates renal retention of sodium and water. Most of these unusual causes of hypertension, which account for less than

5% of all sustained hypertension, are treatable by surgical intervention or medical management.

Regardless of cause, increasing blood pressure levels produce a predictable pattern of end-organ pathologic processes. Echocardiographic studies in borderline hypertension patients show early left ventricular hypertrophy. With sustained hypertension, concentric left ventricular hypertrophy increases. In addition, a progressive hypertensive thickening, remodeling, and degeneration of medium and small arterial vessels (arteriosclerosis) occurs, and is particularly evident in the retina and renal glomerular arterioles, leading to hypertensive retinopathy and nephropathy. Hypertensive cerebral vascular disease and rupture produce catastrophic stroke.

End-organ damage from hypertension usually evolves over many years. Rapid increases in blood pressure, which usually occur in secondary hypertension, may be poorly tolerated, whereas gradual increases in blood pressure and sustained systolic hypertension in older patients may be well tolerated for long periods without morbid events.

Responses to Exercise

The normal pattern of blood pressure response to exercise is characterized by a near-linear increase in systolic pressure combined with a gradual decline in diastolic pressure. Peak blood pressure values at maximal work intensity are in the range of 180-210/60-80. These values may vary considerably, depending on age, weight, and gender. For example, young women may show normal peak blood pressure values of 140/60.

Patients with hypertension usually show systolic and diastolic pressure values that are maintained above the expected normal range. The magnitude of added increase in systolic and diastolic pressure during exercise is usually proportional to the elevation in systolic and diastolic pressure measured at rest. This indicates that blood pressure is "reset" and is maintained at higher levels throughout the spectrum of activity from rest to peak exercise: yet some patients with mild hypertension may dem-

onstrate a normalization of blood pressure during exercise relative to resting values. This normalization is attributed to metabolic vasodilation, which temporarily corrects the elevated peripheral resistance.

Blood pressure responses to exercise may provide additional criteria for diagnosis and management of hypertension. Recent reports reveal that blood pressure values exceeding 180/90 at 50% maximal exercise and maximal blood pressure values exceeding 225/90 are common in patients with mild primary hypertension. A subset of patients with hypertension may show an early rise in systolic pressure to levels of 180 to 200 during submaximal exercise, followed by maximal values in the normal range of 200 to 210. These patients may generate excessively high systolic blood pressures with activities of daily living, although the resting blood pressure and maximal blood pressure values are at the upper limits of normal. Results of studies involving a comparison of blood pressure values during exercise and ambulatory blood pressure monitoring indicate that patients with this pattern of blood pressure response also show evidence of early left ventricular hypertrophy and are at greater risk for the development of fixed hypertension.

The evaluation of blood pressure responses to exercise should involve the use of protocols permitting accurate measurement of blood pressure. A constant speed treadmill protocol (e.g., Balke) is superior to the Bruce protocol, which is commonly used for diagnostic exercise testing. Blood pressure criteria for discontinuation of exercise testing are controversial. In most laboratories, researchers set an arbitrary value of more than 250/120 as a termination point, yet no evidence exists to support these criteria, and in no case reports have hypertensive emergencies been reported to result when subjects exceed these levels.

Treatment

Abundant antihypertensive agents are currently available, including: (1) diuretics, (2) adrenergic blocking agents, (3) vasodilators, and (4) converting enzyme inhibitors. The major classes of antihypertensive agents and their mechanisms of action are summarized in Table 16–1. Selection of a form of antihypertensive therapy should be directed at the underlying pathophysiologic process. Patients with increased plasma volume and high salt intake may benefit from salt restriction and diuretic agents. Persons with hypertension associated with high renin-angiotensin levels are ideally treated with converting enzyme-inhibiting agents. Patients with evidence of high sympathetic activity characterized by increased resting heart rate and rapid increases in heart rate during exercise would benefit from β-adrenergic blocking agents.

Adrenergic blocking agents also include peripheral α-receptor-blockers such as prazosin and doxazosin, which reduce peripheral vasoconstriction mediated by increased sympathetic α-stimulation. Centrally acting adrenergic blocking agents, such as clonidine, attenuate sympathetic outflow at the level of medullary vasomotor centers. The peripheral and central-acting α-adrenergic blocking agents appear to have minimal adverse effects on heart rate, cardiac output, and metabolic responses to exercise.

Vasodilators are also used in the treatment of patients with hypertension. These agents include hydralazine (direct-acting) and the calcium channel-inhibiting agents. The vasodilating agents tend to produce tachycardia secondary to baroreflex responses to lowered blood pressure. They are frequently used in combination with β-adrenergic blocking agents to control the secondary increases in heart rates.

Antihypertensive agents may interact adversely with exercise. Excessive use of most diuretic agents produces hypokalemia, the result of increased loss of urinary potassium. Hypokalemia is associated with skeletal muscle weakness and may aggravate ventricular arrhythmias or ventricular fibrillation. Beta-adrenergic blocking agents restrict heart rate, cardiac output, and maximal oxygen consumption. The combined use of β-blocking agents and vasodilators may cause post-exercise hypotension.

The treatment of athletes or active adults with sustained hypertension is frequently complicated by the side effects of standard antihypertensive therapy. A recent trend in the treatment of hypertension emphasizes the initial use of converting enzyme-inhibiting agents (captopril and enalapril), which have no effect on the sympathetic nervous system and do not produce hypokalemia. The converting enzyme inhibitors are well tolerated and have no adverse effect on exercise performance. Finally, the use of a long-acting transcutaneous form of clonidine may also be a viable alternative. The transcutaneous patches provide 7 days of antihypertensive therapy, which optimizes compliance. In addition, the side effects associated with oral clonidine are minimal.

Exercise Training and Hypertension

Exercise training may be useful in the management of mild hypertension, particularly in young and middle-aged patients. Reductions of 8 to 10 mm Hg systolic and 5 to 8 mm Hg diastolic have been reported in meta-analyses of training studies. Most of the studies that report a favorable effect of dynamic exercise on blood pressure have used training programs involving relatively moderate intensity exercise, usually aerobics, jogging, or bicycling several times per week. Higher intensity or more frequent exercise appears not to offer any ad-

Table 16–1. Major Classes of Antihypertensive Drugs

Drugs	Major Action	Exercise Side Effects
Diuretics	Renal salt and water loss	Hypokalemia
β-blocking	Reduced cardiac output	Reduced $\dot{V}O_{2max}$, fatigue
α-blocking	Vasodilation, reduced vascular resistance	Hypotension
Ca^{2+} blocking	Vasodilation, reduced vascular resistance	Tachycardia, cramps
Vasodilators	Vasodilation, reduced vascular resistance	Reflex tachycardia
Converting enzyme inhibitors	Inhibition of renin-angiotensin, aldosterone, vasodilation, reduced water and salt retention	Excessive hypotension, hyperkalemia

vantage, and may even be less effective at lowering blood pressure.

Significant decreases in blood pressure have been seen as soon as 4 to 5 weeks after initiating of training and persist as long as the active lifestyle is continued. When individuals stop participation in the exercise program, blood pressures often return to pretraining levels.

Research on the mechanisms involved in the effect of exercise on blood pressure have shown that a single bout of dynamic exercise is followed by a sustained decrease in peripheral vascular resistance, which may be caused, at least partly, by a decrease in sympathetic nervous system.

A small number of studies suggest that weight training may also be effective in lowering blood pressure in hypertensive patients. Although more research is needed, an exercise training program that includes circuit weight training appears to be safe and beneficial for patients with mild hypertension.

DIABETES MELLITUS

Diabetes is a complex metabolic disorder with wide-ranging complications, characterized by high levels of plasma glucose and secondary microvascular degeneration which affect the retina, kidneys, and peripheral circulation. Diabetes is classified as insulin-dependent (type I) or noninsulin-dependent (type II). The clinical characteristics of patients with insulin and noninsulin-dependent diabetes are summarized in Table 16–2. Type I diabetes typically oc-

curs in children or young adults under 30 years. The prevalence of insulin-dependent diabetes in the United States is estimated to be 1 in every 300 to 400 persons under 20 years.

Pathophysiology

Insulin-dependent diabetes is caused by acute or gradual loss of the insulin-producing beta cells in the pancreas. This process may involve genetic, viral, or autoimmune factors, either separately or in combination.

Patients with untreated type I diabetes maintain high levels of plasma glucose and are subject to ketoacidosis resulting from the increased metabolism of fat and production of ketone bodies. High levels of plasma glucose cause increased loss of water and sugar through the urine, which leads to secondary thirst, weight loss, and increased appetite.

Insulin-dependent diabetics have multiple systemic complications, including characteristic degeneration of the small arterial vessels within the eye, kidneys, and peripheral arterioles of the lower extremities. Retinal hemorrhage and a high frequency of blindness and progressive renal failure result. Degeneration of peripheral and autonomic nerve function also occurs. The heart and peripheral blood vessels are affected; diabetes accelerates coronary atherosclerosis, and symptomatic coronary disease may develop between the ages of 20 and 40 years. In addition, cardiac function is affected directly, with loss of contractile performance of the ventricles caused by microvascular ischemia, as is the peripheral circulation, which is compromised by similar degenerative changes in distal arterioles. Perfusion of the lower extremities is therefore poor, and frequent complications ensue, including infections of the feet and poor healing of cuts and wounds, which often require amputation because of gangrene.

Type II diabetes typically occurs in overweight adults over 40. These patients also show high levels of circulating plasma glucose, but do not respond with excess fat metabolism and ketosis. The cause of type II diabetes is usually correlated with diminished sensitivity of peripheral insulin re-

Table 16–2. Comparison of Insulin-Dependent (Type I) and Noninsulin-Dependent (Type II) Diabetes

Characteristics	Type I	Type II
Age of onset	<20 yr	>40 yr
Frequency	0.5%	4–5%
Family history	Probable	Frequent
Obesity	±	+ +
Serum insulin level	Low or zero	High (early) Low (late)
Insulin therapy	Always	20 to 30%
Complications	Frequent	Frequent
Life span	Maximum of 40 yr	

ceptors, especially in skeletal muscle and liver. Plasma insulin levels are actually increased because of the excessive release of pancreatic insulin that results from the stimulatory effect of high sustained circulating glucose levels. Eventually, insulin levels fall to subnormal levels because of failure of beta cell function.

Type II diabetics also have frequent cardiovascular complications. The incidence of coronary artery disease is increased and is associated with hyperlipidemia and hypertension, which accompany type II diabetes.

Treatment

Patients with insulin-dependent diabetes are treated with subcutaneous injections of insulin. A typical prescription consists of a mixture of short-acting (crystalline) insulin and longer-acting (sustained release) insulin preparations. Precise control of insulin levels usually requires morning and afternoon insulin doses, which are adjusted according to self-monitored blood glucose determinations. Strict dietary regulation is also mandatory, so that total carbohydrate and calorie intake are maintained to match insulin therapy.

Noninsulin-dependent diabetic patients are treated with a combination of weight loss and oral hypoglycemic agents, which re-establish the sensitivity of peripheral insulin receptors and stimulate the release of insulin from beta cells.

Exercise Training and Diabetes

Exercise may be beneficial in the control of diabetes. Submaximal (60 to 70% of $\dot{V}_{O_{2max}}$) aerobic exercise produces an acute increase in noninsulin-dependent glucose uptake in skeletal muscle. During postexercise recovery, glucose uptake continues as glycogen is resynthesized. In numerous studies, exercise training produced an increase in peripheral sensitivity to insulin in type I diabetics. This effect is only transient and may reverse to pre-exercise insulin sensitivity in only a few days. However, these changes may permit a reduction in the dosage of daily insulin required to control glucose levels during active exercise training. Improvement of several markers of diabetic control have been re-

ported, including lower hemoglobin A-1c levels, which reflect the overall regulation of plasma glucose. The long-term effects of aerobic exercise training in the management of patients with type I diabetes, however, requires further evaluation.

Individuals with type II diabetes show a clear-cut benefit from exercise training. In this group, regular exercise and weight loss may eventually restore near-normal glucose tolerance. Many type II diabetic patients also exhibit a combination of central (abdominal) obesity, hypertension, hyperlipidemia and glucose intolerance caused by insulin resistance. This pattern of metabolic defects has been termed syndrome x. Exercise training is effective in reversing many of these abnormalities because skeletal muscle is a major site of glucose and fatty acid metabolism and peripheral vascular resistance. Exercise training increases insulin sensitivity and lipoprotein lipase activity, and decreases vascular resistance in skeletal muscle. Thus, the combination of dietary and exercise management of patients with type II diabetes and syndrome x is attractive and should be used as initial therapy.

Complications of exercise training in diabetics should be anticipated. The cardiovascular responses to graded exercise may be substantially impaired in type I diabetics. For example, maximal oxygen uptake and maximal attainable heart rate may be as much as 15 to 20% less than those values in age-matched control subjects. In addition, diabetic patients frequently have hypertensive blood pressure responses during exercise as well as post-exertional hypotension. Abnormal cardiovascular responses are attributed to altered autonomic and baroreflex control of heart rate and blood pressure. The incidence of asymptomatic coronary disease is also increased in type I and type II diabetics. Exercise testing is recommended for those patients before an exercise program is prescribed.

Insulin therapy in persons with type I diabetes must be adjusted to compensate for anticipated exercise. This step may require a reduction in the longer-acting insulin dosage, which typically has its peak effect in early to late afternoon. Intake of carbohydrate may also be used to compensate for hypoglycemia that may occur with exercise. The uptake of insulin from subcutaneous injection sites may be influenced by exercise. Several researchers report an increase in insulin uptake from injection in sites that overlie active muscle, such as in the thigh. The increased insulin levels could aggravate hypoglycemia in patients who have an otherwise satisfactory balance of carbohydrate intake and insulin therapy. Most authorities recommend an alternate injection site over the abdomen or in muscle groups that are not involved in vigorous exercise.

END-STAGE RENAL DISEASE

End-stage renal disease (ESRD) affects approximately 100,000 persons in the United States. Its causes include diabetes, hypertension, kidney infections, and a variety of autoimmune and inherited-disorders.

Pathophysiology

ESRD is characterized by a gradual loss of glomerular filtration capacity in the kidney. The result is an accumulation of a variety of circulating waste products, including urea, non-urea nitrogen, and creatinine, which is collectively referred to as "ure-mia." The accumulation of these waste products leads to multisystem dysfunction, including muscle weakness, osteodystrophy, cardiac dysfunction, severe anemia, and endocrine and metabolic imbalance. The composite effects of these systemic disorders result in marked reduction in functional capacity.

Treatment

Three forms of treatment are currently available for chronic renal failure: hemodialysis, peritoneal dialysis, and kidney transplantation. ESRD patients do not survive without treatment, but with therapy they may be sustained for a prolonged period. Not all signs and symptoms are corrected by dialysis, however (Table 16–3). Therefore, life function and activities are severely curtailed by the time required to undergo these procedures. In addition, frequent infections and adverse reactions are associated with dialysis. Renal transplantation, with use of a kidney of a living, related donor or from a properly matched cadaver, usually results in normalization of renal function and lifestyle, although many transplant patients experience side effects from immunosuppressive medications.

Table 16–3. Signs and Symptoms of Uremia

System	Corrected by Dialysis	Not Corrected by Dialysis
Musculoskeletal		Renal osteodystrophy, metastatic calcifications, decreased growth; muscle weakness
Neurologic	Encephalopathy, peripheral neuropathy (early)	Peripheral neuropathy (late)
Cardiopulmonary	Volume-dependent hypertension, pericarditis, pleuritis, pulmonary edema, heart murmur	Hyper-reninemic hypertension, accelerated atherogenesis, calcifications
Hematologic	Platelet and white cell dysfunction	Anemia
Immunologic	Decreased immune responsiveness (?)	
Gastrointestinal	Anorexia, nausea, vomiting, colitis, uremic breath	Peptic ulcer disease
Cutaneous	Pruritus due to uremia, uremic frost	Pruritus due to calcium deposition, pallor
Electrolytes	Hyperkalemia; hyponatremia	Hyperphosphatemia, hypocalcemia, hyperuricemia, metabolic acidosis
Endocrine-metabolic	Carbohydrate intolerance; malnutrition; sexual dysfunction; amenorrhea	Hyperlipidemia, thyroid dysfunction, infertility (women), hyperparathyroidism, vitamin D deficiency

Exercise Training and ESRD

As previously mentioned, ESRD patients show marked impairment of functional capacity in addition to impairment of heart rate and ventricular responses to exercise. This impairment has been attributed to the combined effects of anemia, the effects of circulating uremic products on ventricular function, and autonomic function. The exercise capacity of younger patients with ESRD may be 50% of anticipated normal levels. In addition, the maximal heart rate and cardiac output are attenuated.

Researchers from several institutions have reported experience with moderate exercise training of ESRD patients. In all of these studies, increase in functional capacity was noted, as measured by oxygen consumption, as well as an improvement in subjective tolerance to activities of daily living. Whether routine exercise training affects the uremic state or the secondary complications of uremia is not clear. Some investigators describe an increase in hematocrit and hemoglobin levels in ESRD patients undergoing hemodialysis. These results are difficult to interpret because of the variable effects of hemodialysis on blood volume.

Researchers from some institutions now recommend routine exercise training before and after renal transplantation. Such training may result in improved functional status before and an optimal ability to restore the functional capacity after kidney transplantation. In recent studies, investigators noted that functional capacity may increase by 25%, without exercise training, after successful renal transplantation. This increase in exercise capacity is at least partially attributed to restoration of cardiac output and maximal heart rate as well as normalization of hematocrit. Exercise training after transplantation further increases functional capacity, thus optimizing physical functioning.

CHRONIC OBSTRUCTIVE PULMONARY DISEASE

Chronic obstructive pulmonary disease (COPD) includes a spectrum of airway disorders ranging from asthma and simple bronchitis to chronic obstructive bronchitis and emphysema. The hallmark of COPD is obstruction to airway flow as shown by a variety of dynamic expiratory volume measurements. These parameters include: vital capacity, forced expiratory volume achieved in 1 sec, and the forced expiratory flow rate measured at 25% of forced expiratory volume and at 75% of forced expiratory flow rate. Additional measurements of airway function include pressure-volume loops, which are measured by a simultaneous recording of pressure and volume during maximal inspiration and expiration. In addition, measurements of pulmonary diffusing capacity are determined by the rate of inhaled carbon monoxide uptake. These measurements permit accurate classification of lung disease on the basis of alterations in volume, flow rates, compliance, and capacity for diffusion.

Pathophysiology

Asthma is a common form of reversible bronchospasm elicited by allergy, exercise, infections, or other environmental irritants. The bronchial airways respond with increased secretion of mucus and constriction. This response results in the typical combination of nonproductive cough and wheezing, which is reversible with bronchodilator therapy. Symptoms of asthma may be controlled by the prophylactic administration of oral bronchodilator medication in addition to inhaled bronchodilator preparations as needed. In patients with severe asthma, the use of oral and inhaled steroid preparations is required to control persistent bronchospasm.

Bronchitis is an inflammatory disorder of small airways in the lung (less than 2 mm in diameter). Bronchitis is typically seen in smokers and is characterized by coughing, wheezing, and sputum production. During the initial phases of bronchitis, evidence of impaired lung function as measured by standard spirometry may be minimal. Alterations in "small airways" function is detectable with more sensitive tests. In chronic obstructive bronchitis, forced vital capacity and expiratory flow rates are depressed because of obstruction and dynamic compression of airways at high intrapulmonic pressures. Patients with chronic bronchitis have reduced arterial oxygen saturation and increased arterial CO_2 levels as a result of hypoventilation. Physically, they appear congested and plethoric and are nicknamed "blue bloaters."

Emphysema involves the gradual destruction of lung alveolar cell units and connective tissue stroma in addition to airway inflammation. Most patients with emphysema are longstanding smokers; however, a subgroup of patients have a genetic deficiency of α_1-antitrypsin, which is important in controlling the production of endogenous proteolytic enzymes. Lack of α_1-antitrypsin permits these proteolytic enzymes to destroy lung tissue, leading to enlargement of alveolar units and formation of large (bullous) spaces within the lung. The loss of supporting lung tissue leads to early collapse of airways during expiration and also requires high inspiratory lung volumes to maintain airway patency during inspiration. Accordingly, the total lung volume increases and tidal volume changes are achieved at the peak of inspiratory capacity.

Emphysema and bronchitis also produce arterial desaturation because of the marked disturbance in the matching of ventilation to perfusion within the lung. Arterial CO_2 levels are mildly elevated or normal. Some investigators suggest the use of supplementary oxygen to permit a higher intensity and duration of exercise training for COPD patients. Symptom-limited exercise tests during which supplementary oxygen is used are usually performed for a longer duration, with reduced ventilation and heart rates at submaximal efforts.

Exercise Training and COPD

Most patients with asthma benefit from aerobic exercise training, although the mechanism of this improvement is not clear. In studies of adolescent patients with asthma, exercise tolerance increased and some improvement in airway function with regular exercise training was noted. Exercise training complements the use of bronchodilator agents and may decrease the need for these agents in a few patients.

Some individuals do suffer from a form of "exercise-induced" asthma. In these patients, the onset of asthma is related to epithelial water loss and cooling of the airways. The development of exercise-induced asthma may be prevented by the use of various inhaled bronchodilating agents (β_2-agonists) and other substances (cromolyn sodium) before anticipated exercise.

Patients with chronic bronchitis and emphysema may benefit from prescribed exercise training. Results of most available studies show an increase in exercise tolerance (duration) with minimal or no increase in measured oxygen uptake. This finding is possibly related to increased efficiency of muscle movement or increased tolerance to dyspnea. In studies of airway function and arterial blood gases, patients showed little or no improvement of airway conductance measurements or significant changes in arterial oxygen or carbon dioxide levels after exercise training.

Patients with COPD should be evaluated with symptom-limited exercise testing and measurement of ventilation, electrocardiography, and arterial saturation by ear oximetry. Patients who show marked decreases in saturation may be poor candidates for any form of exercise training. Some of these patients may be able to perform limited exercise with supplementary oxygen. Supraventricular and ventricular arrhythmias are common in patients with COPD who use theophylline-based bronchodilator agents.

Exercise prescription formats for COPD patients vary widely, and no standard is currently available. Some investigators advise repeated intervals of walking to an end point of dyspnea followed by recovery. Other studies have used higher training intensities of 80% maximum tolerated workload for 15 to 20 minutes, twice daily, 5 days per week.

Some recent studies have emphasized upper extremity exercise training (arm, shoulder, chest) to strengthen recruitable nonrespiratory muscle function. This strategy reduces dyspnea (because of dyssynchronous thoracic-abdominal coupling), which is frequently associated with use of the arms during activities of daily living in COPD patients.

PERIPHERAL VASCULAR DISEASE

Obstructive peripheral vascular disease is commonly seen in patients over 50. The usual cause of peripheral vascular disease is atherosclerotic obstruction of the iliac, femoral, and popliteal arteries. Peripheral vascular disease is also a frequent complication of diabetes.

The hallmark symptom of peripheral vascular disease is muscular pain (claudication) during exercise that is relieved by rest. Claudication involves muscular units that are distal to the region of vascular obstruction. Typically, the calf and foot are affected, with obstruction of the femoral and popliteal arteries. Obstruction in a more superior part of the iliac arteries may produce claudication of the buttock and quadriceps group in addition to the gastrocnemius muscles.

Diagnosis

The initial diagnosis of peripheral vascular disease is made on the basis of clinical history and the findings on physical examination. Auscultation of the femoral arteries may reveal bruits and reduced pulse volume on palpation. Measurement of popliteal and ankle systolic pressures are also helpful. The popliteal or posterior tibial systolic pressure is usually 15 to 25 mm Hg higher than the simultaneous brachial artery pressure. A ratio of the posterior tibial to the brachial pressure index of 1 or less suggests peripheral vascular disease. Values of less than 80% are suggestive of moderate peripheral vascular disease, and ratios of less than 50% indicate severe peripheral vascular disease. Exercise testing may be used to amplify these findings. Immediately after exercise, the systolic pressure index may fall to 50% or less in patients with moderate to peripheral vascular disease and less than 15% in persons with severe peripheral vascular disease. The anatomic location and severity of peripheral vascular disease are determined by pulse volume recordings or ultrasonic scanning. Arteriography is necessary for determining possible sites for surgical bypass of obstructive lesions.

Treatment

Medical management of patients with peripheral vascular disease is marginally effective. Various vasodilating agents have achieved variable results. One problem with this approach is the phenomenon of arterial "steal," in which vasodilation of normally perfused segments may shunt blood away from already underperfused areas. Some symptoms of peripheral vascular disease may result from periodic platelet obstruction in the narrowed vascular lumen. The use of antiplatelet agents such as aspirin may be beneficial in these patients. Most patients with peripheral vascular disease are chronic smokers and have other risk factors for coronary artery disease. Discontinuation of smoking and modification of these risk factors is mandatory.

Exercise Training and Peripheral Vascular Disease

Exercise training has been used to improve functional tolerance to exercise and to diminish symptoms of claudication. Some patients show an improvement in walking distance and a delay in onset of claudication symptoms. In several studies, researchers showed that this increase in exercise tolerance is not accompanied by improvement in peripheral blood flow, although they noted an increased oxidative enzyme capacity within skeletal muscle after exercise training. Therefore, an improvement in the efficiency of energy production for muscle contraction may be the basis for symptomatic improvement after exercise training.

Cardiovascular exercise training may be achieved in patients with claudication through the use of combined arm and leg exercise ergometers. Many of the patients achieve a typical training effect with improved oxygen uptake and reduction in the heart rate response to standard exercise testing. The incidence of coronary artery disease in patients with established peripheral vascular disease varies from 50 to 80%. Patients with peripheral vascular disease must be evaluated with upper extremity exercise testing or dipyridamole thallium scintigraphy before beginning an exercise training program.

SUGGESTED READING

Hypertension

Chick TW, Halperin AK, Gacek EM: The effect of antihypertensive medications on exercise performance: A review. *Med Sci Sports Exerc, 20:*447, 1988.

Gordon NF, Scott CB, Wilkinson WJ, Duncan JJ, Blair SN: Exercise and mild essential hypertension. Recommendations for adults. *Sports Med, 10:*390, 1990.

Hagberg JM: Exercise, fitness, and hypertension. In Exercise, Fitness, and Health: A Consensus of Current Knowledge. Edited by Bouchard et al. Champaign, IL: Human Kinetics Books, 1990, pp. 455–466.

Lund-Johanson P: Hemodynamics in essential hypertension. *Clin Sci, 59:*343, 1980.

Tipton CM: Exercise, training and hypertension: An update. *Exerc Sports Sci Rev, 17:*447, 1990.

Diabetes

American Diabetes Association: Clinical Practice Recommendations (1990–1991). Exercise and NIDDM. *Diabetes Care, 1A(Suppl 2):*52, 1991.

Horton ES: Role of and management of exercise in diabetes mellitus. *Diabetes Care, 11:*201, 1988.

Schneider SH, Ruderman NB: Exercise and NIDDM. *Diabetes Care, 13:*785, 1990.

Wallberg-Hendricksson H: Exercise and diabetes. *Exerc Sports Sci Rev, 20:*339, 1992.

End-Stage Renal Disease

Gallager-Lepak S: Functional capacity and activity level before and after renal transplantation. *ANNA J, 18:*378, 1991.

Goldberg AP, Geltman EM, Hagberg JM, et al.: Therapeutic benefits of exercise training for hemodialysis patients. *Kidney Int, 516:*S303, 1983.

Horber FF, Scheidegger JR, Grunig BE, Frey FJ: Evidence that prednisone-induced myopathy is reversed by physical training. *J Clin Endocrinol Metab, 61:*83, 1985.

Kempeneers GLG, Myburgh KH, Wigins T, et al.: The effects of an exercise training programme in renal transplant recipients. *Am J Kidney Dis, 16:*57, 1990.

Lundin AP, Stein RA, Frank F, et al.: Cardiovascular status in long-term hemodialysis patients: An exercise and echocardiographic study. *Nephron, 28:*234, 1981.

Moore GE, Brinker KR, Stray-Gundersen J, Mitchell JH: Determinants of maximal oxygen uptake in patients with end-stage renal disease. Submitted for publication.

Miller TD, Squires RW, Gau GT, et al.: Graded exercise testing and training after renal transplantation: A Preliminary Study. *Mayo Clin Proc, 62:*773, 1987.

Painter PL: Exercise training during hemodialysis: Rates of participation. *Dial Transplant, 17:*165, 1988.

Painter PL, Hanson P, Messer-Rehak DL, et al.: Exercise tolerance changes following renal transplantation. *Am J Kidney Dis, 10:*452, 1987.

Painter PL, Messer-Rehak DL, Hanson P, Zimmerman SW, Glass NR: Exercise capacity in hemodialysis, CAPD and renal transplant patients. *Nephron, 42:*47, 1986.

Shalom R, Blumenthal JA, Williams RS, et al.: Feasibility and benefits of exercise training in patients on maintenance dialysis. *Kidney Int, 25:*958, 1984.

Zabetakis PM, Gleim GW, Pasternak FL, et al.: Long-duration submaximal exercise conditioning in hemodialysis patients. *Clin Nephrol, 18:*17, 1982.

Chronic Obstructive Pulmonary Disease

Carter R, Coast JR, Idell S: Exercise training in patients with chronic obstructive pulmonary disease. *Med Sci Sports Exerc, 24:*281, 1992.

Casaburi R, Wasserman K: Exercise training in pulmonary rehabilitation. *N Engl J Med, 314:*1509, 1986.

Lake FR, Henderson K, Briffa T, Openshaw J, Musk AW: Upper limb and lower limb exercise training in patients with chronic airflow obstruction. *Chest, 97:*1077, 1990.

Swerts PMJ, Kretzers LMJ, Terpstra-Lineman E, et al.: Exercise training as a mediator of increased exercise performance in patients with chronic obstructive pulmonary disease. *J Cardiopulm Rehab, 12:*188, 1992.

Peripheral Vascular Disease

Williams LR, Ekers MA, Collins PS, Lee JF. Vascular rehabilitation: Benefits of a structured exercise-risk modification program. *J Vasc Surg, 14:*320, 1991.

Chapter 17

PHARMACOLOGIC FACTORS IN EXERCISE AND EXERCISE TESTING

Steven P. Van Camp

Medications that affect the exercise response or exercise test are taken by many people who exercise regularly, want to begin an exercise program, or undergo exercise tests. These medications may be administered for noncardiovascular as well as cardiovascular conditions. To understand the exercise response and the exercise electrocardiogram (ECG) of a patient receiving such medications, the actions of these medications must be clearly understood.

Medications may directly affect the exercise response, such as the effects of β-adrenergic blocking agents (beta-blockers) on heart rate, blood pressure, and thus myocardial oxygen consumption. Other medications may affect exercise indirectly; an example is the potential for certain diuretics to produce hypokalemia, which may result in the development of cardiac arrhythmias or false-positive results of an exercise electrocardiogram. In this chapter, we address the importance of medications, their actions and side effects, and considerations relevant to exercise and exercise testing.

The acute and chronic physiologic responses to exercise involve changes in sympathetic and parasympathetic tone, heart rate, blood pressure, myocardial contractility, venous return, arterial resistance, fluid loss, and exercise capacity. Any medication that alters by either inhibiting or exaggerating these responses or the ECG (which is monitored during an exercise test) may affect the exercise response and exercise test of the patient receiving that medication.

As the effects of medications on heart rate, blood pressure, myocardial contractility, cardiac rhythm, electrocardiographic findings, and exercise capacity are considered, the physiologic and pathophysiologic status of the patient must also be considered and understood. An important fact to remember is that medications are usually administered because of pathophysiologic abnormalities such as angina pectoris, congestive heart failure, or arrhythmias rather than for the pathologic conditions (coronary heart disease, valvular heart disease, or congenital heart disease) alone. Patients should not be considered as homogeneous groups of either "normal," "diseased," or cardiac patients. "Normal" and "diseased" patients vary greatly with respect to exercise capacity, autonomic tone, body size, and general medical status, including orthopedic disorders as well as kidney and liver function. Patients with cardiovascular and pulmonary diseases, diabetes mellitus, and renal failure also have a wide range of pathophysiologic responses to exercise. Among these responses are variations in blood pressure, resting and maximal heart rates, left ventricular function, and exercise-limiting pathophysiologic factors (such as myocardial ischemia, poor left ventricular function, arrhythmias, intermittent claudication, bronchospasm and pulmonary insufficiency). Another important factor is the individual variation in response to medication (interpatient variability). These variations may result from metabolic or other unknown factors. All of these individual factors must be considered to understand the role of medications in exercise and exercise testing.

In addition to individual patient responses, pharmacologic factors require consideration. Most medications have dose-related effects. Medications administered in dosages that result in subtherapeutic levels usually have no effects. Within therapeutic ranges, greater effects may occur with larger doses. An adverse response may occur as toxic levels are reached. Many medications interact positively (synergistically) or negatively with other medications. Medications may also induce clinical problems, including arrhythmias, bronchospasm, abnormal ST-T wave responses (the so-called "false-positive" test for myocardial ischemia), hypokalemia, hypovolemia, and depression. Hypokalemia may, in turn, increase the likelihood of cardiac arrhythmias and abnormal ST-T wave changes. Hypovolemia increases the tendency toward orthostatic hypotension, especially in the postexercise period. Depression affects the desire to exercise rather than the hemodynamic elements of exercise or any parameter measured during an exercise test.

The best approach, therefore, to understanding the role of medications in exercise and exercise testing is to:

1. Understand the physiologic and pathophysiologic responses of the individual patient to exercise and exercise testing.
2. Understand the mechanism of action and general actions of the medications, appreciating the individual dose-response factors. To understand the general characteristics of medications within a therapeutic class is important, remember that sometimes medications within these classes may have variable properties (see sections concerning beta blockers and calcium channel blockers).
3. Understand that individual variability occurs in patient responses.
4. Apply the generalities of the properties of the medication and the specifics of a patient's circumstances to the exercise test or exercise prescription.

Remember that the hemodynamic effects of a medication usually occur only if the medication is administered in therapeutic doses. Finally, observation of a response while the patient is receiving medication can confirm suspected responses to identify an individual or idiosyncratic responses.

Medications that can be administered to ambulatory (nonhospitalized) patients are discussed. To consider all medications specifically is impossible, and thus the major categories of medication are discussed, along with relevant examples of specific medications. Understanding of most of those medications not included is possible by considering the class to which they belong. Effects of the medications on heart rate, blood pressure, the ECG, and exercise capacity are indicated when clinically important. Naturally, if a medication results in an increase or decrease in myocardial ischemia, it may have corresponding effects on the symptom of angina pectoris and the electrocardiographic findings.

Generic rather than brand names of medications are used, although it is important to know both terms. For some generic medications, more than one brand name may be available (e.g., Procardia and Adalat are brand names of nifedipine). Some brand names of the generic medications discussed in the chapter are listed in Table 17–1.

Not all side effects are discussed, but an attempt has been made to include those related to exercise testing and prescription.

Medications are often used in combination, so consideration of the pharmacologic actions of all drugs is important when predicting the net effect of simultaneously administered medications.

The effects of medications on heart rate, blood pressure, electrocardiographic findings, and exercise capacity are detailed in Table 17–2. These effects are those typically observed, but the factors mentioned previously must, of course, be considered as well.

Medications that are not administered specifically for cardiovascular conditions may still have effects on resting or exercise heart rate, blood pressure, electrocardiographic findings, or exercise capacity. Therefore, they also merit consideration.

THE β-ADRENERGIC BLOCKING AGENTS

The β-adrenergic blocking agents, or beta-blockers, are used in the treatment of patients with a variety of cardiovascular and other medical conditions including angina pectoris, hypertension, previous myocardial infarction, cardiac arrhythmias, essential (familial) tremors, and migraine headaches.

Table 17–1. Medications Discussed Relative to Exercise and Exercise Testing

Generic Name	Brand Name	Generic Name	Brand Name
Beta-blockers		Enalapril	Vasotec
Acebutolol	Sectral	Fosinopril	Monopril
Atenolol	Tenormin	Lisinopril	Prinivil, Zestril
Betaxolol	Kerlone	Quinapril	Accupril
Metoprolol	Lopressor, Toprol XL	Ramipril	Altace
Nadolol	Corgard		
Penbutolol	Levatol	*α-Adrenergic blocker*	
Pindolol	Visken	Doxazosin	Cardura
Propranolol	Inderal, Inderal LA	Prazosin	Minipress
Timolol	Blocadren	Terazosin	Hytrin
Alpha and beta-blockers		*Antiadrenergic agents without selective*	
Labetalol	Trandate, Normodyne	*blockade of peripheral receptors*	
Nitrates and nitroglycerin		Clonidine	Catapres, Catapres-TTS
Isosorbide dinitrate	Isordil, Sorbitrate,	Guanabenz	Wytensin
	Dilatrate-SR	Guanethidine	Ismelin
Nitroglycerin	Nitrostat, Nitro-Bid	Guanfacine	Tenex
Nitroglycerin ointment	Nitro-Bid, Nitrol ointment	Methyldopa	Aldomet
Nitroglycerin patches	Transderm Nitro, Nitro-	Reserpine	Serapasil
	Dur II, Nitrodisc,		
	Minitran	*Antiarrhythmic agents*	
		Class I	
Calcium channel blockers		Quinidine	Quinidex, Quinaglute
Bepridil	Vascor	Disopyramide	Norpace, Norpace CR
Diltiazem	Cardizem, Cardizem SR,	Procainamide	Pronestyl, Pronestyl SR
	Cardizem CD		Procan SR
Felodipine	Plendil	Moricizine	Ethmozine
Isradipine	DynaCirc	Mexiletine	Mexitil
Nicardipine	Cardene, Cardene SR	Phenytoin	Dilantin
Nifedipine	Procardia, Procardia XL,	Tocainide	Tonocard
	Adalat	Flecainide	Tambocor
Verapamil	Calan, Calan SR	Propafenone	Rhymol
	Isoptin, Isoptin SR	Class III	
	Verelan	Amiodarone	Cordarone
Digitalis		*Bronchodilators*	
Digoxin	Lanoxin	Anticholinergic agents	
	Lanoxicaps	Ipratropium	Atrovent
		Methylxanthines	
Diuretics		Theophylline	Theo-Dur, Uniphyl
Thiazides		Sympathomimetic agents	
Hydrochlorothiazide	Esidrix	Ephedrine	
(HCTZ)		Epinephrine	Primatene
''Loop''		Metaproterenol	Alupent, Metaprel
Furosemide	Lasix	Albuterol	Proventil, Ventolin
Ethacrynic acid	Edecrin	Isoetharine	Bronkosol
Potassium-sparing		Terbutaline	Brethine, Brethaire
Spironolactone	Aldactone	Cromolyn sodium	Intal
Triamterene	Dyrenium		
Amiloride	Midamor	*Hyperlipidemic agents*	
Combinations		Cholestyramine	Questran
Triamterene and	Dyazide, Maxzide	Colestipol	Colestid
hydrochlorothiazide		Clofibrate	Atromid-S
Amiloride and	Moduretic	Dextrothyroxine	Choloxin
hydrochlorothiazide		Gemfibrozil	Lopid
Others		Lovastatin	Mevacor
Metolazone	Zaroxolyn	Nicotinic acid (niacin)	Nicobid
	Diulo	Pravastatin	Pravachol
		Probucol	Lorelco
Nonadrenergic vasodilators		Simvastatin	Zocor
Hydralazine	Apresoline		
Minoxidil	Loniten	*Other*	
		Dipyridamole	Persantine
Angiotensin-converting enzyme (ACE inhibitors)		Warfarin	Coumadin
Benazepril	Lotensin	Pentoxifylline	Trental
Captopril	Capoten		

Table 17–2. Effects of Medications on Heart Rate, Blood Pressure, the Electrocardiogram (ECG) and Exercise Capacity

Medications	Heart Rate Rest	Heart Rate Exercise	Blood Pressure Rest (R) and Exercise (E)	ECG Rest	ECG Exercise	Exercise Capacity
I. Beta blockers (including labetalol)	↓*	↓	↓	↓ HR*	↓ ischemia†	↑ in patients with angina; ↓ or ↔ in patients without angina
II. Nitrates	↑	↑ or ↔	↓ (R) ↓ or ↔ (E)	↑ HR	↑ or ↔ HR ↓ ischemia†	↑ in patients with angina; ↔ in patients without angina; ↑ or ↔ in patients with congestive heart failure (CHF)
III. Calcium channel blockers						
Felodipine Isradipine Nicardipine Nifedipine	↑ or ↔	↑ or ↔	↓	↑ or ↔ HR	↑ or ↔ HR ↓ ischemia†	↑ in patients with angina; ↔ in patients without angina
Bepridil Diltiazem Verapamil	↓	↓	↓	↓ HR	↓ HR ↓ ischemia†	↑ in patients with angina; ↔ in patients without angina
IV. Digitalis	↓ in patients w/atrial fibrillation and possibly CHF. Not significantly altered in patients w/sinus rhythm		↔	May produce nonspecific ST-T wave changes	May produce ST segment depression	Improved only in patients with atrial fibrillation or in patients with CHF
V. Diuretics	↔	↔	↔ or ↓	↔	May cause PVCs and "false positive" test results if hypokalemia occurs. May cause PVCs if hypomagnesemia occurs	↔, except possibly in patients with CHF (see text)
VI. Vasodilators, nonadrenergic vasodilators	↑ or ↔	↑ or ↔	↓	↑ or ↔ HR	↑ or ↔ HR	↔, except ↑ or ↔ in patients with CHF
ACE inhibitors	↔	↔	↓	↔	↔	↔
Alpha-adrenergic blockers	↔	↔	↓	↔	↔	↔
Anti-adrenergic agents without selective blockade of peripheral receptors	↓ or ↔	↓ or ↔	↓	↓ or ↔ HR	↓ or ↔ HR	↔, except ↑ or ↔ in patients with CHF

VII. Antiarrhythmic agents

All antiarrhythmic agents may cause new or worsened arrhythmias (proarrhythmic effect)

Agent	Rest	Exercise	ECG / Comments	Exercise capacity
Class I				
Quinidine	↑ or ↔	↓ or ↔ (R) ↔ (E)	↑ or ↔ HR; May prolong QRS and QT intervals; Quinidine may result in "false negative" test results	↔
Disopyramide				
Procainamide	↕	↕	May prolong QRS and QT intervals; May result in "false positive" test results	↔
Phenytoin / Tocainide / Mexiletine	↕	↕	↔	↔
Flecainide / Moricizine	↕	↕	May prolong QRS and QT intervals	↔
Propafenone	↓ or ↔	↓ or ↔	↓ or ↔ HR	↔
Class II Beta blockers (see I.)				
Class III Amiodarone	→	→	↓ HR	↔
Class IV Calcium channel blockers (see III.)				

VIII. Bronchodilators

Agent	Rest	Exercise	ECG / Comments	Exercise capacity
Anticholinergic agents	↕	↕	↕	↔
Methylxanthines	↑ or ↔	↑ or ↔	↑ or ↔ HR; May produce PVCs	↑ or ↔ HR; May produce PVCs
Sympathomimetic agents	↑ or ↔	↑, ↔, or →	↑ or ↔ HR	↑ or ↔ HR
Cromolyn sodium	↕	↕	↕	↕
Corticosteroids	↕	↕	↕	↕

Bronchodilators ↑ exercise capacity in patients limited by bronchospasm

IX. Hyperlipidemic agents

Clofibrate may provoke arrhythmias, angina in patients with prior myocardial infarction.
Dextrothyroxine may ↑ HR and BP at rest and during exercise, provoke arrhythmias and worsen myocardial ischemia and angina.
Nicotinic acid may ↓ BP.
Probucol may cause QT interval prolongation.
All other hyperlipidemic agents have no effect on HR, BP, and ECG. — ↔

X. Psychotropic medications

Agent	Rest	Exercise	ECG / Comments	Exercise capacity
Minor tranquilizers	May ↓ HR and BP by controlling anxiety. No other effects.			↔
Antidepressants	↑ or ↔	↓ or ↔	(see text); May result in "false positive" test results	↔
Major tranquilizers	↑ or ↔	↓ or ↔	(see text); May result in "false positive" or "false negative" test results	
Lithium	↔	↔	May result in T wave changes and arrhythmias	

(continued)

Table 17–2. (Continued)

Medications	Heart Rate	Blood Pressure	ECG	Exercise Capacity
XI. Nicotine	↑ or ↔	↑	↑ or ↔ HR, May provoke ischemia, arrhythmias	↔, except ↓ or ↔ in patients with angina
XII. Antihistamines	↔	↔	↔	↔
XIII. Cold medications with sympathomimetic agents	Effects similar to those described in sympathomimetic agents, although magnitude of effects is usually smaller			↔
XIV. Thyroid medications Only levothyroxine	↑	↑	↑ HR May provoke arrhythmias ↑ ischemia	↔, unless angina worsened
XV. Alcohol	↔	Chronic use may have role in ↑ BP	May provoke arrhythmias	↔
XVI. Hypoglycemic agents Insulin and oral agents	↔	↔	↔	↔
XVII. Dipyridamole	↔	↔	↔	↔
XVIII. Anticoagulants	↔	↔	↔	↔
XIX. Antigout medications	↔	↔	↔	↔
XX. Antiplatelet medications	↔	↔	↔	↔
XXI. Pentoxifylline	↔	↔	↔	↑ or ↔ in patients limited by intermittent claudication
XXII. Caffeine	Variable effects depending upon previous usage. Variable effects on exercise capacity. May provoke arrhythmias (see text).			
XXIII. Diet pills	↑ or ↔	↑ or ↔	↑ or ↔ HR	(see text)

↑ = increase, ↔ = no effect, ↓ = decrease
* Beta-blockers with ISA lower resting HR only slightly
† May prevent or delay myocardial ischemia (see text)

Actions

These drugs exert their effects by competitively blocking β-adrenergic receptors, thereby limiting their stimulation at rest and during periods of exercise and emotional excitement. The β_1-receptors mediate cardiac stimulation, whereas β_2-receptors mediate relaxation of vascular and bronchial smooth muscle. Beta-blockers act on both of these types of receptors, although "cardioselective" beta-blockers exert a greater effect on β_1-receptors than on β_2-receptors.

The specific effects of beta-blockers on heart rate, blood pressure, and the electrocardiogram are detailed in Table 17–2. Heart rate, blood pressure, and myocardial contractility are decreased at rest and with submaximal or maximal exercise. Therefore, myocardial oxygen consumption is decreased. Additionally, as heart rate decreases, diastolic filling time of coronary arteries increases, thus allowing for increased myocardial oxygen supply in comparison to the "unblocked" state. These changes are responsible for the beneficial effects of beta-blockers observed in patients with angina pectoris.

Use of beta-blockers results in a lower blood pressure, probably by suppressing renin release from the kidneys, decreasing cardiac output, and, possibly, by decreasing central nervous system sympathetic discharge. Other actions include inhibition of platelet aggregation and inhibition of synthesis of thromboxane, a potent vasoconstrictor. Beta-blockers are also useful in the management of certain cardiac arrhythmias by virtue of their direct beta-blocking actions or by a quinidine-like membrane-stabilizing effect. Beta-blockers also appear to improve the prognosis is selected patients after myocardial infarction. The mechanism by which this occurs is unknown, but the antiarrhythmic effects of the beta-blockers are probably instrumental.

Patients for whom exercise capacity is limited by angina pectoris experience improved exercise tolerance while being treated with beta-blockers. These patients are able to perform more exercise before reaching their myocardial ischemic threshold, with its accompanying angina pectoris

and electrocardiographic changes of ischemia. For patients who are not limited by angina pectoris, beta-blocker therapy may decrease exercise capacity if significant fatigue is a side effect of this form of therapy. Patients with significant left ventricular dysfunction with or without angina pectoris may experience a decrease in maximal exercise capacity as a result of the adverse effect of the drugs on myocardial contractility (i.e., negative inotropic effect).

Because beta-blockers are competitive, reversible antagonists of β-adrenergic stimulation; their effects are dose-related, temporary, and dependent upon the endogenous catecholamine concentration of the individual. The general responses are uniform among individuals, but the magnitude of the response varies markedly from patient to patient.

Side Effects

Beta-blockade may produce peripheral arteriolar constriction by blocking β_2-mediated vasodilation, allowing unopposed α-adrenergically mediated vasoconstriction. Worsening of claudication in people with peripheral vascular disease and complaints of cold extremities thus may result. Other possible side effects include coronary artery vasoconstriction and worsening of coronary artery spasm, also resulting from unopposed vasoconstriction; precipitation or worsening of bronchospasm secondary to inhibition of β_2-receptor-mediated relaxation of bronchial smooth muscle; and possible congestive heart failure because of depression of myocardial contractility. Because of their effects on heart rate and atrioventricular (AV) nodal conduction, beta-blockers may result in bradycardia or AV block. Beta-blocker therapy may prove hazardous to patients with diabetes who receive insulin therapy because beta-blockers depress the sympathetic nervous system-mediated response to, and warning signs of, hypoglycemia. These agents inhibit catecholamine-induced glycogenolysis and the signs of hypoglycemia, including nervousness and tachycardia.

Therefore, beta-blocker therapy is generally contraindicated in patients with peripheral vascular disease and claudication, coronary artery spasm, congestive heart failure (or poor left ventricular function), and sinus node disease, as well as patients who receive insulin therapy for diabetes mellitus.

Adverse lipid effects of increased triglycerides and decreased HDL cholesterol have been reported, although these effects are apparently less prominent with cardioselective beta-blockers, and appear to be absent in beta-blockers with ISA. Abrupt withdrawal of beta-blocker therapy may result in acceleration of angina pectoris, tachycardia, myocardial infarction, sudden death, and hypertension (the propranolol withdrawal rebound phenomenon). These effects appear related to increased sensitivity to β-adrenergic stimulation after chronic beta-blocker administration. Bothersome side effects of beta-blockers that affect the central nervous system are fatigue, depression, and vivid or bizarre dreams.

Variable Characteristics

Cardioselectivity is a relative property by which certain beta-blockers exert greater effects on β_1-receptors than on β_2-receptors. Theoretically, this property causes fewer side effects and also allows persons with peripheral vascular disease and bronchospasm to use beta-blockers. Acebutolol, atenolol, betaxolol, and metoprolol are cardioselective beta-blockers. This property is *relative* in that it is lost at higher doses and does not occur to an absolute extent (see Table 17–3).

Beta-blockers with *intrinsic sympathomimetic activity* (ISA) retain their beta-blocking action, but do exert some sympathetic stimulation, primarily at rest. This property results in only a slight decline in resting heart rate and is helpful in treating patients in whom bradycardia would otherwise limit the use of beta blockers. Acebutolol and pindolol are beta-blockers that possess ISA, while penbutolol exhibits a partial ISA effect.

The *lipid solubility* of a beta-blocker determines its duration of action. Beta-blockers with low lipid solubility are metabolized by the liver at slow rates and excreted primarily by the renal route. Additionally, they do not cross the blood-brain barrier. These beta-blockers have the longest duration of action (approximately 24 hours) and theoretically are less likely to cause central nervous system side effects (depression, nightmares, and possibly fatigue) than other beta-blockers.

Labetalol is a medication that exerts both α and β blocking effects. Thus, its actions are a combination of both of these effects, although the beta-blocker effects predominate.

Exercise and Exercise Testing Considerations

Researchers have shown that, although the heart rate and blood pressure response to exercise are blunted in the beta-blocked state, the acute administration of beta-blockers may not decrease maximal oxygen consumption ($\dot{V}O_{2max}$) of maximal exercise

Table 17–3. Characteristics of Beta-Blockers

Specific Beta-Blockers	Cardioselectivity	Intrinsic Sympathomimetic Activity	Lipid Solubility
Acebutolol (Sectral)	+*	+	Low
Atenolol (Tenormin)	+	−	Low
Betaxolol (Kerlone)	+	−	Low
Metoprolol (Lopressor)	+	−	Moderate
Nadolol (Corgard)	−	−	Low
Penbutolol (Levatol)	−	partial	Low
Pindolol (Visken)	−	+	Moderate
Propranolol (Inderal)	−	−	High
Timolol (Blocadren)	−	−	Low

* + = presence of characteristic; − = absence of characteristic.

capacity. The ability of patients receiving beta-blocker therapy to train is controversial, but it appears that a training effect (an increase in $\dot{V}o_{2max}$ or exercise capacity after periods of training) can be achieved despite long-term therapy. Beta-blocker therapy also apparently does not change the relationship between percent $\dot{V}o_{2max}$ and percent of maximal heart rate. Therefore, the usual methods to calculate target heart rate for exercise prescriptions can still be used with reasonable accuracy, with consideration, of course, that the maximal heart rate and thus also the training heart rate will be lower in persons receiving beta-blockers. It is the maximal heart rate with beta-blocker therapy that must be used for prescription purposes. (See the discussion of exercise prescription at the end of this chapter for target heart rate calculation for patients receiving beta-blockers.)

Beta-blockers are said to bring about false-negative results on electrocardiographic tests for myocardial ischemia. A more appropriate way to look at the situation follows. If the level of myocardial oxygen consumption at which a patient develops ischemia is exceeded, he or she will still develop ischemia, even while receiving beta-blocker therapy. Signs of ischemia will be present on the exercise ECG, as in the untreated situation. If beta-blocker therapy prevents the rate pressure product from reaching the point at which myocardial ischemia occurs, neither myocardial ischemia nor electrocardiographic signs of myocardial ischemia will occur. Often the maximal exercise heart rate in patients receiving beta-blocker therapy is blunted to the degree that the tests should be considered *suboptimal* for the purposes of diagnosis rather than negative for the presence of myocardial ischemia. In certain situations, therefore, it may be appropriate to discontinue medication before a diagnostic exercise test is performed (i.e., stop the drug if the test is to be used for diagnosis of CAD; continue the drug if testing efficacy of medical management).

NITRATES

Nitrates are the oldest and most commonly used medications for angina pectoris.

Actions

Nitrates directly relax vascular smooth muscle, exerting their primary effects on the *venous* system and a lesser effect on the arterial system. The resulting venodilation decreases ventricular volume and end-diastolic pressure (preload), and the arteriolar vasodilation decreases systemic vascular resistance and arterial blood pressure (afterload). These specific effects on heart rate, blood pressure, and the electrocardiographic findings are detailed in Table 17–2. An increase in resting heart rate, and to a lesser extent the heart rate during exercise, occurs through a baroreceptor-mediated reflex tachycardia that occurs in response to the arterial vasodilation. Blood pressure declines with the subject at rest and may decline during exercise. At rest, a reflex tachycardia may be noted electrocardiographically. During exercise, ischemic electrocardiographic changes may be prevented, decreased, or delayed. They occur to a lesser extent at similar submaximal workloads when compared with the untreated state; in other words, greater amounts of exercise may be performed before the development of ischemia.

Nitrates are administered in multiple forms and dosages by numerous routes. The hemodynamic effects to be described, as is true for all medications, are seen only if nitrates are administered in therapeutic doses. Nitrates especially may be taken at subtherapeutic doses. This information regarding dosage may be considered when evaluating or anticipating hemodynamic effects.

Patients in whom exercise capacity is limited by angina pectoris show improvement with nitrate administration because of prevention, reduction, or delay in ischemia, and hence angina pectoris. In patients with congestive heart failure, nitrates may improve exercise capacity through reduction in pulmonary venous pressure and aortic impedance. Nitrates have no effect on the exercise capacity of patients without myocardial ischemia, angina pectoris, or congestive heart failure.

The hemodynamic effects of nitrates, in concert, lower myocardial oxygen consumption, an effect of primary clinical importance in the treatment of angina pectoris. Additionally, coronary blood flow to ischemic areas of myocardium may improve because of increased collateral flow or decreased ventricular diastolic pressure with reduced subendocardial vessel compression. Thus, nitrates may increase myocardial supply as well as decrease myocardial oxygen demand in patients with coronary heart disease, although the latter effect is of greater clinical importance. Another hemodynamic effect on nitrates, resulting from their vasodilatory capacity, is the reduction of impedance to ventricular systolic emptying. Although nitrates have no direct effect upon myocardial contractility, they may indirectly improve it by reducing ischemia and impedance to systolic emptying.

By the aforementioned actions, angina pectoris is prevented, reduced, or relieved in patients receiving therapeutic doses of nitrates. Nitrates improve exercise capacity before angina pectoris occurs, and decrease or eliminate electrocardiographic findings of ischemia at submaximal workloads when compared with the untreated state.

The prevention and relief of coronary artery spasm occur with nitrates, but otherwise the net effect on the coronary vasculature is of questionable significance. High-grade coronary artery stenoses are unlikely to be significantly improved with nitroglycerin. Eccentric coronary artery narrowing, however, may be improved by dilation of the uninvolved portion of the vessel. Improvement in congestive heart failure symptoms occurs because of the decrease in preload and decrease in impedance to ventricular systolic emptying.

Forms and Routes of Administration

Nitrates can be administered in multiple forms and by multiple routes: (1) sublingual, (2) oral (long-acting), (3) aerosol oral spray, (4) intravenous, and (5) transdermal (ointments and patches).

Larger doses are necessary when nitrates are administered orally because much of the drug is removed from the blood by the liver before reaching the systemic circulation. These medications may be used to treat angina pectoris on an as-needed basis or administered prophylactically to prevent or to reduce the likelihood of angina.

Typically, medication doses are adjusted until the desired effects are achieved or bothersome side effects occur. Note that marked differences occur between patients with regard to the amount of nitrates that may be required for therapeutic effect or before side effects occur. Patients receiving nitrates on a chronic basis usually develop nitrate tolerance with loss of therapeutic effect unless there is a 10- to 12-hour nitrate-free interval as part of the therapeutic regimen.

Side Effects

Postural hypotension that results from a decrease in systemic blood pressure, headaches related to cerebral blood vessel dilatation, and flushing sensations resulting from peripheral vasodilation are the most bothersome side effects of nitrate usage. These side effects often decrease or disappear in time with continued administration, or a decrease in dosage may be required.

Exercise and Exercise Testing Considerations

Prophylactic use of sublingual nitroglycerin is often effective in preventing angina pectoris. Thus, before an activity that the patient knows might provoke angina, sublingual nitroglycerin may be used to prevent or reduce its occurrence. The possible occurrence of postural hypotension resulting from peripheral vasodilation merits consideration, especially in the postexercise period. Exercise prescriptions involving target heart rates need no alteration if nitrates are administered to a patient because these agents do not significantly affect heart rate response.

CALCIUM CHANNEL BLOCKERS

A recently available category of potent cardiovascular medications is the calcium channel blockers, also known as calcium antagonists or calcium blockers.

Actions

Calcium channel blockers act by blocking various calcium-dependent processes in vascular smooth muscle and myocardial cells. This action occurs through selective blockade of transmembrane calcium flow and the resulting slow inward calcium current. Thus, calcium entry into cardiac and smooth muscle cells is limited.

Although the currently available calcium channel blockers have a similar mechanism of action, they have variable vasodilatory, negative inotropic, and electrophysiologic effects. Generalities will be made in an attempt to understand the clinical effects of the agents. Nicardipine and nifedipine result in the greatest reduction of coronary and peripheral vascular resistance without significant inotropic or electrophysiologic effects. Diltiazem and verapamil have lesser but significant coronary and peripheral vasodilatory effects, with modest negative inotropic and electrophysiologic effects. Newer calcium channel blockers, felodipine and isradipine, have longer half-lives and greater vascular selectivity, resulting primarily in the absence of negative effects on heart rate or myocardial contractility. They are currently approved for the treatment of hypertension. The resultant effects on heart rate, blood pressure, electrocardiographic findings, and exercise capacity are detailed in Table 17–2.

Diltiazem, nicardipine, nifedipine, and verapamil are useful in the treatment of angina pectoris, coronary artery spasm, and hypertension. Their beneficial action in angina pectoris results primarily from a decrease in myocardial oxygen consumption by way of the effects on blood pressure (reduction) and heart rate (reduction). These medications may also increase myocardial oxygen supply when coronary artery spasm plays a role in the myocardial ischemia. Relief or prevention of coronary artery spasm occurs because of direct coronary artery vasodilation. Peripheral vasodilation causes a reduction in blood pressure levels with nicardipine and nifedipine having the greatest and diltiazem the least effects. Whereas diltiazem and verapamil decrease heart rate, the others do not.

Verapamil is the only calcium channel blocker with significantly useful antiarrhythmia properties. It is used primarily in the treatment and prevention of paroxysmal supraventricular tachycardia. Verapamil has also been used in the treatment of patients with hypertrophic cardiomyopathy. Another new calcium channel blocker, bepridil, also affects fast sodium channels. It is approved for chronic stable angina but because of its potential to prolong the QT interval and to provoke serious arrhythmias, it is reserved for patients unresponsive to other medications. It generally produces modest decreases in heart rate and blood pressure at rest and during exercise.

If these medications are administered with other types of medication, including nitrates and beta-blockers, the net effects are related to the sum of the hemodynamic and electrophysiologic effects.

Side Effects

Although no adverse effects result from the coronary vasodilation of calcium channel blockers, the resulting peripheral vasodilation may produce symptoms of headache, flushing, orthostatic hypotension, dizziness, or syncope.

The negative inotropic effects of verapamil and diltiazem are generally counterbalanced by the peripheral vasodilatory effects; thus congestive heart failure is rarely a problem. Verapamil and diltiazem may produce heart block through depression of AV conduction, although this adverse effect is usually limited to patients with conduction system disease.

Thus, the administration of verapamil and diltiazem to patients with poor left ventricular functions, bradycardia, sick sinus syndrome, and high-grade AV block is usually contraindicated. Bepridil is similarly contraindicated in these situations. Its potential to provoke serious arrhythmia has been mentioned earlier.

Constipation may be a bothersome side effect of verapamil, which inhibits intestinal smooth muscle contraction. Peripheral edema may occur with nifedipine use, and less frequently with verapamil, because of their venodilating effects. This edema is usually treated effectively with diuretic therapy. In contrast to beta-blockers, none of the calcium channel blockers cause bronchospasm. Increases in serum digitalis levels are found in patients receiving digitalis and verapamil or felodipine, and may also occur with other calcium channel blockers.

Verapamil and diltiazem should be used with beta-blockers only with caution because all of these medications have negative inotropic and electrophysiologic effects, increasing the likelihood of congestive heart failure, heart block, and bradycardia with combined administration.

Exercise and Exercise Training Considerations

The calcium channel blockers do not limit the ability of an individual to achieve a training effect. Because of their effects on the heart rate and blood pressure response to exercise, an exercise prescription should be calculated ideally by using data from an exercise test performed with the patient following the usual medical regimen.

DIGITALIS

Since its discovery more than 200 years ago by William Withering, digitalis has been used for the treatment of congestive heart failure.

Actions

All digitalis glycosides possess similar positive inotropic and electrophysiologic effects. Digitalis preparations inhibit the magnesium and ATP-dependent, sodium and potassium-activated transport enzyme complex known as Na^+, K^+-ATPase. In so doing, digitalis preparations limit the movement of sodium and potassium across the myocardial cell membrane. Subsequently, as the sodium concentration increases, resulting in increased intracellular calcium concentration. This increase may be responsible for the enhancement of myocardial contractility (positive inotropic action). The electrophysiologic effects of digitalis may also be related to the inhibition of Na^+, K^+-ATPase. Digitalis does not directly affect heart rate or blood pressure at rest or with exercise. Parasympathomimetic (vagal) effects may produce a decrease in heart rate, although typically no significant change in heart rate occurs. Exceptions are the slowing of the ventricular response in patients with atrial fibrillation receiving digitalis, as well as patients with congestive heart failure who experience a decrease in heart rate as the congestive heart failure state improves. The effects of digitalis on heart rate and blood pressure,

the electrocardiographic findings, and exercise capacity are outlined in Table 17–2.

Digitalis has beneficial effects in the treatment of congestive heart failure and atrial arrhythmias. Both the control of the ventricular response in chronic atrial fibrillation or atrial flutter and the prevention of recurrences of paroxysmal atrial fibrillation, atrial flutter, and paroxysmal supraventricular tachycardia occur with digitalis therapy. Multiple forms of digitalis glycosides are available. Digoxin (Lanoxin) is the most commonly used form of digitalis.

Side Effects

The side effects associated with digitalis are almost nonexistent unless serum digitalis levels reach the toxic range. Signs and symptoms of digitalis toxicity include variable neurologic and visual symptoms and, most prominently, cardiac arrhythmias. Almost any cardiac arrhythmia may occur, but classic digitalis toxic arrhythmias include premature ventricular complexes (PVCs), AV junctional escape rhythms, and AV block.

Exercise and Exercise Testing Considerations

Because digitalis preparations do not significantly affect heart rate, blood pressure, or exercise capacity, except as previously indicated, the most important aspect of its use in exercise testing and training is the possible development of false-positive results on the exercise ECG. Digitalis therapy may produce exercise-induced ST-segment depression in patients without coronary artery disease or myocardial ischemia. So that digitalis is not a factor in the exercise test, its use should be stopped 10 to 14 days before the exercise test, if clinically feasible.

DIURETICS

Diuretics increase renal excretion of salt and water and are used primarily for the treatment of hypertension, congestive heart failure, and peripheral edema.

Actions

Diuretics prevent sodium reabsorption at different sites of the nephron, including the proximal and distal tubules and along the loop of Henle. Additionally, some diuretics increase urinary potassium excretion. A reduction of arteriolar sodium content results in decreased peripheral vascular resistance and, subsequently, blood pressure reduction to a mild degree. In congestive heart failure and edematous states, intravascular volume and edema decrease.

The major diuretics include the thiazide diuretics, metolazone, the "loop" diuretics (furosemide and ethacrynic acid), and the potassium-sparing diuretics (spironolactone, triamterene, and amiloride). These diuretics vary in chemical structure, site of action, and potassium-sparing ability. Additionally, combinations of a thiazide (hydrochlorothiazide) and a potassium-sparing diuretic (triamterene) are marketed as Dyazide and Maxzide; the combination of hydrochlorothiazide and amiloride is available as Moduretic.

Diuretics have no effect on heart rate at rest or with exercise, although they may lower blood pressure. If hypokalemia (low serum potassium) results, PVCs and repolarization changes simulating ischemia may occur, resulting in false-positive results of a test for ischemia using the exercise ECG. Diuretics have no effect on exercise capacity, except as they act to control congestive heart failure. A summary of these effects is provided in Table 17–2.

Side Effects

Multiple fluid and electrolyte abnormalities may occur, including decreases in serum levels of potassium, sodium, and magnesium and increases in serum levels of uric acid and glucose. Hypokalemic, hypochloremic alkalosis may also occur. Adverse serum lipid effects of increased cholesterol, low-density lipoprotein (LDL)-cholesterol, and triglycerides have also been reported. Another potential problem is intravascular volume depletion (hypovolemia), resulting in decreases in cardiac output, renal perfusion, and blood pressure.

Exercise Testing and Training Considerations

Because diuretics do not affect heart rate or exercise capacity, no alteration in exercise prescription is necessary. The potential to produce hypokalemia and hypovolemia is the most important characteristic of these drugs in exercise testing and training. As noted previously, PVCs and false-positive test results for ischemia may occur if the patient is hypokalemic at the time of an exercise ECG. Hypokalemia may occur even with the administration of prescription of potassium supplements or the use of potassium-sparing diuretics. Therefore, checking for hypokalemia in patients receiving diuretics, especially before stress tests, is important.

Thiazide diuretics, metolazone, and "loop" diuretics may also result in hypomagnesemia and subsequently an increased risk of ventricular and atrial arrhythmias.

Diuretic-induced hypovolemia may occur, increasing the vulnerability of a patient to hypotension in the post-exercise period when peripheral vasodilation occurs. This side effect is of even greater concern after prolonged periods of exercise, when dehydration may compound the problem.

PERIPHERAL VASODILATORS

Peripheral vasodilators are used in the treatment of hypertension, and in some cases, congestive heart failure. These agents are subsequently discussed according to their mechanism of action.

Nonadrenergic Vasodilators

Nonadrenergic vasodilators, hydralazine and minoxidil, produce direct vascular smooth muscle dilation. The resulting vasodilation lowers blood pressure and may improve left ventricular function in patients with depressed left ventricular function. Thus, these drugs are used primarily in the treatment of hypertension and congestive heart failure. The effects of vasodilators on heart rate and blood pressure, the electrocardiographic findings, and exercise capacity are described in Table 17–2.

Side Effects

Each of these drugs may have multiple side effects. In relation to exercise testing and training, however, the reflex tachycardia that may occur, especially with hydralazine and minoxidil use, is the most important. This tachycardia may cause a worsening of angina pectoris as a result of increased myocardial oxygen demand. The concurrent use of beta-blockers is useful in preventing this side effect. Postexercise hypotension may be accentuated by any of these medications, which lower blood pressure.

Angiotensin-Converting Enzyme (ACE) Inhibitors

Angiotensin-converting enzyme (ACE) inhibitors produce vasodilation via competitive inhibition of angiotensin-converting enzyme, the enzyme responsible for conversion of angiotensin I to angiotensin II. Because angiotensin II is both a potent vasoconstrictor and a stimulator of aldosterone secretion from the adrenal cortex, there is a resultant vasodilation and decrease in arterial blood pressure without associated change in heart rate, cardiac output, or blood volume. ACE inhibitors are used in treatment of hypertension and congestive heart failure. Captopril and enalapril, the first ACE inhibitors released, have been joined by numerous newer ACE inhibitors.

The α-Adrenergic Blockers

Doxazosin, prazosin, and terazosin, α-adrenergic blocking agents, cause peripheral vasodilation and subsequent lowering of blood pressure. Their effects on heart rate and blood pressure, electrocardiographic findings, and exercise capacity are summarized in Table 17–2. They lower blood pressure at rest and during exercise but have no effect on heart rate, the results of the ECG, or exercise capacity.

Antiadrenergic Agents without Selective Blockade of Peripheral Receptors

Medications in this class include methyldopa, clonidine, guanabenz, guanfacine, reserpine, and guanethidine. The first four medications suppress central nervous sympathetic outflow through central α-adrenergic stimulation. Reserpine depletes norepinephrine stored in peripheral nerve endings, and guanethedine directly inhibits norepinephrine release. The effects of these medications on heart rate, blood pressure, electrocardiographic findings, and exercise capacity are summarized in Table 17–2. These medications may decrease resting and exercise heart rate, although the effects are usually slight. Resting and exercise blood pressure levels are diminished. No effect is noted electrocardiographically or in regard to exercise capacity.

Side Effects

Methyldopa, reserpine, and guanethidine have the potential to produce orthostatic hypotension, which may be more serious immediately after exercise. Clonidine typically does not produce orthostatic or exercise-induced hypotension. Reserpine may cause depression, increased fatigue, and decreased desire for exercise.

Exercise and Exercise Testing Considerations

Although a gradual "cool-down" is often helpful in preventing hypotension after exercise, patients receiving medications known to cause hypotension should be monitored closely. The effects of the medications on the exercise prescription are related to their effects on heart rate (see Table 17–2). Ideally, the exercise prescription for patients receiving those medications that affect heart rate should be based on their exercise test results while medicated.

ANTIARRHYTHMIC AGENTS

Antiarrhythmic medications used in the treatment of patients with cardiac arrhythmias are classified by their electrophysiologic effects. Most of these agents do not have significant effects on heart rate, blood pressure, exercise capacity, or exercise training, but they may have effects on the exercise electrocardiogram. Exceptions to this statement include β-adrenergic blocking agents and calcium channel blockers, which were discussed previously. These medications may be used for various arrhythmias. As noted previously, digitalis also may be used in the management of cardiac arrhythmias, primarily supraventricular arrhythmias.

Many antiarrhythmic agents do not have significant direct effects on hemodynamic and exercise parameters; however, indirect effects may occur through medication-induced autonomic nervous system effects. By improving or preventing significant arrhythmias, these drugs may improve a patient's physiologic status and exercise capacity.

Class I antiarrhythmic medications include quinidine, disopyramide, procainamide, moricizine, phenytoin, mexiletine, tocainide, flecainide, and propafenone. These medications have the electrophysiologic effects of decreasing conduction velocity, excitability, and automaticity. They are myocardial depressants, some of which have peripheral vasodilation effects. These drugs have no significant effects on heart rate, with the exception of quinidine and disopyramide, which may elevate heart rates at rest and at low exercise workloads through their parasympatholytic effects; and propafenone, which decreases resting and possibly exercising heart rates. These medications may lower resting blood pressure, but typically they have no effect on exercising blood pressure. These agents may produce prolongation of QRS complex and/or QT interval because of their effects on impulse conduction velocity. Quinidine use can produce false-negative results on exercise electrocardiograms; procainamide has been reported to cause false-positive results on exercise ECGs. Little other information exists concerning the effects of these medications, especially with regard to the newer drugs—flecainide, mexiletine, moricizine, propafenone, and tocainide—on the exercise ECGs.

Class II and IV antiarrhythmic agents, β-adrenergic blockers, and calcium channel blockers, respectively, were previously discussed. Class III antiarrhythmic agents include amiodarone, which slows the heart rate at rest and during exercise through noncompetitive adrenergic inhibition. Amiodarone does not exert significant effects on blood pressure, and no significant effects on the resting or exercise ECG or the exercise capacity are known.

Side Effects

These medications have multiple individual side effects. The possibility of myo-cardial depression and precipitation of congestive heart failure by disopyramide, flecainide, or propafenone is the side effect of greatest clinical importance with regard to exercise testing and training. Any of these antiarrhythmic drugs, however, may have proarrhythmic effects (the capacity to worsen the arrhythmias for which they are administered).

Exercise and Exercise Testing Considerations

Exercise tests for the purpose of exercise prescription need not be performed while the patient is receiving medications, because these antiarrhythmic agents do not significantly affect heart rates, with the possible exception of amiodarone and quinidine. Because of their effect on cardiac rhythm, however, it would be ideal if the patient were receiving these medications at the time of the test.

BRONCHODILATORS

Bronchodilators include anticholinergic, methylxanthine, and sympathomimetic medications. Bronchodilators are administered to correct or prevent bronchial smooth muscle constriction (bronchoconstriction or bronchospasm) in patients with asthma or other forms of pulmonary disease in which bronchospasm occurs. They may be administered by various routes, on a continuous or intermittent basis. By preventing or reversing bronchospasm, these medications increase exercise capacity in patients who are otherwise limited by bronchospasm. They have no effect, however, on exercise capacity of people who are not so limited.

Anticholinergic (parasympatholytic) agents are used in inhaled form to produce bronchodilation. This effect is primarily local, inhibiting vagally medicated reflexes, rather than systemic. No clinically significant heart rate or blood pressure effects are produced.

Methylxanthines, including aminophylline and theophylline, produce bronchodilation by an unclear mechanism. Methylxanthine use may result in increased heart rates and the appearance of cardiac arrhythmias, including PVCs, as well as nausea and vomiting.

Sympathomimetic agents may also be prescribed for patients with bronchospasm. These medications have variable cardiovascular effects depending on their preferential stimulatory effects on β_1 (cardiac) or β_2 (bronchial smooth muscle) receptors. Drugs with primary or significant β_1 effects are likely to produce elevated heart rates and, possibly, hypertension and PVCs. These drugs include ephedrine, epinephrine, and metaproterenol. Drugs with primary β_2 effects are less likely to cause these changes, but may produce systemic vasodilation and compensatory tachycardia. These agents include albuterol, isoetharine, and terbutaline. None of these medications, however, have pure β_1 or β_2 effects.

Cromolyn sodium (a mast cell stabilizer taken by inhalation) and corticosteroids (taken orally or by inhalation) are not true bronchodilators, but are used in the treatment of bronchospasm. They have no effects on heart rate, blood pressure, or electrocardiographic findings, with one exception. Corticosteroids administered in moderate to high oral doses may cause hypertension.

HYPERLIPIDEMIC AGENTS

Hyperlipidemic agents may be administered to patients with and without cardiovascular disease in the treatment of abnormal elevations of serum lipids. Hyperlipidemic medications include cholestyramine, clofibrate, colestipol, dextrothyroxine, gemfibrozil, lovastatin, nicotinic acid, pravastatin, probucol, and simvastatin. They act by a variety of mechanisms, but few have significant hemodynamic or electrocardiographic effects. An exception is dextrothyroxine, which may produce elevations of heart rate and blood pressure, cardiac arrhythmias and, in patients with coronary heart disease, increases in myocardial ischemia and angina. The side effects of nicotinic acid include flushing, decrease in blood pressure, and headaches. Clofibrate has been associated with an increase in arrhythmias, angina, and claudication in patients with previous myocardial infarction. Probucol may cause QT-interval prolongation.

PSYCHOTROPIC MEDICATIONS

Psychotropic medications are used in the treatment of various emotional and psychiatric disorders. They may be categorized as: (1) minor tranquilizers or antianxiety agents, (2) antidepressants, (3) antipsychotic agents, and (4) lithium carbonate.

Minor Tranquilizers

Minor tranquilizers, including diazepam, do not have significant effects on hemodynamics, exercise capacity, or electrocardiographic findings, with the exception of possibly lowering heart rate and blood pressure as they control anxiety.

Antidepressants

Antidepressants include tricyclic antidepressants and monoamine oxidase (MAO) inhibitors. Tricyclic antidepressants appear to act by blocking the uptake of norepinephrine in central nervous system synapses. Their effects include an anticholinergic effect and a quinidine-like effect, which may cause an elevation of heart rate and an increase or decrease in atrial and ventricular arrhythmias, lower blood pressure, and multiple potential electrocardiographic changes including an increase in the PR interval and the QT interval and ST-T wave changes. These medications potentially may produce false-positive results in exercise ECGs. MAO inhibitors act by blocking the breakdown of norepinephrine in the central nervous system. They may produce orthostatic hypotension, but the most serious side effect is a hypertensive crisis, which may occur if these medications interact with certain drugs, including sympathomimetic agents and related compounds or foods with high concentrations of tyramine.

Antipsychotic Medications, Major Tranquilizers

Phenothiazines are the major category of antipsychotic agents or major tranquilizers. These drugs have anticholinergic and direct myocardial depressant effects in addition to producing α-adrenergic blockade. These properties may result in elevated heart rate; decreased blood pressure, especially orthostatic hypotension; and electrocardiographic changes including increased PR and QT intervals, QRS widening, and ST-T wave changes. Various arrhythmias may also occur. These drugs may also have the potential to produce false-positive and false-negative results on exercise ECGs.

Lithium Carbonate

Lithium carbonate is used primarily to treat manic-depressive illnesses. It has a minimal effect on hemodynamic variables. Possible electrocardiographic changes include T-wave changes and arrhythmias. Whether this medication may effect changes on the exercise ECG is not clear.

NICOTINE

Nicotine from cigarette smoking, gum, and transdermal patches, as well as smokeless tobacco, results in the release of epinephrine and norepinephrine. In addition, structures activated by the release of acetylcholine are stimulated by nicotine. The resulting effects include increases in heart rate as well as systolic, diastolic, and pulse pressures. Angina and myocardial ischemia may be exacerbated, with resultant changes evident on the exercise ECG. No evidence exists that nicotine causes false-positive results on the exercise ECG. Additionally, nicotine may produce atrial or ventricular arrhythmias.

ANTIHISTAMINES AND COLD MEDICATIONS

Antihistamines have no effects on hemodynamic variables, the findings of resting or exercise ECGs, or exercise capacity. These medications may, however, be combined with sympathomimetics, such as pseudoephedrine, in some cold remedies. Thus any effects, including elevated heart rates and possibly elevated blood pressure, are related to the sympathomimetic agent. Sympathomimetic agents do not affect electrocardiographic findings or exercise capacity (see Bronchodilators).

THYROID MEDICATIONS

The only thyroid medications that might have an effect on exercise or exercise testing are natural and synthetic forms of levothyroxine. These agents may produce elevations of heart rate and blood pressure, cardiac arrhythmias and, in patients with coronary heart disease, increases in myocardial ischemia and angina.

ALCOHOL

Alcohol may act primarily as a myocardial depressant when ingested on a chronic basis. Chronic alcohol intake may be a contributing factor in the development of hypertension. It may also provoke arrhythmias. Alcohol does not change the results of resting or exercise electrocardiograms, although its use may blunt the appreciation of the symptom of angina on the part of the patient despite the presence of myocardial ischemia.

HYPOGLYCEMIC AGENTS

Hypoglycemic agents, including oral agents and insulin, have no effect on heart rate, blood pressure, electrocardiographic findings, or exercise capacity.

OTHER MEDICATIONS

Oral dipyridamole is currently used for its antiplatelet effects. It does dilate small (resistance) vessels, but has little value in the treatment of myocardial ischemia. These vessels are also acted on by adenosine, an endogenous vasodilator. Dipyridamole has no significant hemodynamic, electrocardiographic, or exercise effects. Other medications that have no effect on hemodynamic variables or electrocardiographic findings include anticoagulants (heparin or warfarin), antigout medications, and antiplatelet medications.

Pentoxifylline has no effect on hemodynamic variables or the electrocardiogram but reportedly increases exercise capacity in patients limited by intermittent claudication. This effect apparently occurs through improved blood flow and oxygenation of ischemic tissue by lowering blood viscosity and improving red blood cell flexibility.

Caffeine, the most widely consumed drug in Europe and North America, is a central nervous system stimulant, chemically a methylated xanthine. Its cardiovascular effects depend on an individual's prior use of it. "Caffeine-naive" persons may experience increases in heart rate and blood pressure, whereas those using it regularly ("caffeine-tolerant" persons) experience little or no change in heart rate or blood pressure. It has no effect on high-intensity, short-term work, and $\dot{V}O_{2max}$, but it may increase endurance capabilities, although research studies are inconclusive. Sensitive individuals may experience ventricular or atrial arrhythmias at high levels of intake.

"Diet pills," drugs used in treatment of obesity, usually consist of sympathomimetic amines, and in some cases, amphetamines. Those containing these two drugs may cause elevations of heart rates and blood pressure, and arrhythmias. Sympathomimetic drugs do not alter exercise capacity. Studies on the effects of amphetamines indicate that they delay fatigue during sustained intense exercise, but studies on endurance capacity have yielded conflicting results. In general, these medications should be discouraged as a poor approach to weight loss, because of the attendant problems of tolerance, psychologic dependence, and social dysfunction.

APPLICATION TO EXERCISE TESTS

When exercise testing is performed, numerous factors must be remembered and considered. First, remember the indication for the exercise test. Is it being performed for diagnostic or prognostic reasons, for the evaluation of treatment, or for exercise prescription purposes? Tests performed for diagnostic or prognostic reasons are often best performed while patients are not taking medications. To understand an individual's response, however, having patients continue their medications at full dosage is often best.

Secondly, the dosage and time of administration of any medication taken before a test should be recorded when that medication is known to affect heart rate, blood pressure, myocardial contractility, and cardiac rhythm. This information is necessary for proper test interpretation and comparison with subsequent tests. Also remember that exercise tests for diagnostic purposes are not 100% accurate, i.e., they are neither 100% sensitive nor specific. Because medications may further alter the sensitivity or specificity of the exercise test, discontinuation of medications before an exercise test merits consideration to enhance specificity or sensitivity. Ideally, exercise tests conducted for prescriptive purposes should be performed while patients are taking the medications that they will receive while training.

A significant change in the medication dosage or schedule may indicate a need for repeat exercise testing for prescription purposes. This need is especially great when the medication has significant effects on the heart rate and blood pressure response to exercise. If it is not feasible to retest a patient after changes in the medical regimen, knowledge of the pharmacologic effects of medications and the clinical status of the patient usually allows appropriate adjustments in target heart rate and exercise prescriptions.

EXERCISE PRESCRIPTION

Modifications of the exercise prescription are not based solely on medication administration, although they may be appropriate for any pathophysiologic state that is incompletely treated, such as reduction in target heart rate to avoid myocardial ischemia. Medications that affect determinants of myocardial oxygen consumption (heart rate, blood pressure, and myocardial contractility) may have significant effects on the exercise prescription. Because most of these effects are dose-related, the exercise prescription can often be calculated by using maximal and resting heart rates obtained from the subject while receiving medications at the time of the exercise test. The exercise prescription is usually not affected if medications do not alter the heart rate or blood pressure response to exercise.

No medications are known to limit the ability to derive a cardiorespiratory training effect. Medications that induce fatigue (e.g., beta-blockers) may limit a person's ability to exercise. Regarding the issue of whether medications enhance exercise capacity and performance, authorities state that exercise capacity is improved only insofar as exercise-limiting, pathophysiologic abnormalities, such as myocardial ischemia, arrhythmias, and bronchospasm, can be eliminated or reduced. Medications do not otherwise improve exercise capacity.

Calculation of target heart rates for patients receiving beta-blockers can be performed in the following manner. Because the relationship between exercise intensity and the percent of maximal heart rate is essentially preserved when a person is receiving beta-blocker therapy, the target heart rate range can be calculated by using resting and maximal exercise heart rates (if the latter is known) during medical therapy. For example, with the use of the Karvonen formula, if the desired target heart rate range is 70 to 85% of the maximal heart rate reserve for a person receiving beta-blocker therapy, who has a resting heart rate of 55 and a maximal exercising heart rate of 135, the calculation is:

Maximal HR	135
Resting HR (RHR)	− 55
HR Reserve	80

70% × 80 = 56   56 + 55 (RHR) = 111
85% × 80 = 68   68 + 55 (RHR) = 123

Thus 70 to 85% of maximal HR reserve during beta-blocker therapy is 111 to 123

(target heart rate range). If the percent of maximal HR is used to calculate the target heart rate range, the following calculation is appropriate:

For 75% of max HR (135),
$$75\% \times 135 = 101$$

The target heart rate ranges are thus lower for persons receiving beta-blockers, but the new ranges are appropriate because they represent the correct percent of maximal capacity for the exerciser.

BIBLIOGRAPHY

1. American College of Sports Medicine: *Guidelines for Exercise Testing and Prescription.* Philadelphia: Lea & Febiger, 1991.
2. Braunwald E: *Heart Disease—A Textbook of Cardiovascular Medicine.* Philadelphia: W.B. Saunders, 1992.
3. Ellestad MH: *Stress Testing—Principles and Practice.* Philadelphia: F.A. Davis, 1986.
4. Wadler GI, Hainline B: *Drugs and the Athlete.* Philadelphia, F.A. Davis, 1989.
5. Wenger NK: Cardiovascular drugs: Effects on exercise testing and exercise training of the coronary patient. In *Exercise and the Heart.* Edited by NK Wenger. Philadelphia: F.A. Davis, 1985.

Section IV

HEALTH APPRAISAL AND EXERCISE TESTING

Chapter 18

HEALTH APPRAISAL IN THE NONMEDICAL SETTING

Neil F. Gordon and Brenda S. Mitchell

It has become clearly apparent that a physically active lifestyle provides partial protection against several major chronic diseases. In particular, there is now convincing evidence that regular exercise is beneficial in the primary prevention of coronary artery disease (CAD) and the reduction of mortality rates after myocardial infarction. Given the high prevalence of sedentary lifestyles and the fact that CAD remains the leading cause of death in Western industrialized countries, there is little doubt that considerable public health benefit would accrue if inactive individuals became more active.

Despite the many potential benefits of a physically active lifestyle, it is essential to realize that to be most efficacious, it must be combined with other positive lifestyle changes, and where applicable, with appropriate medical therapy. Furthermore, although exercise is extremely safe for most individuals, it is prudent to take certain precautions to optimize the benefit-to-risk ratio.

To ensure optimal benefit/risk ratio, the practitioner is encouraged to incorporate some form of health appraisal for use with clients before starting an exercise program. The use of an appropriate health appraisal can assist the practitioner in assessing personal behaviors that pertain to health status, risk factors for CAD, and past and current medical history. The purpose of such an appraisal is to (1) provide information on the safety of beginning exercise, (2) provide information on risk factors and potential future risk for cardiovascular disease so appropriate lifestyle education can be provided, and (3) develop an appropriate exercise prescription and programming that will optimize adherence, minimize risks, and maximize benefits.

It is essential that the health appraisal be both cost-effective and time-efficient so that unnecessary barriers to exercise can be avoided. The precise nature and extent of the appraisal should be determined by the age, sex, and perceived health status characteristics of the participants in the program, as well as the available economic, personnel and equipment resources. Health appraisal can range from a short questionnaire to interviews and sophisticated computerized evaluations.

This chapter presents information that may be incorporated in a health appraisal for (1) safety of exercise, (2) health behaviors and risk factors, and (3) considerations for exercise prescription and programming. It is essential to identify factors that may require consultation with medical or allied health professionals before participation in physical activity or before changing physical activity participation levels, or that affect the precise manner in which exercise is prescribed and therefore require special considerations.

SAFETY OF EXERCISE

Most prospective participants in exercise programs conducted in nonmedical settings are apparently healthy individuals whose goals are to enhance fitness and well-being, reduce weight, and reduce their risk for chronic diseases. For such individuals, the safety goals of a preparticipation health appraisal are the identification of individuals who should receive further medical evaluation to determine whether they have contraindications to exercise or should be referred to a medically supervised exercise program.

According to the guidelines of the American College of Sports Medicine (Table 18–1), it is unnecessary for asymptomatic (Table 18–2), apparently healthy

Table 18–1. Guidelines for Exercise Testing and Participation

	Apparently Healthy		Higher Risk*		
	Younger ≤ 40 years (men) ≤ 50 years (women)	Older	No Symptoms	Symptoms	With Disease[†]
Medical exam and diagnostic exercise test recommended prior to:					
Moderate exercise[‡]	No[§]	No	No	Yes	Yes
Vigorous exercise[#]	No	Yes**	Yes	Yes	Yes
Physician supervision recommended during exercise test:					
Submaximal testing	No	No	No	Yes	Yes
Maximal testing	No	Yes	Yes	Yes	Yes

* Persons with two or more risk factors (see Table 18–3) or symptoms (Table 18–2).
† Persons with known cardiac, pulmonary, or metabolic disease.
‡ Moderate exercise (exercise intensity 40 to 60% $\dot{V}_{O_{2}max}$)—Exercise intensity well within the individual's current capacity and can be comfortably sustained for a prolonged period of time, i.e., 60 minutes, slow progression, and generally noncompetitive.
\# Vigorous exercise (exercise intensity > 60% $\dot{V}_{O_{2}max}$)—Exercise intense enough to represent a substantial challenge and that would ordinarily result in fatigue within 20 minutes.
§ The "no" responses in this table mean that an item is "not necessary." The "no" response does not mean that the item should not be done.
** A "yes" response means that an item is recommended.
Reproduced with permission from American College of Sports Medicine.[1]

men under 40 and women under age 50, with fewer than two CAD risk factors (Table 18–3), to have a medical evaluation by a physician before embarking on a program of vigorous (i.e., exercise intensity above 60% $\dot{V}_{O_{2}max}$) exercise training.[1] It is also considered unnecessary for asymptomatic apparently healthy men and women, irrespective of their age or CAD risk factor status, to have a medical evaluation by a physician before embarking on a program of moderate (i.e., exercise intensity 40 to 60% $\dot{V}_{O_{2}max}$) exercise training.[1] For such individuals, preparticipation screening can be accomplished using validated self-administered questionnaires, such as the Physical Activity Readiness Questionnaire (PAR-Q, Table 18–4).

Although there are many questionnaires available for pre-exercise screening, the PAR-Q has been well developed and found to have a sensitivity of essentially 100% and specificity of approximately 80% for detection of medical contraindications to exercise.[2] (When used in this context, *sensitivity* refers to the percent of persons with medical contraindications to exercise who answer "yes" to one or more questions, and

specificity refers to the percent of persons without medical contraindications to exercise who answer "no" to all questions). The PAR-Q is only one example of a pre-exercise screening questionnaire, and limitations of this questionnaire are discussed below. The responsibility of adding to or modifying the pre-exercise screening tool lies with the director of the exercise program and will be determined by the population served.

The questions included in the PAR-Q are shown in Table 18–4, with significance and clarification of each.

Despite the obvious ease of use and cost-effectiveness of the PAR-Q, several important limitations do exist. These limitations, which should be kept in mind, include: (1) its less than desirable specificity for detecting contraindications to exercise; (2) its limited sensitivity (approximately 35%) and specificity (approximately 80%) for predicting subsequent exercise ECG abnormalities; (3) its inability to screen out persons with two or more major CAD risk factors (who require a medical examination before participation in vigorous exercise); (4) the automatic referral for medical eval-

Table 18–2.   Major Symptoms or Signs Suggestive of Cardiopulmonary or Metabolic Disease*

Symptom: Pain or discomfort in the chest or surrounding areas that appears to be ischemic in nature.
Clarification/Significance: One of the cardinal manifestations of cardiac disease, in particular coronary artery disease. Key features favoring an ischemic origin include:
A.   Character—constricting, squeezing, burning, "heaviness" or "heavy feeling"
B.   Location—substernal; across midthorax, anteriorly; in both arms, shoulders; in neck, cheeks, teeth; in forearms, fingers; in interscapular region
C.   Provoking factors—exercise, excitement, other forms of stress, cold weather, occurrence after meals.
    Key features against an ischemic origin include:
A.   Character—dull ache; "knife-like," sharp, stabbing; "jabs" aggravated by respiration
B.   Location—in left submammary area; in left hemithorax
C.   Provoking factors—after completion of exercise, provoked by a specific body motion.
Symptom: Unaccustomed shortness of breath or shortness of breath with mild exertion.
Clarification/Significance: Dyspnea (defined as an abnormally uncomfortable awareness of breathing) is one of the principal symptoms of cardiac and pulmonary disease. It commonly occurs during strenuous exertion in healthy, well-trained persons and during moderate exertion in healthy, untrained persons. It should be regarded as abnormal, however, when it occurs at a level of exertion that is not expected to evoke this symptom in a given individual. Abnormal exertional dyspnea suggests the presence of cardiopulmonary disorders, in particular left ventricular dysfunction or chronic obstructive pulmonary disease.
Symptom: Dizziness or syncope.
Clarification/Significance: Syncope (defined as a loss of consciousness) is most commonly caused by a reduced perfusion of the brain. Dizziness and, in particular, syncope *during* exercise may result from cardiac disorders that prevent the normal rise (or an actual fall) in cardiac output. Such cardiac disorders are potentially life-threatening and include severe coronary artery disease, hypertrophic cardiomyopathy, aortic stenosis, and malignant ventricular arrhythmias. Although dizziness or syncope shortly *after* cessation of exercise should not be ignored, these symptoms may occur even in healthy persons as a result of a reduction in venous return to the heart.
Symptom: Orthopnea and paroxysmal nocturnal dyspnea.
Clarification/Significance: Orthopnea refers to dyspnea occurring at rest in the recumbent position that is relieved promptly by sitting upright or standing. Paroxysmal nocturnal dyspnea refers to dyspnea, beginning usually 2 to 5 hours after the onset of sleep, which may be relieved by sitting on the side of the bed or getting out of bed. Both are symptoms of left ventricular failure. Although nocturnal dyspnea may occur in persons with chronic obstructive pulmonary disease, it differs in that it is usually relieved after the person relieves himself or herself of secretions rather than specifically by sitting up.
Sign: Ankle edema.
Clarification/Significance: Bilateral ankle edema that is most evident at night is a characteristic sign of heart failure or bilateral chronic venous insufficiency. Unilateral edema of a limb often results from venous thrombosis or lymphatic blockage in the limb. Generalized edema (known as anasarca) occurs in persons with the nephrotic syndrome, severe heart failure, or hepatic cirrhosis. Edema around the eyes and of the face is characteristic of several conditions, including the nephrotic syndrome, acute glomerulonephritis, angioneurotic edema, hypoproteinemia, and myxedema.
Symptom/Sign: Palpitations or tachycardia.
Clarification/Significance: Palpitations (defined as an unpleasant awareness of the forceful or rapid beating of the heart) may be induced by various disorders of cardiac rhythm. These include tachycardia, bradycardia of sudden onset, ectopic beats, compensatory pauses, and accentuated stroke volume due to valvular regurgitation. Palpitations also often result from anxiety states and high cardiac output (or hyperkinetic) states, such as anemia, fever, thyrotoxicosis, arteriovenous fistula, and the so-called idiopathic hyperkinetic heart syndrome.
Symptom: Claudication.
Clarification/Significance: Intermittent claudication refers to the pain that occurs in a muscle with an inadequate blood supply (usually as a result of atherosclerosis) that is stressed by exercise. The pain does not occur with standing or sitting, is reproducible from day to day, is more severe when walking upstairs or up a hill, and is often described as a cramp, which disappears within 1 or 2 minutes after stopping exercise. Coronary artery disease is more prevalent in persons with intermittent claudication. Diabetics are at increased risk for this condition.
Sign: Known heart murmur.
Clarification/Significance: Although some may be innocent, heart murmurs may indicate valvular or other cardiovascular disease. From an exercise safety standpoint, it is especially important to exclude hypertrophic cardiomyopathy and aortic stenosis as underlying causes because these are among the more common causes of exertion-related sudden cardiac death.

---

* These symptoms and signs must be interpreted in the clinical context in which they appear, because they are not all specific for cardiopulmonary or metabolic disease. Adapted with permission from American College of Sports Medicine: *Guidelines for Exercise Testing and Prescription.* (4th ed). Philadelphia: Lea & Febiger, 1991; Braunwald E, Isselbacher KJ, Petersdorf RG, et al. (eds): *Harrison's Principles of Internal Medicine.* New York: McGraw-Hill, 1988; and Braunwald E: The history. *In* Heart Disease. A Textbook of Cardiovascular Medicine. Edited by E. Braunwald. Philadelphia: W.B. Saunders Co, 1988.

Table 18–3.   Major Coronary Risk Factors*

1. Diagnosed hypertension or systolic blood pressure $\geq$ 160 or diastolic blood pressure $\geq$ 90 mmHg on at least 2 separate occasions, or on antihypertensive medication
2. Serum cholesterol $\geq$ 6.20 mmol/L ($\geq$ 240 mg/dL)
3. Cigarette smoking
4. Diabetes mellitus[†]
5. Family history of coronary or other atherosclerotic disease in parents or siblings before age 55

* Reproduced with permission from American College of Sports Medicine.[1]
† Persons with insulin-dependent diabetes mellitus (IDDM) who are over 30 or have had IDDM for more than 15 years, and persons with noninsulin-dependent diabetes mellitus who are over 35 should be classified as patients with disease and treated according to the guidelines in Table 18–1.

uation by a physician of asymptomatic apparently healthy individuals over age 65, even if they intend to participate in moderate exercise; (5) its inability to identify medications that may affect exercise safety; (6) its inability to identify pregnant women, for whom special safety precautions may be required; and (7) from an overall health perspective, the absence of questions aimed at the identification of adverse health behaviors other than sedentary lifestyle.

Recognition of such limitations of the PAR-Q has led to several revisions[2,3] of the questionnaire. The newest version[2] is shown in Table 18–5. This version enhances the specificity for detecting contraindications to exercise and minimizes unnecessary medical referrals. It is important to note differences in how questions are phrased, so customized questionnaires may be developed within various settings that meet the needs of various programs. Customized questionnaires may be developed to address these limitations of the PAR-Q to obtain information about risk factors, personal history, health behaviors, and other information that may warrant special considerations.

PERSONAL HEALTH HISTORY AND CAD RISK FACTORS

In addition to readiness/safety of exercise, it is important for exercise professionals to assess all risk factors for CAD. Because several risk factors for CAD (discussed in Chaps. 14 and 15) are behavior-dependent, health behaviors of participants should be assessed. The PAR-Q touches on several risk factors for CAD; however, it is designed to determine the safety of exercise, not the overall risk for CAD. The following includes risk factors that should be identified to prioritize interventions and encourage changes in lifestyle to reduce disease risk. The information may be important in developing an appropriate exercise prescription or modification of the programming of the exercise.

Personal History

A personal health history can be quite extensive, and may require medically trained professionals for interpretation. As a part of an overall health risk appraisal, the personal history should be tailored to emphasize specific factors that will help to categorize an individual in regard to several broad areas. The most important area is that of *manifestation of symptoms* (symptomatic or asymptomatic). Beyond this stratification is the documentation as to whether a symptom-free individual is at *high risk for the future development of disease* or for participation in an exercise program. Some of this information is identified on the PAR-Q, however, in some instances, more information may be beneficial.

Evidence of *known cardiovascular disease* or of symptoms of cardiovascular disease such as angina pectoris must be documented. Symptoms of peripheral vascular disease, particularly discomfort in one or both legs with walking, should be known and documented.

A history of *respiratory disease* should be determined as well. Seasonal difficulties with breathing or breathing discomfort brought on by physical or emotional stress warrant particular attention.

Diabetes is an independent contributor to the risk of cardiovascular disease development,[4] with the relative risk higher in women than men. This excessive risk includes CAD, peripheral vascular disease and congestive heart failure. Diabetes, of course, is its own metabolic disease and requires specific therapy with diet alone or in combination with prescribed medications

Table 18–4. Physical Activity Readiness Questionnaire (PAR-Q)*

For most people, physical activity should not pose any problem or hazard. PAR-Q has been designed to identify the small number of adults for whom physical activity might be inappropriate or those who should have medical advice concerning the type of activity most suitable.

1. Has your doctor ever said you have heart trouble?
   (**Significance/Clarification:** Persons with known heart disease are at increased risk for cardiac complications during exercise. They should consult a physician and undergo exercise testing before starting an exercise program. The exercise prescription should be formulated in accordance with standard guidelines for cardiac patients. Medical supervision may be required during exercise training.)
2. Do you frequently suffer from pains in your chest?
   (**Significance/Clarification:** A physician should be consulted to identify the cause of the chest pain. If ischemic in origin, the condition should be stabilized before starting an exercise program. Exercise testing should be performed with the patient on his or her usual medication and the exercise prescription formulated in accordance with standard guidelines for cardiac patients. Medical supervision may be required during exercise training.)
3. Do you often feel faint or have spells of severe dizziness?
   (**Significance/Clarification:** A physician should be consulted to establish the cause of these symptoms. Exercise training should not be undertaken until serious cardiac disorders have been excluded.)
4. Has a doctor ever said your blood pressure was too high?
   (**Significance/Clarification:** Persons with more marked elevations in blood pressure (that is, >180/105) should add exercise training to their treatment regimen only after initiating pharmacologic therapy. Medication effects should be considered when formulating the exercise prescription. The exercise prescription should be formulated in accordance with guidelines for hypertensive patients.)
5. Has a doctor ever told you that you have a bone or joint problem such as arthritis that has been aggravated by exercise, or might be made worse with exercise?
   (**Significance/Clarification:** Existing musculoskeletal disorders may be exacerbated by inappropriate exercise training. Persons with forms of arthritis known to be associated with a systemic component (for example, rheumatoid arthritis) may be at an increased risk for exercise-related medical complications. A physician should be consulted to determine whether any special precautions are required during exercise training.)
6. Is there a good physical reason not mentioned here why you should not follow an activity program even if you wanted to?
   (**Significance/Clarification:** A physician should be consulted to determine whether the condition/factor requires special precautions during exercise training or contraindicates exercise training.)
7. Are you over age 65 and not accustomed to vigorous exercise?
   (**Significance/Clarification:** Persons over age 65 are at increased risk for certain chronic diseases. The exercise prescription may need to be modified for elderly persons.)

If a person answers yes to any question, vigorous exercise or exercise testing should be postponed. Medical clearance may be necessary.

---

* With permission from PAR-Q Validation Report. British Columbia Department of Health, June 1975 (Modified Version).

(see Chap. 7 in Guidelines for Exercise Testing and Prescription).

Overfatness continues to be a common problem in this country. Overweight or obesity is an independent risk factor for the development of CAD.[5] Obesity is frequently a predecessor of Type II diabetes. Measurement of body composition is thoroughly discussed in Chapter 19. The health professional must be able to identify the individual who is at risk for weight-related problems, and appropriately intervene (or refer) for weight management with diet and exercise (see Chap. 38).

Elevated blood pressure is associated with stroke, heart failure and heart attack. This relationship is discussed in Chapter 14. Blood pressure measurement and categorization of blood pressure elevations have been standardized (see Appendix B). National guidelines for the follow-up and management of persons with high blood pressure are also available.[6] Individuals with hypertension should be under medical care. Exercise training and dietary modifications may be a very important part of the medical management of the condition.

Table 18–5.   Physical Activity Readiness Questionnaire: Matching Questions of Original and Revised Versions*

Original	Revised
1. Has your doctor ever said you have heart trouble?	1. Has a doctor ever said you have a heart condition and recommended only medically supervised physical activity?
2. Do you frequently have pains in your heart and chest?	2. Do you have chest pain brought on by physical activity?
3. Do you often feel faint or have spells of severe dizziness?	4. Do you tend to lose consciousness or fall over as a result of dizziness?
4. Has a doctor ever said your blood pressure was too high?	6. Has a doctor ever recommended medication for your blood pressure or a heart condition?
5. Has your doctor ever told you that you have a bone or joint problem such as arthritis that has been aggravated by exercise or might be made worse with exercise?	5. Do you have a bone or joint problem that could be aggravated by the proposed physical activity?
6. Is there a good physical reason not mentioned here why you should not follow an activity program even if you wanted to?	7. Are you aware, through your own experience or a doctor's advice, of any other physical reason against your exercising without medical supervision?
7. Are you over 65 and not accustomed to vigorous exercise?	(No matching question)
(No matching question)	3. Have you developed chest pain within the past month?

* With permission from Shephard RJ, Thomas S, Weller I: The Canadian Home Fitness Test. *Sports Med, 11:*358, 1991.

Abnormalities in blood lipid levels are known to be at the basis of the atherosclerotic process (see Chaps. 14 and 15).[7] Individuals with abnormal lipid profiles are encouraged to modify their diet to reduce the intake of saturated fats and cholesterol. These individuals should be identified and encouraged to maintain control of their dietary fat intake (see Chap. 39).

Heart disease runs in families. There is an independent association of a positive *family history* for heart disease and its development.[8] This history goes beyond the measured risk factors such as cigarette smoking, excess weight, nutritional factors, and physical inactivity. Therefore, genetic predisposition to the development of CAD seems to be very important. The family history should identify any first-degree relatives (parents, siblings, and children). The risk of developing a heart attack is particularly high when the family history documents heart attack in a first-degree relative with its onset under the age of 60.[8] In these instances, the identification of the patterns of blood lipids (especially lipoprotein levels) is important because blood lipid levels are more likely to be elevated in the offspring of parents whose first event related to CAD occurred before age 60.

Family history of other diseases, specifically diabetes mellitus and certain types of cancer, may be important in emphasizing dietary change in certain individuals.

Health Behaviors

There is a clear linkage between *dietary habits* and the development of several disease states. Most clear is a linkage between saturated fat and cholesterol content of a diet and the development of narrowed arteries—the atherosclerotic process (see Chap. 15). Diets high in cholesterol and saturated fat must be modified to decrease the risk of progressive atherosclerosis.[9] Diets high in sodium can lead to persistent elevation of systemic blood pressure, contributing to the ravages of hypertension, including heart attack, heart failure, stroke, and kidney failure.

Diets deficient in complex carbohydrates and fiber have been linked with excessive rates of development of carcinomas of the gastrointestinal tract.

Appraisal of diet should ideally include documentation and analysis of usual dietary choices as they pertain to total caloric intake, saturated fat, cholesterol, sodium and types of carbohydrates. Appraisal of dietary intake can range from a simple evaluation of dietary preferences to computer-scored instruments that analyze 24-hour dietary patterns, 3-day food records, and even 7-day food records.

Relating dietary analysis to objective measures of health (i.e., excessive calories in overweight individuals, excess sodium and overweight in hypertensive individuals) can be an excellent starting point for changing dietary patterns to improve health status (see Chaps. 38 and 39).

Although it is essential to identify individuals who may be at risk when exercising (Tables 18–6 and 18–7; see also Chap. 29),

Table 18–6. Pathologic Conditions Possibly Associated with Sudden Cardiac Death During Exercise*

Conditions Resulting in Myocardial Ischemia
  Atherosclerotic coronary artery disease
  Coronary artery spasm
  De novo coronary artery thrombus
  Myocardial bridging
  Hypoplastic coronary artery
  Anomalous coronary arteries
Structural Abnormalities
  Hypertrophic cardiomyopathy
  Idiopathic concentric left ventricular hypertrophy
  Right ventricular cardiomyopathy
  Mitral valve prolapse
  Other valvular heart disease
  Marfan's syndrome
  Congenital cardiac defects
Conduction Abnormalities
  Wolff-Parkinson-White syndrome
  Lown-Ganong-Levine syndrome
  QT interval prolongation syndrome
Miscellaneous
  Heat stroke
  Myocarditis
  Sarcoidosis

* With permission from Sadaniantz A, Thompson PD: The problem of sudden death in athletes as illustrated by case studies. *Sports Med, 9*:199, 1990. Kohl HW, Powell KE, Gordon NF, et al: Physical activity, physical fitness and sudden cardiac death. *Epidemiol Rev, 14*: 37, 1992.

Table 18–7. Patient Characteristics Associated with an Increased Risk for Cardiac Events During Exercise*

Clinical Status
  Multiple myocardial infarctions
  Poor left ventricular function (ejection fraction <40% at rest)
  History of chronic congestive heart failure
  Rest or unstable angina pectoris
  Complex dysrhythmias
  Left main coronary artery or three-vessel atherosclerosis on angiography
Exercise Test Response
  Low exercise tolerance (<4 METs)
  Low peak heart rate off drugs (<120 beats·min^{-1})
  Severe ischemia (ST >2 mm)
  Angina pectoris at low heart rate or workload
  Inappropriate systolic blood pressure response (decrease with increasing workloads)
  Complex cardiac dysrhythmias, especially in patients with poor left ventricular function
Exercise Training Participation
  Exercises above prescribed limits

* With permission from American College of Sports Medicine.[1]

identification of past *exercise habits* also will assist the practitioner in developing appropriate prescriptions and programming that will have realistic goals, maximize adherence, and be safe for the individual. The appraisal of exercise habits must include past history of vigorous physical activity, current physical activity habits (both leisure and on the job), and documentation of physical symptoms associated with activity, particularly discomfort in the chest and/or disproportionate development of shortness of breath related to physical activity. Any muscle or joint discomfort associated with or aggravated by exercise should be identified.

Cigarette smoking is one of the best established risks to maintenance of optimal health.[10] Cigarette smoking is most dramatic in the areas of cardiovascular disease and lung cancer. (In 90% of persons with carcinoma of the lung, the disease is attributable to smoking.) The rate of smoking in young women and adolescents is increasing.

Chapter 14 thoroughly discusses the cardiovascular risk of smoking. In addition to the increased risk for developing CAD, the

Table 18–8. Health-Related Factors That Can Potentially Affect The Exercise Prescription

Factor: Alcohol and other substance abuse.
Implications/Significance: Alcohol intake may elevate the heart rate response to submaximal effort, impair exercise tolerance, promote dehydration, and increase the risk for heat injury. Habit-forming drugs such as cocaine may accentuate the risk for cardiac complications during exercise.
Factor: Cigarette smoking.
Implications/Significance: Acutely, cigarette smoking may elevate the heart rate, respiration, and blood pressure response to exercise, increase the susceptibility toward ventricular arrhythmias, increase platelet aggregability (and the risk for thrombosis), and predispose to coronary artery spasm. Chronically, cigarette smoking accentuates the risk for atherosclerosis.
Factor: Diet/nutrition.
Implications/Significance: Dietary content, especially total fat, saturated fat and cholesterol intake, impacts serum lipids and lipoproteins and, thus, the risk for coronary artery disease. When an individual is on a calorie-restricted diet, care should be taken to ensure that adequate carbohydrates are consumed to replenish muscle glycogen stores that may be depleted during exercise. Resistance training may be of particular benefit when it comes to preserving lean body mass and minimizing a decline in resting metabolic rate during dieting.
Factor: Diseases.
Implications/Significance: Chronic diseases such as coronary artery disease, diabetes mellitus, hypertension, cerebrovascular disease, AIDS, cancer, osteoporosis, renal disease, arthritis, and COPD all require special consideration when compiling an exercise prescription. For patients with such conditions, the exercise prescription should be individualized in accordance with standard guidelines.
Factor: Eating disorders, such as anorexia nervosa.
Implications/Significance: Care should be taken to de-emphasize weight loss and, possibly, high caloric expenditure exercise, where appropriate. To preserve lean body mass, resistance training should be emphasized.
Factor: Environmental considerations.
Implications/Significance: The environment in which the individual intends exercising must be considered when compiling an exercise prescription. In particular, weather (heat, humidity, cold), altitude, and air pollution (carbon monoxide, ozone) should be factored into the design of the exercise prescription.
Factor: Family history.
Implications/Significance: Family history of premature cardiovascular disease increases the risk for such diseases in a given individual.
Factor: Medications.
Implications/Significance: Certain medications may alter the heart rate and/or blood pressure response to exercise, evoke electrocardiographic abnormalities, and alter exercise capacity. (See Chapter 12.)
Factor: Obesity.
Implications/Significance: Emphasis should be placed on increasing caloric expenditure and minimizing the risk for muscle soreness, orthopedic injury, or other discomfort. Initially, lower-intensity exercise of longer duration should be emphasized.
Factor: Past and present exercise history.
Implications/Significance: Previous history of exercise experiences, in particular exertion-related orthopedic injuries and reasons for noncompliance, should be considered. Present exercise participation is of importance when decisions are made about the type, frequency, intensity, and duration at which exercise training should be commenced with.
Factor: Personality/behavior pattern.
Implications/Significance: May influence compliance with exercise guidelines and decisions regarding individual or group training.
Factor: Pregnancy and breast feeding.
Implications/Significance: Exercise should be prescribed in accordance with accepted guidelines for pregnant and lactating women. Avoid overheating, overexertion, and dehydration; maintain heart rate <140 beats/minute; and adjust caloric intake according to the amount of physical activity.

risk of sudden death (defined as death within 1 hour in an apparently healthy individual) occurs five times more commonly among pack-per-day smokers compared to nonsmokers. Smoking is also associated with an unfavorable and significant reduction in HDL-cholesterol levels.

Such bleak statistics are counterbalanced by the encouraging and well-documented benefits of smoking cessation. Within 2 years of stopping cigarette smoking, the excess risk of cardiovascular disease drops dramatically. This decline in cardiovascular risk is a dose-response phenomenon; the heavier the prior habit, the more dramatic the benefits. The rate of progression of atherosclerosis is likely to decline in the ex-smoker as well.

Every effort should be made to provide smoking participants with clear and persuasive information regarding the risks associated with continuing smoking and the benefits of cessation. Chapter 40 discusses various strategies for smoking cessation.

The *type A behavior* pattern is believed to be a contributor to the overall risk of developing CAD.[11] The original description and identification of type A behavior required a difficult and elaborate technique of structured interview. Subsequent means of evaluating type A behavior are more objective and streamlined. One of these methods may be included as a component of an appraisal of health behavior. Identification of participants whose behavior pattern places them at high risk for heart attack is important, and counselling should be provided to lower that risk (see Chap. 41).

HEALTH-RELATED FACTORS REQUIRING SPECIAL CONSIDERATION

The PAR-Q has been recommended as a minimum pre-exercise screening standard for entry into low to moderate intensity physical activity programs.[1] Once an individual has been provided with medical clearance to participate in an exercise program (by virtue of either the PAR-Q or a medical examination), it is important for the exercise professional to determine if there are any additional health-related factors that require special consideration. Although potential risks are associated with exercise participation, the most important is precipitation of sudden cardiac death. The risk of sudden death with exercise is discussed in Chapter 29. In adults, several studies have now clearly shown that the transiently increased risk of cardiac arrest that occurs during vigorous exercise results largely from the presence of pre-existing cardiac abnormalities, in particular CAD (Table 18–6).

Other health-related conditions that might affect the exercise prescription (or program) are discussed in Table 18–8. The significance and clarification in exercise prescription and programming are also presented. These factors should be viewed as "red flags" because their presence may indicate a change in the type, frequency, intensity, duration, and/or progression of the exercise to make it most appropriate for the given individual.

It is essential that the exercise professional obtain as much information about his or her participants as possible to best meet their individual needs and make the exercise most beneficial. A regular evaluation of health status and health behaviors should be incorporated into long-term programs to update the prescriptions and programs according to changing needs.

REFERENCES

1. American College of Sports Medicine: *Guidelines for Exercise Testing and Prescription.* 4th ed. Philadelphia: Lea & Febiger, 1991.
2. Shephard RJ, Thomas S, Weller I: The Canadian home fitness test. 1991 Update. *Sports Med, 11:*358, 1991.
3. Fitness Safety Standards Committee: Final Report to the Minister of Tourism and Recreation on the Development of Fitness Safety Standards in Ontario (Canada). February, 1990.
4. Kannel WB, McGee DL: Diabetes and cardiovascular disease: The Framingham study. *JAMA, 241:*2035, 1979.
5. Kannel WB, et al.: Obesity as an independent risk factor for cardiovascular disease: A 26-year follow-up of participants in the Framingham Heart Study. *Circulation, 67:* 968, 1983.
6. National High Blood Pressure Education Program. The fifth report of the Joint National Committee on Detection, Evaluation, and Treatment of High Blood Pressure (JNCV). Ann Int Med 1993 (In press).
7. National Institutes of Health: Lowering

blood cholesterol to prevent heart disease. NIH Consensus development conference statement. *JAMA, 253:*2080, 1985.

8. Snowden CB, et al.: Predicting coronary disease in siblings—a multivariate assessment: The Framingham Heart Study. *Am J Epidemiol, 115:*217, 1982.

9. Lewis B, et al.: Towards an improved lipid-lowering diet: Additive effects of changes in nutrient intake. *Lancet, 2:*1310, 1981.

10. Fielding JE: Smoking: Health effects and control. *N Engl J Med, 313:*491, 1985.

11. Haynes SG, Feinleib M, Kannel WB: The relationship of psychosocial factors to coronary heart disease in the Framingham study III. *Am J Epidemiol, 111:*37, 1980.

Chapter 19

FITNESS TESTING

Larry R. Gettman

The term "fitness testing" in this manual refers to evaluating the four main health-related areas of physical fitness: (1) cardiovascular-respiratory function; (2) body composition; (3) muscular strength and muscular endurance; and (4) flexibility. As described in the fourth edition of the ACSM Guidelines for Exercise Testing and Prescription,[1] the definition of physical fitness is:

> "A set of attributes that people have or achieve that relates to the ability to perform physical activity."[2]

and the definition offered for health-related fitness is

> "A state characterized by (a) an ability to perform daily activities with vigor and (b) the demonstration of traits and capacities that are associated with low risk of premature development of hypokinetic diseases."[3]

Periodic testing of health-related fitness shows the participants how they stand relative to normal fitness levels. The results can then be used to emphasize the importance of having an active lifestyle to achieve and maintain high levels of cardiovascular and respiratory function, low amounts of body fat, sufficient muscular strength and endurance, and flexibility, especially in the lower back, hips and legs. Results from fitness tests should be viewed both as the means to an end and as an end in themselves. The results of fitness tests should be used in the exercise prescription. They provide a picture (snapshot) of present health and fitness status and can be motivators for improvement and reinforcers for fitness maintenance. Five ways in which test results can be effectively utilized include:

1. Strength and weakness identification. Scores of the fitness tests can be used to identify strengths and weaknesses within the individual. Appropriate counseling can aid those individuals who need to improve identified weaknesses.

2. Achievement of individual goals. Periodic fitness tests can be used to verify the degree of achievement of individually established goals.

3. Educational purposes. Test results can be used to stimulate further interest in health-related topics. For example, cardiovascular-respiratory fitness tests can be used to teach concepts of heart and lung function, work capacity, efficiency, and the importance of minimizing risks related to cardiovascular disease. Body composition tests can be used to teach concepts in nutrition and weight control. Muscular strength and endurance tests may be used to illustrate their importance for accomplishing daily tasks involving lifting and carrying. Flexibility tests demonstrate the degree of mobility for work and play and for preventing and controlling joint pain such as in the low-back region.

4. Motivation. Most individuals are inherently curious about their physical capabilities and how their fitness scores compare with those of other individuals and how they may change over time. By becoming aware of how they compare with criterion standards and with other individuals, participants may become motivated to improve their scores or at least maintain a desired level. Participants may also be motivated by seeing improvement in their fitness scores as a result of regular activity.

5. Program evaluation. Test results can be also used to determine if a fitness program is achieving desired goals. The average score for an individual

or group can be compared to a determined normal value or the changes in average scores can reflect the amount of fitness change resulting from the program.

PREPARTICIPATION HEALTH APPRAISAL

Tests of physical fitness and programs to enhance health-related fitness are usually conducted in nonmedical settings on apparently healthy people. For safety reasons, it is important to screen fitness participants for risk factors before attempting any vigorous exercise either in a fitness test or in a fitness program. The purposes of a preparticipation health appraisal[1] are to:

1. Identify and exclude individuals with medical contraindications to exercise.
2. Identify persons with clinically significant disease conditions who should be referred to a medically supervised exercise program.
3. Identify individuals with disease symptoms and risk factors for disease development who should receive further medical evaluation before starting an exercise program.
4. Identify persons with special needs for safe exercise participation (e.g., elderly persons, pregnant women).

To obtain the above information, a health/medical questionnaire is administered to the participant. A thorough health/medical questionnaire should contain questions to assess the conditions as discussed in Chapter 18. A widely used, well accepted short-form health/medical questionnaire, called the Physical Activity Readiness Questionnaire or PAR-Q, is discussed in detail in Chapter 18.

Identification of major health risks in the health/medical questionnaire or answering YES to any question on the PAR-Q requires postponing fitness testing until medical clearance is obtained. After medical clearance has been approved by a physician, informed consent is obtained before fitness testing commences.

INFORMED CONSENT

After the appropriate health history information has been reviewed and any necessary medical clearance obtained, informed consent should be presented to the participant before any fitness testing is activated. The essential elements of informed consent consist of the following[1]:

1. Explain the procedures used in the fitness tests
2. Outline the potential risks and discomforts of participating in tests of fitness
3. State the responsibilities of the participant which includes the reporting of unusual feeling or discomfort during the tests
4. Describe the expected benefits of the fitness tests
5. Solicit inquiries from the participant and make sure all questions are satisfactorily answered before starting the test procedures
6. Offer freedom of consent. Participation in fitness testing is voluntary, and the participant has the right to refuse participation in any test or to stop a test at any time.

The legal issues surrounding informed consent are discussed in Chapter 44.

RESPONSIBILITIES OF THE FITNESS PROFESSIONAL

After health history information, medical clearance, and informed consent are obtained, the series of fitness tests may be initiated. It is the responsibility of the fitness professional to:

1. Recognize valid test results
2. Recognize abnormal responses
3. Recognize and respond to emergency situations
4. Assume responsibility for equipment maintenance and calibration, testing forms and supplies, and environmental factors (maintain a temperature of 22°C and humidity under 60%)

Descriptions for calibrating treadmills and cycle ergometers appear in Chapter 45. A suggested list of laboratory equipment and supplies for basic fitness testing is listed in Table 19-1.

A fitness professional should also demonstrate the ability to interpret results of

Table 19–1. Laboratory Equipment and Supplies

1. Recording forms
   a. Cardiovascular-respiratory (including PWC graph)
   b. Body composition
   c. Muscular strength and muscular endurance
   d. Flexibility
   e. Norms for all tests
2. Stopwatch
3. Stethoscope
4. Sphygmomanometer—calibrated
5. ECG recording device—(if needed)
6. Cycle ergometer (or treadmill)—calibrated
7. Metronome—calibrated
8. Spirometer—calibrated
9. Skinfold calipers—calibrated
10. Anthropometric measuring tape
11. Weight machines or free weights for strength—calibrated
12. Sit-up mat or board
13. Hand grip dynamometer—calibrated
14. Sit-and-reach box (or other flexibility equipment)

fitness evaluations with regard to norms and standards. Most fitness scores and categories are stratified by age and gender and are based on normal distribution around the mean. One option for presenting norms is to use five categories based on the standard deviation.

Rating	Standard Deviation (std. dev.)
Excellent	+ 0.5 std. dev. from good
Good	+ 0.5 std. dev. from average
Average	± 0.5 std. dev. from mean
Fair	− 0.5 std. dev. from average
Poor	− 0.5 std. dev. from fair

TESTS FOR CARDIOVASCULAR-RESPIRATORY FUNCTION

After all preliminary information has been obtained and preparations have been made, the assessment of cardiovascular-respiratory function may begin. At a basic level, these fitness tests involve the measurement of resting heart rate, resting blood pressure, and a physical work capacity test on a calibrated cycle ergometer or treadmill.

Measuring Heart Rate

Resting (pre-exercise) heart rate should be counted for 60 seconds. Counting heart rate for any time interval less than 60 seconds introduces an error of measurement at rest (because of the relatively slower rate than during exercise). The error of measurement at rest increases as the time interval decreases. During exercise, shorter intervals of counting should be employed (10 to 15 seconds) because of the faster heart rates. The error of measurement during exercise increases as the time interval increases.

Chest auscultation using a stethoscope is the most accurate technique of counting heart rate at rest and during exercise when the heart sounds are heard clearly and the trunk is stable (such as in cycle ergometry). To count heart rate using chest auscultation, place the stethoscope over the left aspect of the sternum or over the sixth rib under the left pectoralis muscle and anterior to the left axillary line for best auscultation of heart sounds during exercise. It is difficult to hear the heart sounds if the stethoscope is placed over fat or muscle tissue. Press firmly on the stethoscope to prevent movement of its membrane across the skin, which causes noise artifact.

Radial pulse palpation is another technique used to count heart rate. It is the best palpation technique to use during exercise if the arm and hand can be held steady (such as in cycle ergometry). To count heart rate using the radial pulse palpation technique, place the fingertips of your first and second fingers over the radial artery on the lateral (thumb) side of the forearm at the distal (lower) end of the radius. Gently compress the artery against the anterior surface of the distal end of the radius. Do not press too hard. This might cut off the circulation and no pulse will be felt.

When it is difficult to obtain heart rate from chest auscultation or radial pulse palpation, carotid palpation may be attempted if the neck region is stable during exercise. Using the fingertips of the first and second fingers, palpate over the carotid artery (either right or left) by pressing inward and backward along the larynx at a level corresponding to the thyroid cartilage (laryngeal prominence). Avoid excessive massage or pressure on the carotid artery because this stimulates the baroreceptors to decrease blood pressure and slow heart rate. The person may get dizzy and faint.

The fitness professional should be aware that many factors affect resting heart rate. Smoking, caffeine, high temperature, high humidity, stress, food digestion, medications (stimulants), and acute exercise affect heart rate leading to a higher than normal resting heart rate. Some medications (depressants and some antihypertensive medications) may cause lower than normal resting heart rate.

Measurement of Blood Pressure

Sphygmomanometry is the technique used to measure blood pressure. Standards for the measurement of blood pressure are published by the American Society on Hypertension[4] (Appendix B) and should be followed. For a resting pressure, the participant should assume a seated position with the left arm (or right arm) placed horizontally on a table that is preferably the same height as the heart level. A stethoscope and sphygmomanometer are used to indirectly measure the systemic arterial blood pressure.

A sphygmomanometer consists of an inflatable cuff connected by rubber tubes to a manometer (either mercury or aneroid) and a rubber bulb to regulate air during inflation and deflation of the cuff. To correctly perform sphygmomanometry, palpate the brachial artery 1 cm below the elbow joint on the medial side of the forearm. Wrap the deflated cuff snugly around the upper arm with the lower edge of the cuff 1 inch above the antecubital fossa and the arrow on the cuff directly over the brachial artery. The stethoscope is placed firmly over the brachial artery below the lower edge of the cuff.

The cuff must fit the upper arm properly, based on arm girth. A normal sized cuff is 12 to 14 cm (5 to 5.5 inches) in width and 30 cm (12 inches) in length. Narrow cuffs give an artificially high blood pressure reading. A cuff that is too wide gives artificially low blood pressure readings. Guidelines on fitting a cuff are described in the American Society on Hypertension

Guidelines for Measurement of Blood Pressure.[4] (Appendix B).

Measurement of blood pressure during exercise requires significant practice. It is essential to isolate and support the arm to minimize movement and competing sounds. It may be advantageous to tape the cuff and stethoscope in position to concentrate on the measurement process.

After pumping the cuff to 5 mm Hg above the anticipated systolic pressure (120 to 160 mm Hg at rest), deflate the cuff at a rate equal to 2 mm Hg per one beat of the heart. Thus, the faster the heart rate, the faster the deflation rate. If the rate of deflation is too fast, a large auscultation gap is created, resulting in a large error of blood pressure measurement. A slow deflation rate is uncomfortable to the participant (remember, blood flow is being restricted through the arm). It is important to keep vision perpendicular to the mercury or aneroid scale to prevent parallax error.

The fitness professional should be aware that many factors affect resting blood pressure. Smoking, caffeine, cardiac output, peripheral vascular resistance, stress, medications (stimulants), and acute exercise (work and proprioception) affect blood pressure, leading to higher-than-normal values. Some medications (depressants) may cause a lower-than-normal resting blood pressure.

Measurement of Physical Work Capacity

Cardiovascular-respiratory fitness may be assessed through various forms of physical work capacity tests. Tests of maximal cardiovascular-respiratory function traditionally involve maximal efforts on a treadmill or cycle ergometer in a testing laboratory or maximal efforts outside while performing a 1-mile run, 1.5-mile run, 12-minute walk/run, or 1-mile walk.

The best way to determine the maximal ability of the cardiovascular-respiratory system is to measure it under the stress of maximal work. Open circuit spirometry is used to directly measure maximal oxygen uptake ($\dot{V}O_{2max}$) during a treadmill or cycle ergometer test. $\dot{V}O_{2max}$ is considered the "gold standard" for representing maximal cardiovascular-respiratory function (see

Chap. 20). Maximal time performance on a treadmill or maximal time performance on a 1-mile run, 1.5-mile run, or 1-mile walk have also been used to estimate $\dot{V}O_{2max}$. Heart rate, blood pressure, and electrocardiogram (ECG) may be readily monitored during the laboratory tests, which makes them valuable as prime tests of physical work capacity. These measurements are not only expensive, but are not usually available during outside track performances on the 1-mile run, 1.5-mile run, 12-minute walk/run, or 1-mile walk.

Estimation of $\dot{V}O_{2max}$ can also be done using a submaximal test of physical work capacity using a cycle ergometer, treadmill, or step bench. These submaximal tests are based on the linear relationship between submaximal heart rate and submaximal workload (described in Chap. 7) and the assumption of an age-predicted maximal heart rate. In each protocol, the relationship between submaximal heart rate and the submaximal workload (power) is examined and a maximal workload corresponding to the predicted maximal heart rate is estimated. $\dot{V}O_{2max}$ is then estimated from the calculated $\dot{V}O_2$ at the predicted maximal workload.

Three cycle ergometer submaximal cardiovascular-respiratory tests are described in the ACSM Guidelines for Exercise Testing and Prescription (4th edition).[1] The reader is referred to the ACSM Guidelines for more information on these protocols. Additionally, the YMCA Cycle Ergometer test[5] is a popular test used to estimate $\dot{V}O_{2max}$. The test is described thoroughly in *Y's Way to Physical Fitness*,[5] and the reader is referred to that text for exact procedures.

Submaximal tests that estimate $\dot{V}O_{2max}$ are less expensive and are safer for the participants. Use of a cycle ergometer allows more accurate heart rate and blood pressure measurements because there is less movement than when one is using a treadmill. The bench step test is least accurate of all because heart rate is recorded after the work test has been completed and not during the test. Estimation of $\dot{V}O_{2max}$ from recovery heart rate after a step test is not as accurate as monitoring physical parameters during a submaximal or maximal physical work capacity test.

Standard values for $\dot{V}O_{2max}$ are presented in Table 19–2. Two problems are associated with submaximal estimation of $\dot{V}O_{2max}$:

1. Errors may occur in predicting maximal heart rate from age (220 − age) because the standard error of prediction is ± 10 beats.
2. Abnormally high maximal workloads (and thus $\dot{V}O_{2max}$) are predicted when using heart rates lower than 110 beats per minute because the slope of

Table 19–2. Standard Values for $\dot{V}O_{2max}$ in mL/kg/min*

Rating	Age (yrs)				
	20–29	30–39	40–49	50–59	60+
Men					
Excellent	>51	>48	>46	>42	>40
Good	49–51	46–48	44–46	40–42	38–40
Average	42–48	39–45	37–43	33–39	31–37
Fair	39–41	36–38	34–36	30–32	28–30
Poor	<39	<36	<34	<30	<28
Women					
Excellent	>42	>39	>37	>33	>33
Good	40–42	37–39	35–37	31–33	31–33
Average	33–39	31–36	29–34	25–30	25–30
Fair	30–32	28–30	26–28	22–24	22–24
Poor	<30	<28	<26	<22	<22

* With permission from Gettman LR: Personal Fitness Profile Database. National Health Enhancement Systems. Phoenix, AZ, 1987.

the relationship between heart rate and workload is nonlinear and less steep than heart rates greater than 110 beats per minute.

Parameters that may be monitored during cardiovascular-respiratory tests include heart rate, blood pressure, rated perceived exertion (RPE), electrocardiogram (ECG), lactic acid, and oxygen uptake ($\dot{V}O_2$).

Heart Rate: Heart rate is the easiest parameter to monitor. Chest auscultation or radial pulse techniques may be used. Heart rate reflects the intensity of the workload.

Blood Pressure: Blood pressure is more difficult to obtain during exercise than heart rate, but it is a very valuable measurement. It reflects the resistance in the blood vessel system that the heart faces. Systolic blood pressure multiplied by the heart rate reflects the myocardial oxygen demand. This is called the "double product" or "rate pressure product."

Rated Perceived Exertion (RPE): The original Borg scale is used to estimate how the participant perceives the intensity of the exercise. The original scale relates closely to the heart rate of the participant. This scale is easy to use and should be posted at the exercise testing station and in the exercise workout area.

Electrocardiogram (ECG): ECG is monitored to evaluate the electrical activity in the heart conduction system and muscle. Conduction blocks, arrhythmias, irregular heartbeats, and ischemic responses can be detected through the ECG recordings.

Lactic Acid: Lactic acid is measured to reflect the anaerobic component and "anaerobic threshold" of the exercise test. It requires blood sampling and expensive equipment and is usually used in research experiments.

Oxygen Uptake $\dot{V}O_2$: $\dot{V}O_2$ is monitored to reflect the aerobic component of the exercise workload. This is time-consuming and requires expensive equipment.

The purpose of the test and the population being tested determine which parameters are measured during the test.

MEASUREMENT OF BODY COMPOSITION

The term body composition refers to dividing the body into two main components consisting of lean body weight (LBW) and fat weight (FW). It is known that a high amount of fat weight (obesity) is a risk factor for heart disease, diabetes, cancer, and other health problems. Excess fat weight makes movement inefficient and difficult. On the other hand, a high lean body weight allows the body to accomplish work efficiently and expend more calories even at rest. Thus, a high LBW makes it easier to control body weight within a desired range.

It is important to distinguish between being "overweight" and being "overfat" (obese). Overweight is defined as exceeding the normal or standard weight for a specific height and skeletal frame size, when grouped by sex. As an example, if the recommended weight range for a man 5 feet 10 inches tall is 135 to 176 pounds, any weight in excess of that range is considered overweight. Any weight under this range is considered underweight.

No consideration is given to the levels of body fat or lean body mass in these definitions. Individuals who are overweight might be carrying too much fat or may have above average lean body mass development. Most football players could be considered overweight by the aforementioned definition because they usually have very high levels of lean body mass. The term overweight is not necessarily undesirable, especially when the lean body mass is high. Measuring body density and calculating fat weight and lean body weight allows a more accurate method of estimating desired weight rather than using height/weight tables, which do not determine fat and lean weight.

Obesity is defined as having excess body fat. There is no universal agreement on which percent body fat level constitutes obesity because there is no universal agreement on which technique should be used to establish body fat standards. Grade 1 through 3 levels of obesity have been assigned to body mass index scores (see the section describing body mass index), but these do not account for the body fat percentage.

Standard values for percent body fat,

based on the normal distribution, are found in Table 19–3.

The assessment of body composition ranges from a simplistic view of weight for height to sophisticated, expensive measurement techniques. All techniques have the goal of determining desired body weight. Perhaps the most reasonable way to estimate a desired weight is to measure actual percent body fat and compare the result with an average or good reference point on a statistically normal distribution of body fat scores (Table 19–3). Then, select a more desirable percent body fat score on that statistical distribution of body fat scores and calculate the total weight change needed to achieve the desired level. This will be explained further in a subsequent section.

Body Mass Index

The simplest way to examine body weight status is to calculate the body mass index (BMI) or Quetelet Index. BMI is calculated by dividing the body weight in kilograms by the height in meters squared (kg/m^2). It examines body weight relative to height. As the BMI increases, mortality from heart disease, cancer, and diabetes also increases.[6]

The following BMI standards for both men and women have been used to classify obesity[7]:

Rating	BMI (kg/m^2)
Desirable	20.0–24.9
Grade 1 Obesity	25.0–29.9
Grade 2 Obesity	30.0–39.9
Grade 3 Obesity	40.0–up

Waist-to-Hip Ratio

Subcutaneous body fat levels in the upper body (represented by the waist measurement) and lower body (represented by the hip measurement) are distributed differently by gender, age, body type, and activity levels. For example, inactive people store more total fat than active people. Adult women tend to store fat in the arms and thighs, whereas adult men store fat mainly in the abdomen. Both male and female endomorph body types store fat in the middle and lower body. Ectomorph body types store fat in an even fashion throughout the body. Mesomorphs store very little body fat when they are young, but tend to store it in the upper body with increasing age and/or inactivity.

Fat distributed in the abdomen (upper body or android obesity) is associated with greater morbidity and mortality than is fat distributed below the waist (lower body or gynoid obesity).[8] Ideally, the waist circumference (representing upper body or android fat distribution) should be smaller than the hip circumference (representing

Table 19–3. Standard Values for Percent Body Fat

Rating	Age (yrs)				
	20–29	30–39	40–49	50–59	60+
Men*					
Excellent	<11	<12	<14	<15	<16
Good	11–13	12–14	14–16	15–17	16–18
Average	14–20	15–21	17–23	18–24	19–25
Fair	21–23	22–24	24–26	25–27	26–28
Poor	>23	>24	>26	>27	>28
Women†					
Excellent	<16	<17	<18	<19	<20
Good	16–19	17–20	18–21	19–22	20–23
Average	20–28	21–29	22–30	23–31	24–32
Fair	29–31	30–32	31–33	32–34	33–35
Poor	>31	>32	>33	>34	>35

* With permission from Jackson AS, Pollock ML: Generalized equations for predicting body density of men. *Br J Nutr,* 40:497–504, 1978.

† With permission from Jackson AS, Pollock ML, and Ward A: Generalized equations for predicting body density of women. *Med Sci Sports Exerc,* 12:175–182, 1980.

lower body or gynoid fat distribution). The waist-to-hip measurement ratio is therefore recommended as one way to counsel participants on their fat distribution and associated risks of morbidity and mortality.

The waist circumference is measured in a horizontal plane at the narrowest portion of the torso (usually 2 to 3 inches above the umbilicus). The hip circumference is measured in a horizontal plane at the level of the projections of the greater trochanters, which usually coincide with the greatest protrusion of the gluteal muscles. If these two do not coincide, measure the largest circumference around the buttocks to represent the hip measurement.

The average waist/hip ratio for women aged 17 to 39 is 0.80. The ratio increases with age to above 0.90. The average waist/hip ratio for men aged 17 to 39 is 0.90. The ratio increases with age to above 0.98. It is recommended that the waist/hip ratio be below 1.00 for both women and men.[8]

Measurement of Body Composition

The most direct way to measure body composition is to do a chemical analysis of the whole body to determine the amount of water, fat, protein and minerals. In humans, most measurements are based on a "two component" system described by Behnke.[9] The two components are lean body mass or fat-free weight, and body fat. The lean body mass encompasses all of the body's nonfat tissues, including the skeleton, water, muscle, connective tissue, organ tissues, and teeth. The body fat component includes both the essential and nonessential fat stores. Essential fat includes fat incorporated into organs and tissues, with nonessential fat being primarily within adipose tissue. There are several techniques available for determination of body composition, many which are limited in their usefulness because of (1) lack of sufficient research to determine reliability and validity, (2) the expense in terms of equipment and personnel, and (3) the complexity of the methods. Many rely on the different properties of the two body components, such as differences in photon absorption, sound wave or electromagnetic wave transmission, x-ray absorption, electrical conductivity, or electrical impedance.

Whatever the technique, the measurement obtained is that of body density (density of either lean body mass or fat mass). Density is a measure of compactness and it is known that the density of fat and muscle and the ratios of skeletal weight and body water to lean body weight are extremely constant. Density is equal to the mass divided by the volume. The two most common techniques for determining body density are hydrostatic (underwater) weighing and measurement of skin fold thickness.

Hydrostatic Weighing

This technique is the standard and the criterion technique by which other methods are validated. It is based on the knowledge that fat has a density less than that of water, and thus will float. Lean tissue has a density greater than that of water and will sink in water. Thus, fat people tend to float and weigh less underwater, whereas lean people tend to sink and weigh more underwater. At a given body weight, a fat person has a larger volume than a thin one and thus a smaller density.

In this procedure, the subject is submerged and weighed underwater. This technique requires special equipment for submerging and weighing the subject underwater and for determining the residual volume of air in the lungs (which would buoy the body in water, thus affecting the results). It requires significant training and cooperation by the subject in assuming a still position underwater and exhaling air from the lungs.

The technique is reproducible with trained subjects and technicians, but has some possible errors: accurate measurement of residual volume, assumptions of the densities of fat and muscle, and possible collection of air in the intestines. These variations, as well as the normal biologic variability in the fat-free mass in a given population, result in estimations of body fat within ±2.5% of the "true" value.[10]

Skin Fold Thickness

This is the most practical technique for estimating body fat. This technique relies on the observation that, within any population, a certain fraction of the total body fat lies just under the skin (subcutaneous fat), and if one could obtain a representative sample of that fat, overall body fatness (density) could be predicted. Investigators have found that the subcutaneous fat represented a variable fraction of total fat (20 to 70%), depending on age, sex, overall fatness, and the measurement technique used. Generalized equations have been developed for predicting body fat in men and women by Jackson and Pollock[11] and Jackson, Pollock, and Ward.[12] These equations include the sum of skin folds and age, thus reducing the variability associated with age. The original samples of subjects used to generate these equations for men and women represented adults aged 20 to 60 years, racial and ethnic proportions equal to the American population, fit and unfit, athletic and nonathletic and large and small people. The equations have been cross-validated with independent samples and can be used in the generalized population of the United States.

The body density equations for men and women use the sum of 3 or the sum of 7 skin folds. To be accurate and valid, you must use the exact skin fold techniques that were used to derive the equations. The seven measurements used in the derivation of the equations are described in Table 19–4 and pictured in Chapter 1. In accomplished and well-trained technicians, estimates of percent body fatness from skinfold measures has an error of about 3.7%.[10]

Bioelectrical Impedance

This popular method is based on differences in resistance to electrical current in lean body mass and fat mass. A harmless 50 k Hz current is sent through the subject, and the impedance is measured. Body water (primarily found in the lean body tissue) conducts the electrical current, and the higher the body water content, the better the conductance (less impedance). This impedance is then converted (using impedance equation) to lean body mass, which is then used to calculate fat mass, and thus percent body fat.

This technique has been found reliable, but not valid, meaning that the results obtained in the same person are consistent; However, it is shown that individuals who have high fat measurements in hydrostatic weighing show low body fat estimates by bioelectrical impedance, and those with low fat measurements by hydrostatic weighing, show high body fat estimates by bioelectrical impedance. Additionally, the individual's hydration level, alcohol intake, previous exercise, skin resistance, and medication intake may affect the readings.

Table 19–4. Descriptions of the Seven Skin Folds used in the Jackson and Pollock[11] and Jackson, Pollock, and Ward[12] equations

All measurements are taken on the right side of the body.

Chest	Diagonal fold midway between the anterior axillary line and the nipple for men and one third of the distance for women
Axilla	Vertical fold on the midaxillary line at the level of the xyphoid process
Triceps	Vertical fold midway between the olecranon and acromion processes on the midline with arm hanging straight down
Subscapular	Diagonal fold just below and following the inferior angle of the scapula
Abdomen	Vertical fold measured 2 cm on the right side of the umbilicus
Suprailiac	Diagonal fold following the natural contour of the skin fold above the iliac crest at the anterior axillary line
Thigh	Vertical fold on the front midline of the thigh halfway between the knee and hip joints

Men[10]

$$\text{Density} = 1.1093800$$
$$- 0.0008267(\text{sum3})$$
$$+ 0.0000016(\text{sum3})^2$$
$$- 0.0002574(\text{age})$$

Sum of chest, abdomen, and thigh

%Fat = (495/D − 450)

Women[11]

$$\text{Density} = 1.0994921$$
$$- 0.0009929(\text{sum3})$$
$$+ 0.0000023(\text{sum3})^2$$
$$- 0.0001392(\text{age})$$

Sum of triceps, suprailiac, and thigh

%Fat = (495/D − 450)

Although this technique is easy to perform, it requires expensive equipment and has not been found to be accurate in the extreme body fat levels.

Dual X-Ray Absorptiometry (DEXA)

This technique is a new and exciting method for evaluating body composition. It involves exposure to very low levels of x rays of two different energy levels. The body is scanned from head to toe, and the attenuation of the x ray through the various body components is calculated. Lean body mass and fat mass absorb the x ray to different degrees; thus relative percentages can be calculated. This technique is valid, and is being studied in a wide variety of individuals against standard techniques to determine its reliability.

Other Techniques

Radiography

An x ray of a limb allows the measurement of the widths of fat, muscle, and bone, and has been used to trace the growth of these tissues over time. It is very accurate, but requires exposure to high levels of radiation and is very expensive.

Ultrasound

Sound waves are transmitted through tissues, and the echoes are received and analyzed. This technique has been used to measure the thickness of subcutaneous fat. The method is promising, but requires a well-trained operator and expensive equipment. Reliability and validity data are not complete.

Nuclear Magnetic Resonance (NMR)

Electromagnetic waves are transmitted through tissues. Select nuclei absorb and release the energy at a particular frequency (resonance). The resonant frequency characteristics are related to the type of tissue. The computer analysis of the signal can provide detailed images and calculate the volumes of specific tissues.

Potassium-40 Count

Potassium is located primarily within the cells, and a portion of this potassium is a naturally occurring radioactive isotope of potassium: ^{40}K. The ^{40}K can be measured in a whole-body counter and is proportional to the mass of lean tissue. This technique is very expensive, although considered valid and reliable.

Musculoskeletal Diameters

Measurement of structural dimensions with a measuring tape have not been shown to be an accurate measure of determining body fat. There appears to be no relationship between skeletal muscle size or skeletal size and the amount of fat weight.

Circumferences (Body Girth)

Measurement of body girths may be reasonably accurate in estimating body fat (from prediction equations) in unfit subjects. However, these measurements do not detect changes in body composition over time when lean tissue increases and fat mass decreases. Thus, for consistent evaluation of body fat percentage, they appear to be impractical.

Calculation of Desired Body Weight

After the percentage of body fat is calculated for an individual, it may be compared to standard values (see Table 19–3). The norms in Table 19–3 are based on the average fat percentage levels of 308 men and 249 women from studies conducted by Jackson and Pollock[11] and Jackson, Pollock, and Ward.[12] The norms were calculated by using multiple units of the standard error of estimate from the mean in each age decade.

The recommended body fat levels for men and women in the various age groups could be defined as the best value in the average range of scores for each sex and age group. On the basis of the norms detailed in Table 19–3, the recommended percent body fat levels for men and women are:

	Age in years				
	20–29	30–39	40–49	50–59	60+
Men	14	15	17	18	19
Women	20	21	22	23	24

The establishment of one recommended body fat level for all men or for all women is difficult because of the aging effect, and because there are no data supporting a given level of body fat as being a "cut-off" for health risk. The desired body weight for each person should be derived with realistic goals, and the assumption that body composition will change normally with age.

The desired body weight may be defined as the weight at which the body fat percentage is equal to or lower than the recommended fat level for the sex and age of the individual. For competitive athletes, the desired weight may be synonymous with "playing weight," which is equivalent to the average fat level for the playing position in that sport. As an example, the calculation of the desired weight for a 42-year-old man weighing 210 lbs with a current body fat level of 29.0% follows.

Step 1. Calculate current fat weight in pounds.
Current body weight (lbs) × current body fat (%) = current fat weight (lbs)
Example: 210 lbs × 0.29 = 61 lbs of current fat weight

Step 2. Calculate current LBW in pounds.
Current body weight (lbs) − current fat weight (lbs) = current LBW (lbs).
Example: 210 lbs − 61 lbs = 149 lbs of current LBW (or 71% of the total body weight)

On the assumption that LBW can be at least maintained in a program of regular exercise and a calorically restricted diet, the desired weight is calculated by adding 17.0% fat to the LBW. (The value 17.0% is the best value of the average range of scores for men aged 40 to 49 years. See Table 19–3.) The logic of this procedure is subsequently illustrated.

Step 3. Calculate the desired weight by using a constant LBW.
Desired weight (100%) = desired fat weight (17.0%) + desired LBW (83%)
Example: LBW (lbs) = 83.0% of desired body weight
149 lbs = 0.83 × desired body weight

Desired body weight (lbs) = 149 lbs/0.83
Desired body weight = 180 lbs

Therefore this man should lose 30 pounds (a reduction from 210 to 180 lbs) to achieve his desired weight. Any percent fat level can be selected as the recommended level for the desired weight. The main consideration is to be realistic when selecting a recommended fat level and to consider the individual's age and physical activity level.

Some clinicians recommend that all men should attain 15% or 16% body fat and all women should attain 19% or 22% as the ideal level. Following this procedure may not be appropriate because the norms listed in Table 19–3 indicate that body fat increases normally with age and no "fixed" average fat level exists. Another problem with using a fixed value involves individuals who are already under those values. The 15% or 16% fat goal for men would necessitate a gain in weight for individuals who are already below these levels. For men to be lower than 15% or 16% fat is not necessarily unhealthy. In fact, most men below those levels are probably at a desirable body weight and may not need to change.

Athletes are prime examples of individuals with low body fat levels associated with high fitness levels. The concept of recommending a desired weight or "playing weight" for an athlete can follow the same logic as the previous example. For instance, a football player weighing 280 lbs with 15% fat may want to play at the 13% fat level. If his LBW is maintained at 238 lbs, his playing weight would be 273 lbs (playing weight = 238/0.87). Thus, a desired weight can be calculated for any individual when sex, age, and fitness level are considered.

MUSCULAR STRENGTH AND MUSCULAR ENDURANCE ASSESSMENT

Possession of superior muscular strength enables the individual to perform any task involving strength with greater ease and control. Superior muscle endurance allows an individual to perform muscular tasks for a long period without undue fatigue. The measurement of total body strength and total muscle endurance is difficult because of the numerous muscles and muscle groups, each of which is unique in fiber type and function, making strength and endurance muscle and muscle group specific. The tests recommended in this chapter were selected on the basis of their practicality and appropriateness for use in adult fitness programs.

Muscular Strength Assessment

Strength is defined as the muscular force exerted against movable and immovable objects. Strength is best measured by tests that require one maximal effort on a given movement or position. The types of muscular contraction (isotonic, or dynamic and isometric) are described in Chapter 26.

Isotonic testing protocols usually include calisthenic or weight-lifting exercises. Isometric strength is measured using dynamometers or cable tensiometers. Isokinetic machines offer accommodating resistance and can be used to record the force exerted throughout an entire range of motion in a muscle group. These devices are usually expensive because they involve electronic recording mechanisms.

The principle of specificity (see Chap. 9) must be considered when administering strength tests. If participants are training isotonically with calisthenics and weight training, isotonic strength tests should be given to assess isotonic strength changes. Isometric or isokinetic strength testing may not be sufficiently specific to assess isotonic strength changes resulting from an isotonic training program. Although some transfer of isotonic strength to isometric or isokinetic testing occurs, the isometric or isokinetic tests are not as specific in evaluating isotonic strength.

Isotonic strength can be easily assessed by the one-repetition maximum (1RM) weight lifting test. Weight training machines are usually used for isotonic strength tests because the weights are easily and quickly selected in the testing protocol and the weights are safely secured in the apparatus. Because no additional spotters are required with machine weights, the test is efficient in terms of time and staffing.

In the 1RM testing protocol, the subject has a series of trials to determine the greatest weight that can be lifted just once for that particular movement. The procedure starts with a low weight that can be easily and safely lifted. Weight is added gradually until the lift can be performed correctly just one time. The subject should be encouraged to breathe freely with each lift and discouraged from breath-holding or performing the Valsalva maneuver.

A 1RM isotonic strength measure can be obtained for any weight training exercise. For practical purposes, the 1RM bench press (chest press) and leg press tests described by Jackson, Watkins, and Patton[13] are recommended for assessment of upper and lower body strength. These authors reported that the 1RM bench press and military press (shoulder press) tests are the most valid measures of upper body strength and that the upper leg press and lower leg press tests are the most valid measures of lower body strength when using Universal Gym equipment.

After the 1RM is determined for the bench press tests, the 1RM weight in pounds is divided by the participant's body weight in pounds to obtain strength represented per pound of body weight (1RM lb/body weight lb). The result is then compared to the standards presented in Table 19–5. The same procedure is used for calculating the leg press results; standard values for this test are presented in Table 19–6.

In the past, the hand grip strength test was used to assess isometric muscular strength. It was thought that grip strength was an indicator of general body strength. However, the results of these tests were variable and not reliable because of inconsistent testing protocols. The principle of specificity applies to the grip strength test just as it applies to the bench press and leg press tests. Grip strength norms for the Ishiko[14] method are presented in Table 19–7.

Muscular Endurance Assessment

Muscular endurance involves the ability of a muscle or muscle group to repeat identical movements (dynamic) or to maintain a certain degree of tension over time (static).

Table 19–5. Standard Values for Bench Press Strength in 1 RM lb/lb Body Weight*

Rating	Age (yrs)				
	20–29	**30–39**	**40–49**	**50–59**	**60 +**
Men					
Excellent	>1.25	>1.07	>0.96	>0.85	>0.77
Good	1.17–1.25	1.01–1.07	0.91–0.96	0.81–0.85	0.74–0.77
Average	0.97–1.16	0.86–1.00	0.78–0.90	0.70–0.80	0.64–0.73
Fair	0.88–0.96	0.79–0.85	0.72–0.77	0.65–0.69	0.60–0.63
Poor	<0.88	<0.79	<0.72	<0.65	<0.60
Women					
Excellent	>0.77	>0.65	>0.60	>0.53	>0.54
Good	0.72–0.77	0.62–0.65	0.57–0.60	0.51–0.53	0.51–0.54
Average	0.59–0.71	0.53–0.61	0.48–0.56	0.43–0.50	0.41–0.50
Fair	0.53–0.58	0.49–0.52	0.44–0.47	0.40–0.42	0.37–0.40
Poor	<0.53	<0.49	<0.44	<0.40	<0.37

* Adapted with permission from The Institute for Aerobics Research. 1985 Physical Fitness Norms. [Unpublished Data.] Dallas, TX, 1985.

Muscular endurance tests may be relative or absolute. In a relative endurance test, the muscles work with a proportionate amount of the maximal strength load. An absolute endurance test requires a set load for all subjects without a definite relationship to the maximal strength of each individual. The three types of muscular endurance tests are:

1. Dynamic: identical repetitions of a movement are repeated over time, such as in the sit-up and push-up tests.
2. Static repetitive: the number of times a force equal to a certain percentage of maximal strength or body weight is registered against a static measuring device.
3. Static timed: the amount of time a muscle contraction is maintained, such as in the flexed arm hang test.

The sit-up and push-up tests are perhaps the easiest and most practical tests to use for evaluation of dynamic muscle endurance. Static repetitive and static timed tests require special equipment and may involve time-consuming procedures.[5]

Muscular endurance tests primarily tax

Table 19–6. Standard Values for Upper Leg Press Strength in 1 RM lb/lb Body Weight*

Rating	Age (yrs)				
	20–29	**30–39**	**40–49**	**50–59**	**60 +**
Men					
Excellent	>2.07	>1.87	>1.75	>1.65	>1.55
Good	2.00–2.07	1.80–1.87	1.70–1.75	1.60–1.65	1.50–1.55
Average	1.83–1.99	1.63–1.79	1.56–1.69	1.46–1.59	1.37–1.49
Fair	1.65–1.82	1.55–1.62	1.50–1.55	1.40–1.45	1.31–1.36
Poor	<1.65	<1.55	<1.50	<1.40	<1.31
Women					
Excellent	>1.62	>1.41	>1.31	>1.25	>1.14
Good	1.54–1.62	1.35–1.41	1.26–1.31	1.13–1.25	1.08–1.14
Average	1.35–1.53	1.20–1.34	1.12–1.25	0.99–1.12	0.92–1.07
Fair	1.26–1.34	1.13–1.19	1.06–1.11	0.86–0.98	0.85–0.91
Poor	<1.26	<1.13	<1.06	<0.86	<0.85

* Adapted with permission from The Institute for Aerobics Research. 1985 Physical Fitness Norms. [Unpublished Data.] Dallas, TX, 1985.

Table 19–7. Standard Values for Grip Strength—Dominant Hand (kg)*

Rating	Age (yrs)				
	20–29	30–39	40–49	50–59	60+
Men					
Excellent	>54	>53	>51	>49	>49
Good	51–54	50–53	48–51	46–49	46–49
Average	43–50	43–49	41–47	39–45	39–45
Fair	39–42	39–42	37–40	35–38	35–38
Poor	<39	<39	<37	<35	<35
Women					
Excellent	>36	>36	>35	>33	>33
Good	33–36	34–36	33–35	31–33	31–33
Average	26–32	28–33	27–32	25–30	25–30
Fair	22–25	25–27	24–26	22–24	22–24
Poor	<22	<25	<24	<22	<22

* With permission from Ishiko T: The Organism and Muscular Work. In *Fitness, Health, and Work Capacity: International Standards for Assessment.* Edited by LA Larson New York: Macmillan Publishing Co., 1974.

the anaerobic metabolism of skeletal muscles and differ from cardiovascular-respiratory endurance tests, which mainly tax the heart and lungs and the aerobic metabolism of skeletal muscles. As with muscular strength tests, muscular endurance tests are specific to the muscles and muscle groups tested. Because most muscular endurance tests involve a subjective end point that depends upon motivation and technique, the examiner should be consistent in offering any type of verbal motivation to subjects.

In the 1-minute sit-up test, the subject assumes a supine position with the hands interlocked behind the neck and knees bent to a 90 degree position (heels are approximately 18 inches from the buttocks for most people). A partner or the tester holds the ankles to give support. Within a one minute period, the subject performs as many correct situps as possible (elbows touching knees). The subject should not hold the breath during this test, but rather should breathe freely with each repetition. Standard values for adults appear in Table 19–8.

The pushup test is administered with

Table 19–8. Standard Values for 1-min Situp Endurance*

Rating	Age (yrs)				
	20–29	30–39	40–49	50–59	60+
Men					
Excellent	>47	>39	>34	>29	>24
Good	43–47	35–39	30–34	25–29	20–24
Average	37–42	29–34	24–29	19–24	14–19
Fair	33–36	25–28	20–23	15–18	10–13
Poor	<33	<25	<20	<15	<10
Women					
Excellent	>43	>35	>30	>25	>20
Good	39–43	31–35	26–30	21–25	16–20
Average	33–38	25–30	19–25	15–20	10–15
Fair	29–32	21–24	16–18	11–14	6–9
Poor	<29	<21	<16	<11	<6

* With permission from Pollock ML, Wilmore JH, Fox SM: *Health and Fitness through Physical Activity.* New York: John Wiley & Sons, 1978.

male subjects in the standard "up" position and female subjects in the modified "knee" position. When testing male subjects, the tester places a fist on the floor beneath the subject's chest and the subject must lower his body to the floor until the chest touches the tester's fist. The fist method is not used for female subjects, and no criteria are established for determining how the chest must touch the floor for the proper pushup. For both men and women, however, the subject's back must be straight at all times and the subject must push up to a straight arm position. The maximal number of push-ups performed consecutively without rest is counted as the score, and the result is compared to normal values detailed in Table 19–9.

Descriptions of static repetitive, static timed, and other dynamic muscle endurance tests (e.g., chin-ups, squat thrusts, and dips) are provided in textbooks detailing physical education tests and measurements. Definite guidelines must be followed when scoring muscular endurance tests because correct (or incorrect) form influences final results. As mentioned previously, motivational factors greatly affect results, and motivation procedures must therefore be standardized. Because muscle endurance tests are specific, dynamic endurance tests should be used to evaluate dynamic muscle endurance, and static tests should be used to determine static muscle endurance.

FLEXIBILITY MEASUREMENT

Flexibility refers to the ability to move the body parts through a wide range of motion without undue strain to the articulations and muscle attachments. Flexibility measurements include flexion and extension movements. No general test is available that provides representative values of total body flexibility; tests are specific to each joint and muscle group and connective tissue area.

The most accurate tests of flexibility are those in which a goniometer is used to measure the actual degrees of rotation of the various joints. A goniometer is a protractor type of instrument that is used to measure the joint angle at both extremes in the total range of movement. The goniometer has two arms that attach to two body parts with the center of the instrument over the center of the joint tested. The center of the goniometer must be placed carefully over the exact center of the joint tested. The arms of the goniometer should be taped over each midline on the bones emanating from the joint center. The difference between the joint angles recorded at both extremes in the total range of movement of the joint indicates the number of degrees of movement possible.

An electrogoniometer has a potentiometer that replaces the protractor of the goniometer. The potentiometer provides an electric signal proportional to the angle of

Table 19–9. Standard Values for Push-up Endurance*

Rating	Age (yrs)				
	20–29	**30–39**	**40–49**	**50–59**	**60+**
Men					
Excellent	>54	>44	>39	>34	>29
Good	45–54	35–44	30–39	25–34	20–29
Average	35–44	25–34	20–29	15–24	10–19
Fair	20–34	15–24	12–19	8–14	5–9
Poor	<20	<15	<12	<8	<5
Women					
Excellent	>48	>39	>34	>29	>19
Good	34–48	25–39	20–34	15–29	5–19
Average	17–33	12–24	8–19	6–14	3–4
Fair	6–16	4–11	3–7	2–5	1–2
Poor	<6	<4	<3	<2	<1

* With permission from Pollock ML, Wilmore JH, Fox SM: *Health and Fitness through Physical Activity*. New York: John Wiley & Sons, 1978.

the joint. This device can give continuous readings of the degrees of rotation of the joint tested. Because continuous recordings of joint movement are possible with the electrogoniometer, it is used to assess flexibility during physical activity; the assessment of functional flexibility is much more accurate and realistic. The goniometer and electrogoniometer techniques, however, can be time-consuming and expensive. More practical tests have been developed to estimate general flexibility of joints, such as the trunk flexion, shoulder elevation, trunk extension, and ankle flexibility tests.

Before flexibility performance tests are administered, the person should gently stretch the muscles being tested to "warm up" and prevent injury. It is also desirable to have the subject practice the flexibility test to determine the best possible performance.

Because lower back problems are prevalent in the adult population, the sit-and-reach test (trunk flexion) is used to assess lower back flexibility. It is easily administered and requires minimal equipment. Actually, the sit-and-reach test also involves the extensibility (or tightness) of the hamstring musculature, buttocks, lower back, upper back, and shoulders.

In the sit-and-reach test, the subject sits on the floor with legs extended straight in front and against a 12-inch-high box with a measuring stick or tape secured on top.

The 15-inch mark of the measuring tape should be at the edge of the box. The person then places the index fingers of both hands together and slowly reaches forward as far as possible on the measuring tape, holding the position for 1 second. The score is the most distant point reached by the fingertips in the best of three trials. The knees must be straight and in contact with the floor at all times. Bouncing into the stretch position is not allowed and the movement must be slow and gradual. Normal values for adults are listed in Table 19–10.

Shoulder elevation, trunk extension, and ankle flexibility tests are also used in general flexibility assessment. The shoulder elevation test measures the ability to elevate the shoulders. From a prone position with the arms straight and shoulders wide apart, the subject raises a stick upward as high as possible while keeping the chin on the floor and the elbows and wrists straight. The examiner measures the distance from the bottom of the stick to the floor, and the best measurement from three trials is recorded. The best measurement in inches is then multiplied by 100, and the product is divided by arm length measured in inches. The arm length is defined as the distance between the acromion process and the upper surface of the stick, which is held with the arms hanging downward. The shoulder elevation measurement should be taken at the highest vertical point at which

Table 19–10. Standard Values for Trunk Flexion in Inches*

Rating	Age (yrs)				
	20–29	30–39	40–49	50–59	60+
Men					
Excellent	>21	>20	>19	>18	>17
Good	19–21	18–20	17–19	16–18	15–17
Average	13–18	12–17	11–16	10–15	9–14
Fair	10–12	9–11	8–10	7–9	6–8
Poor	<10	<9	<8	<7	<6
Women					
Excellent	>23	>22	>21	>20	>19
Good	22–23	21–22	20–21	19–20	18–19
Average	16–21	15–20	14–19	13–18	12–17
Fair	13–15	12–14	11–13	10–12	9–11
Poor	<13	<12	<11	<10	<9

* Adapted with permission from Golding LA, Myers CR, Sinning WE (eds): *The Y's Way to Physical Fitness*. Rosemont, IL: YMCA of the USA, 1982.

Table 19–11. Standard Values for Shoulder Elevation*

Rating	Shoulder Elevation Score (inches)
Men	
Excellent	106–123
Good	88–105
Average	70–87
Fair	53–69
Poor	35–52
Women	
Excellent	105–123
Good	86–104
Average	68–85
Fair	50–67
Poor	31–49

* With permission from Johnson BL, Nelson JK: *Practical Measurements for Evaluation in Physical Education.* Minneapolis: Burgess Publishing, 1969.

Table 19–13. Standard Values for Ankle Flexibility*

Rating	Ankle Flexibility Score (degrees of movement)
Men	
Excellent	77–99
Good	63–76
Average	48–62
Fair	34–47
Poor	15–33
Women	
Excellent	81–89
Good	68–80
Average	56–67
Fair	43–55
Poor	32–42

* With permission from Johnson BL, Nelson JK: *Practical Measurements for Evaluation in Physical Education.* Minneapolis: Burgess Publishing, 1969.

the stick is held momentarily. Normal values for men and women are provided in Table 19–11.

In the trunk extension test, the subject lies on the mat with the feet and hips secured by the examiner. With the hands resting on the lower back, the subject raises the trunk as far upward and backward as possible. The vertical distance between the mat and suprasternal notch is measured to the nearest 1/4 inch. This measurement is multiplied by 100 and the product is di-

Table 19–12. Standard Values for Trunk Extension*

Rating	Trunk Extension Score (inches)
Men	
Excellent	50–64
Good	43–49
Average	37–42
Fair	31–36
Poor	28–30
Women	
Excellent	48–63
Good	42–47
Average	35–41
Fair	29–34
Poor	23–28

* With permission from Johnson BL, Nelson JK: *Practical Measurements for Evaluation in Physical Education.* Minneapolis: Burgess Publishing, 1969.

vided by trunk length measured in inches. Trunk length is defined as the vertical distance between the suprasternal notch and the floor while the subject is seated with the back against a wall. Standard values for men and women are provided in Table 19–12.

Extreme caution is required when administering the trunk extension test, because pressure is exerted on the posterior areas of the lumbar vertebrae. Individuals with existing or suspected back problems should not attempt this test.

The average ankle flexibility test measures the ability to flex and extend the ankle. The subject sits on the floor or on a table with the back of the knee touching the surface. Keeping the heel stationary, the foot is dorsiflexed as much as possible. The angle of this foot position is recorded on a protractor placed at the side of the foot. The subject then extends (plantar flexes) the foot as far as possible, and the angle of the foot position is noted. The difference between the position in dorsiflexion and plantarflexion is the average ankle flexibility score in degrees of movement. Normal values for average ankle flexibility are provided in Table 19–13.

REFERENCES

1. American College of Sports Medicine: Guidelines for Exercise Testing and Pre-

scription. Fourth Edition. Philadelphia: Lea & Febiger, 1991.

2. Casperson C, Powell KE, and Christenson GM: Physical activity, exercise and physical fitness: Definitions and distinctions for health-related research. *Public Health Reports, 100:*126, 1985.

3. Pate RR: The evolving definition of physical fitness. *Quest, 40:*174, 1988.

4. American Society on Hypertension: Recommendations for Routine Blood Pressure Measurement by Indirect Cuff Sphygmomanometry. *Am J Hypertens, 5:*207, 1992.

5. Golding LA, Myers CR, and Sinning WE (eds.): Y's Ways to Physical Fitness, 3rd Edition. Champaign, IL: Human Kinetics Publishers, 1989.

6. Bray GA, Gray DS: Obesity Part 1—Pathogenesis. West J Med, *149:*429, 1988 (in Nieman DC: Physical Activity and Obesity. Fitness and Sports Medicine: An Introduction, Palo Alto, CA: Bull Publishing Co., 1990).

7. Jequier E: Energy, Obesity, and Body Weight Standards. Am J Clin Nutr *45:* 1035, 1987 (In Nieman DC: *Body Composition Measurement. Fitness and Sports Medicine: An Introduction.* Palo Alto, CA: Bull Publishing Co., 1990).

8. Shimokata H, et al: Studies in the distribution of body fat: I. Effects of age, sex, and obesity. *J Gerontology, 44:*M66, 1989.

9. Behnke, AR, Feen BG, and Welham WC: The specific gravity of healthy men: Body weight/volume as an index of obesity. *JAMA 118:*495–498, 1942.

10. Powers SK, Howley ET: Exercise Physiology Wm C. Brown Publishers, 1990. pp 381–388.

11. Jackson AS, Pollock ML: Generalized equations for predicting body density of men. *Br J Nutr, 40:*497, 1978.

12. Jackson AS, Pollock ML, Ward A: Generalized equations for predicting body density of women. *Med Sci Sports Exerc, 12:*175, 1980.

13. Jackson A, Watkins M, Patton R: A factor analysis of twelve selected maximal isotonic strength performances on the Universal Gym. *Med Sci Sports Exerc, 12:*274, 1980.

14. Ishiko T: The Organism and Muscular Work. In *Fitness, Health, and Work Capacity: International Standards for Assessment.* Edited by LA Larson. New York: Macmillan Publishing Co., 1974.

BIBLIOGRAPHY

Institute for Aerobics Research: 1985 Physical Fitness Norms. [Unpublished Data.] Dallas, TX, 1985.

Johnson BL, Nelson JK: Practical Measurements for Evaluation in Physical Education. Minneapolis, MN: Burgess Publishing, 1969.

Pollock ML, Wilmore JM, Fox SM: *Health and Fitness through Physical Activity.* New York: John Wiley & Sons, 1978.

Chapter 20

FUNDAMENTALS OF CARDIORESPIRATORY EXERCISE TESTING

Robert G. Holly

The heart and lungs work together as a unit to supply oxygen to the tissues in relation to their needs. As tissue needs for oxygen increase (as they do in muscle during exercise), there are certain predictable responses in individuals with normally functioning heart and lungs. Furthermore, when disease is present in either the cardiovascular or respiratory system, there are also more or less predictable deviations from the normal responses. Exercise tests, with measurements of both cardiovascular and respiratory responses, can be called cardiorespiratory exercise (CRX) tests. Such tests can provide valuable information noninvasively about the functioning of both the cardiovascular and respiratory systems. In this chapter, we:

1. review the meaning of the maximal oxygen uptake,
2. discuss the importance of the lactate threshold and other variables obtained during CRX testing,
3. consider how the results obtained during CRX testing can be used in the diagnosis of cardiovascular and respiratory disease,
4. discuss the general characteristics of appropriate modes and protocols,
5. describe briefly the calculation of oxygen uptake, and
6. present an overview of methods of measurement of oxygen uptake.

MAXIMAL OXYGEN UPTAKE

The maximal oxygen uptake may be defined as the maximal rate at which oxygen can be taken up, distributed, and used by the body in the performance of exercise that utilizes a large muscle mass. A high level depends on the proper functioning of three important systems within the body: the respiratory system, which takes up oxygen from inspired air and transports it into the blood; the cardiovascular system, which pumps and distributes this oxygen-laden blood throughout body tissues; and the active muscles of the musculoskeletal system, which use this oxygen to convert stored substrates into work and heat during physical activity.[1] Maximal oxygen uptake is most often abbreviated $\dot{V}O_{2max}$, where $\dot{V}$ represents the volume taken up per minute, O_2 represents oxygen, and max represents maximal conditions. Thus, $\dot{V}O_{2max}$ is the maximal volume of oxygen used by the body per minute. It is the measure of the maximal aerobic (or oxygen-requiring) metabolism of the body, and for this reason is often referred to as the maximal aerobic capacity or maximal aerobic power. Although the former term is frequently used, the latter term is more accurate. Because $\dot{V}O_{2max}$ is a measure of energy flow, it is a measure of power rather than of volume or capacity. For this reason, $\dot{V}O_{2max}$ is referred to as maximal aerobic power or maximal oxygen uptake (where uptake means the rate at which O_2 is taken up).[2]

Except for steady-state exercise at light to moderate work rates, there is a variable component to the total metabolism from anaerobic processes. At maximal exercise, the total metabolism or rate of energy transfer is the sum of maximal aerobic power ($\dot{V}O_{2max}$) and maximal anaerobic power. Various tests of anaerobic power have been described[3] and will not be considered further here. However, it is important to realize that aerobic metabolism is only one component of the total metabolic rate at maximal exercise.

Maximal aerobic power is measured for many reasons ranging from an assessment of cardiorespiratory function in heart failure patients to the prediction of performance in world class athletes. Appendix D, "Metabolic Calculations" in the *Guidelines*,[4] presents an approach to estimating oxygen uptake under standardized, steady-state conditions. However, these equations are thought to have limited utility in estimating maximal aerobic power in nonsteady state conditions (such as those occurring during ramp or rapidly advancing incremental tests and at peak exercise). In various situations such as scientific studies, the assessment of athletes, and in clinical evaluations where it is desirable to have an accurate measure of maximal aerobic power rather than an estimate, the measurement of $\dot{V}O_{2max}$ is preferred. Historically, the measurement of $\dot{V}O_{2max}$ has been a costly, laborious, and time-consuming operation, primarily confined to research laboratories.[5,6] With the advent of reasonably priced and rapidly responding gas analyzers, accurate volume-measuring devices, and associated computer technology, the measurement of $\dot{V}O_{2max}$ is now accessible to more scientists, clinicians, and fitness personnel than ever before.

As work rate increases on an ergometric device (e.g., speed and grade on a treadmill or resistance and tempo on a cycle ergometer), so also does $\dot{V}O_2$.[1] If the subject is not limited by prior signs or symptoms of exertional intolerance, $\dot{V}O_2$ increases with increasing work rate until it peaks or plateaus. After this point, rate may continue to increase briefly with no further increase in $\dot{V}O_2$. This is the $\dot{V}O_{2max}$ and represents a physiologic limit. Although work rate may continue to increase following a plateau of $\dot{V}O_2$, this increase is accomplished anaerobically. The magnitude of this increase in work rate beyond the start of the plateau does not affect the measurement of $\dot{V}O_{2max}$, but instead relates to the subject's anaerobic power and motivation. The $\dot{V}O_{2max}$ is a reliable measurement with a test-retest correlation coefficient of 0.959 and a standard error of the estimate of 0.094 L/min or 2.2% of the overall mean.[7]

From the early work of Taylor et al.,[8] a plateau in $\dot{V}O_{2max}$ was presumed to occur when there was less than a 150 mL/min (2.1 mL/kg/min) increase in $\dot{V}O_{2max}$ with an increase in grade of 2.5% at a speed of 7 mph. Thus, there would be an increase of less than 0.6 METs or about 25% of the expected increase of 2.5 METs. Other criteria for achievement of $\dot{V}O_{2max}$ in well-motivated subjects include a respiratory exchange ratio (R) of greater than 1.0 and a blood lactate concentration greater than 8 mmol/L. In several studies involving both younger and older subjects, less than 50% of these individuals attained a plateau in $\dot{V}O_2$ at maximal workrates. Thus, it seems reasonable to accept alternate criteria for $\dot{V}O_{2max}$ as long as the subject is well motivated. This is discussed more fully in the review by Davis.[6]

In older, sedentary, and/or diseased populations, a common finding is that neither a plateau nor another criterion of $\dot{V}O_{2max}$ is reached. This occurs because the subject ceases exercise before $\dot{V}O_{2max}$ due to a limiting sign or symptom such as angina, fatigue, blurred vision, or ST segment depression, among others. In this instance, the peak $\dot{V}O_2$ measured is more representative of a limiting disease or condition rather than a physiologic limit and is often referred to as a symptom-limited $\dot{V}O_{2max}$ ($\dot{V}O_{2max_{SL}}$) or functional capacity to differentiate it from a physiological $\dot{V}O_{2max}$.

CARDIORESPIRATORY RESPONSES TO GRADED EXERCISE

Heart rate (HR), blood pressure and the electrocardiogram (ECG) are typically measured in cardiac patients during exercise testing. Normal and abnormal responses of these variables to graded exercise have been fully described elsewhere (see Chapter 7). Briefly, HR and systolic blood pressure (SBP) increase regularly with work rate. Very rapid increases in HR may indicate, among other things, paroxysmal tachycardia, inadequate increase in stroke volume secondary to heart disease, poor physical conditioning, vasoregulatory asthenia, and anxiety. Conversely, inadequate increases in HR and SBP may indicate second- or third-degree heart blocks, sinus node disease, and significant cardiac dysfunction, among other problems. Changes in the ECG may help distinguish among these different possibilities. Similarly, in evaluating patients with poor work tolerance and/or difficulty in breathing, assessing respiratory responses to exercise (in addition to cardiovascular variables) may aid in the differential diagnosis. How CRX tests may aid in this process is the topic of the next section. Here we review the remaining basic cardiorespiratory responses to graded exercise.

In response to exercise on a cycle ergometer, which increments at the rate of 15 watts/min (Fig. 20–1),[9] minute ventilation ($\dot{V}_E$), $\dot{V}_{O_2}$, and the rate of CO_2 output ($\dot{V}_{CO_2}$) increase in concert with the linear increase in work rate. A clinically relevant and useful relationship is that, under most circumstances, the increase in these ventilatory and gas exchange variables is linear until the onset of blood lactate accumulation (OBLA) or lactate threshold (LT). This is the point at which the rate of production and passage of lactate into the blood exceeds its rate of removal. At this time, both $\dot{V}_E$ and $\dot{V}_{CO_2}$ begin to increase more rapidly, whereas the increase in $\dot{V}_{O_2}$ remains linear. The stimulus for this change in $\dot{V}_E$ and $\dot{V}_{CO_2}$ apparently comes from the buffering of lactic acid. Once lactic acid is formed in the working muscles, it quickly dissociates into H^+ and La^-. The H^+ is then buffered by the bicarbonate buffering system as follows:

$$H^+ + HCO_3^- \Leftrightarrow H_2CO_3 \Leftrightarrow H_2O + CO_2.$$

The CO_2 produced by this reaction must be cleared by the lungs. Hence, both $\dot{V}_E$ and $\dot{V}_{CO_2}$ increase at a steeper rate above the LT, while the bicarbonate buffer begins to fall. These responses become the basis for the noninvasive estimation of the LT.[10] This point has also been called the anaerobic threshold (AT)[3,9] or ventilatory threshold (T_{vent}).[4] As a percent of $\dot{V}_{O_2max}$, it can be reliably measured with a test-retest correlation coefficient of 0.91 and a standard error of the estimate of 3.08%.[11] Despite some concern as to exactly what the ventila-

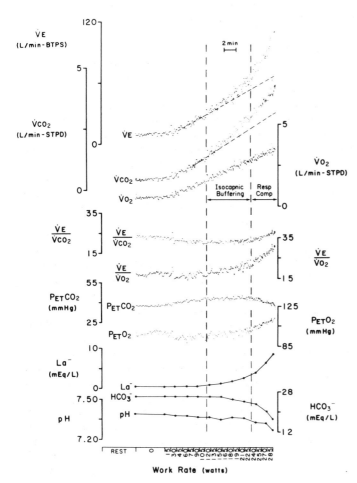

Fig. 20–1. Breath-by-breath measurements of minute ventilation ($\dot{V}_E$), CO_2 output ($\dot{V}_{CO_2}$), O_2 uptake ($\dot{V}_{O_2}$), $\dot{V}_E/\dot{V}_{O_2}$, $\dot{V}_E/\dot{V}_{CO_2}$, end tidal partial pressures of CO_2 (P_{ETco2}) and O_2 (P_{ETo2}), arterial lactate (La^-) and bicarbonate (HCO_3^-) concentrations, and pH for a one-minute incremental work test on a cycle ergometer. The lactate threshold (LT) occurs when lactate increases (first dashed line). This is accompanied by a fall in HCO_3^- concentration and generally an increase in $\dot{V}_E/\dot{V}_{O_2}$, whereas $\dot{V}_E/\dot{V}_{CO_2}$ remains essentially constant. These respiratory variables are characteristic of the ventilatory threshold (T_{vent}). "Isocapnic buffering" refers to the period when $\dot{V}_E$ and $\dot{V}_{CO_2}$ increase curvilinearly at the same rate without an increase in $\dot{V}_E/\dot{V}_{CO_2}$, thus retaining a constant P_{ETco2}. After the period of isocapnic buffering (second dashed line). P_{ETco} decreases, reflecting respiratory compensation for the metabolic acidosis of exercise. With permission from Wasserman K, Hansen JE, Sue DY, Whipp BJ: *Principles of Exercise Testing and Interpretation.* Philadelphia: Lea & Febiger, 1987.

tory response at the LT represents,[12] its clinical utility seems valid.[9,13]

The most valid method currently used to estimate the LT noninvasively (and, thus, to determine T_{vent}) is the V-slope method of Beaver et al.[10] In this method, $\dot{V}_{CO_2}$ is plotted against $\dot{V}_{O_2}$ as shown in Figure 20–2. During the first part of the graded exercise test (GXT), the relationship between the two gas exchange variables is linear. However, at the LT, $\dot{V}_{CO_2}$ begins to increase at a faster rate than $\dot{V}_{O_2}$, which results in a departure in the previously linear relationship. The $\dot{V}_{O_2}$ at which this occurs is the LT determined noninvasively or T_{vent}. Other, less specific characteristics of T_{vent} are described in detail in the excellent text by Wasserman et al.[9] (In the literature, some use the term lactate threshold (LT)

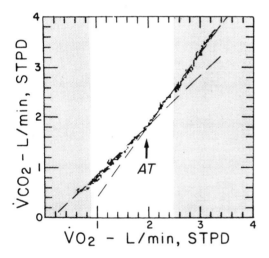

Fig. 20–2. V-slope method of determining the noninvasive lactate or anaerobic threshold (AT). Continuous measurements of CO_2 output are plotted against O_2 uptake during a CRX. The lactate, ventilatory or anaerobic threshold (AT) occurs at the point where the relationship between the two variables diverges from linearity as $\dot{V}_{CO_2}$ begins to increase more rapidly than $\dot{V}_{O_2}$. Data in the shaded areas are ignored in the analysis because of nonlinearity in the kinetics at the start of the work rate increment and hyperventilation for CO_2 at the upper end. The data in the nonshaded area are analyzed by least squares statistical methods to obtain the best fit to a two component model. The intersecting point is the T_{vent}. With permission from Wasserman K, Hansen JE, Sue DY, Whipp BJ: *Principles of Exercise Testing and Interpretation.* Philadelphia: Lea & Febiger, 1987.

when the actual breakpoint in blood lactate is measured as a function of $\dot{V}_{O_2}$, and lactic acidosis threshold (LAT) when the threshold is determined noninvasively from gas exchange responses (including the V-slope method) resulting as a consequence of the acidosis-induced additional $\dot{V}_{CO_2}$.)

As lactate concentration increases above LT, there may be a period of isocapnic buffering (constant arterial P_{CO_2}), characterized by a constant end tidal partial pressure of CO_2 ($P_{ET}CO_2$), even in the presence of continually increasing blood lactate concentration (Fig. 20–1). $P_{ET}CO_2$ is the level of CO_2 at end expiration and is indicative of both alveolar and arterial CO_2 content. During this period, there is a constant relationship between $\dot{V}_E$ and $\dot{V}_{CO_2}$, characterized by a constant ventilatory equivalent for CO_2 ($\dot{V}_E/\dot{V}_{CO_2}$). However, because $\dot{V}_E$ is increasing more rapidly than $\dot{V}_{O_2}$, the ventilatory equivalent for O_2 ($\dot{V}_E/\dot{V}_{O_2}$) is increasing as well. Finally, as work rate continues to increase, the rising lactic acid concentration is incompletely buffered by the bicarbonate system, so pH falls. $\dot{V}_E$ now increases more rapidly than $\dot{V}_{CO_2}$ in response to the increase in acid drive to respiration. As a consequence $P_{ET}CO_2$ decreases (because the subject is now blowing off CO_2 more rapidly than it is produced by the combination of aerobic and anaerobic metabolism) and $\dot{V}_E/\dot{V}_{CO_2}$ increases for the same reason. This is respiratory compensation for the metabolic acidosis of strenuous exercise.

As seen in Figure 20–3, the LT can be used to characterize the responses of various populations to the GXT.[1] It is higher in physically conditioned than in sedentary subjects because trained individuals can accomplish a higher work rate before lactate begins to accumulate in the blood. It is lower in patients with cardiovascular disease because anything that limits blood flow to a muscle (decreased stroke volume/cardiac output in coronary artery disease or decreased blood flow in peripheral vascular disease) will be likely to cause the early onset of lactate accumulation and, thus, a lower LT and T_{vent}.

As described by Wasserman et al.,[9] further information can be derived from the measurement of LT. It represents the $\dot{V}_{O_2}$

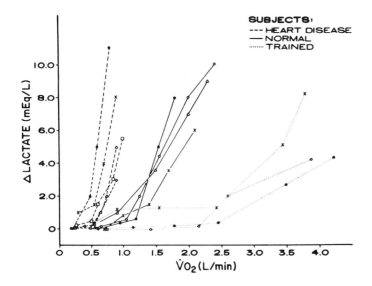

SUBJECTS:
--- HEART DISEASE
— NORMAL
.... TRAINED

Fig. 20–3. Lactate concentration in arterial blood as related to oxygen consumption for trained normal subjects, normal sedentary subjects, and patients with primary heart disease. With permission from Wasserman K, Whipp BJ: Exercise physiology in health and disease. *Am Rev Respir Dis, 112:*219, 1975.

above which there is a delay in reaching a steady state in $\dot{V}O_2$; it represents the work rate above which $\dot{V}_E$ increases with time even with a constant work rate; and it represents the work rate above which it is difficult to sustain exercise for longer than an hour. Furthermore, it may be useful in exercise prescription. An intensity between the LT and point of respiratory compensation (i.e., the period of isocapnic buffering) (see Fig. 20–1) has been suggested as appropriate (JE Young, personal communication).

DIAGNOSTIC UTILITY OF CARDIORESPIRATORY EXERCISE TESTS

The results of CRX tests may be used as a diagnostic aid in conjunction with other information. Zavala[14] has presented a flow chart for interpreting the CRX test in the evaluation of dyspnea that is based on the approach of Wasserman[15] (Fig. 20–4). $\dot{V}O_{2max}$ is measured and is considered normal if it is above 85% predicted $\dot{V}O_{2max}$ based on work rate. Predicted $\dot{V}O_{2max}$ can be determined from tables[4] or nomograms.[4,9] A normal $\dot{V}O_{2max}$ may be expected in those without disease and in obesity and mild heart or lung disease. If $\dot{V}O_{2max}$ is low, the LT is assessed either directly or noninvasively as T_{vent}. If this is below 40% of predicted $\dot{V}O_{2max}$, evidence of circulatory impairment exists; i.e., O_2 delivery to the tissues is less than expected.

Thus, there would be an early onset of lactate accumulation (see Fig. 20–3). However, if the LT is at or above 40%, breathing reserve (see below) should be assessed. A normal breathing reserve at this point may indicate poor effort, poor conditioning, or mild coronary artery disease. A low breathing reserve (less than 0.3) is indicative of ventilatory impairment; i.e., there is a ventilatory limitation to exercise. Breathing reserve (BR) is defined as:

$$BR = (MVV - \dot{V}_{Emax})/MVV$$

$$= 1 - (\dot{V}_{Emax}/MVV),$$

where MVV is the maximal voluntary ventilation and is typically measured by breathing as rapidly, deeply and forcibly as one can for 12 to 15 seconds and multiplying by 5 or 4, respectively, to obtain a measure in L/min. An indirect estimate of MVV can be obtained by multiplying forced expiratory volume in 1 second (FEV_1) by 40.[9] MVV is typically at least 15 L/min greater than $\dot{V}_{Emax}$ except in extremely fit individuals and those with primary lung disease.[9] If $\dot{V}_{Emax}$ is close to MVV, this is an indication of a low breathing reserve and of a possible ventilatory limitation to exercise. For more information on the diagnostic approach to CRX testing, the interested reader is referred to texts on this subject by Wasserman et al.,[9] Jones,[16] Weber and Janicki,[13] and Zavala.[14]

DIAGNOSTIC APPROACH TO CARDIORESPIRATORY EXERCISE TESTING

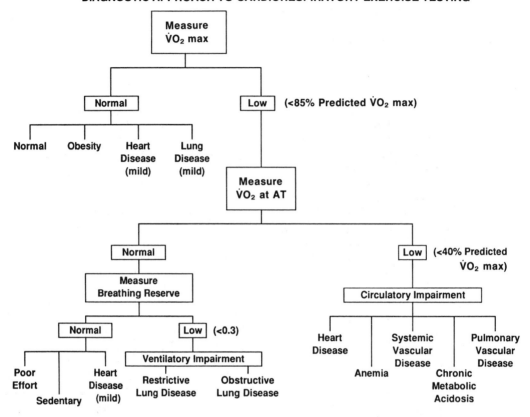

Fig. 20–4. In the differential diagnosis of dyspnea, $\dot{V}_{O2max}$ is first evaluated. If $\dot{V}_{O2max}$ is <85% of predicted $\dot{V}_{O2max}$, then assess LT or T_{vent}. If LT or T_{vent} is <40% of the subject's predicted $\dot{V}_{O2max}$, circulatory impairment is indicated. If LT or T_{vent} is normal but breathing reserve is low (<0.3), ventilatory impairment is indicated. Adapted with permission from Zavala DC: *Manual on Exercise Testing.* Third Edition. Iowa City, IA: University of Iowa Publications, 1987.

MODES AND PROTOCOLS

Most investigators have noted that $\dot{V}_{O2max}$ is approximately 10% higher when assessed on the treadmill compared to the cycle ergometer.[6] Buchfuhrer et al.[17] found that the $\dot{V}_{O2}$ at the LT determined noninvasively was lower on the cycle ergometer than on the treadmill by about 13%; however, as a percentage of $\dot{V}_{O2max}$, it was similar on both modes (approximately 50%). $\dot{V}_{O2max}$ appears to be most accurately determined by protocols lasting between 8 and 12 minutes[6,7] with shorter, smaller work intervals or a ramp. This topic has been recently reviewed in detail by Davis.[6]

CALCULATION OF OXYGEN UPTAKE

$\dot{V}_{O2}$ can be calculated from either cardiovascular or respiratory variables. For example, a common relationship is

$$\dot{V}_{O2} = \dot{Q} \times (a\text{-}\bar{v}O_2 \text{ difference}), \quad (1)$$

where $\dot{Q}$ is cardiac output (in L/min) and a-$\bar{v}O_2$ difference is the difference in oxygen concentration between arterial blood (commonly written C_{aO2}) and mixed venous blood ($C_{\bar{v}O2}$). It is expressed as a fraction (e.g., 5 mL O_2/100 mL blood = 0.05). Although this relationship is a good example of the interplay between the cardiovascular and respiratory systems, it does little to help us calculate $\dot{V}O_2$ because neither $\dot{Q}$ nor $a\text{-}\bar{v}O_2$ difference is readily measured noninvasively.

A more helpful relationship is

$$\dot{V}O_2 = (\dot{V}_I \times F_{IO2}) - (\dot{V}_E \times F_{EO2}), \quad (2)$$

where $\dot{V}_I$ is the rate at which air is inspired, F_{IO2} is the fraction of oxygen in the inspired air, $\dot{V}_E$ is the rate at which air is expired (minute ventilation) and F_{EO2} is the fraction of oxygen in the expired air.[2,17] Thus, $\dot{V}O_2$ simply represents the difference between the rates at which oxygen is inspired and expired. Recall that $\dot{V}_I$ only equals $\dot{V}_E$ when the respiratory exchange ratio, $R = \dot{V}CO_2/\dot{V}O_2$, equals 1.00 (i.e., when the rates of CO_2 output and O_2 uptake are equal and when the volumes are considered dry (i.e., water vapor has been subtracted). Only when $R = 1.00$ can equation 2 be rewritten

$$\dot{V}O_2 = \dot{V}_E \times (F_{IO2} - F_{EO2}). \quad (3)$$

Because the concentration or fraction of oxygen in inspired air ($F_{IO2} = 20.93\% = 0.2093$) is known, $\dot{V}O_2$ can be calculated from equation 2 by using two volume-measuring devices to determine the inspired and expired volumes and an oxygen analyzer to measure oxygen concentration in mixed expired air. Thus, the four factors on the right side of equation 2 would be known and $\dot{V}O_2$ could be calculated. However, this calculation is sensitive to even slight variations in the calibration of the inspiratory and expiratory devices, and thus is not routinely performed.

More typically, $\dot{V}O_2$ is calculated as follows[18]: $\dot{V}_E$ and F_{EO2} are measured using a volume measuring device and an oxygen analyzer, respectively. F_{IO2} is known. $\dot{V}_I$ is then calculated from the following relationship. Because nitrogen is neither produced nor consumed during metabolism, $\dot{V}_{N_2}$, the rate of nitrogen production or consumption is equal to zero, or

$$\dot{V}_{N_2} = (\dot{V}_I \times F_{IN2})$$
$$- (\dot{V}_E \times F_{EN2}) = 0. \quad (4)$$

Therefore,

$$\dot{V}_I \times F_{IN2} = \dot{V}_E \times F_{EN2}, \quad (5)$$

or

$$\dot{V}_I = (\dot{V}_E \times F_{EN2})/F_{IN2}. \quad (6)$$

The fraction of N_2 in inspired air (F_{IN2}) is known and is equal to $79.04\% = 0.7904$. The fraction of N_2 in the expired air (F_{EN2}) can be calculated from the relationship,

$$F_{EN2} = 1.0000 - F_{EO2} - F_{ECO2}, \quad (7)$$

as long as dry gases are being analyzed (see below). Note that the difference in concentration of nitrogen in inspired and expired air is a consequence of the differences in the inspiratory and expiratory volumes and not caused by production or consumption of nitrogen. For example, if more oxygen is being consumed than carbon dioxide is being produced ($R < 1.00$), $\dot{V}_I$ is greater than $\dot{V}_E$ and nitrogen now occupies a greater fraction of the expiratory volume than inspiratory volume ($F_{EN2} > F_{IN2}$). Using equation 7 and the value for F_{IN2}, we can solve for $\dot{V}_I$ in equation 6:

$$\dot{V}_I = [\dot{V}_E \times (1.0000 - F_{EO2}$$
$$- F_{ECO2})]/0.7904. \quad (8)$$

If we now recall equation 2,

$$\dot{V}O_2 = (\dot{V}_I \times F_{IO2}) - (\dot{V}_E \times F_{EO2}), \quad (2)$$

we can solve for $\dot{V}O_2$ by substituting equation 8 and the value for F_{IO2} (0.2093) into equation 2:

$$\dot{V}O_2 = \dot{V}_E \times [0.265 \times (1.0000 - F_{EO2}$$
$$- F_{ECO2}) - F_{EO2}]. \quad (9)$$

The value contained within the brackets in equation 9 is called the True O_2 and represents the fraction of oxygen consumed for any $\dot{V}_E$. By inspecting equation 9, we see that $\dot{V}O_2$ can be calculated by using a volume-measuring device to determine $\dot{V}_E$ and by using gas analyzers to measure the expired fractions of oxygen and carbon dioxide (F_{EO2} and F_{ECO2}, respectively).

Whereas $\dot{V}_E$ is measured under ambient conditions, i.e. at **A**mbient **T**emperature, **P**ressure, and **S**aturated with water vapor (ATPS), in metabolic calculations, by convention, it is expressed relative to **S**tandard conditions of **T**emperature (273° K), **P**ressure (760 mm Hg), and **D**ry (i.e., no water vapor) (STPD) so that these flow rates may be compared in environmental conditions varying as to altitude, heat and humidity. $\dot{V}_E$ (ATPS) may be converted to $\dot{V}_E$ (STPD) as follows[18]:

$$\dot{V}_E(STPD) = \dot{V}_E(ATPS)$$
$$\times [(P_B - WVP)/760 \text{ mm Hg}]$$
$$\times [273° K/(273° K + T_G)], \quad (10)$$

where P_B is ambient barometric pressure and WVP is the water vapor pressure at the gas temperature (T_G) in the volume-measuring device. T_G is in °C and WVP can be found in standard tables.[18]

MEASUREMENT OF OXYGEN UPTAKE

To obtain accurate, reproducible, and valid results, it is necessary to have properly calibrated and functioning equipment.[16] Calibration gases must be of known concentration. One cannot assume this, but must have the gas certified against a primary gravimetric standard, chemical gas analyzer, or read against a gas chromatograph, mass spectrometer, or other calibrating instrument which has, itself, been calibrated against a primary gravimetric

standard or chemical gas analyzer. Calibrate gas analyzers immediately before each test with the calibration gas. Analyzers of unknown or questionable stability should not be used. Before each testing session, check all respiratory hoses and connections for airtightness. On a routine (monthly to quarterly) basis, calibrate ergometric devices, thermistors, and volume measuring devices; check stability of analyzers. Closely monitor respiratory valves for proper functioning and ensure that the dessicant (used to dry gases) is fresh. If using a mouthpiece, ensure that a nose clip is placed securely on the nose and that the mouth seals well around the mouthpiece.

$\dot{V}_{O_2}$ can be measured manually,[5] semiautomatically[19] or automatically with a microprocessor-based system.[20] The generality of the approach is first illustrated by describing a system for manual or semiautomatic measurement of $\dot{V}_{O_2}$ (Fig. 20–5), followed by a brief discussion of on-line (microprocessed) data collection (Fig. 20–6).

Operation of the Manual or Semiautomatic System for $\dot{V}_{O_2}$ Measurement

General:

1. Volumes and gas fractions are measured.
2. Volumes to be measured are:
   a. Portion of $\dot{V}_E$ through the volume-measuring device.
   b. Additional ventilation or the portion of $\dot{V}_E$ drawn off by the gas

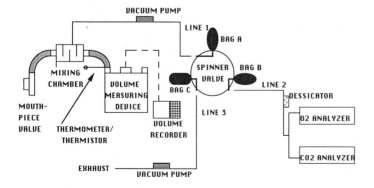

Fig. 20–5. System configuration for manual or semi-automatic measurement of pulmonary gas exchange ($\dot{V}_{O_2}$, $\dot{V}_{CO_2}$, $\dot{V}_E$, etc.).

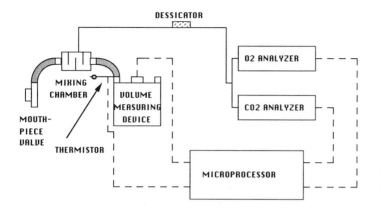

Fig. 20–6. System configuration for on-line (microprocessed) measurement of pulmonary gas exchange. Note that in breath-by-breath analysis, the sampling gas line would connect directly to the mouthpiece and there would be no need for a mixing chamber.

sample (vacuum) pump that fills the gas sample bag.

3. Mixed expired gas fractions to be measured are:

    a. F_{EO2}

    b. F_{ECO2}.

4. To measure gas composition of dry expired gases, the gases being sampled by the analyzers are passed through a dessicant.

5. To convert $\dot{V}_E$ in ATPS to STPD conditions, record gas temperature (at the volume-measuring device) and barometric pressure.

System configuration (Fig. 20–5)

1. Air is drawn in through the one-way mouthpiece valve (i.e., flapper valves are placed in the mouthpiece so that air can only flow into the mouth from the room and out of the mouth into the mixing chamber). On expiration, air is blown out through the mixing chamber (which mixes the gases), past the thermometer or thermistor, and through the volume-measuring device, which records $\dot{V}_E$ (minus "additional ventilation" as described below) on a calibrated chart recorder.

2. The mixed gas sample for analysis (i.e., additional ventilation) is drawn off through a sampling port on the mixing chamber by a vacuum pump and passes through a three-way spin-

ner valve and into a 2 L gas collecting bag (A). In the absence of the spinner valve, gases can be measured in a similar fashion, as described below, using the three hoses shown: line 1 to vacuum pump, line 2 to analyzers, and line 3 to gas bag being sampled.

3. There are 3 bags on the valve at any one time. One bag is collecting gas (bag A on line 1), a second bag is being analyzed (bag B on line 2), and a third bag is being evacuated (bag C on line 3) so that bag C can be filled again with a new gas sample when it is rotated onto line 1 in the next minute. Thus, the spinner valve is turned from line 1 to 2 to 3 to 1, etc., so that after sample collection, the sample is next analyzed and then the bag is evacuated. Note that the two other bags are also being either filled, analyzed, or evacuated simultaneously so that all of these processes are essentially continuous, just from different bags.

Precollection procedures

1. Determine barometric pressure.
2. Fill desiccant column with new desiccant.
3. Ensure that all equipment is operating, warmed up, and calibrated.
4. Measure additional ventilation by collecting a sample of room air for exactly 1 minute from line 1 (see Fig.

20–1). Limit flow through the vacuum pump to 1 to 1.5 L/min with a hose clamp. Using the gas sample port on spirometer, empty this bag into the spirometer to measure the volume of gas that this system draws off in 1 minute. This is additional ventilation.

5. Shortly before starting gas collection (within 1 to 3 minutes), calibrate gas analyzers.

6. To fill a bag with calibration gas, first evacuate and flush bag with calibration gas twice. Next turn on calibration gas, insert tip of gas bag firmly into gas line, and open valve on gas bag. When the bag is full, close valve first, then remove bag from gas line and turn off calibration gas valve.

Collection procedures

1. Have subject place mouthpiece securely in mouth and check seal. Adjust for comfort and put on nose clip.
2. At time t = 0,
   a. Start stopwatch.
   b. Mark $\dot{V}_E$ recorder accurately.
   c. Switch a new bag to gas collection port.
3. At each minute of exercise,
   a. Mark $\dot{V}_E$ recorder accurately.
   b. Rotate or place evacuated bag onto gas collection port.
   c. Analyze gas previously collected. Record this value after readings have stabilized.
   d. Read gas temperature at volume measuring device.
   e. Evacuate bag for next minute's gas collection.
4. At end exercise
   a. Accurately mark $\dot{V}_E$ recorder. If less than 1 full minute of exercise, you will need to calculate what $\dot{V}_E$ would have been for that minute. For example, if the subject stopped at 8 minutes 47 seconds of exercise, the correction to your recorded ventilation volume in the last 47 seconds is:

$$\dot{V}_E = [(60 \text{ sec/min})/47 \text{ sec}]$$

$$\times \text{ ventilation volume.}$$

This gives $\dot{V}_E$ in units of L/min versus L/47 seconds.
   b. Rotate gas sample to analyzer and record values.
   c. Upon completion of gas collection, evacuate bags, turn off vacuum pumps, place analyzers in standby, turn off other equipment, and blow room air through volume-measuring device to dry the internal components. Wash and disinfect respiratory equipment (mouthpiece and hoses).

Calculate $\dot{V}_{O_2}$ from Equation 9:

1. Calculate total $\dot{V}_E$ (ATPS) = $\dot{V}_E$ measured + additional ventilation. (Note that $\dot{V}_E$ measured may need to be adjusted by a calibration factor, according to the last calibration of the volume-measuring device).
2. Convert $\dot{V}_E$ (ATPS) to $\dot{V}_E$ (STPD), using Equation 10.
3. Solve for $\dot{V}_{O_2}$ using Equation 9:

$$\dot{V}_{O_2} = \dot{V}_E \times [0.265 \times (1.0000$$

$$- F_{EO_2} - F_{ECO_2}) - F_{EO_2}] \quad (9)$$

Operation of an On-Line (Microprocesser-based) System for $\dot{V}_{O_2}$ Measurement

1. The theory and operation of $\dot{V}_{O_2}$ measurement using computers are analogous to manual collection. A block diagram is shown in Figure 20–6. The interested reader is directed to the article by Jones.[20]
2. On-line data collection and analysis greatly speed $\dot{V}_{O_2}$ measurement; however, care must be taken to ensure that the system is operating correctly. An effective initial check of system operation is to observe that reasonable values are being recorded for respiratory variables.
3. On-line data collection and analysis also make breath-by-breath $\dot{V}_{O_2}$ measurement possible. In this configuration, the sampling gas line would connect directly to the mouthpiece and there would be no need for a mixing chamber. Actual gas fractions, not mixed gases, would be analyzed. The temporal alignment of respiratory

variables is critical for accurate breath-by-breath measurements. Huszczuk et al.[21] describe a gas exchange simulator for such purposes. It is currently available commercially (Medical Graphics, St. Paul, MN). Although breath-by-breath analysis is important in scientific metabolic studies and clinical testing of cardiorespiratory patients as reviewed here, the greater initial expense perhaps argues against such measurement in general fitness testing where the measurement of $\dot{V}O_{2max}$ is typically sufficient.

ACKNOWLEDGEMENTS

The author gratefully acknowledges the many helpful and insightful suggestions and the critical review of this manuscript by James A. Davis, Ph.D.

REFERENCES

1. Wasserman K, Whipp BJ: Exercise physiology in health and disease. *Am Rev Respir Dis, 112:*219, 1975.
2. Bartels H, Dejours P, Kellogg PH, Mead J: Glossary on respiration and gas exchange. *J Appl Physiol, 34:*549, 1973.
3. Lamb DR: *Physiology of Exercise.* New York: MacMillan, 1984, pp. 294–299.
4. American College of Sports Medicine: *Guidelines for Exercise Testing and Prescription.* Fourth edition. Philadelphia: Lea & Febiger, 1991.
5. Consolazio CF, Johnson RE, and Pecora LJ: *Physiological Measurements of Metabolic Functions in Man.* New York: McGraw-Hill, 1963, pp. 1–98.
6. Davis JA: Direct determination of aerobic power. In *Physiological Assessment of Human Fitness.* Edited by PJ Maud and C Foster. Champaign IL: 1992. Human Kinetics. In press.
7. McArdle WD, Katch FI, Pechar GS: Comparison of continuous and discontinuous treadmill and bicycle tests for max $\dot{V}O_2$. *Med Sci Sports Exerc, 5:*156, 1973.
8. Taylor HL, Buskirk E, and Henschel A: Maximal oxygen uptake as an objective measure of cardiorespiratory performance. *J Appl Physiol, 8:*73, 1955.
9. Wasserman K, Hansen JE, Sue DY, Whipp BJ: *Principles of Exercise Testing and Interpretation.* Philadelphia: Lea & Febiger, 1987.
10. Beaver WL, Wasserman K, Whipp BJ: A new method for detecting anaerobic threshold by gas exchange. *J Appl Physiol, 60:*2020, 1986.
11. Davis JA, Frank MH, Whipp BJ, Wasserman K: Anaerobic threshold alterations caused by endurance training in middle-aged men. *J Appl Physiol, 46:*1039, 1979.
12. Brooks GA: Anaerobic threshold: Review of the concept and directions for future research. *Med Sci Sports Exerc, 17:*22, 1985.
13. Weber KT, Janicki JS: *Cardiopulmonary Exercise Testing.* Philadelphia: WB Saunders, 1986.
14. Zavala DC: *Manual on Exercise Testing.* Third Edition, Iowa City, IA: University of Iowa Publications, 1987.
15. Wasserman K: The anaerobic threshold measurement in exercise testing. *Clinics Chest Med, 5:*77, 1984.
16. Jones NL: *Clinical Exercise Testing.* Philadelphia: W.B. Saunders, 1988.
17. Buchfuhrer MJ, Hansen JE, Robinson TE, et al.: Optimizing the exercise protocol for cardiopulmonary assessment. *J Appl Physiol, 55:*1558, 1983.
18. McArdle WD, Katch FI, Katch VL: *Exercise Physiology.* Third edition. Philadelphia: Lea & Febiger, 1991, pp. 796–803.
19. Wilmore JH, Costill DL: Semiautomated systems approach to the assessment of oxygen uptake during exercise. *J Appl Physiol, 36:*618, 1974.
20. Jones NL: Evaluation of a microprocessor-controlled exercise testing system. *J Appl Physiol, 57:*1312, 1984.
21. Huszczuk A, Whipp BJ, Wasserman K: A respiratory gas exchange simulator for routine calibration in metabolic studies. *Eur Respir J, 3:*465, 1990.

Chapter 21

BASIC ELECTROCARDIOGRAPHIC ANALYSIS

J. P. Schaman

Electrocardiographic (ECG) interpretation can be simple at times and at other times complex. The evaluation of ECG findings is always best in the light of clinical information, if available. For example, ST segment elevation in a patient with chest pain could well indicate an acute myocardial infarction, whereas the same tracing in a young, healthy, asymptomatic man is most likely the normal variant, "early repolarization ST segment elevation." Our knowledge of the ECG has known limitations, and occasionally even experienced interpreters have differing opinions. Occasionally, tracings must be considered "borderline" or "nonspecific," and are therefore not helpful and are frankly dissatisfying. We must also realize that ECG findings do not necessarily provide the data to predict the ultimate outcome of the patient. A patient with a normal ECG may die suddenly of a heart attack, whereas a patient with grossly abnormal ECG findings may live many years without apparent difficulty.

Despite these shortcomings, ECG interpretation can be most rewarding and enjoyable, particularly if approached somewhat as a game rather than as an academic struggle. By following the rules and "game plan" presented in this chapter, most ECGs can be evaluated accurately with pleasure rather than with frustration.

BASIC ELECTROPHYSIOLOGY

The resting myocardial cell is in a "polarized" state, i.e., the resting potential is about -90 mV, when comparing the inside and the outside of the cell. This resting state is regularly interrupted by a jolt of electric activity that causes the cell membrane to become permeable. A rapid ionic shift and the development of a positive potential of approximately $+30$ mV result.

This reaction is called phase 0 of the action potential (Fig. 21–1), or the depolarization phase. Phases 1 to 3 represent the three phases of repolarization, with phase 2 being the "plateau," which is usually slightly positive or close to 0 mV. Phase 4 is the period of electric diastole. In nonpacemaker cells, this phase is flat; in pacemaker cells, this phase is gradually unsloping until it reaches a threshold level, at which time phase 0 depolarization follows.

The cell interior usually has a preponderance of potassium ions and only a small number of sodium ions. Considerably more negative charge is inside the cell and more positive charge is outside the cell. The cell exterior has primarily sodium ions. During depolarization, the membrane becomes more permeable and sodium rushes into the cell, increasing the total intracellular amount of sodium. Sodium carries positive charges and hence creates a positive environment intracellularly. During repolarization, sodium and potassium pumps return the ions to their previous resting locations, and the myocar-

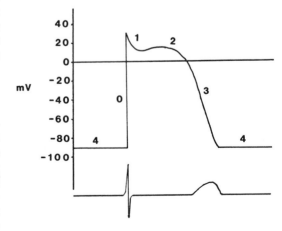

Fig. 21–1. Action potential.

dium is prepared for the next depolarization and contraction.

WAVES, LEADS, AND AXIS

The ECG tracing is a plot of the electric activity of the heart in millivolts against time. The ECG graph paper is divided into small 1-mm squares and larger 5-mm squares (Fig. 21–2). Horizontally, each small square is equivalent to 0.04 sec (with standard paper speed of 25 mm/sec), and each large square is equivalent to 0.2 sec. Vertically, each small square is 0.1 mV (with a calibration of 10 mm/mV).

A normal, single heartbeat consists of five major waves: P, Q, R, S, and T (Fig. 21–3). The P-wave is the electric impulse associated with contraction of the atria. The Q-, R-, and S-waves are considered as a unit, representing the depolarization of the ventricles. These waves are known as the QRS complex. The T-wave is produced by repolarization of the ventricles.

The 12-lead ECG comprises three groups of leads: (1) bipolar limb leads I, II, III; (2) unipolar limb leads aVR, aVL, aVF; and (3) precordial or chest leads V_{1-6}. Each bipolar limb lead has a negative or ground electrode and a positive exploring electrode. In lead I, the positive electrode is on the left arm and the negative electrode is on the right arm. In lead II, the positive electrode is on the left leg and the negative electrode is on the right arm. Lead III has the positive electrode on the left leg and the negative electrode on the left arm. These three leads form the sides of Einthoven's triangle (Fig. 21–4). When these three leads are moved so that they intersect at a

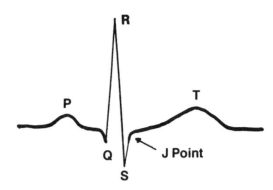

Fig. 21–3. Major waves of normal electrocardiographic pathway.

common point, a useful axis system results (Fig. 21–5).

One of the most important concepts in electrocardiography is the relationship between the direction of travel of the electric impulse and a given lead. If the impulse travels toward the positive pole (electrode), an upward deflection in the ECG tracing results. If the impulse travels toward the negative pole, a downward deflection results.

The unipolar or augmented leads have the positive electrode on one of the limbs: R-right arm, L-left arm, and F-left foot. The ground electrode consists of all of the remaining electrodes. The axis system formed by these leads differs from the bipolar limb leads (Fig. 21–6). By combining the two groups, however, a total axis system for the limb leads results (Fig. 21–7). This system can be used to determine the mean electric axis of ventricular depolarization. By plotting the mean QRS deflection,

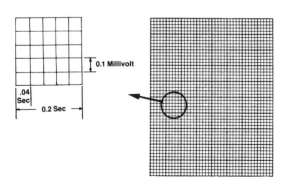

Fig. 21–2. Electrocardiogram graph paper.

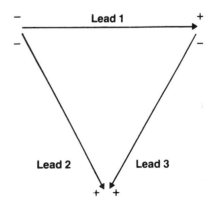

Fig. 21–4. Einthoven's triangle.

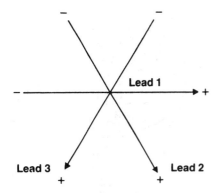

Fig. 21–5. Axis system incorporating leads I, II, and III.

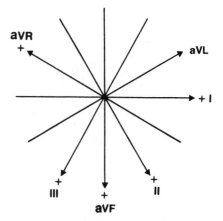

Fig. 21–7. Total axis system.

either negative or positive, of two perpendicular leads, the interpreter can plot the axis of depolarization. Using this principle, a short-cut estimation of axis can be made, because the axis is perpendicular to the lead that has a zero mean QRS deflection (i.e., R = Q + S).

If, for example, the height of the R-wave equals the sum of the heights of the Q- and S-waves in lead I, this lead has a zero mean QRS deflection. By plotting the axis on Figure 21–7, we see that the QRS axis is perpendicular to lead I, i.e., along lead aVF, either upward or downward. The next step is to inspect lead aVF to determine whether the QRS is primarily positive or negative. If positive, the axis will be +90° (Fig. 21–8); if negative, the axis will be −90°. The normal electric axis is thought to be from −30 to

+120°. Left axis deviation refers to a mean QRS frontal axis between −30 and −120°, which may result from a horizontal position assumed by the heart, the upward displacement of the diaphragm (as occurs with pregnancy, tumors, ascites, and so forth), left bundle branch block, left anterior hemiblock, left ventricular hypertrophy, inferior myocardial infarction, cardiomyopathy, and other causes. Right axis deviation refers to a QRS axis between +120 and +180°, which may result from a vertical position assumed by the heart, downward displacement of the diaphragm (as occurs with inspiration or emphysema), right ventricular hypertrophy, right bun-

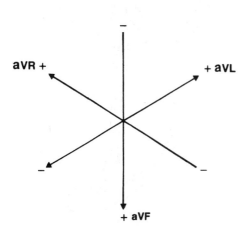

Fig. 21–6. Axis system incorporating leads aVR, aVL, and aVF.

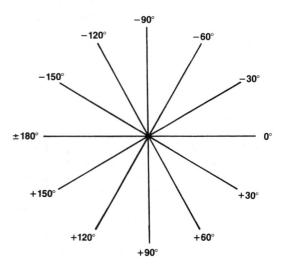

Fig. 21–8. Axis frame.

dle branch block, and anterior myocardial infarction.

The limb leads, bipolar and unipolar, give information about the electric activity of the heart in only the frontal plane (Fig. 21–7). The precordial leads, V_{1-6}, give information in the precordial plane, which is perpendicular to the frontal plane. The appropriate positioning of the positive electrode in the precordial leads follows:

V_1: Right sternal border in the fourth intercostal space

V_2: Left sternal border in the fourth intercostal space

V_3: Equally spaced between V_2 and V_4

V_4: Midclavicular line in the fifth intercostal space

V_5: Anterior axillary line in the fifth intercostal space

V_6: Midaxillary line in the fifth intercostal space.

Correct lead placement in electrocardiography is critical. Any variation from correct lead placement results in tracings other than the "standard 12 ECG." For example, in exercise stress testing, patients are frequently prepared with a 12-lead ECG during exercise. Because standard limb lead placement results in considerable movement artifact, the limb leads are frequently placed at the anterior aspects of the shoulders and at the right and left lower costal margins. Thus adjustment allows useful and "readable" tracings to be obtained, yet it does not give a "standard 12-lead ECG." Therefore, recording a 12-lead ECG with standard limb lead placement before rewiring the leads to the exercise placement is important.

THE ELECTRIC CONDUCTION SYSTEM

The interpretation of an ECG tracing necessitates an understanding of the electric conduction system of the heart (Fig. 21–9). The impulse originates in the sinoatrial (SA) node and travels through the atrial tracts to the atrioventricular (AV) node. During this time, the atria are depolarized and a P-wave is inscribed on the ECG tracing (Fig. 21–3). After a brief pause at the AV node (PR interval), which allows time for the atria to contract and to eject their contents into the ventricles, the impulse

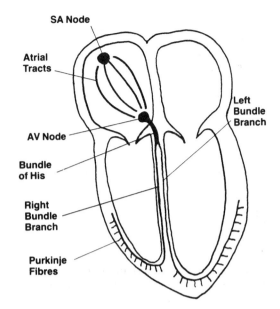

Fig. 21–9. Electric conduction system.

travels down the bundle branches to depolarize the ventricles by way of the Purkinje fibers (QRS complex).

By referring to the electric conduction system of the heart, an electrophysiologic explanation for all ECG abnormalities is possible. Figure 21–10 illustrates the var-

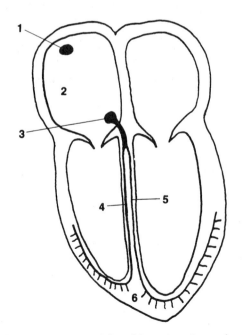

Fig. 21–10. Potential problem areas in conduction system.

Table 21–1.   Relationship of Potential ECG Problems to the Electric Conduction System

Problem Area	Potential Problem
Sinoatrial node	Sinus arrhythmia
	Sinus tachycardia
	Sinus bradycardia
	SA block—incomplete
	—complete
	Sinus arrest
	Sick sinus syndrome
Atria	Atrial premature beats
	Paroxysmal atrial tachycardia
	Wandering atrial pacemaker
	Atrial flutter
	Atrial fibrillation
	Right or left atrial hypertrophy
	Intra-atrial block
Atrioventricular node	Nodal premature beats
	Nodal tachycardia
	Pre-excitation (Wolff-Parkinson-White syndrome)
	AV block—1st degree
	—2nd degree—Mobitz Type I (Wenckebach)
	—Mobitz Type II
	—3rd degree
	AV dissociation
Right bundle branch	Right bundle branch block
	Aberrant conduction
Left bundle branch	Left bundle branch block
	Fascicular block—Left anterior hemiblock
	—Left posterior hemiblock
	Aberrant conduction
Ventricles	Premature ventricular contractions
	Ventricular tachycardia
	Ventricular flutter
	Ventricular fibrillation
	Myocardial ischemia
	Myocardial infarction
	Right or left ventricular hypertrophy

ious locations of potential problems. In Table 21–1, these areas are correlated to most known ECG abnormalities. Before discussing many of these conditions, a game plan is needed that will facilitate almost without fail the accurate interpretation of any ECG tracing.

PRACTICAL RULES IN ECG EVALUATION

Even an inexperienced electrocardiographer can interpret most ECG tracings by memorizing and systematically following, preferably in the order listed, nine points:

1. Rate
2. Rhythm
3. P-waves
4. PR interval
5. QRS complex:
   a. Duration
   b. Configuration
   c. Axis
6. ST segment
7. T-waves
8. U-waves
9. QT interval

Rate

Rate can be determined by using an ECG Heart Rate ruler or several other techniques, such as

$$\text{Rate} = \frac{300}{(\text{Number of large squares between two R-waves})}$$

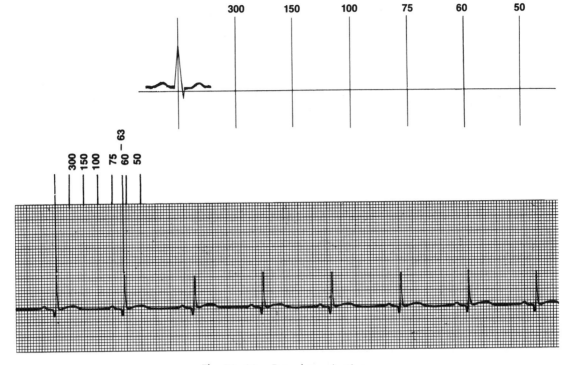

Fig. 21–11. Rate determination.

or the (300 – 150 – 100 – 75 – 60 – 50) technique (see Fig. 21–11).

Rhythm

Regular rhythm usually refers to ventricular rhythm and implies equal R-R intervals. Such is the case in normal sinus rhythm (Fig. 21–12); however, equal R-R intervals can also occur in such rhythms as paroxysmal atrial tachycardia or idioventricular rhythm (Figs. 21–13, 21–14).

An irregularity in rhythm is called an arrhythmia, but a better term would be dysrhythmia, because arrhythmia implies no rhythm at all. An arrhythmia can have a certain degree of system to the irregularity, as in respiratory sinus arrhythmia, bigeminy, or Wenckebach AV block (Figs. 21–15 to 21–17). The arrhythmia could also appear randomly, as in scattered extrasystoles or premature beats (Fig. 21–18), or with complete irregularity, as in atrial fibrillation or ventricular fibrillation (Figs. 21–19, 21–20).

P-Waves

A necessary step in analysis is to note the shape, duration, and amplitude of P-waves,

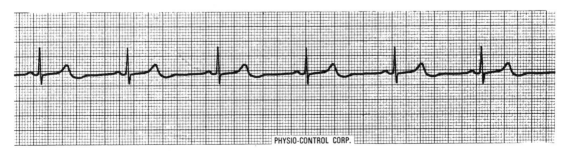

Fig. 21–12. Normal sinus rhythm.

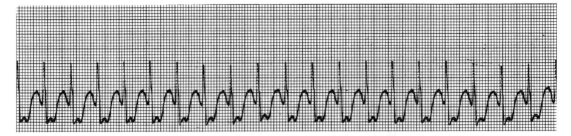

Fig. 21–13. Paroxysmal atrial tachycardia (PAT).

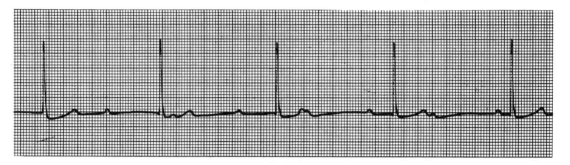

Fig. 21–14. Idioventricular rhythm.

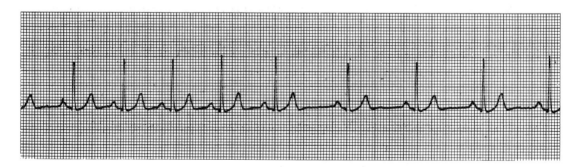

Fig. 21–15. Sinus arrhythmia.

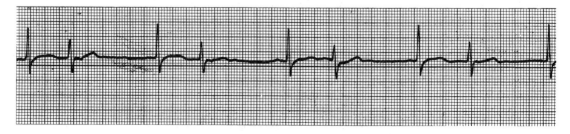

Fig. 21–16. Bigeminy.

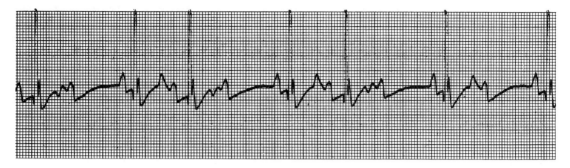

Fig. 21–17. Wenckebach phenomenon.

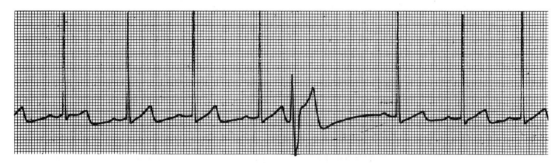

Fig. 21–18. Premature ventricular contractions (PVCs).

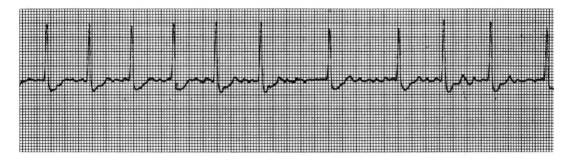

Fig. 21–19. Atrial fibrillation.

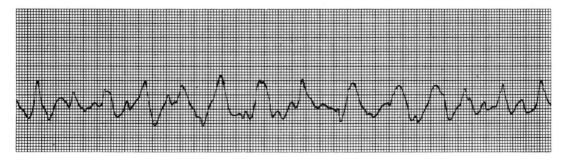

Fig. 21–20. Ventricular fibrillation.

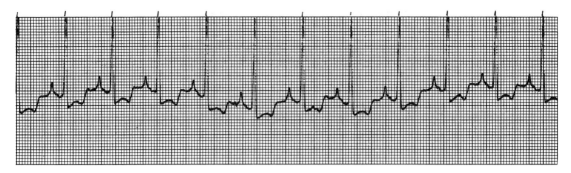

Fig. 21–21.   Tall and narrow P-waves suggestive of right atrial hypertrophy.

as well as to determine whether a QRS complex follows each P-wave and if a P-wave precedes each QRS complex. P-wave duration is usually less than 0.11 sec. In right atrial hypertrophy, the P-waves are tall and narrow (Fig. 21–21); in left atrial hypertrophy, the P-waves are wide and often notched (Fig. 21–22). In atrial flutter, the P-waves take on a "sawtoothed pattern," which characterizes flutter waves (Fig. 21–23). In atrial fibrillation, no identifiable P-waves are seen, and the rhythm is said to be "irregularly irregular" (Fig. 21–24). In essence, the R-R intervals do not have pattern or regularity.

PR Interval

The PR interval is measured from the beginning of the P-wave to the beginning of the QRS complex. It is normally not shorter than 0.12 sec and not longer than 0.20 sec. This amount of time is required to allow the atria to eject blood into the ventricles before ventricular contraction. A shortened PR interval is noted in Wolff-Parkinson-White (W-P-W) (Fig. 21–25) syndrome (pre-excitation), in which abnormal conduction pathways bypass the AV node, or occasionally in nodal rhythm, in which retrograde conduction through the atria occurs. The PR interval is prolonged in first-degree AV block (Fig. 21–26). An important step is to determine if the PR interval is constant and if the P-waves are related to the QRS complexes. Occasionally, the atria and ventricles can beat independently (third-degree AV block), but appear to be related. In Figure 21–27, every second QRS complex is preceded by a P-wave with a constant PR interval. In actual fact, three P-waves occur for every two QRS complexes, and the atria beat independently of the ventricles. The atrial rate is 84 and regular and the ventricular rate is 56 and regular.

QRS Complex

Duration

The duration of the normal QRS complex is less than 0.12 sec. A widened QRS

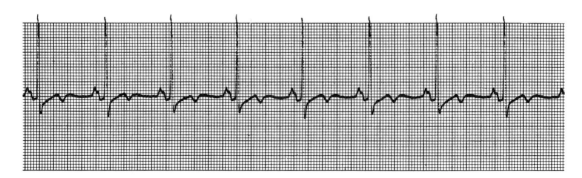

Fig. 21–22.   Wide and notched P-waves suggestive of left atrial hypertrophy.

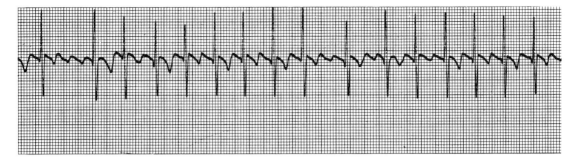

Fig. 21–23. Atrial flutter.

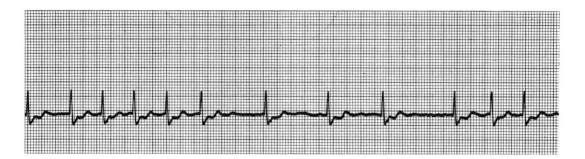

Fig. 21–24. Atrial fibrillation.

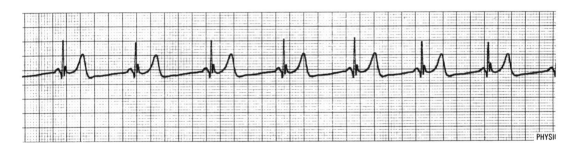

Fig. 21–25. Short PR interval.

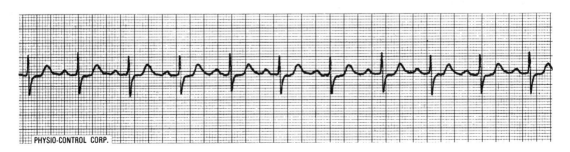

Fig. 21–26. Prolonged PR interval (0.22 sec) in first-degree block.

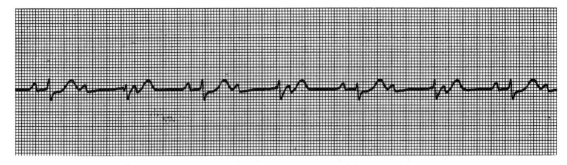

Fig. 21–27. Third-degree atrioventricular block with two QRS complexes for every three P-waves.

complex can occur in right and left bundle branch block (Table 21–2, Fig. 21–28), pre-excitation syndrome (W-P-W), left ventricular hypertrophy, aberrant conduction, premature ventricular contractions, ventricular tachycardia, and hyperkalemia.

Configuration

When assessing the configuration of the QRS complex, its nature, constant or varying, should be noted. Slight changes in QRS amplitude can occur during respiration because of changes in the position of the heart (Fig. 21–29). During exercise, this change in amplitude can be significant. The presence of premature ventricular contractions (PVCs) with varying QRS configuration is indicative of multifocal extrasystoles, which are more significant findings than unifocal extra beats (Figs. 21–30, 21–31).

That the relative amplitudes of Q-, R-, and S-waves are helpful in diagnosing ventricular hypertrophy (Table 21–3) has become a matter of controversy. The theory relating to ventricular hypertrophy is based on the premise that if the ventricular wall is thicker than normal, the impulse will take longer to traverse it and the voltage of the QRS complexes will increase in leads that overlook the hypertrophied ventricular muscle. The various criteria proposed for the diagnosis of ventricular hypertrophy are not reliable, with poor sensitivity but good specificity.

Axis

The determination of the frontal plane electric axis was previously discussed. Axis deviation can be important in the diagnosis of ventricular hypertrophy as well as left anterior and posterior hemiblocks (Tables 21–3, 21–4). The left bundle branch comprises the anterior and the posterior fascicles. Left anterior hemiblock is common and is not usually of major significance; left posterior hemiblock rarely occurs and is usually indicative of a significant disease process.

Table 21–2. Comparison of ECG Findings in Bundle Branch Block

ECG Findings	
Right Bundle Branch Block	**Left Bundle Branch Block**
M-shaped QRS complex in V_{1-2} and broad S in lead I	M-shaped QRS complex in V_{5-6} and broad S in lead III
ST depression and T inversion in lead III, V_{1-2}	ST depression and T inversion in lead I, aVL, V_{5-6}

Table 21–3. Comparison of ECG Findings in Ventricular Hypertrophy

ECG Findings	
Right Ventricle	**Left Ventricle**
Tall R or R' in V_{1-2}; small S in V_{1-2}; deep S in V_{5-6}	Tall R in V_{5-6} (>25 mm); deep S in V_{1-2} (>25 mm)
ST depression and T-wave inversion in leads II, III, V_{1-3}	ST depression and T-wave inversion in lead I, aVL, V_{5-6}
Right axis deviation	Left axis deviation
QRS duration usually normal	QRS duration 0.9 sec or more

Left　　　　　　　　**Right**

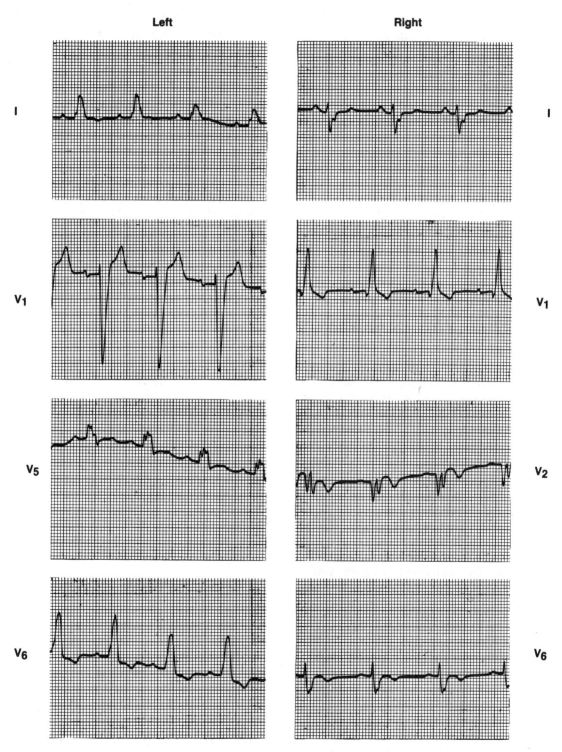

Fig. 21–28. Bundle branch block.

Table 21–4. Comparison of ECG Findings in Hemiblock

ECG Findings	
Left Anterior Hemiblock	**Left Posterior Hemiblock**
Left axis deviation ($-60°$)	Right axis deviation ($+120°$)
Small Q in lead I; small R in lead III	Small R in lead I; small Q in lead III
Normal QRS duration	Normal QRS duration
	No evidence of right ventricular hypertrophy

ST Segment

Changes in the ST segment are important in the diagnosis of myocardial ischemia or infarction. The ST segment level is compared to the isoelectric line, which is the level of the segment from the T-wave to the P-wave of the following beat. For instances in which this level is not well defined, especially during exercise, the isoelectric line is considered the level of the PR interval immediately preceding the QRS complex. The ST segment is discussed more fully in *Myocardial Infarction and Ischemia*.

T-Waves

In assessing T-waves, an important step is to note their direction and amplitude. They can be upright (Fig. 21–32A), inverted (Fig. 21–32B), flattened (Fig. 21–32C), or diphasic (Fig. 21–32D). T-waves are usually upright in leads I, II, and V_{5-6}, and are inverted in aVR. Inverted or diphasic T-waves can be seen in normal subjects in leads III and V_{1-2}. T-wave changes, either alone or with ST segment changes, are frequent ECG abnormalities. These findings can often be normal variants or may result from a wide range of physiologic conditions (posture changes, respiration, drugs, mental factors, and so forth). Because of the high correlation of T-wave changes with coronary heart disease, however, they should be treated with respect. The amplitude of the T-wave is also extremely variable. Very tall, tented T-waves are a feature of hyperkalemia (Fig. 21–32E).

U-Waves

The U-wave is usually of low amplitude, and immediately follows the T-wave. The U-wave is usually in the same direction as the T-wave. This wave is most easily seen

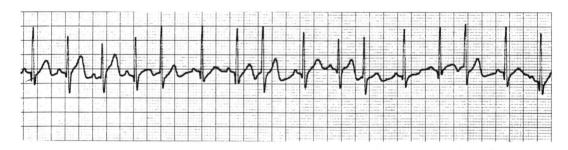

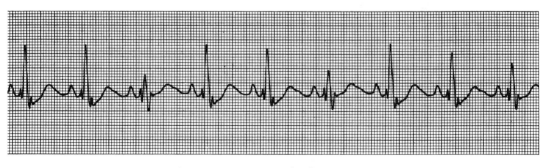

Fig. 21–29. QRS amplitude variation.

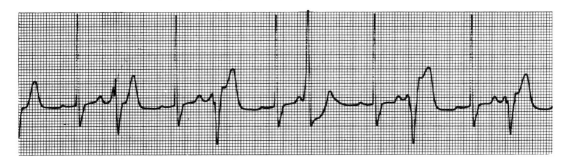

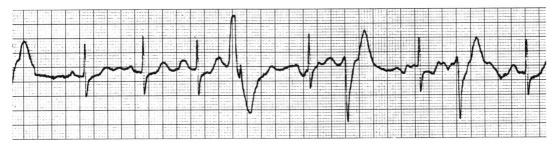

Fig. 21–30. Multifocal PVCs.

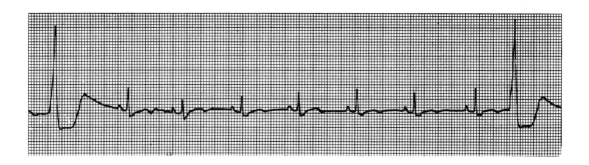

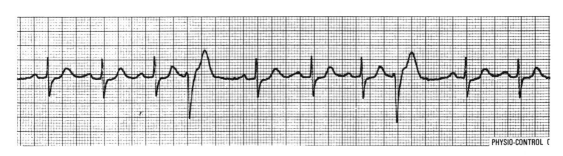

Fig. 21–31. Unifocal PVCs.

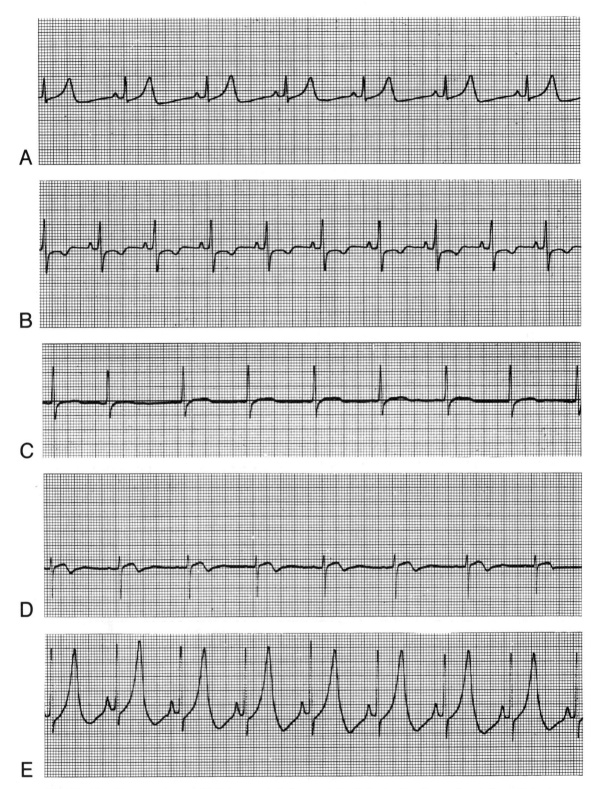

Fig. 21–32. T-waves. **A,** upright; **B,** inverted; **C,** flattened; **D,** diphasic; **E,** tall tented, as in hyperkalemia.

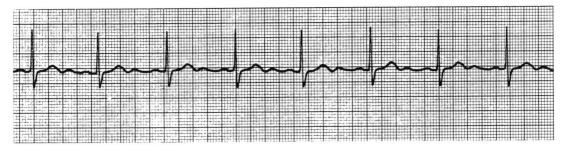

Fig. 21–33. U-waves.

Table 21–5. Normal QT Intervals at Various Heart Rates

Heart Rate (Beats/Min)	QT Interval (Sec)
40	0.42–0.50
50	0.36–0.46
60	0.33–0.43
70	0.30–0.40
80	0.29–0.38
90	0.28–0.36
100	0.27–0.35
110	0.26–0.33
120	0.25–0.32
150	0.23–0.28

in the middle precordial leads (V_{2-4}) and is more pronounced in patients with hypokalemia (Fig. 21–33).

QT Interval

This segment is measured from the beginning of the QRS complex to the end of the T-wave. It correlates well with the ejection time of the heart (systole). The normal range is from 0.35 to 0.45 sec, although this segment varies greatly with heart rate (Table 21–5). Prolonged QT intervals occur in patients with myocardial ischemia, myocardial infarction, ventricular dysfunction, bundle branch block, left ventricular hypertrophy, hypokalemia, and hypocalcemia.

ARRHYTHMIAS (VENTRICULAR AND SUPRAVENTRICULAR)

Premature Contractions

A premature beat is one that comes before the expected normal sinus-node originating beat. In other words, the interval from the preceding normal beat to the abnormal beat is less than the normal RR interval. The premature contraction can be supraventricular, either atrial or junctional (previously called nodal), or ventricular. Making the distinction between ventricular and supraventricular premature contractions is important. Table 21–6 is a list of various criteria that are often, but not al-

Table 21–6. Supraventricular versus Ventricular Premature Beats

ECG Criteria	Premature Beats	
	Supraventricular	Ventricular
QRS complex of beat in question	Normal duration (<0.12 sec); same configuration as normal beat	Increased duration (≥0.12 sec); bizarre configuration compared to normal beat
P-wave preceding beat in question	Usually present (sometimes difficult to see in nodal premature contractions)	Absent
Interval between two normal beats on either side of beat in question	Less than two normal RR intervals (i.e., <2/RR/)	Equal to two normal RR intervals (see Fig. 21–35)

Normal Complexes

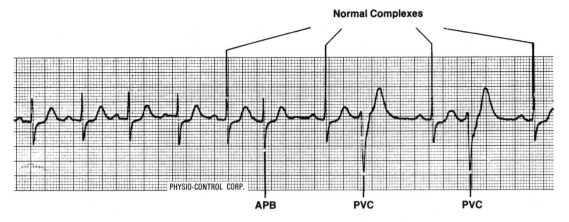

APB   PVC   PVC

Fig. 21–34. PVC versus atrial premature beats (APB).

ways, helpful in distinguishing ventricular and supraventricular premature beats. Use of these criteria is illustrated in Figure 21–34; examples of premature beats are illustrated in Figures 21–35 and 21–36. A particular challenge arises when premature beats of supraventricular origin are conducted with aberrant conduction. In aberrant conduction, the electric impulse takes a different route through the conduction system, which usually results in QRS complexes that are wide and different in configuration when compared to regular beats. In this instance, the QRS criteria are no longer helpful, however, the other criteria can be useful in the diagnosis of this conduction disturbance.

Occasionally, premature beats are frequent and occur with a predictable regularity. If every second beat is premature, this rhythm is called bigeminy. Similarly, if the premature beat occurs every third beat, the rhythm is labeled trigeminy (Fig. 21–37). A premature ventricular contraction (PVC)

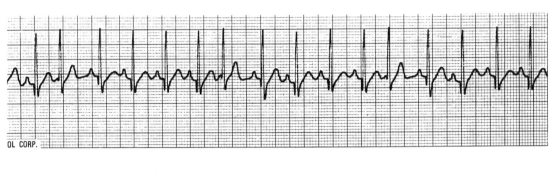

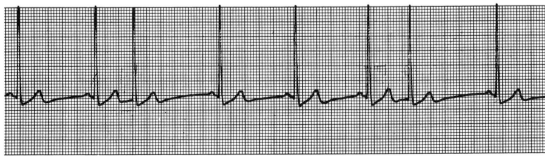

Fig. 21–35. Supraventricular premature contractions.

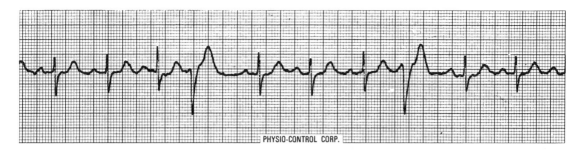

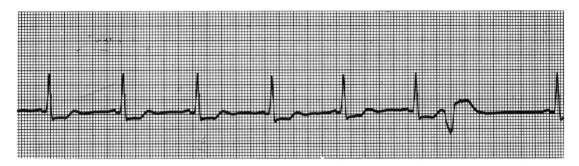

Fig. 21–36. Premature ventricular contractions.

A

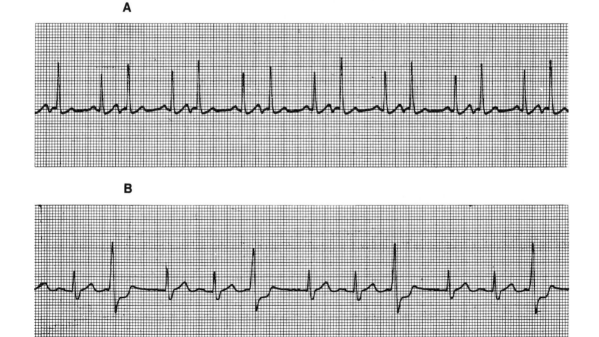

B

Fig. 21–37. A, bigeminy; **B,** trigeminy.

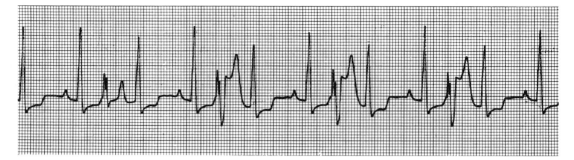

Fig. 21–38. Interpolated PVCs.

that occurs at the same time as or close to the preceding T-wave is significantly more dangerous, because ventricular tachycardia or fibrillation can develop. Similarly, multifocal PVCs are more ominous than unifocal PVCs (Figs. 21–30, 21–31). Interpolated PVCs are exceptions to the rules (Fig. 21–38). They are interposed between two normal sinus beats without disturbing the basic rhythm. They occur only in persons with a slow heart rate.

Supraventricular Tachycardias

Paroxysmal supraventricular tachycardias are characterized by sudden onset and abrupt termination (Fig. 21–39). They are usually initiated by a premature beat and the rate is generally between 130 and 220 beats/min. This common dysrhythmia, frequently called PAT (paroxysmal atrial tachycardia), often occurs in people with structurally normal hearts.

Atrial Flutter and Fibrillation

People with atrial flutter usually exhibit a regular atrial rate of between 250 and 320 beats/min, with varying degrees of AV block. A characteristic "sawtoothed" pattern results (Fig. 21–40). Atrial flutter can occur in individuals with normal hearts; in patients with chronic obstructive lung disease, pulmonary embolism, hyperthyroidism, alcoholism, mitral valve disease, myocardial infarction; and in association with thoracic and cardiac surgical procedures.

Atrial fibrillation is characterized by totally chaotic atrial activity, with no discernible P-waves, at a rate of 350 to 500 beats/min. The ventricular response is always "irregularly irregular" at a rate of 140 to 170 beats/min, if not treated (Fig. 21–41). Treatment is digitalization, and a ventricular rate of 70 to 90 beats/min is considered adequate control. The cause of atrial fibrillation is similar to that for atrial flutter.

Pre-excitation Syndromes

Pre-excitation is present when the ventricle is activated by atrial impulses earlier than if the impulses were to reach the ventricles by the normal conduction pathway. Several abnormal AV "bridges" have been described, the most common probably being that described by Wolff, Parkinson,

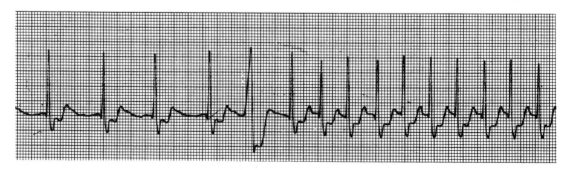

Fig. 21–39. Development of paroxysmal supraventricular tachycardia.

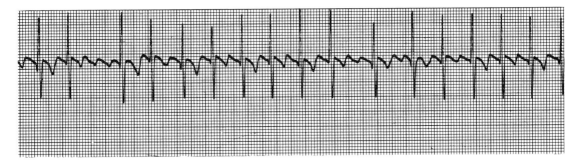

Fig. 21–40.   Atrial flutter.

and White (W-P-W). The ECG shows a short PR interval followed by a wide QRS complex with a delta wave. The delta wave is a slurred initial deflection of the QRS complex.

Ventricular Tachycardia, Flutter, and Fibrillation

Ventricular tachycardia is a rhythm of ventricular origin consisting of three or more consecutive premature beats at a rate of 120 to 200 beats/min (Fig. 21–42). Occasionally, if the tachycardia is slow, atrial fusion beats can be seen. Fusion beats occur when normally conducted sinus beats "fuse" or merge with ventricular ectopic beats. Ventricular tachycardia is common in patients with coronary artery disease, particularly with ischemia and acute infarction. The pattern of ventricular flutter is more rapid than that of normal ventricular tachycardia (Fig. 21–43). To distinguish between ventricular arrhythmias and supraventricular arrhythmias with aberrant interventricular conduction is difficult if not impossible. Because this distinction is important, clinicians sometimes need to perform electrophysiologic (EP) studies, which involve intracardiac and His bundle electrocardiography.

Ventricular fibrillation is fatal unless it can be reversed by defibrillation (Fig. 21–44). Ventricular fibrillation frequently occurs with acute myocardial infarction, ischemia, and as the end stage in heart failure. Ventricular asystole has complete absence of ventricular activity and appears as a straight line on the ECG tracing (Fig. 21–45).

Myocardial Infarction and Ischemia

Acute myocardial infarction is caused by a sudden occlusion of a major branch of a coronary artery, usually the result of a thrombus forming at the site of an atheromatous plaque. Myocardial infarction is the death of heart muscle that results from a deficiency in the oxygen supply. Characteristic ECG changes are usually, but not always, seen. The ST segment is the most important component of the ECG when diagnosing acute myocardial infarction or myocardial ischemia. The three ECG changes that are indicative of myocardial

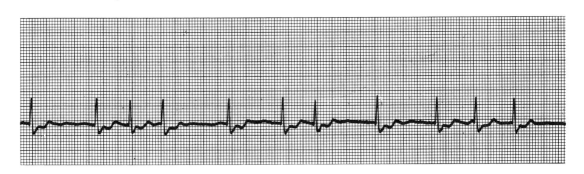

Fig. 21–41.   Atrial fibrillation.

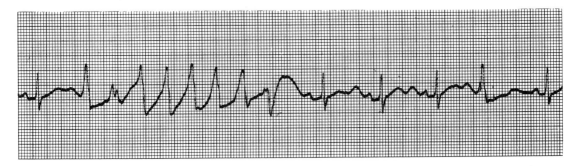

Fig. 21–42.   Paroxysmal ventricular tachycardia.

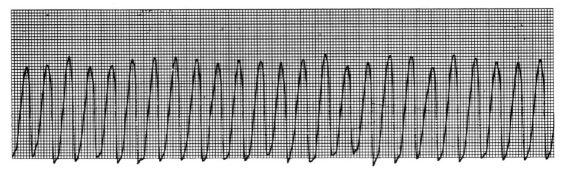

Fig. 21–43.   Ventricular flutter.

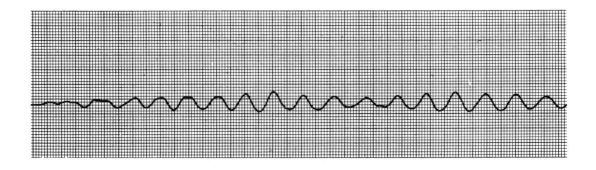

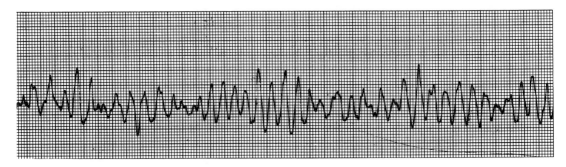

Fig. 21–44.   Ventricular fibrillation.

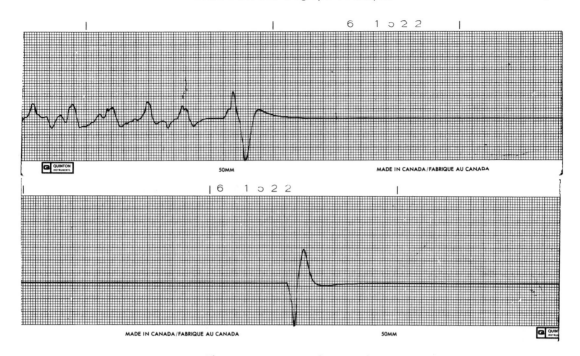

Fig. 21–45.   Ventricular asystole.

infarction are: (1) pathologic Q-wave, which is characterized by a width of 0.04 sec or more, a depth greater than 2 mm, or both; (2) ST segment elevation; and (3) T-wave inversion (Fig. 21–46). Only about 33% of persons with myocardial infarction develop pathologic Q-waves. These Q-waves are said to be a sign of a true transmural infarction. If only ST segment and T-wave changes are noted, the infarction is said to be nontransmural or subendocardial. This distinction is not always hard and fast.

These changes can help in the decision

as to whether an infarction is acute, recent, or old (Table 21–7). Localization of a myocardial infarction is possible because of the ECG changes occur in leads that point in the direction of the infarction (Table 21–8).

Myocardial ischemia occurs when the heart muscle starves for oxygen, usually because of insufficient blood flow that results from coronary atherosclerosis. During times of ischemia, the patient develops chest pain, or angina. Most patients with ischemic heart disease have normal ECG findings in the absence of chest pain. Signs of an old myocardial infarction and occasionally "nonspecific T-wave changes" might be evident. These changes consist of

Table 21–7.   Staging of Myocardial Infarction

| Stage | ECG Change | | |
	ST Segment	T-Wave	Q-Wave
Acute	Elevated	Normal or inverted	Sometimes present
Recent	Normal	Usually inverted	Present
Old	Normal	Usually normal	Present

Table 21–8.   Localization of Myocardial Infarction

Area of Infarction	Leads Showing Changes
Inferior	II, III, aVf
Anterior	V_{1-3}
Lateral	I, aVL, V_{4-6}
Posterior	Look for reciprocal changes in V_{1-2}

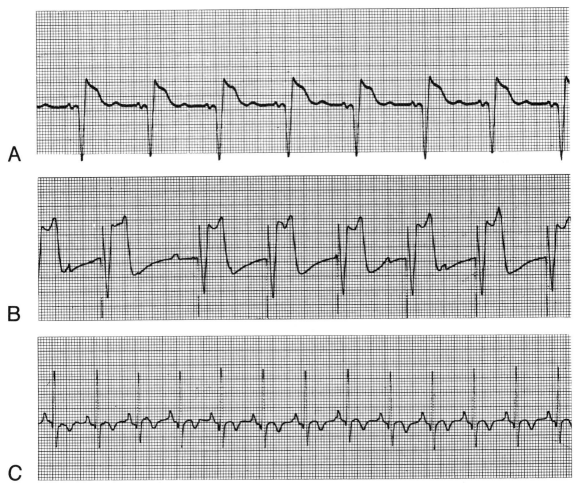

Fig. 21–46. Characteristic changes associated with myocardial infarction. **A,** pathologic Q-waves. **B,** ST segment elevation. **C,** T-wave inversion.

T-wave flattening and inversion, and are not diagnostic, only suggestive, of ischemia. ST depression is the usual ECG change noted in individuals with acute ischemia. An ECG obtained during exercise is helpful when assessing a patient for ischemic heart disease. Myocardial ischemia may be reflected in the exercise ECG by the following changes:

1. ST segment depression
2. T-wave inversion or flattening
3. Prolongation of the QT interval
4. Appearance of ventricular or supraventricular arrhythmias
5. Conduction disturbances (AV block, bundle branch block, etc.)
6. Inappropriate heart rate increase
7. Increase in R-wave amplitude

Not all ST segment depression is considered pathologic; rather it depends on the depth of depression and on the configuration of the ST segment, whether horizontal, upsloping, or downsloping (Fig. 21–47). The exercise ECG and the significance of the changes noted is discussed in Chapter 22.

Other Conduction Disturbances

SA Block, Sinus Arrest, and Sick Sinus Syndrome

Sinus arrest implies nonfunction of the SA node, an occurrence that usually cannot

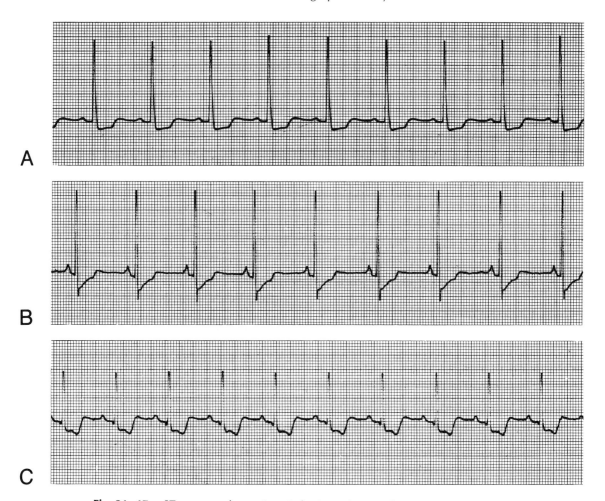

Fig. 21–47. ST segment depression. **A,** horizontal; **B,** upsloping; **C,** downsloping.

be distinguished from SA block, which implies exit block of the impulse from the SA node to the atria. SA block can be incomplete (Fig. 21–48A) or complete (Fig. 21–48B). In the former, an occasional absence of P-QRS-T sequence is noted. In the latter, P-waves are absent (depending on the site of the ectopic pacemaker); the QRST sequence is slow; and the QRS interval is normal or prolonged, depending on the site of the ectopic pacemaker.

The designation sick sinus syndrome or "tachy-brady syndrome," is applied to rhythms characterized by severe bradycardia and irregular atrial tachycardia. The cause is a diseased sinus node, which is usually the result of ischemic heart disease. Pa-

tients with this condition often require a permanent pacemaker.

Intra-Atrial Block

A P-wave duration of longer than 0.11 second and notched P-waves are indicative of intra-atrial (IA) block (Fig. 21–49). This condition is common and is seen most often in individuals with coronary artery disease as well as in association with left ventricular hypertrophy. On occasion, IA block may actually represent left atrial enlargement, in which case it is not a true block.

AV Block

AV block is an abnormal delay or failure of conduction at the AV node, which must

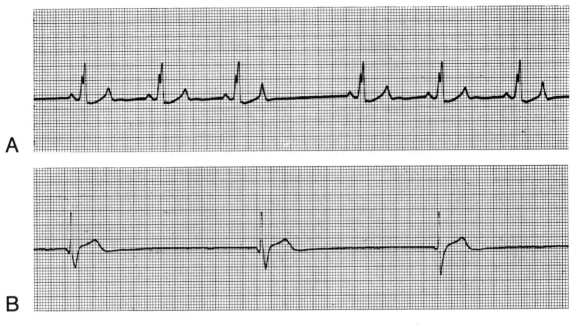

A

B

Fig. 21–48.   Sinoatrial block. **A,** incomplete; **B,** complete.

be kept distinct from normal delay or conduction failure that is the result of physiologic refractoriness. The three degrees of
AV block are:

> *First degree:* prolongation of the PR inter-
> val beyond 0.20 sec (Fig. 21–50A)
> *Second degree:* dropped QRS complexes
> (Fig. 21–50B)
>> Mobitz Type I: progressive lengthen-
>> ing of the PR intervals until a beat is
>> dropped   (Wenckebach   phe-
>> nomenon)
>> Mobitz Type II: consecutively con-
>> ducted beats with constant PR inter-
>> vals before the dropped beat
> *Third degree:* complete AV block with a

slower ventricular rhythm unrelated
to the P-waves (Fig. 21–50C)

AV block can also result from conduction
failure related to physiologic refractoriness, as is often seen in rapid supraventricular tachycardias (Fig. 21–50D). In this situation, the AV node is usually not diseased.

Aberrant Conduction

In aberrant ventricular conduction, a supraventricular impulse arrives so early that
parts of the bundle of His are refractory
after the preceding beat; a bundle branch
block pattern then develops (Fig. 21–51).
In 85% of individuals, the result is a right

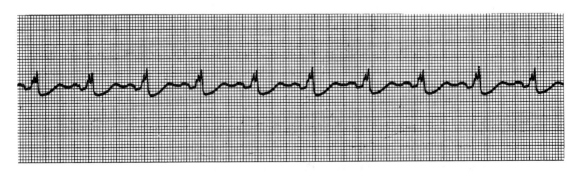

Fig. 21–49.   Intra-atrial block. Note wide (0.12 sec) notched P-wave.

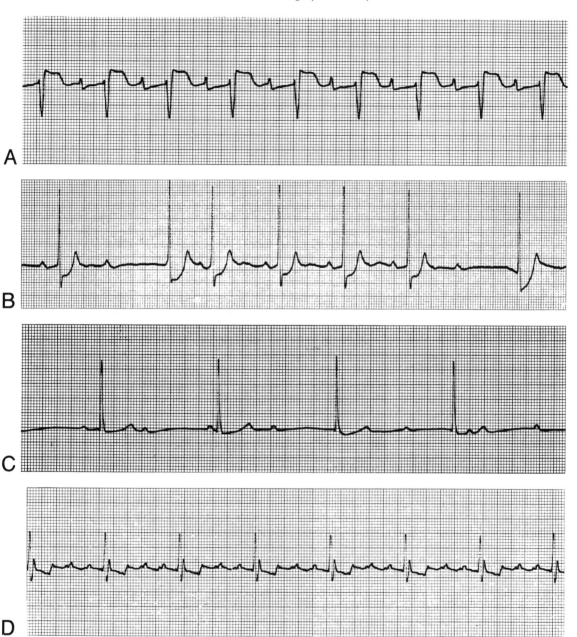

Fig. 21–50. Atrioventricular block. **A,** first-degree; **B,** second-degree, Mobitz type I (Wenckebach); **C,** third-degree; **D,** atrial tachycardia with 4:1 block.

bundle branch block pattern. This finding is often overlooked, with the result that supraventricular arrhythmias are frequently misdiagnosed as ventricular. Such a misdiagnosis has important therapeutic implications. A tracing of lead V_1 with two aberrantly conducted beats of right bundle branch block configuration is illustrated in Figure 21–51.

Drug Effects on the ECG

Drugs can cause various alterations in the resting ECG. Digitalis has the most

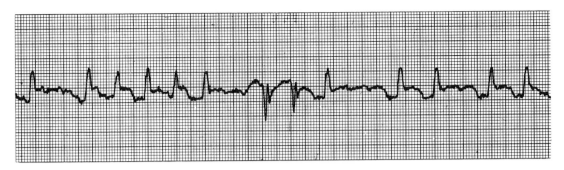

Fig. 21–51. Aberrant ventricular conduction.

prominent effect, producing changes that mimic heart disease and causing many blocks and arrhythmias. Digitalis causes depression of the ST segment as well as flattening and inversion of T-waves. The ST segment develops a characteristic "sag" which is upwardly concave. The arrhythmias associated with digitalis toxicity can be life-threatening.

The antiarrhythmic agent quinidine also affects the ECG, with ST-T wave changes as well as potentially life-threatening SA blocks. Many diuretics cause hypokalemia, which can cause arrhythmias as well as pro-

longation of the QT interval. Tricyclic antidepressant drugs increase the tendency to develop arrhythmias and also cause T-wave inversion. Beta-blockers cause negative chronotropic effects and, in combination with nitrates and calcium channel blockers, may delay the onset of ischemia and create a possible false-negative ECG response to exercise. The effects that drugs may have on the ECG are extensive and variable. Therefore, a review of the specific effects of those drugs taken by an individual patient is useful, particularly if ECG abnormalities are noted in that patient.

Chapter 22

ADDITIONAL DIAGNOSTIC TESTS: SPECIAL POPULATIONS

Barry A. Franklin, Darlene Fink-Bennett, Vicky Savas, Gregory Pavlides, and Robert D. Safian

Over the past decade, several advances have been made in the diagnosis and treatment of coronary artery disease (CAD). Developments in nuclear cardiology, including myocardial perfusion imaging and ventricular function testing, have yielded greater accuracy in diagnosing the presence of CAD when compared with conventional exercise electrocardiography. Clinicians now recognize the value of serial noninvasive testing in predicting the likelihood of disease through the application of Bayesian analysis. The need for noninvasive assessments for patients unable to exercise has led to the development of pharmacologic stress tests. Transesophageal echocardiography, an ultrasound examination of the heart using sound waves similar to sonar, can now provide important information relative to myocardial structure and function. Such tests have markedly improved the objectivity of clinical decision-making regarding the need for coronary arteriography. This chapter is an overview of these additional diagnostic tests, with specific reference to their clinical utility, risk, indications and contraindications, and advantages and limitations.

LIMITATIONS OF THE EXERCISE ELECTROCARDIOGRAM: DEVELOPMENT OF RADIONUCLIDE METHODS FOR CAD DETECTION

Exercise tolerance testing is one of the most common methods performed in the evaluation of the patient with suspected CAD. The test is based primarily on the electrocardiographic (ECG) response to exercise, with 1 mm or more ST-segment depression used as an indicator of myocardial ischemia (Fig. 22–1). The conventional exercise ECG, however, has significant limitations in the diagnosis of occult CAD.[1] In some instances, exercise-induced ST-segment depression may be suggestive of underlying heart disease when, in fact, no disease is present. This situation occurs predominantly in populations with a low prevalence of CAD (e.g., young, asymptomatic women). Conversely, a lack of exercise-induced ST-segment depression may imply that CAD is absent when disease may actually be present.

Although the predictive accuracy of the exercise ECG seems reasonable, with an approximate 75% sensitivity and an 85% specificity, the 25% false-negative rate and 15% false-positive rate highlight its limitations in detecting occult CAD and its use as a screening procedure.[2] These limitations have led to the development of two noninvasive radionuclide methods for CAD detection: those that assess myocardial perfusion and those that assess ventricular function.

Assessing Myocardial Perfusion with Thallium-201

Thallium-201 is one of the radionuclides that can be used to assess regional myocardial perfusion. Its distribution after intravenous injection is proportional to myocardial blood flow, after which it is extracted by normal myocardial cells in a manner analogous to potassium. Normally perfused myocardium reaches a maximum thallium-201 uptake within minutes after its injection. It is not permanently affixed within the myocyte and, therefore, re-enters (washes out) the circulation with time. In persons without obstructive CAD, the distribution of thallium-201 throughout the myocardium is relatively homogenous; however, myocardium supplied by a compromised (stenotic) coronary artery is underperfused at peak exercise and thallium-201 accumulation within the myocardial cells supplied by that vessel is reduced. This

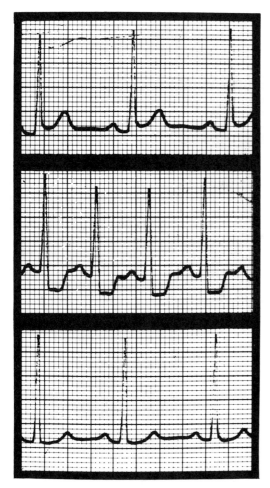

Fig. 22–1. *Top,* resting electrocardiogram (ECG) (V$_5$) before exercise testing. *Middle,* after several minutes of exercise test. Subject concurrently experienced mild angina pectoris. Myocardial ischemia verified further by significant ST-segment depression. *Bottom,* resting ECG 6 minutes after exercise, again representative of a "normal" ECG.

scenario provides the clinical rationale for the injection of thallium-201 at near-maximal exercise, with imaging scheduled as soon as possible in recovery (within approximately 10 minutes) and again several hours after exercise to assess for redistribution.

Exercise and Myocardial Perfusion Imaging Procedures

Myocardial perfusion imaging with thallium-201 has been used primarily in conjunction with exercise tolerance testing to detect areas of ischemia or myocardial scar secondary to total coronary artery occlusion. Exercise testing is generally performed on a treadmill following standard protocols (e.g., Balke or Bruce) and using routine ECG and blood pressure monitoring. At near-maximal exertion, however, the patient is injected with a small intravenous dose of thallium-201 (3 mL of saline containing 2 mCi of thallium-201 chloride), and is instructed to continue to exercise for an additional 60 seconds. Planar or single photon emission computed tomographic (SPECT) gamma camera imaging is then performed within 10 minutes of the thallium-201 injection. Planar images of the heart are obtained in anterior, 45° LAO and 70° LAO projections. SPECT images are acquired by rotating a gamma camera around the heart. The acquired data is then reconstructed using computer algorithms similar to CT and displayed in short, horizontal, and vertical long axes. Planar imaging of thallium-201 myocardial perfusion is limited by the super imposition of one portion of the myocardium over the other, whereas SPECT imaging permits the myocardium to be viewed in multiple sections (slices), a technique that has enhanced myocardial perfusion imaging's ability to detect small areas of ischemia or infarction.

The patient is then re-imaged with or without an additional 1 mCi of thallium-201 (booster dose) to determine if any redistribution (change in thallium uptake) has occurred from the exercise image.

Differentiating Areas of Exercise-Induced Ischemia from Myocardial Scar Tissue

Images obtained shortly after exercise pictorially depict regional myocardial perfusion at the time of stress. If the coronary arteries are normal, all portions of the myocardium receive approximately the same amount of isotope and the images have a homogenous/uniform appearance. If, however, one or more of the coronary arteries is/are obstructed, the portions of myocardium supplied by them show reduced thallium uptake, called "cold spots," representing areas of stress-induced ischemia or myocardial scar tissue. A second set of images called "the redistribution scan," taken several hours after exercise, helps to differentiate regions of decreased isotopic uptake as being either a manifestation of exercise-induced ischemia or scar from a prior myocardial infarction. If the area is only transiently hypoperfused, as is ischemic tissue, the redistribution scan shows a normalization of the stress-induced perfusion defect (Fig. 22–2); in contrast, infarcted tissue is manifested by persistent and unchanged regions of diminished activity, or "fixed defects" (Fig. 22–3).[3] Partial redistribution is seen in areas of infarction if adjacent or surrounding areas of ischemia are present.

Significance of Lung Uptake

Increased lung uptake on postexercise images, particularly in conjunction with exercise-induced perfusion defects, indicate extensive CAD and impaired left ventricular function. The uptake in the lung is not located within the blood pool, but a manifestation of increased pulmonary thallium extraction from the circulation.

Assessing Coronary Anatomy

The location of the perfusion defect can be used to predict the site of individual coronary stenoses. Septal and anterior defects are suggestive of left anterior descending CAD (sensitivity, 75%; specificity, 90%); inferior defects signify right coronary artery stenosis (sensitivity, 69%; specificity, 86%); and posterolateral defects imply left circumflex artery obstruction (sensitivity, 38%; specificity, 91%).[4] Predicting which vessel is involved when inferolateral thallium-201 defects occur is difficult because of considerable interindividual variation in myocardium perfused by the right and circumflex coronary arteries. Although simultaneous defects in the anterior, septal, and lateral vascular beds are highly sensi-

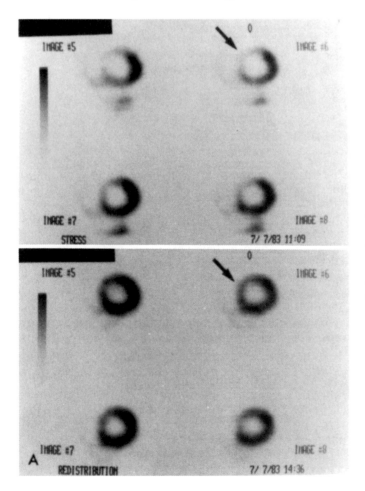

Fig. 22–2. Thallium images immediately after exercise (*top*) and during redistribution phase 4 hours later (*bottom*). *Arrow*, anteroseptal defect during exercise stress that exhibits redistribution, signifying viable but transiently ischemic myocardium.

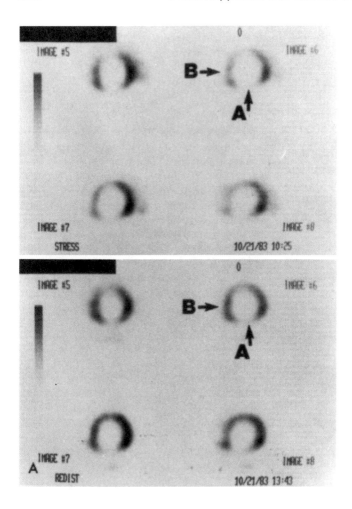

Fig. 22–3. Thallium stress (*top*) and redistribution (*bottom*) images are shown in a patient with a previous myocardial infarction in the inferior wall (A) with ischemia in the anteroseptal wall (B).

tive (92%) for left main coronary artery stenosis, similar perfusion abnormalities may occur with double or triple vessel disease. Consequently, many false-positive findings result (specificity, 15%) with this pattern.[5]

Accuracy in Comparison with Exercise ECG Findings

In numerous clinical studies, researchers have compared exercise thallium-201 myocardial perfusion imaging with conventional exercise ECG testing as a means of defining the presence or absence of CAD. In most studies, stress thallium-201 scintigraphy was superior to exercise electrocardiography in terms of sensitivity, specificity, and predictive accuracy, particularly when quantitative approaches were employed in conjunction with visual image interpretation.[6]

The overall sensitivity and specificity of planar or SPECT myocardial perfusion imaging for the detection of CAD ranges from 82 to 98% (90%) and 43 to 91% (70%). Detection of individual vessel stenoses, however, is generally low if planar myocardial perfusion imaging is performed with sensitivities of 55 to 78% for left anterior descending, 50 to 78% for right coronary artery, and 21 to 45% for left circumflex disease, whereas SPECT sensitivity and specificity for left anterior descending, left circumflex, and right coronary artery disease is of 78 to 80% and 82 to 92%; 66 to 88% and 84 to 91%; 75 to 94% and 62 to 99%, respectively.[2,7] The improved sensitivity and specificity of myocardial perfusion imaging in comparison with exercise stress electrocardiography is attributed to the fact that imaging can reveal regions of diminished radionuclide activity when the exercise ECG is uninter-

Table 22–1. Causes of "False-Positive" Exercise ECG Responses

1. Female gender
2. Left ventricular hypertrophy
3. Drugs (e.g., digitalis, antianxiety, and antidepressants)
4. ST-segment abnormality at rest
5. Hypertension
6. Sudden intense exercise
7. Valvular heart disease—aortic stenosis, aortic insufficiency, and mitral valve prolapse syndrome
8. Left bundle branch block
9. Anemia
10. Hypoxia
11. Vasoregulatory abnormalities
12. Wolff-Parkinson-White syndrome and other conduction defects
13. Pectus excavatum ± mitral valve prolapse
14. Hypokalemia
15. Cardiomyopathy
16. Pericardial disorders

pretable for ischemia or when suboptimal levels of exercise fail to elicit ischemic ST-segment depression. The improved specificity is a result of the fact that the primary cause of thallium perfusion defects is coronary artery stenosis, whereas there are numerous causes of ST-segment displacement with exercise other than myocardial ischemia (Table 22–1). Although the results of myocardial perfusion studies are uniformly better than those obtained with exercise electrocardiography alone, these studies do require the application of Bayesian analyses.[2,4,8] Accordingly, noninvasive tests have the greatest impact in patient groups with an intermediate pretest likelihood of disease.

Estimating Pretest Likelihood of Heart Disease

Clinicians now use three variables to estimate the risk of heart disease even before the exercise test is conducted. These variables, including age, sex, and symptoms, define a person's pretest risk or likelihood of disease (Table 22–2).[8] The risk of disease may be even further defined by complementary information regarding blood pressure, smoking status, and serum cholesterol profile.

In general, the incidence of heart disease increases with advancing age. Moreover, at any given age, men are at a higher risk than women. Individuals who have anginal symptoms also have a greater pretest probability of disease than those who are free of symptoms. For example, an asymptomatic 45-year-old woman has only a 1% chance of having significant CAD (see Table 22–2). A 55-year-old man with atypical angina has a 59% pretest probability of heart disease, whereas a 65-year-old man with typical angina has a very high (94%) pretest risk of heart disease.

Determining Post-test Likelihood of Disease

The results of the exercise test are considered along with the pretest risk to determine the post-test likelihood of disease. When the pretest risk of CAD is either very high or very low, a normal or abnormal exercise ECG response has minimal impact on the post-test likelihood of disease. Thus, for the aforementioned 45-year-old woman or 65-year-old man, any findings from an exercise ECG would be of limited additional value in the diagnosis of CAD.

Table 22–2. PreTest Likelihood of CAD (Percentage) in Patients by Age, Sex, and Symptoms*

Age (yr)	Asymptomatic		Nonanginal Chest Pain		Atypical Angina		Typical Angina	
	Men	Women	Men	Women	Men	Women	Men	Women
35	1.9	0.3	5.2	0.8	21.8	4.2	69.7	25.8
45	5.5	1.0	14.1	2.8	46.1	13.3	87.3	55.2
55	9.7	3.2	21.5	8.4	58.9	32.4	92.0	79.4
65	12.3	7.5	28.1	18.6	67.1	54.4	94.3	90.6

* Adapted with permission from Diamond GA, Forrester JS: Analysis of probability as an aid in the clinical diagnosis of coronary artery disease. N Engl J Med 300:1350, 1979.

On the other hand, when the pretest risk of heart disease is in the intermediate range, the exercise test results may substantially alter the post-test likelihood of disease. For example, the 55-year-old man with atypical angina has an approximate 59% likelihood of having significant CAD before any testing is done ("pretest likelihood of disease"). After an exercise ECG, his likelihood of having significant CAD ("post-test likelihood of disease") separates to about 90% if the test results are abnormal, demonstrating significant ST-segment depression, and about 30% if the test yields normal findings (Fig. 22–4).[2]

Selection of Patients

The results of exercise thallium-201 testing have the greatest impact in patients with an intermediate likelihood of CAD, that is, in the 30 to 70% range of pretest probability. These patients demonstrate the greatest degree of change in the post-test probability of disease. Thus, the middle-aged or elderly patient with atypical angina receives the greatest benefit from thallium-201 scintigraphy (see Table 22–2), because by considering the clinical history alone, the physician has already determined a moderate pretest likelihood of disease.

Rationale for Employing Multiple Noninvasive Studies

Most asymptomatic patients with exercise-induced ST-segment depression do not require exposure to the risk (albeit small) and expense of coronary arteriography, but further investigation of the possible presence of significant CAD is advisable. For these individuals, serial noninvasive testing appears warranted, because each test offers independent and additive data concerning the presence of disease.[1] Thus, an individual with a 10% pretest likelihood of CAD has a 30% likelihood after a "positive" exercise ECG. Figure 22–5 shows how this 30% likelihood becomes the pretest likelihood for the second test. When a thallium-201 exercise myocardial perfusion scan is used as the second test, abnormal results increase the likelihood of disease to about 80%, whereas normal findings reduce the likelihood of disease to less than 5%.[2] In the first instance, cardiac catheterization may be advisable; in the second instance, it is not recommended. Thus, with the use of exercise thallium-201 scintigraphy in conjunction with the conventional exercise ECG, the need for coronary arteriography can be defined more intelligently.

Clinical Uses

In several clinical situations, a thallium-201 exercise myocardial perfusion scan may be particularly useful. Thallium-201 imaging should be considered for use in patients with chest pain who fail to achieve 85% of the age-predicted maximal heart rate because of dyspnea, fatigue, or beta blockade therapy and in whom the exercise ECG shows no ischemic ST-segment

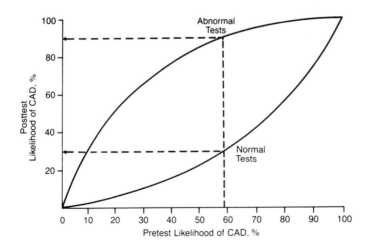

Fig. 22–4. Impact of 59% pretest likelihood of CAD on post-test likelihood of disease when exercise ECG is normal, 30%, or abnormal, 90%. Sensitivity of exercise ECG is 75%; specificity 85%. Adapted with permission from Epstein SE: Implications of probability analysis on the strategy used for noninvasive detection of coronary artery disease. *Am J Cardiol,* 46:491, 1980.

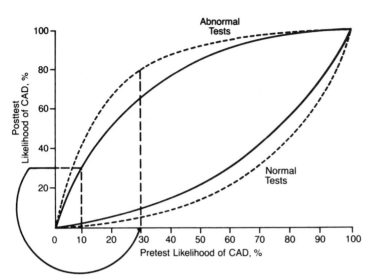

Fig. 22–5. Use of two noninvasive tests in predicting existence of CAD. Pretest likelihood of coronary disease of 10% yields likelihood of 30% after abnormal exercise ECG. This 30% likelihood becomes pretest likelihood for second test-exercise thallium myocardial perfusion scintigram. Abnormal scintigraphic findings increase likelihood of disease to about 80%; normal findings reduce likelihood of disease to less than 5%. *Solid lines,* exercise ECG (sensitivity, 75%; specificity, 85%); *broken lines,* thallium exercise myocardial perfusion scan (sensitivity, 85%; specificity, 90%). Adapted with permission from Epstein SE: Implications of probability analysis on the strategy used for noninvasive detection of coronary artery disease. *Am J Cardiol, 46:491,* 1980.

depression.[6] Experience shows that thallium-201 scintigraphy maintains both sensitivity and specificity in this setting, approximating 80% and 90%, respectively.[9] This occurs because exercise-induced thallium abnormalities can appear at a lower heart rate than stress-induced ECG findings of ischemia. Extent of disease, however, is probably underestimated because of the individual's inability to reach 85% of his or her age-predicted maximal heart rate. Another group of patients in whom thallium-201 imaging can be of value includes individuals who are asymptomatic but have "positive" exercise ECGs.

Thallium-201 exercise scintigraphy may also be of particular value in patients with ECG abnormalities that develop during exercise and are uninterpretable with respect to evidence of ischemia, e.g., in the presence of digitalis, significant ST-segment depression at rest, right or left ventricular hypertrophy, left bundle branch block, interventricular conduction delays (Wolff-Parkinson-White Syndrome), previous myocardial infarction, electrolyte imbalance, and pre-excitation syndromes. Finally, thallium-201 scintigraphy may be used to assess coronary anatomy and severity of disease, predict residual CAD after myocardial infarction, and evaluate patients after percutaneous transluminal coronary angioplasty or coronary artery bypass graft surgery. Such information has important prognostic and therapeutic implications.[3]

Limitations

Despite the improved accuracy of stress thallium-201 scintigraphy over the conventional exercise ECG, radionuclide imaging techniques have certain deficiencies. Major drawbacks include variability in imaging techniques and the qualitative visual interpretation of planar thallium-201 images. False-negative results may occur in some patients with triple vessel CAD because thallium-201 chloride distribution reflects regional blood flow to the myocardium, not coronary anatomy. If an individual has triple vessel CAD in conjunction with good collateral flow to the affected areas, the distribution of thallium-201 throughout the myocardium will be homogenous without a discernible perfusion defect ("cold spot"). The stress ECG results, along with the patient's clinical status, usually serve to identify these patients. Severe left ventricular hypertrophy and/or the inability of a patient to achieve at least 70% of his or her age-predicted maximal heart rate can also result in a false-negative study.[6] For this reason, beta-blocking drugs should be discontinued at least 48 hours before the myocardial perfusion scan as they can prevent the patient from achieving the rate-pressure product required to detect ischemic myocardium. Nitrates should also be discontinued for 48 hours before testing to maximize the sensitivity and specificity of myocardial perfusion imaging. Functional coronary collateral vessels represents another important cause of false-negative thallium-201 studies, affording some protection during exercise to myocardium perfused by critically stenosed coronary arteries.[10] Finally, small defects, left circumflex arterial obstructions, and perfusion abnormalities in the distribution of vessels with a moderate stenosis may at times not be detected. Clinically significant lesions, producing angina pectoris, ischemic ST-segment depression, or both, usually exceed 75% of the vessel lumen (Fig. 22–6).[11,12]

Because the normal myocardial perfusion scan depends on both adequate coronary perfusion and normal functioning myocardium, disorders other than CAD may elicit abnormal findings. False-positive studies can result from coronary spasm, myocardial bridge(s), coronary anomalies, aortic stenosis, and left bundle branch block.[3] False-positive studies can also result from attenuation of thallium-201's low energy photons, as occurs in large-breasted women (anterior wall) or by the diaphragm (inferior wall). Breast artifacts can usually be recognized if the images reveal well-defined areas of reduced perfusion along the anterior wall of the left ventricle. To avoid this problem, the breasts should be taped above the region of the heart during image acquisition. Diaphragmatic attenuation of the inferior wall can be differentiated from ischemia or infarction by performing a right lateral decubitus image. By placing the patient with his or her left side up, the diaphragm is moved away from the heart, permitting its visualization. Patients with a left bundle branch block may demonstrate reduced perfusion within the septum—a finding that is not necessarily a manifestation of ischemia, but more likely to be attributed to asynchronous impulse conduction. In such cases, pharmacologic stress myocardial perfusion imaging with dipy-

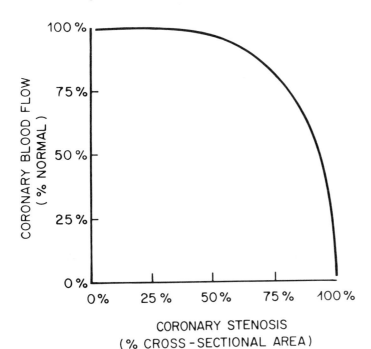

Fig. 22–6. Relationship between myocardial perfusion and coronary artery stenosis. Coronary blood flow is not significantly impaired until stenosis exceeds 75% of cross-sectional area of vessel. With permission from Dehn M, et al.: Clinical exercise performance. In *Clinics in Sports Medicine*. Edited by B Franklin and M Rubenfire. Philadelphia: WB Saunders Co.., 1984.

ridamole or adenosine can be employed. The septum may also appear abnormal in patients with aortic stenosis because of localized calcification or fibrosis.

New Radioactive Imaging Agents

Thallium-201 chloride has limitations as a myocardial perfusion imaging agent because its physical properties are not well suited to scintillation gamma camera imaging. Thallium-201's low 67-80 keV mercury x-ray photons are attenuated by overlying soft tissue (breast, diaphragm) and its long half-life ($T\frac{1}{2}$) of 73 hours limits the total dose of thallium-201 that can be administered to 3 to 4 mCi. Because of these limitations, investigators have sought myocardial perfusion imaging agents that could be labeled with technetium-99m (Tc-99m), a radionuclide with optimal physical characteristics for gamma camera imaging. Technetium-99m's short half-life permits the administration of large doses of this radionuclide and its 140 keV photon is ideally suited to imaging with a scintillation camera. Technetium-99m sestamibi (Cardiolite) and Tc-99m teboroxime (Cardiotec) are two Tc-99m labeled myocardial perfusion imaging agents that are now available for routine use.[13,14]

Technetium-99m sestamibi, like thallium-201, accumulates within the heart in proportion to regional blood flow. Once there, however, it becomes affixed to mitochondria within the cells and, in contrast to thallium-201, does not redistribute. This feature permits image acquisition flexibility in that images may be recorded up to 6 hours after injection. This image flexibility in conjunction with Tc-99m's optimal physical imaging characteristics has resulted in the creation of a superior myocardial perfusion imaging agent for the evaluation of both chronic and acute disorders of the cardiovascular system.[13]

Technetium-99m sestamibi can be used to detect the presence and extent of CAD. It may also be used to determine the efficacy of medical/interventional therapy, identify salvageable myocardium or myocardium at risk, triage patients in the Emergency Room with acute chest pain, confirm the presence of an acute myocardial infarc-

tion, identify significant CAD in patients clinically suspected of unstable angina, and determine the efficacy of thrombolytic therapy.[15-21]

Technetium-99m sestamibi myocardial perfusion imaging to detect CAD is performed using either a 1-day rest-stress or 2-day stress-rest protocol. To perform a 1-day rest-stress Tc-99m sestamibi myocardial perfusion scan, the patient is given 8 to 9 mCi of Tc-99m sestamibi intravenously. Myocardial perfusion rest images are then obtained at 60 to 90 minutes. The stress myocardial perfusion images are performed 30 minutes to 4 hours after rest image acquisition following the intravenous administration of an additional 22 to 25 mCi of Tc-99m sestamibi at near peak exercise. To facilitate maximal uptake, the patient is asked to continue to exercise for an additional minute. Planar or SPECT gamma camera images of the myocardium are generally taken at 30 to 60 minutes; however, these images can be obtained at any time up to 6 hours post radiotracer administration.

The 2-day stress-rest protocol is similar to the 1-day rest-stress protocol differing only in that the stress portion of the examination is performed prior to the rest study. Because there is a 24-hour hiatus between the two studies, larger doses of Tc-99m sestamibi, for example, 15 to 30 mCi, can be used for each.[13,18]

The sensitivity and specificity of Tc-99m sestamibi in detecting CAD is similar to thallium-201. Technetium-99m's optimal imaging characteristics, however, result in myocardial perfusion images that are more easily interpreted than thallium-201 scans because of increased spatial resolution, decreased scatter, and a higher myocardial to background ratio. Moreover, the radiation exposure to the patient from Tc-99m sestamibi myocardial perfusion imaging is similar to that afforded by thallium-201. Breast and diaphragmatic attenuation artifacts are fewer and, if present, can be easily distinguished from ischemia/infarction because of the agent's lack of redistribution and "image acquisition flexibility." If an area of decreased perfusion is present in the region of the anterior wall of a large-breasted woman, reimaging can be performed with the breast in a different position. If following this maneuver, radiotracer is demonstrated within the anterior wall, ischemia is excluded. If a diaphragmatic attenuation artifact is suspected, it can be differentiated from ischemia/infarction by simply reimaging the patient in the right decubitus position.

Technetium-99m sestamibi's lack of redistribution permits imaging the acutely ill patient because time is available between tracer administration and myocardial perfusion image acquisition. The tracer can be injected, the patient stabilized, and then the image acquired.[15,17]

The sensitivity and specificity of myocardial perfusion imaging in confirming the presence or absence of an acute myocardial infarction and/or unstable angina is 97%, 92%, 96%, and 80%, respectively. Technetium-99m sestamibi flexibility also permits evaluation of the efficacy of thrombolytic therapy. If the pre- and post-thrombolytic myocardial perfusion scans are unchanged, thrombolysis has probably failed; in contrast, improved images suggest that reperfusion has occurred.[7,16,18,19]

Technetium-99m teboroxime (Cardiotec) is the other new myocardial perfusion imaging agent that has been labeled with Tc-99m pertechnetate. Its myocardial uptake, like that of Tc-99m sestamibi and thallium-201 chloride, is also proportional to regional blood flow. Teboroxime is very rapidly extracted from the circulation by myocardial cells so that an image of regional myocardial blood flow can be obtained in as little as 2 minutes from the time of its intravenous administration. Its washout, however, is rapid, so that within 15 minutes, little to no teboroxime remains within the myocardium. Myocardial perfusion acquisition time therefore must be completed within 20 minutes of its administration. This time constraint has limited teboroxime's role in the detection of CAD. It is difficult to complete a stress/myocardial perfusion scan in such a short time unless dipyridamole or adenosine is used. The sensitivity and specificity of Tc-99m teboroxime myocardial perfusion imaging in detecting both acute and chronic disorders of the cardiovascular system is reported to be similar to those of Tc-99m sestamibi and thallium-201 imaging.[14]

ASSESSING VENTRICULAR FUNCTION WITH RADIONUCLIDE ANGIOCARDIOGRAPHY

Cardiac blood-pool imaging facilitates the evaluation of cardiac function at rest and during exercise, including the rapid sequential assessment of the left ventricular ejection fraction, regional wall motion, ventricular volumes, and diastolic filling rates. The left and right ventricles can be visualized by the intravenous injection of the radioisotope technetium-99m so that it binds to the red blood cells and remains in the blood pool during scintigraphy. With the use of a computer, rapid serial images of the heart can be obtained.

Exercise and Radionuclide Angiocardiography

Radionuclide angiocardiography is an accurate and reproducible method that correlates well with cardiac catheterization for the determination of left ventricular ejection fraction. Because it is a noninvasive technique, it has the advantage of allowing low-risk serial studies of the effect of interventions such as exercise, medication, or coronary artery reperfusion, for example, after percutaneous transluminal coronary angioplasty or coronary artery bypass surgery.[5] Two approaches to exercise radionuclide angiocardiography have emerged: the "first-pass" method and the "gated equilibrium" method; in both, Tc-99m is used as a tracer.[6] In first-pass studies, the tracer is injected as a bolus, and activity is recorded with a scintillation camera during the initial passage of the tracer through the heart. A time-activity curve is constructed, and the ejection fraction is calculated by determining the number of radioactive counts in the area of the left or right ventricle at end-diastolic and end-systolic silhouettes, cine-like movies, and functional images.

Equilibrium blood-pool imaging differs slightly in that the isotope is allowed to equilibrate within the vasculature. The cardiac cycle is divided into 12 to 28 frames, with the R-wave of the ECG used as a reference point. Images are obtained during several hundred cardiac cycles to generate a multigated radionuclide cineangiogram (MUGA). The left ventricular ejection fraction can be calculated in a manner similar to that with the first-pass technique.

Exercise Testing: Methods and Protocol

During exercise, the subject uses a cycle ergometer while in the supine, upright, or semi-upright position,[22] and the camera is positioned to obtain a 45 to 50° left anterior oblique image. The initial workload (warm-up) generally involves pedaling at power outputs of 300 kilopond-meters per minute (kpm/min) or less; thereafter, workload increments average 100 to 150 kpm/min every 3 minutes, to attainment of peak physical exertion (optimal rate-pressure product more than 250) or until clinical signs, symptoms, or volitional fatigue occur. Measurements of the ejection fraction and regional wall motion at rest and during exercise are compared.

Interpretation of Results

The radionuclide angiocardiogram is evaluated for ejection fraction, regional wall motion, and end-diastolic and end-systolic volumes. Mean normal values ($\pm$ SD) for left and right ventricular ejection fraction at rest are 62.3% $\pm$ 6.1 and 52.3% $\pm$ 6.2, respectively.[23] Damage from a previous myocardial infarction is evident as either akinesis or hypokinesis of a segment of the myocardium in the distribution of the obstructed coronary artery.

The ejection fraction and wall motion response to exercise can be a sensitive indicator of left ventricular performance. In patients with ischemic CAD, ventricular function may be normal at rest; with the increased stress of exercise, however, a portion of the wall may become transiently ischemic and exhibit impaired contractility. Thus, abnormal exercise responses that are highly sensitive for the presence of CAD include the development of new regional wall motion abnormalities, an increase in end-systolic volume, and an inability to augment the ejection fraction by at least 5%.[24]

Clinical Uses

Exercise radionuclide angiocardiography may be used to diagnose the presence of CAD (sensitivity $\geq$ 85%), to assess the severity and extent of CAD, to evaluate prognosis after myocardial infarction, to clarify the risk of open heart surgery, and to identify viable but ischemic myocardium that may respond favorably to percutaneous transluminal coronary angioplasty or coronary artery bypass grafting.[24,25] Radionuclide angiocardiography can also be used to assess the effects of medication and exercise therapy in patients with CAD; however, numerous reports indicate that ejection fraction and regional wall motion remain unchanged after physical conditioning programs.[26]

Comparison with Thallium-201 Myocardial Perfusion Imaging

Myocardial perfusion imaging and radionuclide angiocardiography offer the physician readily available and clinically valuable noninvasive techniques in the evaluation of CAD. These techniques provide information that complements and sometimes replaces that previously obtained through cardiac catheterization. Moreover, both methods appear to have comparable sensitivity and specificity for CAD detection, in the range of 85 to 90%.[25]

Limitations

Problems encountered with exercise radionuclide angiocardiography include patient difficulty in achieving prolonged ($\geq$ 2 minutes) optimal stress levels to obtain statistically valid counts, observer variance in the qualitative evaluation of regional wall motion and the quantitation of left ventricular ejection fraction, and the lack of specificity for ejection fraction diminution with exercise stress.[6] Many patients with nonischemic-induced left ventricular dysfunction, including those with hypertension, valvular heart disease, chronic obstructive pulmonary disease, and dilated cardiomyopathy, demonstrate an unchanged (flat) or decreased ejection fraction with exercise. Abnormalities other than major coronary artery stenosis may also be important in false-positive responses; for example, microvascular disease may play a role.[27]

PHARMACOLOGIC STRESS TESTS

Exercise stress testing is a well-accepted means of identifying CAD. Unfortunately, many patients at risk for developing CAD are unable to exercise. Obesity, sedentary lifestyle, peripheral vascular occlusive disease, and debilitative orthopedic problems such as arthritis often prohibit attainment of adequate cardiac stress ($\geq 85\%$ of age-predicted maximal heart rate). Yet, patients with these conditions often have coronary disease. The need for noninvasive assessments for patients unable to exercise led to the development of pharmacologic stress tests.[28,29] This section discusses dipyridamole thallium scintigraphy but subsequently focuses on two tests that may be overtaking it in popularity: adenosine thallium scintigraphy and dobutamine echocardiography.

Dipyridamole Thallium Scintigraphy

Thallium imaging undertaken after oral administration or intravenous dipyridamole infusion can be used as a means of inducing regional myocardial perfusion abnormalities in patients who are unable to perform sustained exercise. This potent vasodilator markedly enhances blood blood flow to normally perfused myocardium, whereas myocardium fed by stenotic coronary arteries demonstrates relative hypoperfusion and diminished thallium activity. The approach assesses coronary flow reserve, in contrast to exercise-induced ischemia, and appears comparable to exercise thallium-201 imaging for CAD detection. Sensitivity and specificity of thallium-201 scintigraphy using intravenous dipyridamole infusion average 85% and 91%, respectively.[28] Other uses include predischarge risk stratification of patients after acute myocardial infarction,[30–32] preoperative evaluation of candidates undergoing surgery for peripheral vascular or aortic disease,[33–35] differentiation of ischemic myocardium from scar tissue,[36] and determining restenosis risk following coronary angioplasty.[37]

Methodology varies according to the route of dipyridamole administration. Thallium-201 is injected 45 minutes after oral dipyridamole administration (generally 300 to 375 mg); images are obtained immediately after thallium injection and again 3 hours later. The intravenous form is administered at a dosage of 0.56 mg/kg given over 4 minutes, followed by thallium-201 injection.

Although dipyridamole thallium imaging has proven useful in detecting CAD, the vasodilator's relatively long half-life and difficulty in managing side effects has discouraged greater acceptance. Oral dipyridamole has a duration of action lasting several hours. Gastrointestinal side effects and a variable rate of absorption[38] when dipyridamole is given orally prompted development of an intravenous form. The intravenous drug has a 15- to 30-minute duration of action, prohibiting dosage titration as a method of symptom management. Minor side effects from intravenous dipyridamole include chest pain, headache, and dizziness.[39] Major side effects include cardiac arrhythmias, acute myocardial infarction, and sudden death.[40–42] The side effects can be reversed with intravenous aminophylline,[43] which directly competes with adenosine at the receptor sites; however, because of dipyridamole's long half-life, symptoms may recur after discontinuation of aminophylline.

Adenosine Thallium Scintigraphy

Interest in adenosine as a method of pharmacologic stress occurred because of the problems associated with dipyridamole. Adenosine's mechanism of action is similar to that of dipyridamole because the latter works indirectly by elevating levels of endogenous adenosine. Once in the circulation, adenosine crosses the cell membrane, binding to A_1 or A_2 receptors.[44] At the A_1 receptors, it inhibits sinoatrial and atrioventricular nodal conduction. The latter property has been clinically advantageous for treatment of paroxysmal supraventricular tachycardia.[45] At the A_2 receptors, adenosine causes intense vasodilation in all vascular beds that do not contain critical stenoses, except hepatic veins and the preglomerular arterioles of the kidney.[46] Similar to what occurs with dipyridamole, after adenosine administration, thallium-201 is taken up preferentially in regions perfused by dilated vessels that do not contain significant stenoses. Thus, the adequacy of adenosine testing, in contrast to conventional exercise stress, does not rely on pronounced increases in the rate-pressure product.

The major use of adenosine thallium imaging has been to evaluate for the presence of CAD. Verani et al.[47] recently found an overall sensitivity and specificity of 83% and 84%, respectively. The sensitivity for one-vessel disease was 73%; for two-vessel disease, 90%; and three-vessel disease, 100%. Nguyen et al.[48] had a similar experience, with an overall sensitivity of 92% and specificity of 100%. As occurs with other methods of stress used with thallium scintigraphy, breast attenuation of the scintigraphic signals and diaphragm motion unfavorably influence test results by causing false-positives.

The methodology at our center calls for obtaining a baseline blood pressure and an ECG, followed by a 6-minute continuous intravenous infusion of adenosine at a dosage of 140 mcg/kg/min. Adenosine's side-effects and short half-life, less than 2 seconds,[49] warrant the use of an infusion pump for accurate dosing. Blood pressure determinations and 12-lead electrocardiography are repeated every minute during the infusion. Blood pressures should not be obtained from the arm receiving the adenosine infusion, since cuff inflation may interrupt the action of this short-lived agent and deflation may produce a transient bolus. Moreover, separate intravenous sites should be used for adenosine and thallium to avoid causing an adenosine bolus due to thallium flush. Thallium is injected 3 minutes after the initiation of the adenosine infusion, and imaging occurs after 3 additional minutes and again in 3 hours.

The side effects of adenosine infusion are generally well tolerated and include chest pain,[47] which occurs in 50% of patients, flushing, headache, shortness of breath, dizziness, and lightheadedness.[29] In situations in which the side effects are poorly tolerated, the short half-life allows titration of the dose to lower levels to prevent adverse reactions. Major side effects include heart block, hemodynamic changes, and ischemia. A recent series found a 10% incidence of first-degree and 3.5% incidence of second-degree heart block.[47] We have found heart block generally to be transient; it often resolves spontaneously before any change in the adenosine infusion can be made.

As with conventional exercise testing, adenosine thallium imaging is contraindicated in patients with unstable angina, poorly controlled hypertension or hypotension, Class III or IV congestive heart failure, aortic stenosis, or recent myocardial infarction. In addition, patients with second- or third-degree heart block (without a pacemaker), sick sinus syndrome, or a history of severe bronchospasm should not be challenged because of the potential for exacerbation of these conditions.[29,50,51] Patients should not be tested with adenosine within 24 to 36 hours of taking dipyridamole because severe and prolonged side effects may result.[52] Methylxanthines such as caffeine and theophylline should be avoided a minimum of 12 hours before adenosine administration to limit interference with coronary artery vasodilation.

Almost all adverse effects of adenosine can be managed by simply reducing or halting the infusion. As with dipyridamole, prolonged symptoms are best managed with aminophylline. Additional adjunctive medical therapy includes atropine for heart block and nitroglycerin for ischemia. However, in our experience, complications are rare and very short-lived, usually obviating the need for treatment.

Dobutamine Echocardiography

Like nuclear imaging techniques, echocardiography has been used with various pharmacologic agents to evaluate the presence of CAD in patients who are unable to exercise. Berthe et al.[53] were the first to use echocardiography to detect ischemic wall motion abnormalities induced by dobutamine. In contrast to dipyridamole or adenosine stress, the mechanism by which dobutamine causes ischemia is related to increased oxygen demand secondary to increases in heart rate and contractility.

Dobutamine echocardiography has been used most commonly to identify patients with suspected CAD. Using wall motion abnormalities as the indicator, sensitivity ranges from 86 to 89% and specificity from 86 to 88%.[53–56] Structural information used in the evaluation of valvular and ventricular pathologies is revealed by echocardiography; moreover, wall motion abnormalities at a given heart rate in response to incremental dobutamine doses can be used to grade disease severity.[57] An additional indication for dobutamine echocardiography is the identification of hibernating myocardium. In one investigation, patients treated with thrombolytic reperfusion therapy underwent evaluation of myocardial viability by dobutamine echocardiography and positron emission tomographic (PET) scanning. The studies were found to have a concordance of 79%.[58]

The methodology of dobutamine echocardiography includes incremental infusions of dobutamine along with blood pressure, ECG, and echocardiographic monitoring (Table 22–3).[29] Although a standard protocol may be used, the dosage and duration of dobutamine infusion can be varied depending on the index of suspicion for CAD. Endpoints for the infusion include severe hypotension or hypertension, ischemic ST-segment depression, echocardiographic wall motion abnormalities, or significant arrhythmias. Echocardiographic detection of new wall motion abnormalities has been greatly facilitated by the use of computer-based digital acquisition, which allows continuous-loop, side-by-side display of ventricular images.[59]

Side effects are generally well tolerated during dobutamine echocardiography. Minor side effects include flushing, facial tingling, dyspnea, headache, and chest pain. Major complications resulting from ischemia can generally be avoided if the indications for test termination include echocardiographic detection of new wall motion

Table 22–3. Protocol: Dobutamine Echocardiography

1. Baseline blood pressure, 12-lead ECG, and echocardiogram
2. Begin dobutamine infusion (5 or 10 μg/kg/min), increasing the dose by 5 or 10 μg/kg increments every 5 minutes until 40 μg/kg/min is achieved
3. Repeat blood pressure, 12-lead ECG, and echocardiogram immediately before the conclusion of each 5-minute stage

abnormalities.[29] Arrhythmias occur approximately 15% of the time[54,56] and generally resolve spontaneously after discontinuation of the dobutamine infusion. Management of complications includes discontinuation of the dobutamine infusion. Persistent or severe ischemia can be managed with nitroglycerin or intravenous beta-blockers.

In addition to the usual exclusion criteria for any stress test, there are those specific to dobutamine echocardiography. Because dobutamine facilitates atrioventricular conduction, patients with atrial fibrillation should not be tested unless their ventricular rate is well controlled. Patients with a history of ventricular ectopy, poor left ventricular function, or both, should also be considered for alternative methods of study.

Which Method?

Pharmacologic stress testing is generally reserved for patients with neurologic, vascular, or orthopedic impairment of the lower extremities. The above-referenced drugs (dipyridamole, adenosine, dobutamine) have comparable sensitivities and specificities for detecting CAD. Nevertheless, dipyridamole is declining in popularity because of its side effect profile and long duration of action. A comparison of the advantages and disadvantages of adenosine thallium versus dobutamine echocardiography is shown in Table 22–4, with specific reference to test time, side effects, cost, sensitivity and specificity.[29]

In a crossover, blinded trial, Martin et al.[60] compared dipyridamole, adenosine, and dobutamine stress echocardiography in 40 patients; 25 had angiographically documented CAD and the remaining 15 did not. The sensitivity of dobutamine stress echocardiography (76%) was significantly higher than that of adenosine echocardiography (40%) and that of dipyridamole echocardiography (56%). This was attributed, at least in part, to the rate-pressure product, which was more than 50% higher with dobutamine compared with adenosine or dipyridamole, suggesting that myocardial oxygen demand was higher with dobutamine. Adenosine testing had a significantly higher specificity (93%) com-

Table 22–4. Pharmacologic Stress Testing: Advantages and Disadvantages of Adenosine Thallium Versus Dobutamine Echocardiography

	Adenosine Thallium	Dobutamine Echocardiography
Test time	Several hours	60 minutes
Side Effects		
Major	Heart block, bradyarrhythmias	Tachyarrhythmias
Minor	Similar, more frequent	Similar, less frequent
Ischemia	Less likely	More likely
Cost	More expensive	Less expensive
Sensitivity	90%	89%
Specificity	84%	88%
Advantages	Less likely to induce ischemia	Graded study; can detect disease severity
	Very short half-time	Detection of hibernating myocardium
		Structural information

pared with dobutamine (60%) and dipyridamole (67%). Adverse symptoms were significantly more frequent in patients taking adenosine (100%) compared with those taking dipyridamole (88%) or dobutamine (80%). Treatment for persistent symptoms was required in more patients after dipyridamole (40%) than after dobutamine or adenosine (12% and 0%, respectively). More patients preferred dobutamine (48%) or dipyridamole (40%) echocardiography to adenosine echocardiography (12%). The authors concluded that dobutamine stress echocardiography is more sensitive and better tolerated than adeno-

sine or dipyridamole echocardiography, whereas adenosine echocardiography is more specific and results in fewer persistent side effects. These data may influence the choice of drug for pharmacologic stress echocardiography.

TRANSESOPHAGEAL ECHOCARDIOGRAPHY

Transesophageal echocardiography (TEE) is a relatively new technique that has numerous clinical applications. Simply defined, TEE is two-dimensional and Doppler echocardiography of the heart and

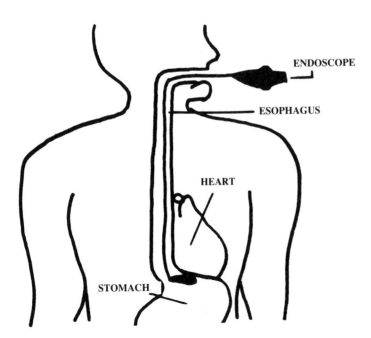

Fig. 22–7. Transesophageal echocardiography is an ultrasound examination of the heart using sound waves similar to sonar. It is performed by inserting a flexible tube through the mouth into the esophagus. The instrument used is similar to a gastroscope, which is frequently used for examination of the esophagus, stomach, and upper bowel. The technique provides important information regarding the structure of cardiac muscle, heart valves and major arteries.

thoracic great vessels, performed through the esophagus and stomach by a modified gastroscopy probe (echo-probe) with one or two ultrasound transducers at its tip (Fig. 22–7).

The historical and technologic evolution of TEE started in 1976, when M-mode transesophageal echocardiography was first performed in the U.S.[61] Although mechanical two-dimensional echo transducers were used for TEE in the late 70s,[62] the modern era of TEE started in 1982, when German investigators used TEE probes with phased-array transducers.[63] In 1987, color Doppler transducers were introduced, and in 1989, biplanar imaging by means of two transducers in the echo probe with color and continuous wave Doppler became possible, and is the standard technique of today. The latest technologic advance is the multiplane echo probe, which allows an infinite number of planes to be obtained in a span of 360 degrees. The multiplane echo probes will soon be available for routine clinical use.

Compared to standard transthoracic echocardiography (TTE), TEE has several distinct advantages. First, it provides better image resolution because of the closer proximity of the ultrasound transducer to cardiac structures, and the higher frequency transducers routinely used (5 MHz for TEE versus 2.5 MHz for TTE). Second, TEE provides superior images of posterior cardiac structures, like left and right atria, left atrial appendage, atrial septum, left main coronary artery, pulmonary arteries and veins, and thoracic aorta. Third, TEE allows continuous echocardiographic imaging during operations or cardiac interventions without interfering with the procedure.

Technique

The technique of TEE is fairly simple and similar to the method gastroenterologists used for years for upper gastrointestinal endoscopy. The procedure is explained to the patients in detail, and informed consent is obtained. The evaluation is deferred if there is a history of dysphagia or esophageal disorder. An intravenous line is desirable but not essential. Intravenous sedation is optional; although it increases the accep-

tance of the procedure, the potential side effects and the need for postprocedure observation should be considered. The only exception is with suspected aortic dissection, in which intravenous sedation should be used. Endocarditis prophylaxis is not routinely required. The high incidence of procedural bacteremia reported in early studies, was not confirmed by later larger series, and there are no reported cases of infective endocarditis attributed to TEE.[64]

Transesophageal echocardiography is an invasive procedure that is remarkably safe. The failure rate among 10,419 patients from a number of European Centers was 1.9%, with rare complications and only one death.[65] In our own experience of approximately 1000 cases, the failure rate was less than 1% and no complications or deaths occurred.

Indications

The clinical conditions in which TEE can be of clinical value are listed in Table 22–5. There are, however, several conditions in which TEE may provide the diagnostic method of choice, including the detection of intracardiac masses and thrombi, suspected infective endocarditis, evaluation of prosthetic cardiac valves, aortic dissection, and congenital heart disease in adolescents and adults. A great number of TEE studies are performed to detect intracardiac sources of emboli; however, the value of TEE in that setting remains controversial.

Intracardiac Masses and Thrombi

Echocardiography is the most readily available technique for detection of intracardiac masses or thrombi. Transesophageal echocardiography is superior to TTE in detecting and characterizing intracardiac masses and thrombi. In a recent European study involving 32 patients, TEE detected lesions in all cases (100% sensitivity) versus 26 (81%) by TTE.[66] More importantly, TEE can have an impact on patient management. In a recent report from the Mayo Clinic, TEE provided additional information in most diagnoses of intracardiac mass, and influenced treatment in a substantial proportion.[67]

Table 22–5. Clinical Application of Transesophageal Echocardiography

I. Diagnostic Applications
  A. Transthoracic echocardiogram (TTE) of inadequate quality (chronic obstructive lung disease, early post-open heart surgery, obesity, chest deformities and intubated patients in the intensive care units, including trauma patients)
  B. Transthoracic echocardiography of acceptable quality
    1. Mitral regurgitation, when quantitation by TTE is difficult.
    2. Conditions where anatomical detail of the mitral valve and perivalvular tissue is important (mitral stenosis prior to valvuloplasty, mitral valve prolapse).
    3. Suspected aortic valve deformities.
    4. Abnormalities of left ventricular outflow tract.
    5. Suspected or diagnosed infective endocarditis.
    6. Suspected atrial thrombus.
    7. Suspected or diagnosed intracardiac masses.
    8. Evaluation of prosthetic cardiac valves.
    9. "Cryptogenic" stroke.
    10. Congenital heart disease in adolescents and adults.
    11. Thrombus detection in the main pulmonary arteries.
    12. Dissection of the thoracic aorta.
II. Monitoring Applications
  A. Intraoperatively
    1. Assessing results of mitral valve reconstruction.
    2. Monitoring left ventricular function during high-risk noncardiac surgery.
  B. In the cardiac catheterization laboratory
    1. Monitoring left ventricular function during intervention
    2. During balloon mitral valvuloplasty

Infective Endocarditis

Infective endocarditis remains a diagnostic and therapeutic challenge. Diagnosis of infective endocarditis is generally based on the patient's clinical picture and positive blood cultures; nevertheless, the confirmation of a vegetation by echocardiography is important. Transesophageal echocardiography probably constitutes the greatest advance in identifying infective endocarditis over the last few years. Traditionally, the TTE sensitivity in detecting intracardiac vegetations has been between 60 and 80%. Transesophageal echocardiography has been found consistently to have a sensitivity over 90%.[68,69] The enhanced sensitivity with TEE becomes more impressive when the vegetations are smaller than 10 mm.[70] Additionally, TEE made possible the antemortem diagnosis of perivalvular abscesses, which appear to be more common than previously thought. Recently, Daniel et al.[71] reported their findings in 46 patients with infective endocarditis and perivalvular abscess confirmed either by autopsy or surgery. These patients were from a larger cohort of 118 patients with infective endocarditis, signifying that 39% of the patients had abscesses. Of the 46 abscesses, TTE detected 13 (28%) versus 40 (87%) detected by TEE.

Prosthetic Cardiac Valves

About 50,000 prosthetic cardiac valves are implanted each year in the U.S. Unfortunately, several problems associated with prosthetic valves can emerge, with the most important being prosthetic cardiac valve dysfunction. Transesophageal echocardiography is now recognized as the method of choice in examining prosthetic cardiac valves, especially in the mitral position.[72] The following characteristics explain why: (1) TEE has 100% sensitivity in detecting prosthetic mitral regurgitation, whereas suboptimal images are often obtained by TTE due to the acoustic "back shadow" of the valve; (2) TEE can accurately differentiate valvular from perivalvular mitral insufficiency; (3) TEE provides superior imaging of bioprosthetic valve leaflets; (4) TEE accurately displays disc excursion in low profile mechanical valves; (5) TEE is accurate in detecting valvular thrombi, vegetations and perivalvular abscesses; and (6) TEE detects left atrial thrombus in patients with mitral valve prosthesis.

Aortic Dissection

Aortic dissection (AD) is a very serious condition that must be promptly diagnosed and treated to reduce the risk of death. Untreated AD carries a 60 to 75% risk for death within 2 weeks. The diagnosis of AD remains difficult and requires a high level

Table 22–6. Aortic Dissection—Diagnostic Techniques

	Chest X Ray	CT with Contrast	Aorta-gram	TTE	TEE
Cost	Low	Mod	High	Low-Mod	Low-Mod
Patient Transport	No	Yes	Yes	No	No
Time Required	Little	Mod	Mod	Little	Little
Invasive	No	Yes	Yes	No	Semi
IV Dye	No	Yes	Yes	No	No
Sensitivity	50–60%	90%	>95%	70%	98%
Specificity	Low	>95%	>90%	90%	99%

TTE = transthoracic echocardiogram; TEE = transesophageal echocardiography; CT = computed tomography.

of suspicion. Traditionally, AD has been diagnosed by computed tomography of the thorax, whereas aortography has been the accepted standard. However, TEE, with its unique ability to image the thoracic aorta, has now become the method of choice for the diagnosis of AD.[73,74] Table 22–6 shows the merits and limitations of several common tests used to diagnose AD. Accordingly, TEE provides an accurate assessment that can be applied in the Emergency Department, without time delay or patient transfer. It requires no intravenous dye injection and provides additional information about blood flow between true and false lumen by Doppler examination. When available, it should be the first test in patients with suspected AD.

Summary

Transesophageal echocardiography is a relatively new diagnostic cardiac technique, with already established clinical indications. It is fairly simple and carries little risk in experienced centers. For many clinical conditions including intracardiac masses and thrombi, infective endocarditis, prosthetic cardiac valves, aortic dissection and congenital heart diseases in adults, TEE can be considered the diagnostic technique of choice. The technique is also emerging as the preferred method for other conditions involving the aorta, like atheromatous disease or thrombus. More importantly, TEE appears to influence the patient's treatment as well as diagnosis.[75]

CARDIAC CATHETERIZATION

More than 70 years ago, Dr. Werner Forssmann first performed cardiac catheterization in a living subject, when he passed a catheter through his own antecubital vein into the right atrium under fluoroscopic guidance. Forssmann's primary goal was to develop a therapeutic technique for intracardiac drug delivery for the management of cardiac arrest. Since that time, others have applied Forssmann's technique for diagnostic purposes, including measurements of right heart pressures and cardiac output, left heart catheterization, and selective coronary arteriography. Most recently, there has been a return to cardiac catheterization as a therapeutic modality, particularly for the purpose of percutaneous interventional procedures such as balloon angioplasty, coronary atherectomy, intravascular stent placement, and laser revascularization.

Technical Aspects of Cardiac Catheterization

Logistics

The cardiac catheterization laboratory consists of several components. Each laboratory must have high-quality radiographic equipment for acquiring images of high resolution and for permanent image recording. In addition, modern laboratories must be equipped with physiologic recorders to measure intracardiac pressures and cardiac output. Finally, all catheterization laboratories should be capable of functioning like intensive care units, with arrhythmia monitoring and an emergency cart. Although most cardiac catheterization laboratories are located within the hospital, freestanding facilities and mobile catheterization laboratories are becoming more popular. Many hospitals perform diagnostic cardiac catheterization procedures in an outpatient setting, whereas most interventional therapeutic procedures are performed in an inpatient setting.

Technique of Cardiac Catheterization

In general, there are three approaches to the cardiac catheterization technique. The femoral arterial approach, the most common technique employed today, is performed by percutaneous entry of the femoral vein and artery. Right-heart catheterization may be performed by advancing the right-heart catheter (such as a balloon-flotation Swan-Ganz catheter) from the femoral vein to the right side of the heart. Left-heart catheterization may be performed by retrograde passage of the left heart catheter from the femoral artery to the ascending aorta and left ventricle.

A second technique is the brachial approach, which may be performed by either percutaneous or cutdown entry of the brachial vein and artery. Right and left heart catheterization are performed as described for the femoral approach.

The third technique is transseptal left heart catheterization, which requires right heart catheterization from the femoral vein followed by passage of a small needle across the intra-atrial septum into the left atrium. Once access to the left atrium is achieved, a catheter may be placed antegrade from the left atrium to the left ventricle, to measure pressures and perform angiography.

Regardless of the technique used, cardiac catheterization is performed under local anesthesia after mild sedation.

Hemodynamic Assessment of the Patient

Pressure Measurements

In routine cardiac catheterization, fluid-filled catheters are connected to external pressure transducers to measure pressures at the tip of the catheter. Characteristic pressure waveforms are associated with each of the cardiac chambers and great vessels for each phase of the cardiac cycle. The interpretation of the pressure waveforms, as well as the magnitude of pressures, is important to the understanding of various disease states such as valvular stenosis, valvular regurgitation, congestive heart failure, and pericardial disorders.

Cardiac Output

In the cardiac catheterization laboratory, cardiac output is generally measured in one of two ways. With the Fick method, pulmonary blood flow is determined by measurement of the arteriovenous oxygen difference across the pulmonary circulation and by measurement of the pulmonary oxygen consumption. In the absence of an intracardiac shunt, the pulmonary and systemic blood flow are virtually identical. The Fick method may also be applied in the presence of an intracardiac shunt, in which case the pulmonary and systemic arteriovenous oxygen differences are different, and the extent of the shunt can be easily calculated.

The second common method of cardiac output determination is the thermodilution method. This technique relies on two thermistors on the shaft of the right heart catheter (one in the vena cava and one in the pulmonary artery). By injecting saline into the proximal port in the vena cava, one can determine the cardiac output by measuring the blood temperature at the distal port in the pulmonary artery.

Detection and Localization of Intracardiac Shunts

Cardiac catheterization techniques can be used to detect, localize, and quantitate congenital or acquired intracardiac shunts. Left-to-right shunts may be localized by sampling blood oxygen saturations from several points along the course of a routine right heart catheterization, looking for an inappropriate increase in oxygen saturation. For example, oxygen saturations can be measured at any point in the vena cava, right atrium, right ventricle, and pulmonary artery, and the site of a significant "step-up" in oxygen saturation can be identified. If there is a significant "step-up" in the right atrium, this is usually consistent with the presence of a congenital atrial septal defect. For patients with recent acute myocardial infarction, the presence of a step-up in the right ventricle is usually due to an acquired ventriculoseptal defect. The magnitude of the shunt can be calculated using the Fick method, and has a major impact on the decision to surgically repair the defect. Right-to-left shunts may also be detected and localized by determining the site of arterial desaturation ("step-down") during left heart catheterization.

Determination of Vascular Resistance

Vascular resistance for the pulmonary and systemic circulations can be easily calculated if the appropriate pressures and cardiac output have been determined. Vascular resistance is directly proportional to pressure, and inversely proportional to cardiac output.

Calculation of Valve Areas

In many cases, patients undergo cardiac catheterization to evaluate the severity of valvular stenosis. The valve area can be calculated on the basis of the pressure gradient across the valve and the blood flow across the valve during that phase of the cardiac cycle. In general, valve area is proportional to the cardiac output and inversely proportional to the pressure gradient across the valve.

Angiographic Assessment of the Patient

Coronary Angiography

Coronary angiography may be performed by the retrograde femoral or bra-chial arterial approach. The development of preformed catheters for selective coronary angiography has greatly simplified these techniques. The major epicardial coronary arteries and their branches can be easily identified by positioning the catheter in the left or right coronary artery, followed by manual injection of radiocontrast material through the catheter. By positioning the x-ray equipment in different angles, it is possible to study most of the major vessels and their branches.

The most common use of coronary angiography is to identify significant stenoses in the coronary arteries (Fig. 22–8), which could guide further therapy including adjustment of medical therapy, application of percutaneous interventional procedures (such as balloon angioplasty), or the need for coronary artery bypass surgery. Coronary angiography may also be used to detect less common disorders of the coronary circulation, including vasospasm, congenital defects, and other structural anomalies such as myocardial bridging. Coronary angiography and bypass graft angiography are also being used with increasing frequency in patients with recurrent angina following coronary bypass surgery.

Many noninvasive studies can identify patients with CAD, and several can identify

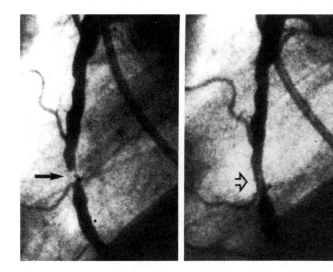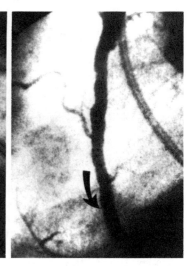

Fig. 22–8.   Selective coronary angiogram in the lateral projection demonstrates a focal, eccentric 90% stenosis in the mid-right coronary artery (left panel, black arrow). After balloon angioplasty, there is a mild residual stenosis with a focal linear dissection (middle panel, arrowhead). Six months later, repeat angiography demonstrates no significant residual stenosis, and the focal dissection has healed completely (right panel, black arrow).

which vessels are involved. However, coronary angiography is the most sensitive method for detecting coronary artery stenoses. Furthermore, the morphology of the stenosis (eccentricity, length, calcification, thrombus) and the location of the stenosis (aorto-ostial, origin lesion, bifurcation) bear directly on the success of treatment, and this information can be obtained only by coronary angiography.

Left Ventriculography

Left ventriculography may be performed by using special angiographic catheters (which can also be used for pressure measurements), and should be a routine part of cardiac catheterization. Opacification of the left ventricle is accomplished by injection of radiocontrast using a power injector. Left ventriculography is useful for detecting global or regional abnormalities of ventricular wall motion (hypokinesis, akinesis, or dyskinesis), abnormalities of ventricular contour (thrombus, aneurysm), and abnormalities of the mitral valve (mitral prolapse, mitral regurgitation). Full assessment of left ventricular function also includes determination of volumes (end-diastolic volume, end-systolic volume, and stroke volume) and ejection fraction.

Application of Cardiac Catheterization

Indications

The decision to perform cardiac catheterization is usually based on several factors, including the age of the patient, the clinical diagnosis, and the ability of other noninvasive tests to support the diagnosis. The most common indication is to confirm the presence and severity of a clinically suspected condition, and to identify other associated conditions. The decision to proceed with cardiac catheterization is most compelling when the physician determines that the patient is likely to require special intervention, such as balloon angioplasty or cardiac surgery (Fig. 22–8). For example, in a patient with angina pectoris in whom noninvasive studies suggest significant reversible ischemia despite medical therapy, cardiac catheterization, coronary angiography, and left ventriculography are generally indicated. Similarly, in an elderly patient with syncope and aortic stenosis, catheterization is indicated to define the severity of aortic stenosis and to identify other associated conditions, such as CAD.

A second general indication for cardiac catheterization is in the diagnosis of clinical syndromes of uncertain cause. A good example might be a middle-aged woman with atypical chest pain who requires frequent admission to the hospital. Cardiac catheterization and coronary angiography can help the patient, family, and physician by identifying the presence or absence of CAD, or by establishing an unsuspected cause of chest pain (such as constrictive pericarditis).

A third general indication for cardiac catheterization is the diagnosis and immediate treatment of selected patients with acute myocardial infarction and/or shock. Early diagnosis and treatment (which might include pharmacologic therapy, intra-aortic balloon counterpulsation, emergency angioplasty, or emergency surgery) may offer the best opportunity for survival.

Contraindications

There are few, if any, absolute contraindications to cardiac catheterization. In the last 10 years, cardiac catheterization and coronary angiography have been performed safely in patients with cardiogenic shock, aortic dissection, acute myocardial infarction, and bacterial endocarditis. Certainly, in elective situations, other associated medical conditions (e.g., fever, electrolyte disturbances, anemia) should be corrected first, if possible.

Complications of Cardiac Catheterization

Although the incidence of complications is low, it is always prudent to weigh the relative risks and benefits of the procedure for each patient. Risk factors for death from cardiac catheterization include extreme age (neonates and the very elderly), patients in functional class IV, the presence of left main CAD, the presence of critical aortic stenosis, left ventricular ejection fraction less than 30%, and other serious noncardiac disorders (renal failure, respiratory failure, cerebrovascular disease). The actual risk of death for most patients is approximately 0.1%, but may increase more than tenfold in the presence of one or more of these risk factors.[76]

Other complications of diagnostic cardiac catheterization are myocardial infarction (less than 0.1%), cardiac perforation (less than 0.1%), neurologic events (0.1%), serious arrhythmia (0.3%), vascular injury requiring transfusion or vascular repair (1.6%), vasovagal reactions (2.1%), and allergic reactions to the radiocontrast agent (2.1%). For cardiac catheterization procedures associated with interventional therapies, the risks of the procedure may be increased.[77]

ACKNOWLEDGMENT

The authors gratefully acknowledge the assistance of Brenda White in the preparation of this manuscript.

REFERENCES

1. Laslett LJ, Amsterdam EA: Management of the asymptomatic patient with an abnormal ECG. *JAMA, 252:*1744, 1984.
2. Epstein SE: Implications of probability analysis on the strategy used for noninvasive detection of coronary artery disease. *Am J Cardiol, 46:*491, 1980.
3. Willens HJ: Advances in cardiac diagnosis: Nuclear cardiology. In *Clinics in Sports Medicine.* Edited by B Franklin and M Rubenfire. Philadelphia: WB Saunders, 1984.
4. Berman DS, Garcia EV, Maddahi J: Thallium-201 myocardial scintigraphy in the detection and evaluation of coronary artery disease. In *Clinical Nuclear Cardiology.* Edited by DS Berman and DT Mason. New York: Grune and Stratton, 1981.
5. Rigo P: Value and limitations of segmental analysis of stress thallium myocardial imaging for localization of coronary artery disease. *Circulation, 61:*973, 1980.
6. Beller GA: Radionuclide techniques in the evaluation of the patient with chest pain. *Mod Concepts Cardiovasc Dis, 50:*43, 1981.
7. Nuclear Cardiology. Assessment of ischemia, viability, and prognosis. Thallium-201 SPECT offers advantages in assessment of CAD. April 1992.
8. Diamond GA, Forrester JS: Analysis of probability as an aid in the clinical diagnosis of coronary artery disease. *N Engl J Med, 300:*1350, 1979.
9. Iskandrian AS, Segal BL: Value of exercise thallium-201 imaging in patients with diagnostic and non-diagnostic electrocardiograms. *Am J Cardiol, 48:*233, 1981.
10. Rigo P, et al.: Influence of coronary collateral vessels on the results of thallium-201 myocardial stress imaging. *Am J Cardiol, 44:*452, 1979.
11. Dehn MM, Blomqvist CG, Mitchell JH: Clinical exercise performance. In *Clinics in Sports Medicine.* Edited by B Franklin and M Rubenfire. Philadelphia: WB Saunders, 1984.
12. Borer JS, et al.: Effect of nitroglycerin on exercise-induced abnormalities of left ventricular regional function and ejection fraction in coronary artery disease. *Circulation, 57:*314, 1978.
13. Berman DS: Introduction—Technetium-99m myocardial perfusion imaging agents and their relation to thallium-201. *Am J Cardiol, 66:*1E, 1990.
14. Johnson LL, Seldin DW: Clinical experience with Technetium-99m Teboroxime, a neutral, lipophilic myocardial perfusion imaging agent. *Am J Cardiol, 66:*63E, 1990.
15. Boucher CA: Detection and location of myocardial infarction using technetium-99m sestamibi imaging at rest. *Am J Cardiol, 66:*32E, 1990.
16. Wackers FJ: Thrombolytic therapy for myocardial infarction: Assessment of efficacy by myocardial perfusion imaging with technetium-99m Sestamibi. *Am J Cardiol, 66:*36E, 1990.
17. Gregoire J, Theroux P: Detection and assessment of unstable angina using myocardial perfusion imaging: Comparison between Technetium-99m Sestamibi SPECT and 12-lead electrocardiogram. *Am J Cardiol, 66:*42E, 1990.
18. Maddahi J, et al.: Myocardial perfusion imaging with Technetium-99m Sestamibi SPECT in the evaluation of coronary artery disease. *Am J Cardiol, 66:*55E, 1990.
19. Gerson MC: Nuclear cardiology in the investigation of chronic coronary artery disease. *JAMA, 250:*2037, 1983.
20. Iskandrian AS, Hakki AH: Thallium-201 myocardial scintigraphy. *Am Heart J, 109:*113, 1985.
21. Berman DS, et al.: Comparison of SPECT using technetium-99m agents and thallium-201 and PET for the assessment of myocardial perfusion viability. *Am J Cardiol, 66:*72E, 1990.
22. Bonzheim SC, et al.: Physiologic responses to recumbent versus upright cycle ergometry, and implications for exercise prescription in patients with coronary artery disease. *Am J Cardiol, 69:*40, 1992.

23. Pfisterer ME, Battler A, Zaret BL: Range of normal values for left and right ventricular ejection fraction at rest and during exercise assessed by radionuclide angiocardiography. *Eur Heart J, 6:*647, 1985.

24. Okada RD, Boucher CA, Strauss HW, Pohost GM: Exercise radionuclide imaging approaches to coronary artery disease. *Am J Cardiol, 46:*1188, 1980.

25. Meizlish JL, Berger HJ, Zaret BL: Exercise nuclear imaging for the evaluation of coronary artery disease. In *Exercise and the Heart.* 2nd Ed. Edited by NK Wenger. Philadelphia: FA Davis, 1985.

26. Jensen D, et al.: Improvement in ventricular function during exercise studies with radionuclide ventriculography after cardiac rehabilitation. *Am J Cardiol, 46:*770, 1980.

27. Opherk D, et al.: Reduced coronary reserve and ultrastructural changes of the myocardium in patients with angina pectoris but normal coronary arteries. *Circulation, 59:*11, 1979.

28. Beller GA: Pharmacologic stress imaging. *JAMA, 265:*633, 1991.

29. Savas V, Grines CL, Juni J, O'Neill WW: Pharmacologic stress tests: Dobutamine echo vs adenosine-thallium scintigraphy. *Cardiology 8:*40, 1991.

30. Leppo JA, et al.: Dipyridamole-thallium-201 scintigraphy in the prediction of future cardiac events after acute myocardial infarction. *N Engl J Med, 310:*1014, 1984.

31. Younis LT, et al.: Prognostic value of intravenous dipyridamole thallium scintigraphy after an acute myocardial ischemic event. *Am J Cardiol, 64:*161, 1989.

32. Gimple LW: Predischarge dipyridamole thallium predicts the frequent events occurring before late testing and identifying risk after uncomplicated acute myocardial infarction. *Am J Cardiol, 64:*1243, 1989.

33. Eagle KA: Dipyridamole-thallium scanning in patients undergoing vascular surgery. *JAMA, 257:*2185, 1987.

34. Boucher CA, et al.: Determination of cardiac risk by dipyridamole-thallium imaging before peripheral vascular surgery. *N Engl J Med, 312:*389, 1985.

35. Leppo J, et al.: Noninvasive evaluation of cardiac risk before elective vascular surgery. *J Am Coll Cardiol, 9:*269, 1987.

36. Eichhorn EJ, et al.: Usefulness of dipyridamole-thallium-201 perfusion scanning for distinguishing ischemic from nonischemic cardiomyopathy. *Am J Cardiol, 62:*945, 1988.

37. Jain A, et al.: Clinical significance of perfusion defects by thallium-201 single photon emission tomography following oral dipyridamole early after coronary angioplasty. *J Am Coll Cardiol, 11:*970, 1988.

38. Homma S, et al.: Usefulness of oral dipyridamole suspension for stress thallium imaging without exercise in the detection of coronary artery disease. *Am J Cardiol, 57:*503, 1986.

39. Ranhosky A, Kempthorne-Rawson J, and the Intravenous Dipyridamole Thallium Imaging Study Group: The safety of intravenous dipyridamole thallium myocardial perfusion imaging. *Circulation, 81:*1205, 1990.

40. Josephson MA, et al.: Noninvasive detection and localization of coronary stenosis in patients: Comparison of resting dipyridamole and exercise thallium-201 myocardial perfusion imaging. *Am Heart J, 103:*1008, 1982.

41. Bayliss J, Pearson M, Sutton GC: Ventricular dysrhythmias following intravenous dipyridamole during stress myocardial imaging. *Br J Radiol, 56:*686, 1983.

42. Friedman HZ, Goldberg SF, Hauser AM, O'Neill WW: Death with dipyridamole thallium imaging. *Ann Intern Med, 109:*990, 1988.

43. Afonso S: Inhibition of coronary vasodilating action of dipyridamole and adenosine by aminophylline in the dog. *Circ Res, 26:*743, 1979.

44. Londos L, Cooper DMF, Wolff J: Subclasses of adenosine receptors. *Proc Nat Acad Sci USA, 77:*2551, 1980.

45. DiMarco JP, et al.: Adenosine: Electrophysiologic effects and therapeutic use for terminating paroxysmal supraventricular tachycardia. *Circulation, 68:*1254, 1983.

46. Fenton RA, Bruttig SP, Rubio R, Berne RM: Effect of adenosine in calcium uptake by intact and cultured vascular smooth muscle. *Am J Physiol, 252:*H598, 1987.

47. Verani MS, et al.: Diagnosis of coronary artery disease by controlled coronary vasodilatation with adenosine and thallium-201 scintigraphy in patients unable to exercise. *Circulation, 82:*80, 1990.

48. Nguyen T, Heo J, Ogilby JD, Iskandian AS: Single photon emission computed tomography with thallium-201 during adenosine-induced coronary hyperemia. Correlation with coronary arteriography, exercise thallium imaging and two-dimensional echocardiography. *J Am Coll Cardiol, 16:*1375, 1990.

49. Moser GH, Schrader J, Deussen A: Turnover of adenosine in plasma of human and dog blood. *Am J Physiol, 256:*C799, 1989.

50. Homma S, Gilliland Y, Gviney TE, Strauss HW: Safety of intravenous dipyridamole for stress testing with thallium imaging. *Am J Cardiol, 59:*152, 1987.

51. Cushley MJ, Tatterfield AE, Holgate ST: Inhaled adenosine and guanosine on airway resistance in normal and asthmatic subjects. *Br J Clin Pharmacol, 15:*161, 1983.

52. Conradson TBG, Dixon CMS, Clark B, Barnes PJ: Cardiovascular effects of infused adenosine in man. Potentiation by dipyridamole. *Acta Physiol Scan, 129:*387, 1987.

53. Berthe C, et al.: Predicting the extent and location of coronary artery disease in acute myocardial infarction by echocardiography during dobutamine infusion. *Am J Cardiol, 58:*1167, 1986.

54. Sawada SG, et al.: Echocardiographic detection of coronary artery disease during dobutamine infusion. *Circulation, 83:*1605, 1991.

55. Cohen JL, et al.: Dobutamine digital echocardiography for detecting coronary artery disease. *Am J Cardiol, 67:*1311, 1991.

56. Savas V, et al.: Dobutamine stress echocardiography. An alternative to thallium scintigraphy. *Circulation, 82:*III-744, 1990.

57. Brown SE, et al.: Detection of coronary stenosis using dobutamine stress echocardiogram: Correlation with quantitative angiography. *Circulation, 80:*II-337, 1989.

58. Pierard LA, Delandsheere CM, Berthe C: Identification of viable myocardium by echocardiography during dobutamine infusion in patients with myocardial infarction after lytic therapy. Comparison with positron emission tomography. *J Am Coll Cardiol, 15:*1021, 1990.

59. Armstrong WF, O'Donnell J, Ryan T, Feigenbaum H: Effect of prior myocardial infarction and extent and location of coronary disease on accuracy of exercise echocardiography. *J Am Coll Cardiol, 10:* 531, 1987.

60. Martin TW, et al.: Comparison of adenosine, dipyridamole, and dobutamine in stress echocardiography. *Ann Intern Med, 116:*190, 1992.

61. Frazin L, et al.: Esophageal echocardiography. *Circulation, 54:*102, 1976.

62. Hisanaza K, et al.: A new transesophageal real-time two-dimensional echocardiographic system using a flexible tube and its clinical application. *Pro Jpn Soc Ultrson Med, 32:*43, 1977.

63. Schlüter M, et al.: Transesophageal cross-sectional echocardiography with a phased array transducer system. Technique and initial clinical results. *Br Heart J, 48:*67, 1982.

64. Melendez LJ, et al.: Incidence of bacteremia in transesophageal echocardiography: A prospective study of 140 consecutive patients. *J Am Coll Cardiol, 18:*1650, 1991.

65. Daniel WG, et al.: Safety of transesophageal echocardiography: A multicenter survey of 10,419 examinations. *Circulation, 83:*817, 1991.

66. Mügge A, Daniel WG, Haverich A, Lichtlen PR: Diagnosis of noninfective cardiac mass lesions by two-dimensional echocardiography. Comparison of the transthoracic and transesophageal approaches. *Circulation, 83:*70, 1991.

67. Reeder GS, Khandheria BK, Seward JB, Tajik AJ: Transesophageal echocardiography and cardiac masses. *Mayo Clin Proc, 66:* 1101, 1991.

68. Mügge A, Daniel WG, Frank G, Lichtlen PR: Echocardiography in infective endocarditis: Reassessment of prognostic implications of vegetation size determined by the transthoracic and the transesophageal approach. *J Am Coll Cardiol, 14:*631, 1989.

69. Taams MA, et al.: Enhanced morphological diagnosis in infective endocarditis by transesophageal echocardiography. *Br Heart J, 63:*109, 1990.

70. Erbel R, et al.: Improved diagnostic value of echocardiography in patients with infective endocarditis by transesophageal approach. A prospective study. *Eur Heart J, 9:* 43, 1988.

71. Daniel WG, et al.: Improvement in the diagnosis of abscesses associated with endocarditis by transesophageal echocardiography. *N Engl J Med, 324:*795, 1991.

72. Khandheria BK, et al.: Value and limitations of transesophageal echocardiography in assessment of mitral valve prostheses. *Circulation, 83:*1956, 1991.

73. Erbel R, et al.: Echocardiography in diagnosis of aortic dissection. *Lancet, 1:*457, 1989.

74. Treasure T, Raphael MJ: Investigation of suspected dissection of the thoracic aorta. *Lancet, 338:*490, 1991.

75. Pavlides GS, et al.: Contribution of transesophageal echocardiography to patient diagnosis and treatment: A prospective analysis. *Am Heart J, 120:*910, 1990.

76. Grossman W: Complications of cardiac catheterization: Incidence, causes, and prevention. In *Cardiac Catheterization, Angiography and Intervention.* 4th Edition. Edited by W Grossman and DS Baim. Philadelphia: Lea & Febiger, 1991.

77. Wyman RM, et al.: Current complications of diagnostic and therapeutic cardiac catheterization. *J Am Coll Cardiol, 12:*1400, 1988.

Section V

EXERCISE PROGRAMMING

Chapter 23

DECISION MAKING IN PROGRAMMING EXERCISE

Patricia L. Painter and William L. Haskell

The accumulation of information, experience, and knowledge in the science of exercise physiology has resulted in the widespread incorporation of exercise training as adjunctive therapy for individuals with documented heart disease, those at high risk for its development, and those interested in its prevention. The rapid growth of preventive and rehabilitative programs may result in a haphazard or "cookbook" approach to exercise prescription in which exercise staff members use only minimal information when developing an exercise prescription according to a set of guidelines that may not, in all cases, be appropriate. Decision making in preventive and rehabilitative exercise programming should be a logically consistent and comprehensive approach to developing and implementing exercise programs and life-style modifications. Such an approach increases the chances of achieving the goals of (1) individualized exercise prescription, (2) ensuring safety for participants, and (3) facilitating regular participation in lifelong activity.

We present a model for decision making in preventive and rehabilitative exercise programs. This model is developed from extensive clinical experience in cardiac rehabilitation, although it is applicable when developing and implementing exercise for any population. When using this model, we emphasize the use of the *Guidelines for Exercise Testing and Prescription* as a starting point, making modifications for individuals according to sound clinical judgment and common sense. The *Guidelines* are not intended to provide final answers for all situations encountered in exercise prescription or programming, because a vast amount of information on the optimal relationships between frequency, intensity, and duration for developing cardiovascular fit-

ness, modifying risk factors, assisting in weight control, or affecting psychologic status remain unknown and are subject to further study.

DEVELOPING POLICY AND MAKING DECISIONS

To ensure the safety of all who participate in exercise (participant, staff, and facility), program policy must be firmly established and followed. This policy must address all phases of the participant/program interactions shown in Table 23–1: (1) screening for exercise; (2) developing the exercise prescription; (3) implementing the exercise prescription; and (4) maintenance of appropriate exercise. Good policy development should be based on available scientific and clinical principles of exercise testing, prescription, and training; facilitate flexibility and guidance in decision making by exercise program staff members and participants; protect and provide for the safety of the participant; and protect the program and exercise personnel.

The development of program policy and the decision making on the part of the exercise staff require consideration of several factors at all levels of the participant/program interaction. Each of these factors for consideration is actually a continuum of possibilities (Table 23–2); for example, the health status of individuals interested in exercise training ranges from normal, healthy individuals with no risk factors for disease to persons with multisystem disease processes. Similarly, program settings can range from the community health club or recreation department to the medical center research exercise laboratory.

The focus of this discussion is the importance of each of these considerations in developing policy and making decisions con-

Table 23–1. Phases of Program/Participant Interactions

Screening
  Exercise
  No exercise
  Further evaluation → no exercise
  Further evaluation → exercise
Exercise prescription development
  Type of activity
  Frequency
  Duration
  Intensity
  Progression
Implementation of the exercise prescription
  Exercise setting
  Time of exercise
  Level of monitoring
  Level of supervision
  Group or individual exercise
  Emergency plans
Maintenance
  Progression
  Periodic evaluation
  Supervision levels
  Motivational techniques

cerning exercise programming. Whatever policy is developed for an exercise program, the program personnel must understand the reasons behind the policies and be comfortable with their implementation. Exceptions to any policy should be kept to a minimum and then only with documented rationale.

PHASES OF PROGRAM/PARTICIPANT INTERACTIONS (Table 23–1)

Screening is the process by which the determination is made whether a participant will exercise in a given exercise program. Screening results in a decision to (1) reject an individual for exercise; (2) refer the individual for further medical evaluation and/or treatment before acceptance for exercise; (3) refer the individual to a program with more appropriate levels of supervision; or (4) accept the individual for exercise. The *Development of an Exercise Prescription* is the process of integrating information obtained from the medical and/or health history and exercise assessment into an individualized exercise program, with specific prescription of the ap-

Table 23–2. Factors to Consider at Every Level of Program/Participant Interaction

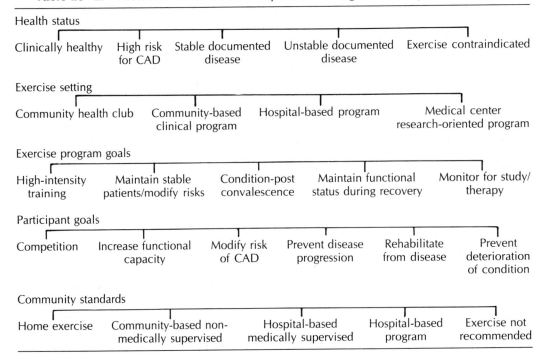

Health status				
Clinically healthy	High risk for CAD	Stable documented disease	Unstable documented disease	Exercise contraindicated

Exercise setting			
Community health club	Community-based clinical program	Hospital-based program	Medical center research-oriented program

Exercise program goals				
High-intensity training	Maintain stable patients/modify risks	Condition-post convalescence	Maintain functional status during recovery	Monitor for study/ therapy

Participant goals					
Competition	Increase functional capacity	Modify risk of CAD	Prevent disease progression	Rehabilitate from disease	Prevent deterioration of condition

Community standards				
Home exercise	Community-based non-medically supervised	Hospital-based medically supervised	Hospital-based program	Exercise not recommended

propriate type, frequency, duration, and intensity of activity. The *Implementation of the Exercise Prescription* phase is the manner in which the participants follow their unique exercise prescription. The variable factors in successful implementation of exercise include the time of exercise, the physical setting, level of monitoring, levels of staff supervision and qualifications of staff, group or individual exercise, the use of resistance and upper body exercise, and emergency plans to ensure safety for the participant and the program. Successful implementation of exercise facilitates regular participation, enjoyment, and safety for all participants. The *Maintenance or Continuation of the Exercise Program* phase is the process of keeping a participant involved in appropriate levels of physical activity for a lifetime. This process involves periodic evaluation of a participant's responses to exercise, modification of the exercise (increasing or decreasing duration or intensity), re-evaluation of the levels of supervision and/or monitoring, and developing motivational techniques to increase adherence and enjoyability.

Screening

The *health status* of the individual participant is of major importance in all levels of exercise programming. An individual may become involved in an exercise program at any point on a continuum (see Table 23–2). Therefore, to know that for certain medical conditions there are definite contraindications to exercise is essential. For these patients, any benefits that may be derived from exercise training are outweighed by the potential risk of medical complications and possible death when exercise is applied (see page 13 in *Guidelines for Exercise Testing and Prescription*. 3rd Ed.). In addition, certain conditions exist in which the individual is at risk of medical complications and/or death with exercise, but the benefits of exercise training (either physiologic or possibly psychologic) may outweigh the risks. Careful screening and subsequent placement into appropriate programs can reduce the risks of acceptable levels.

The *exercise setting* also determines whether an individual's participation in a given exercise program is appropriate. A hospital-based exercise program that is medically supervised with ECG monitoring capabilities and has rapid in-house emergency response time is most appropriate for individuals at high risk of medical complications with exercise (i.e., low ejection fraction, poorly controlled dysrhythmias, and angina). For participants with documented disease who demonstrate stable responses to exercise, a program with less supervision and less of a "medical" environment may be most appropriate to decrease dependency on the clinical team, decrease costs, and encourage individual responsibility in the rehabilitation process. Interaction with normal, healthy individuals in a well-controlled environment may be beneficial for many of these patients.

Program goals and *participant goals* for exercise must also be considered in the screening process. If the goals of the program and the participant are compatible, acceptance into the program is appropriate. For example, if a program is designed solely for maintaining cardiovascular fitness, and an individual's goal is to train for competition, a more appropriate gesture is to refer the individual to a program that can assist in meeting that goal (if that goal is appropriate considering the patient's health status).

Community standards may also be considered in the screening process, although this factor should not dictate the criteria for entry into the program. Respecting community attitudes, even if somewhat conservative, is important, especially when starting a program. Experience and careful implementation and documentation assists in molding community standards as long as there is well-documented clinical data to support a more progressive approach to screening for exercise.

The screening process must assess the risk-benefit ratio of exercise not only for the individual participant, but also for the exercise program. Appropriate screening of individuals for entrance into a program is a major step in avoiding potential legal problems with the exercise, which can have serious financial and public relations consequences. Program staff members should never hesitate to request further evaluation and/or treatment from the referring physician before accepting a participant into the exercise program. They also should not hesitate to refer individuals to another program if they believe the individual requires a higher level of medical monitoring and supervision than they are able to provide. Program personnel should also be willing to refer an individual to a program with lower levels of supervision in an attempt to decrease dependence on the clinical staff.

Development of the Exercise Prescription

The *health status* of the individual is a major consideration when developing an exercise prescription. Examples include special concern for the type of activity when a subject has orthopedic limitations and exclusion of patients with poor left ventricular function in strength training activities. As indicated in the *Guidelines*, the health status of the individual also determines the intensity and duration of exercise. The rate of progression of exercise is also affected by health status. For example, individuals at a higher risk stratification level are expected to progress more slowly because of a more conservative exercise prescription (i.e., lower intensity) and often as a result of the physiologic limitations imposed by the disease. Likewise, individuals who have been somewhat active should progress faster in their exercise program than sedentary individuals whose slower progression is primarily to avoid injuries and to ensure appropriate adaptation in previously unused muscles.

The *exercise setting* clearly affects the exercise prescription—activities depending on facilities, equipment, and emergency responses available. *Program goals* and *participant goals* must be assessed carefully when developing the exercise prescription. Ideally, an exercise program is established with the goals of improving health status, including exercise tolerance and reducing risk factors for heart disease. A program designed to develop strength with minimal cardiovascular training (i.e., high-intensity, short-duration cardiovascular training) is inappropriate for a participant who has a primary goal of losing weight. That participant should be referred to a program that offers aerobic exercise at lower intensity and longer duration as well as dietary counseling.

The *goals of the participant* are of paramount importance when developing an exercise prescription. Little is gained by developing an exercise prescription of aerobic exercise 3 times a week for 30 minutes at an intensity of 60 to 70% of maximal capacity if the individual's goal is to change from a totally sedentary lifestyle and maybe get some social interaction as well. The closer the prescribed exercise is to meeting the goals of the individual, the more likely the individual is to adhere to the exercise and possibly become interested in more structured exercise at the frequency, intensity, and duration that result in positive health benefits in the future.

Epidemiologic evidence exists that only 15 to 20% of the general population exercises regularly, according to the recommended "ideal" exercise prescription. In most cases, getting the individual to initiate some form of acceptable activity is of benefit, as is spending time identifying barriers that may exist to incorporating regular activity into their lifestyle. Such barriers may include previous experiences with exercise that either were not enjoyable or were unsuccessful; time demands placed on the individual by job, family commitments, and the like; and cultural background and socioeconomic status, which dictate acceptable and feasible activity patterns. Identification of such "barriers" should assist program staff members and the participant to be creative in developing plans to overcome the barriers and to optimize the potential for success with the exercise program.

Community standards for exercise prescription may vary widely; often, any deviation from the typical 3 days per week for 30 min at 60 to 70% of maximal capacity may be questioned. It is well worth the efforts of the program staff to document compliance to exercise and physiologic responses to the exercise prescriptions to demonstrate safety and efficacy of variations in the typical exercise prescription.

Implementation of the Exercise Prescription

The *health status* of the participants has significant bearing on how exercise is implemented; it determines the levels of monitoring, supervision (numbers of staff and qualifications necessary), as well as necessary emergency procedures. The organization of the actual exercise session also is affected by the health status of participants; for example, those persons requiring careful monitoring would not be involved in group activities.

Assessment of participants before the exercise session varies according to health status. At certain times, an individual should not exercise, and reasons for temporarily deferring physical activity on a given day are listed in Table 23–3. In some instances, the exercise staff may allow a participant to exercise—with a modified prescription (i.e., decreased intensity) and/or with increased levels of supervision or monitoring—depending on established policy as well as the personnel and resources available for the exercise session.

The regular assessment of the participant's response to exercise is an essential part of implementing the exercise prescription. Such an assessment may: (1) indicate the need to modify the exercise prescription (i.e., increase duration and/or

Table 23–3. Reasons to Temporarily Defer Physical Activity*

Recurrent illness
Progression of cardiac disease
Abnormally elevated blood pressure
Recent changes in symptoms (see Table 23–4)
Orthopedic problem
Emotional turmoil
Severe sunburn
Alcoholic hangover
Cerebral dysfunction—dizziness or vertigo
Sodium retention—edema or weight gain
Dehydration
Environmental factors
   Weather (excessive heat or humidity)
   Air pollution (smog or carbon monoxide)
Overindulgence
   Heavy, large meal within 2 hours
   Coffee, tea, Coke (xanthines and other stimulating beverages)
Drugs
   Decongestants
   Bronchodilators
   Atropine
   Weight reduction agents

* Modified from the American Heart Association.

Table 23–4. Signs and Symptoms of Excessive Effort

During and/or immediately after exercise:
   Anginal discomfort
   Ataxia, lightheadedness, or confusion
   Nausea or vomiting
   Leg claudication
   Pallor or cyanosis
   Dyspnea persisting for more than 10 min
   Dysrhythmia
   Inappropriate brachycardia
   Decrease in systolic blood pressure
Delayed:
   Prolonged fatigue (24 hr or more)
   Insomnia
   Weight gain due to fluid retention—salt and water overload; heart failure
   Persistent tachycardia

intensity in an individual who may not be achieving an appropriate training stimulus); (2) reveal symptoms or signs of excessive effort (Table 23–4); and (3) reveal inappropriate responses to exercise, which may be indicative of a progression of disease and/or the appearance of symptoms that may in turn indicate the development of new medical problems. Levels of concern about such signs depends on the health status of the participant involved. Often a decrease in the intensity of exercise may alleviate the symptoms; however, persistence of such signs and/or symptoms should prompt discontinuation of exercise and referral to the physician for further evaluation (Table 23–5).

Remember that healthy individuals participating in an exercise program may also experience changes in their physiologic status with exercise and/or over time, which may be indicative of early signs and/or pro-

Table 23–5. Indications to Discontinue Exercise Program

Orthopedic problems aggravated by activity
Progression of cardiac illness unresponsive to medical therapy
Development of new systemic disease aggravated by exercise
Major surgery
Psychiatric decompensation
Acute alcoholism

gression of subclinical disease. Examples of such signs and symptoms are listed in Table 23–6. All exercise staff members should be aware of these symptoms and should be prepared to refer the individual to a physician should they appear.

The *program goals* determine not only the equipment and staffing requirements, but also the actual structure of the exercise sessions. The implementation of the exercise prescription in programs designed to monitor medically high-risk individuals differs from implementation in those programs that provide a supervised setting for stable patients with documented disease. The level of responsibility placed on the individual in an exercise program should be determined by the program goals. For example, a program designed to return the participant to an active job places emphasis on individual responsibility (with staff support and encouragement) to help promote a sense of independence and a healthy lifestyle, which includes a program of lifelong exercise. In contrast, the staff of a program designed to monitor high-risk patients need to observe ECG and blood pressure responses to exercise carefully and to document any signs or symptoms of "maladaptation" in the physiologic responses for further evaluation and treatment by the physician. This setting requires higher staffing ratios, and the participant's involvement in implementing the exercise prescription may be minimal.

Successful implementation of the exercise prescription also necessitates evaluation of the participant goals and needs. For most participants, convenient access to the

Table 23–6. Indications of a Change in Physiologic Status or Progression of Disease

Excessive fatigue
Shortness of breath
Angina (or change in typical angina patterns)
Change in cardiac rhythm
Dramatic increase in weight
Swelling of extremities
Unexplained restlessness or fatigue
Unexplained change in blood pressure at rest or during exercise
Reduction in physical working capacity

exercise setting is important. Timing of the exercise sessions should meet the needs of the participants involved and not only those of the staff or facility. Participants who work full-time and/or odd shifts may be excluded from programs that are unable to offer flexible hours. To have participants feel rushed or stressed getting to the exercise session is undesirable, especially for individuals who use the exercise as a part of a stress management program.

Patient expectations should also be considered when organizing exercise classes. For example, participants who are interested in efficient use of time may want to complete the exercise sessions with little social interaction; individual exercise on a treadmill or other exercise equipment may be appropriate for these individuals. People who are interested in a variety of activities and peer interaction may be most compliant to a program that provides group or game activities. Patients for whom the primary goal is to return to work and/or leisure time activities, such as gardening, hunting, and the like that require significant use of the upper body, benefit from the incorporation of resistance training and upper body activities as a part of their program. Circuit training involving the use of a variety of types of apparatus may be well suited for these individuals (see Chapter 25).

Community standards may dictate some aspects of exercise implementation. Communities with a limited number of programs available have to accommodate a wide variety of participants (and therefore medical conditions) in the same setting. This spectrum complicates the organization of the sessions, staffing requirements, and possibly the monitoring procedures. Other factors affected by community standards include: (1) levels of monitoring required for various patient groups; (2) use of resistance exercise in clinical populations; (3) qualifications of the staff for various patient populations; (4) levels of physician involvement in the exercise program; and (5) emergency procedures. The variable expectations and attitudes of referring physicians in the community must be addressed when developing and implementing the exercise prescription.

Maintenance

Once the exercise program is initiated, the challenge to the exercise staff is to motivate the participants to continue to try to keep physical activity as an integral part of the lifestyle. The health status of an individual may determine how this task is accomplished. We recommend some form of periodic evaluation of exercise responses in all participants. Participants at high risk for developing heart disease and those with documented disease should be evaluated for ECG and blood pressure responses, either during an exercise stress test or at their prescribed exercise intensity. As described in the previous section, such periodic evaluations may result in modification of the exercise prescription, decreased or increased levels of supervision, referral to the personal physician for further evaluation and/or treatment, discontinuation of the exercise program, or referral to a more appropriate exercise setting. In community-based adult fitness programs, field testing or submaximal exercise testing can be used to demonstrate progress. Periodic evaluations track progress with the exercise and may be used for motivational purposes.

Motivational techniques, such as distance records, noncompetitive games, low-level competitions, and predicted time runs, challenge the staff to be creative and keep participants involved and satisfied with their program.

The *exercise setting* often determines the long-term outcome of an exercise program. For example, a hospital-based, monitored exercise program often is not able to accommodate those individuals who "graduate" to nonmonitored exercise; these participants should be referred to a less-supervised exercise program. Another example is the participant in a jogging program who is injured and thus requires the use of facilities to perform other activities.

Similarly, the *exercise program goals* determine which participants continue to exercise in their program. As long as the exercise program goals and the *participant goals* are in accord and the health status does not change, the participant can continue to exercise. These goals must also be reassessed periodically to ensure that all parties involved remain satisfied with the current program.

The consideration of *community standards* in maintenance of the exercise program is similar to that discussed in *Implementation of the Exercise Prescription*. Because of the lack of third-party payments for some exercise programs, many physicians refer their patients to community-based programs, or advise home exercise. This practice is reasonable for normal healthy individuals or for persons with risk factors for development of coronary artery disease. Low-risk patients with stable exercise responses can maintain their exercise programs at home or in unmonitored and minimally supervised programs. The key factor in this approach is identification of patients who are at high risk for complications during exercise before advising continuation of exercise outside the monitored setting.

Exercise training is a valuable tool in the management of patients, as well as in improving the health and functional status of the healthy population. Exercise can, however, have deleterious effects if participants are inappropriately screened; if the exercise prescription is developed and implemented from inadequate information (medical and individual); or if the exercise staff members are unaware of changes in a participant's health status. Exercise is, in itself, a physiologic stress to the individual, which is only beneficial when applied to individuals who are in a stable medical and physiologic state. The benefits of exercise training are cumulative with time. Therefore, to defer exercise for evaluation (and possible follow-up treatment) is reasonable when a change in medical status is suspected, instead of continuing exercise when the individual is not stable and therefore is placed at undue risk.

Decisions must be made by the exercise program staff at each of the possible participant/program interactions. These decisions should be made based on sound clinical judgment with consideration of the factors discussed in this chapter. Program policy must support this decision-making process. The decisions made by the exercise program staff are actually risk and benefit evaluations. In decision making, the exercise staff should ask, "what are the risks to the participant," and "what would result in the greatest short- and long-term benefit to the participant?" A risk-benefit evaluation must also be made for the program. For example, in the screening process, the staff should ask, "what risks are associated with involving this individual in our exercise program," and "what short- and long-term benefits can we provide for this individual?" This framework of policy devel-opment and decision making aids the exercise staff in meeting the goals of providing a safe, beneficial, and enjoyable exercise program for all persons involved.

ACKNOWLEDGMENTS

The authors thank Neil Oldridge, Steve Blair, and William Allen for their ideas, review, and support in preparing this chapter.

Chapter 24

EXERCISE LEADERSHIP: KEY SKILLS AND CHARACTERISTICS

Patricia J. McSwegin and Cynthia L. Pemberton

The popular image of an exercise leader is that of an energetic individual with a fit body and loud voice. Those characteristics contribute to an exercise leader's effectiveness, but they are not the key factors in leadership. An effective exercise leader has the skills of a good teacher. Both are knowledgeable about their subject, adjust their leadership style to meet the objectives of their situation, communicate effectively, organize activities to maximize participation and safety, observe specific behaviors to provide individual feedback, and create a positive motivational climate. Other chapters in this book cover the exercise knowledge base; this chapter describes the key concepts and techniques of creating a positive motivational climate, developing interpersonal communication skills, understanding leadership styles, using organizational strategies, and providing feedback, all of which underlie effective leadership in exercise situations.

CREATING A POSITIVE MOTIVATIONAL CLIMATE

The key to successful exercise leadership is the creation of a positive motivational climate, an atmosphere that provides opportunities for clients to participate successfully in various experiences. The exercise leader must be aware that success can be defined in a number of different ways, depending on the needs and perceptions of individual clients.[1] A positive environment should be warm (clients feel welcome and respected), interesting (clients learn facts and how to apply those facts in ways that are meaningful in their personal lives), and effective (clients engage in activities that move them toward achievement of their goals).

Current research[2] suggests that exercise clients need to establish lifelong activity habits (which requires them to become responsible decision makers); thus exercise leaders must provide more than a model of how to do specific exercises. They must help clients establish beneficial habits in exercise, diet, and stress control by getting them involved in experiences that increase their knowledge, enhance their movement skills, and move them toward intrinsic (self) motivation. Having clients simply follow the routines demonstrated by a floor leader will not contribute to their becoming self-sufficient. Skill development and motivation both require the leader to observe individual behavior and provide appropriate feedback on how to improve that behavior.

Both the client who is recovering from some type of cardiovascular event and the one merely exercising to lose weight need to be motivated to engage regularly in appropriate physical activity. One step in helping clients enhance motivation is to improve their understanding of the hows, whys, and whats of exercise. Such information can be delivered in special lectures, independent of activity time, or as an integral, ongoing part of activity sessions. Client motivation to continue exercising can be enhanced also by helping them learn how to move appropriately and to discover how to make modifications for their own situations and conditions. A third step in enhancing client motivation is to provide a positive, encouraging environment through words and gestures which recognize client achievements, suggest ways to improve further, and offer support for continued effort.

INTERPERSONAL COMMUNICATION SKILLS AND CONCEPTS

Clarity of communication is a major factor in establishing an effective motivational climate and requires specific knowledge and skills. The first step in developing communication skills is to understand the various aspects of oral communication: verbal/nonverbal, sending/receiving, content/emotion.[3] An effective communicator formulates messages with an understanding of how they may be received, including the messages that might be seen as well as heard, and then listens to responses from, and watches reactions of, the listener to evaluate the effectiveness of the message sent.

During the process of communication, the primary focus of most individuals is on formulation of their message (content) into words (verbal) to be sent (sending), ignoring the nonverbal, receiving, and content aspects. Failure to recognize how the receiver might interpret the nonverbal and emotional aspects of the message often leads to misunderstanding. For example, exercise leaders usually greet clients with some inquiry like "How are you?" and then, expecting an automatic "I'm okay," often do not attend to the client's answer. Yet the client's response (verbal or nonverbal), might relay a message (through content or emotion) that this person needs attention, wants to talk more, or is not well and is seeking help on how to modify his or her activity that day.

That same simple message ("How are you?") serves as an example of the importance of planning for nonverbal as well as verbal aspects of communication. Body language, proxemics, and paralanguage are non-verbal aspects of communication.[3] The messages sent by body language, (eye contact, posture, and gestures) are often different, and more powerful, than the words themselves. Establishing eye contact, leaning toward the client, having alert posture, and using gestures of openness (hands turned upward) are consistent with a sincere inquiry regarding one's health. *Proxemics* refers to spatial relationships among people. The exercise leader must be careful not to invade personal space, that is, not to get too close physically to clients (other than when offering technical support that requires manipulation). Conversely, keeping a physical distance conveys coldness and lack of individual caring. Hall, cited in Martens,[3] suggests 4 to 12

feet as the appropriate distance for social situations. *Paralanguage* refers to qualities of voice, such as pitch and tempo, which convey meaning beyond the meaning of the words spoken. It refers also to the emotional aspects of the message conveyed by various characteristics of the voice and speech patterns used.[3] A listless, weak, flat "How are you?" might be worse than ignoring the client because the message received is one of not really caring. The voice qualities used—pitch, richness, enunciation, speed, loudness, and rhythm—have a major effect on the message. In fact, the emotional, nonverbal aspects of a verbal communication can override the content, distorting what was meant to be conveyed. To be an effective leader, one must practice blending the listening, nonverbal, and emotional elements of oral communication with the sending, verbal and content aspects.

Martens[3] offers several guidelines on how and what to practice to improve message delivery. Key among those guidelines are the need to:

1. Deliver a direct, specific message with no hidden meanings. (e.g., "Do not allow the weights to bang. Banging the weights indicates lack of control, which is dangerous to you and to the equipment.")

2. Deliver a clear, consistent message—focus on one thing and repeat it. (e.g., "Warm-up is the first part of a good exercise routine. Be sure to warm up before starting vigorous activity.")

3. Separate fact from opinion—(e.g., "Too much fat in the diet is not healthful, but in my opinion it is okay to eat ice-cream once a week.")

4. Make sure that verbal and nonverbal aspects of your message match each other and your meaning. (e.g., a smile, eye contact, and an extended hand should accompany "Welcome to class!")

5. Check to find out if the listener understands the message as it was meant to be conveyed. (e.g., "Do you have any questions?" or "Try that move while I check your form.")

LEADERSHIP STYLES

Communication skills are important to develop, no matter what leadership or teaching style is used, but the particular style used in delivering the program (i.e., leadership style) is important also. Leadership can be discussed from many perspectives, the leader as strategist, motivator, facilitator, arbiter, or scholar. Because exercise leaders need to be teachers as well as leaders, and because the leadership elements of teaching encompass all of the perspectives identified above, this section addresses leadership styles as they relate to the teaching role of an exercise leader. (An exercise leader might also have other roles, such as those related to public relations, budgeting, maintenance, etc.)

In general, there are two basic teaching or leadership styles: direct and indirect.[4] In the *direct* or command style, clients are told exactly what to do, when, and how. They have little opportunity to make decisions regarding their behavior. This style is particularly effective when organizing large groups and for ensuring that immediate safety needs are met. It is not as effective if a program goal is for clients to develop self-responsibility and decision-making skills.

The *indirect* style provides clients with more opportunity to explore (movements, concepts, machines, etc.) and make decisions for themselves regarding how, when, and where they will participate. The leader's role in an indirect style is to arrange experiences that encourage clients to explore, e.g., selecting aerobic dance music, designing their own weight training program, and working with partners or in groups for encouragement and sharing of knowledge. Using the indirect style does not mean that the leader simply watches clients do whatever they choose; this leader creates opportunities for clients to learn, but in a manner that allows each client to have a role in determining the pace, direction, and shape of the learning. There is more individualization of both learning and participation in the indirect style. In reality, many leaders use a combination of teaching styles, creating a continuum from direct to indirect style. Teaching styles fall along the continuum depending on the situation, clients, type of class, expectations of clients, and goals of the class, including how much choice should be given to the clients as compared to how much control should be asserted by the leader. Table 24–1[4] describes the strengths of teaching styles.

In selecting a leadership style, one must first consider how comfortable he or she will feel in carrying out the responsibilities of leadership required by that style. Second, and just as important, one must consider the program objectives in regard to clients. If the objective is simply to teach clients certain activity routines and exercise techniques, the direct style can be effective. The leader models activity and the clients follow, gaining knowledge about the activity and benefit from the participation. But if the objective is more complex (e.g., to gain skill in analyzing one's own needs, to figure out how to accomplish fitness goals in a variety of manners, or to strengthen one's attitude toward an active lifestyle), the indirect style is particularly good. In this case, the leader poses questions, devises challenging scenarios, and encourages clients to participate at individual paces in various activities, with the intent of gaining insight into themselves. Using a command (direct) style is usually easier for a beginning leader with a large group, but even a new leader can combine elements of

Table 24–1. Strengths of Teaching Styles*

Direct	Indirect
Objectives set by leader	Methods chosen by client
Tasks chosen by leader	Cognitive learning increased
Evaluation chosen by leader	Learning individualized
Safety maximized	Problem solving encouraged
Time used efficiently	
Large groups managed effectively	
Learning of simple tasks maximized	

* Adapted with permission from Kirchner G: *Physical Education for Elementary School Children.* Dubuque: William C. Brown, 1992; and from Graham G, Holt-Hale S, Parker M: *Children Moving.* Mountain View, CA: Mayfield, 1987.

the two styles to fit the particular needs of the situation. Given the diverse nature of exercise programs and of learner preference, it is recommended that exercise leaders be familiar with various teaching styles and become adept at using the style appropriate to the situation.[4]

Organizational Skills

To give attention to each client individually, the leader must be positioned in a manner that allows each client to see and to be seen. Usually such positioning requires the leader to move around and through the class. However, some organizational patterns, such as stations, systematically move the clients so that each can be observed without much leader movement. The exercise leader should be prepared to employ a variety of organizational patterns to provide for clear observation of clients and to ensure that clients also have a clear view and sufficient movement space. Table 24–2[4] describes various organizational patterns and identifies uses of each.

The exercise leader must also consider what to look and listen for when surveying the clients. Too often, leaders merely scan the group and ignore sounds. Is there a hum of activity in the weight training room? Are the clients moving from machine to machine? Do the sounds and movement patterns indicate that lots of activity is occurring? A scan of the room can answer those questions, but while scanning, the leader needs to look and listen for specific actions and sounds: full extension on bench presses, backs firmly supported during overhead presses, metallic clicks from weight machines, chin tucked on sit-ups, etc. To quickly and accurately notice such points, the leader must first have clearly in mind the key actions desired and then focus on searching for those actions while looking or walking about the exercise facility. (The exercise leader draws upon his or her knowledge base to determine key actions and to make decisions about corrective procedures.)

In addition to looking at and listening for specific actions, the leader must attend to individuals, even when leading a large group. During scanning, the leader can pause frequently to look at various individuals, to make eye contact with each in turn, and to ask each client how they are doing. The leader should focus on one client long enough to pick up on nonverbal messages that may indicate discomfort or concern.

Feedback Considerations

Having made specific observations, the leader then needs to provide appropriate feedback to groups and to individuals. This feedback can be of a general or specific nature, but positive feedback appears to be more effective in increasing motivation.[5] *General feedback* acknowledges good effort and encourages clients to continue their activity. A pat on the back, a smile, the thumbs-up sign, and a hearty "Good job" are all examples of general feedback. General feedback can be given during the activity and/or as a summary statement at the end of the workout: "Great effort today!" or "You really kept those feet moving today!" General feedback is important for individuals as well as groups because it provides emotional support to each participant.

However, specific feedback may be needed to help participants learn how to do exercises for themselves or to learn enough to be able to independently follow exercise prescriptions properly. *Specific feedback* provides information about the exercise being done. For example, are knees bent and feet flat during sit-ups, is footfall heel-to-toe in jogging, are elbows kept in front of the pelvic bones on arm curls? Using technique reminder cues for the group is acceptable, but ultimately each client needs to discover if he/she is doing the activity correctly and, if not, how to correct it.

In providing feedback, especially specific feedback, the leader applies knowledge about exercising to the actual situation as it occurs with each client. For example, the aqua-aerobics leader is likely to have instructed the group on the importance of moving as vigorously as possible without bouncing hard off of the pool floor. Having scanned the class, the leader comments on the group's good effort (general feedback) and then reminds a given individual to bend the knees when landing to reduce the impact with the pool floor (specific

Table 24–2. Organizational Patterns

Formation	Explanation	Uses
Circle X X X X X X X X X X	Form circle by having clients follow leader as leader circles. Other methods include joining hands and forming a circle, or having the class take position on a circle printed on the floor or exercise area.	Warm-up exercises Mimetics Teaching simple stunts Teaching basic dance steps Simple games Circle relays
Line X X X Y X X	Place client for each line desired equidistant apart, then signal the class to line up behind these individuals. The first client in each line may move out in front of the line or shift to the side as illustrated.	Roll taking Teaching basic skills Teaching stunts on floor or mats Simple games Relays

Fan
 	
   X
X
X
X   Y
X
   X
    X
	The fan formation is used for small group activities. Arrange clients in a line facing their leader, then have them join hands and form a half-circle.	Mimetics
		Simple floor stunts
		Teaching dance skills
		Relays

Shuttle
  6 X
  4 X
  2 X
    1 X
  3 X
  5 X
	Arrange clients in two, three, or more equal lines, then separate lines the distance required for the activity. Client 1 performs his skill, then shifts to the rear of the opposite line; client 2 performs and shifts to the rear of the opposite line, etc.	Activities requiring close observation by teacher
		Tumbling activities from opposite ends of mat
		Teaching skills
		Relays

Zigzag 1 X⟶X 2 3 X⟷X 4 5 X⟷X 6	Arrange class or squads into two equal lines with partners facing each other. Client 1 passes to 2, 2 passes to 3, 3 passes to 4, until the last client is reached	Throwing, catching and kicking skills

Scattered
 	
  X
X   X
   X
X   X
   X
X   X
   X
   X
	Allow clients to find a spot in the exercise area. Have each client reach out with his arms to see if he can touch another person. Require the clients who can touch others to shift until they are free of obstructions.	Warm-up exercises
		Mimetics
		Simple floor stunts
		Creative activities

* Adapted with permission from Kirchner G: *Physical Eduction for Elementary School Children.* Dubuque: William C. Brown Publishing, 1992.

feedback). Comments like "Extend your arms," "Bend your knees," "Tuck your chin," and "Keep your elbows in," are all examples of specific feedback, which helps clients correct their technique.

Specific feedback can include reminders about training guidelines as well as about movement techniques. For example, the principle of specificity and the concept of warm-up suggest that stretching-type actions be used for enhancing flexibility and be combined with aerobic-type actions as a part of warm-up. The exercise leader must be alert to give specific feedback to individuals whose behavior shows lack of understanding about, or unwillingness to comply with, training guidelines.

Finally, feedback should include acknowledgment of correct behavior, not just errors. Examples of positive feedback include: "Good technique in lowering the weights slowly to prevent banging." or "You did jumping jacks and stretches before starting your weight training. That shows an understanding of warm-up."

Summary on Feedback

General Feedback (addresses emotional needs):
1. Given to individuals and to groups
2. Conveys recognition of effort ("Good job!")
3. Provides pleasant, positive atmosphere (Smile!)
4. Encourages continued effort ("Try one more rep!")
5. Reminds participants of general information: ("Warm up slowly!", "Feel the motion!", "Go at your own pace!")

Specific Feedback: (addresses technique and cognitive needs)
1. Given to individuals and to groups (cues and key points)
2. Offers suggestions on how to improve action ("Shorten your stride," "Relax your shoulders," "Lift your head")
3. Avoids negative ("Keep your chin tucked" versus "Don't arch")
4. Is based on actions of client: observation of individuals
5. Focuses on one aspect; is short, concise
6. Is provided immediately

EFFECTIVE ORGANIZATION

Program philosophy and teaching styles influence and are influenced by several other factors that contribute to effective organization. According to Kirchner,[4] those factors include client characteristics (e.g., age, skill, fitness status), class size, time allotted per class, schedule (time of day), availability of aides, equipment and facilities available.

Client Characteristics and Class Size

To individualize exercise variables such as intensity, duration, and type, the exercise leader must know the fitness status of each client. Sometimes this information is provided by exercise specialists, test technologists, or program specialists who have administered and/or interpreted fitness test scores and relayed their recommendations to the exercise leader. Sometimes little client information is available beyond the screening information required before entry into an exercise program. In these cases, it is wise to note each client's age and sex and then observe his or her skill and effort in various low-intensity activities. This information can provide insight into the homogeneity of the group as well as the status of each client.

Group homogeneity is as important as class size and time allotted per class when deciding how to individualize exercise observation and feedback. Even a large group of clients (40 +) can be provided with individual feedback if they are divided into sub-groups of similar characteristics (aerobic fitness level, interest, pace, body composition, etc.). The exercise leader can then formulate a plan for, and monitor, each subgroup, either at stations, by location in the workout area, or through task cards with specific directions for the group. A large, homogeneous group can exercise together, in parallel lines or in a circle, with the exercise leader circulating to assist and encourage individuals (see Table 24-2[4]).

Scheduling and Time Allotted Per Class

The daily routines of clients also influence their exercise habits. Exercise can be effective at any time of the day, but clients have personal preferences and individual schedule needs. Thus, it is important to have exercise facilities and programs available at various times. Proximity to meals, need to rush to or from other appointments, speed in changing clothes, and other such scheduling conflicts should be considered in setting-up exercise class times.

The length of an exercise class period is usually 30 to 60 minutes, but the amount of time a client exercises independently can vary from a few minutes to 2 or 3 hours. Programs set up by the exercise leader should be at least 30 minutes, with a short time for warm-up and cool-down. The decision to establish a longer exercise class time must reflect the fitness and skill levels of the targeted clients. Less fit, less skilled individuals need to start with shorter, less intense exercise periods, whereas more fit, more skilled individuals can sustain (and need) longer, more intense exercise periods.

Availability of Aides

When available, aides can assist the leader with various tasks. They can provide individual feedback, run record players, monitor pulses, record data, or simply serve as models during group exercise. To be most effective, aides must be trained to fulfill their responsibilities correctly.

Equipment and Facilities

Availability of equipment and facilities influences several of the above factors, especially schedule, time allotted, and class size. The number, size, and type of rooms or workout areas available clearly dictates the number, size, and types of classes/activities which can be offered. The amount and type of equipment available influence not only the number of classes to be offered but *also* the type of classes (e.g., beginner to advanced; aqua versus land aerobics; free versus machine weights, etc.) It is helpful to have sufficient equipment to allow all clients to be active simultaneously, but only if each client has been taught proper use of the equipment. Selection of equipment is itself influenced somewhat by the skill, fit-

ness status, and interests of the individuals expected to participate.

The effectiveness of the exercise experience will increase to the extent that the exercise leader incorporates these factors into the exercise plan. Rules, routines, and policies, such as the following, should reflect these factors:

- Stay in rotation with other clients while working out on the weight machine circuit (rule)
- Start your weight training sets at a workload that allows you to complete at least 15 reps (routine)
- If late, be sure to warm up for 5 minutes before joining an aerobics class in session (routine)
- If you have a cardiovascular health problem, you must have physician consent to enter an exercise program (policy).

ACCOMMODATING DIFFERENCES: CHILDREN, OLDER ADULTS, AND VARIOUS FITNESS LEVELS

The exercise leader is faced with special challenges when working with children, older adults, or any group of clients in which there is a wide difference in fitness level. Such situations are not unusual; therefore, all exercise leaders should be prepared to accommodate the special needs of those clients. Consider the following in making plans for working with such groups:

Children Need:
- Opportunity to set their own pace
- A wide choice of activities
- Short bouts of activity with frequent rest breaks
- Lower intensity than adults
- Clear instructions in language they can understand
- Demonstrations as well as words
- Frequent feedback, both general and specific
- Equipment that fits and matches their fitness levels
- Modification of game rules to encourage participation and focus activity on specific outcomes
- Use of games, music, challenging tasks to motivate them

Older Adults Need:

- Opportunity to set their own pace
- Gradual progression from start of a workout to peak and from workout to workout
- Modification of activities for special conditions such as obesity, arthritis, or orthopedic problems, which interfere with mechanics of activity
- Systematic monitoring and frequent feedback, general and specific
- Thorough warm-up with stretching and aerobic activity
- Equipment appropriate to their fitness (low starting weights)

Less Fit Clients Need:

- Opportunity to set their own pace
- Organizational patterns that allow them to participate as members of the group, but with freedom to go at their own rate: stations (do as many reps as possible in 30 seconds); task groups (do a specific activity until done); fitness groups (exercise routines differ for high versus medium versus low levels); entire class (with modifications suggested to allow different efforts: kick versus jump, empty hands versus hand weights, low versus high step)
- Instruction and experience in judging their exercise effort (develop a realistic feel for how hard they are exercising)
- Frequent encouragement
- Assistance in setting realistic goals

Highly Fit Clients Need:

- The same opportunities given to less fit clients but designed to allow them increased effort within realistic limits
- To recognize when to rest and that rest is okay.

All Clients Need:

- To learn to take responsibility for monitoring themselves.
- To assist in the care of equipment.
- To behave in ways that are safe for themselves and others.

SUMMARY

If a facility or program exists simply to provide a safe place for clients to use up-to-date equipment largely on their own, the exercise leader's role focuses on supporting the client's decisions. If, however, development of decision-making skills and self-responsibility are program objectives, it is incumbent on the exercise leader to be more than an activity role model. The exercise leader needs to communicate clearly, provide corrective and motivational feedback, and organize the exercise environment so that clients can practice decision making while participating vigorously.

It is the exercise leader's responsibility to help clients meet their individual needs: some clients are motivated, others need constant encouragement; some know good lifting, running, or calisthenic techniques, others need much instruction; some learn well through verbal messages, others need visual or manipulative signals. An effective leader recognizes the various needs and designs a plan to help clients improve—in knowledge, in skill, and in attitude as well as in fitness. To fulfill those responsibilities, the exercise leader must care about people, stay current on exercise information, have skill in teaching, and be fit enough to demonstrate personal commitment to an active lifestyle and to have the energy to carry out all of these responsibilities.

REFERENCES

1. Roberts G (ed): *Motivation in Sport and Exercise*. Champaign, IL: Human Kinetics, 1992.
2. Casperson C: Physical inactivity and coronary heart disease. *Phys Sports Med, 15:* 43–44, 1987.
3. Martens R: *Coaches Guide to Sport Psychology*. Champaign, IL: Human Kinetics, 1987.
4. Kirchner G: *Physical Education for Elementary School Children*. Dubuque: William C. Brown, 1992.
5. Gill D: *Psychological Dynamics of Sport*. Champaign, IL: Human Kinetics, 1987.

Chapter 25

FLEXIBILITY/RANGE OF MOTION

Wendell Liemohn

Flexibility contributes to total fitness because efficient body movement depends on having functional range of motion (ROM) at all joints of the musculoskeletal system. This chapter presents a dialogue on terms and concepts, a discussion of basic biomechanics, and a commentary on guidelines in evaluating and prescribing stretching activities, as they relate to flexibility and ROM.

TERMS AND CONCEPTS

The terms flexion and flexibility are sometimes used in a manner that tends to confound their intended meaning. Although a neophyte might talk about flexing muscles, those with practical knowledge in exercise understand that muscles are contracted, and that the terms flexion and flexibility relate to movements occurring at joints. Flexion is defined as the act of bending or being bent and flexibility relates to the ability to bend without breaking.[1] In the context of its use in applied anatomy, the term flexion is used to denote a bending movement in the sagittal plane as two body segments are moved in approximation to each other. In Figure 25–1, the individual performing the fingertips-to-floor test is demonstrating flexion at both iliofemoral (hip) joints as well as some at the intervertebral joints of the spine. If she were to return to her neutral or starting position, the movement would be called extension. However, if she were to continue extending in the sagittal plane to her end-ROM position, the movement would be called hyperextension.

The individual in Figure 25–2 is demonstrating an exceptional degree of hyperextensibility. Nevertheless, because the movement meets the criteria for the definition of flexion, she is also demonstrating an extraordinary degree of flexibility. However, there is potential confusion in describing an individual's ability to hyperextend as being indicative of flexibility. Thus the acronym ROM is mostly used in this chapter in place of the term flexibility in discussing this important fitness component. First, the term ROM is not laden with potential semantic problems such as those alluded to previously. A second reason is that most movements are not initiated from an end-ROM position (e.g., maximum flexion, maximum medial rotation, etc.); but rather, movement is usually initiated at some point between the end-ranges of joint excursion, and it is often desirable to measure ROM in both directions.

Having "good flexibility" implies demonstrating functional ROM at *all* joints. Flexibility is, however, joint-specific. Thus, because one has good ROM at one joint does not guarantee that he or she has good ROM at others. A second problem in portraying ideal flexibility is that ROM is somewhat dependent on several demographic variables, and hence normative data are limited. For example, adults tend to have less ROM as they get older. However, it is uncertain as to how much of this diminution in ROM is caused by aging per se or to the reduced physical activity related to aging. Although gender differences exist, these differences are often joint-specific and do not always favor women.[2,3] Moreover, some research suggests that male asymmetry with respect to ROM (i.e., less ROM in dominant limb than in nondominant one) accounts for some of the gender differences seen.[4] Genotype would be another consideration. Not all young women, regardless of training regimen, could attain the posture demonstrated by the gymnast in Figure 25–2. Thus, even though flexibility is somewhat of an individual mat-

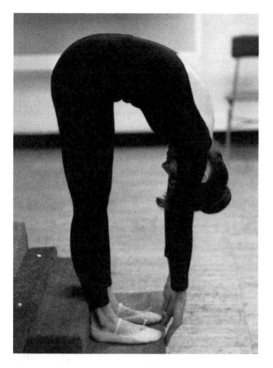

Fig. 25–1. Fingertips-to-floor. In the performance of this activity, once the lumbar curve is straightened, remaining movement occurs at the iliofemoral joint.

ter, significant decrements in ROM can preclude attaining a satisfactory degree of physical fitness. For example, having good ROM at the iliofemoral joint and in the articulations of the spine is paramount to having a healthy back.

Most of the illustrations and much of the discussion in succeeding sections of this chapter center on movements relating to the spine. Although this was done inten-

tionally because many concerns relate to ROM exercises for the spine, the concepts that will be raised can often be generalized to limb movement as well. Exceeding end-ROM through a careless ballistic movement can put stress on a synovial joint, whether it be in the spine or in an extremity. A ballistic movement is (1) initiated by forceful muscle contraction of one or more agonists or prime-movers (unopposed by contraction of the antagonistic muscles), (2) followed by relaxation of the agonist(s) resulting in an inertial or coasting phase, and (3) usually ended with eccentric contraction of the antagonists to slow down the movement. *If* the antagonists do not control the final stage of the movement and the momentum of the body part is great enough, the body part may exceed its end-ROM and injure soft tissues. In either case, this stress, particularly if repeated frequently, can have a deleterious effect on ligaments, articular cartilage, and/or other soft tissue structures of the joint capsule.

BASIC BIOMECHANICS

Postural Considerations

Spinal carriage is functionally integrated to all movements because all movements emanate from the spine. A strong argument has also been made that the spine and its associated tissues are the primary engine of locomotion in our species[5]; any acceptance of this view would necessitate an appreciation of the importance of the maintenance of good spinal mobility. Figure 25–3 shows that there is a limited degree of spinal mobility in the sagittal and coronal

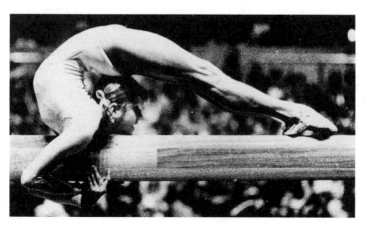

Fig. 25–2. Hyperextension. This figure is presented for demonstration purposes only; for although it may suggest the epitome of flexibility, the long-term effects of the attainment of postures such as this warrant further study. With permission from White AA, Panjabi MM: Physical properties and functional biomechanics of the spine. In *Clinical Biomechanics of the Spine.* 2nd edition. Philadelphia: JB Lippincott, 1990, p. 85.

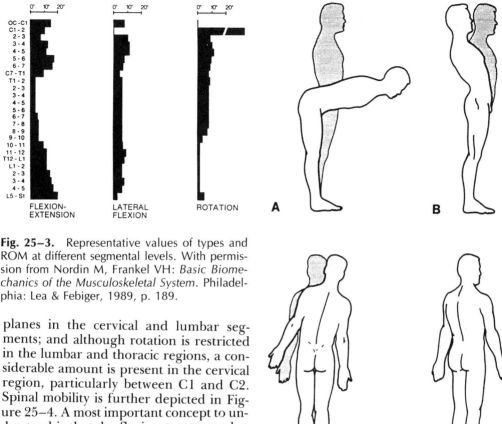

Fig. 25–3. Representative values of types and ROM at different segmental levels. With permission from Nordin M, Frankel VH: *Basic Biomechanics of the Musculoskeletal System.* Philadelphia: Lea & Febiger, 1989, p. 189.

planes in the cervical and lumbar segments; and although rotation is restricted in the lumbar and thoracic regions, a considerable amount is present in the cervical region, particularly between C1 and C2. Spinal mobility is further depicted in Figure 25–4. A most important concept to understand is that the flexion movement between L1 and S1 is actually a straightening of one's "normal" lordotic curve.

The muscles crossing the hip joint can be viewed as "guy wires" bracing the pelvis. If any of these "guy wires" are too tight, the abdominal musculature may not be able to control pelvic positioning. Because the sacral portion of the pelvis is the foundation for the "kinetic chain" of 24 vertebra "stacked" on it, pelvic positioning plays an important role in the integrity of the spine. For example, tightness in the hip extensors (hamstrings) or flexors (iliopsoas) can severely affect the ability of the abdominal muscles to help dissipate forces imposed on the spine. This could (1) compromise the bioenergetics of gait, (2) adversely affect other biomechanical functions of the spine, (3) damage soft tissues (e.g., discs and ligaments), and/or (4) set the stage for low back pain.

Lengthening Connective Tissue

To voluntarily move body segments, muscles must contract. Likewise, muscles

Fig. 25–4. A depiction of ranges of movement occurring in the sagittal, frontal, and transverse planes. With permission from White AA, Panjabi MM: Physical properties and functional biomechanics of the spine. In *Clinical Biomechanics of the Spine.* 2nd edition. Philadelphia: JB Lippincott, 1990, p. 63.

opposite or antagonistic to contracting muscles must lengthen sufficiently to permit movement. However, if the musculotendinous units antagonistic to the contracting units are shortened and/or unusually strong, ROM is reduced. Because the musculotendinous units that are short are the ones that must be lengthened if ROM is to be improved, these muscles (and their associated connective tissue) are often called "target muscles."[7] It should be noted that, if these contractile elements are relaxed, the tendon and its associated connective tissue (i.e., endomysium, perimysium, and epimysium) are usually the major deterrents to good ROM (Fig. 25–5).[8] One way to decrease the resistance of the target musculature is to increase the length of its viscoelastic tendon and associated connective tissue.

In the scientific literature, force on a tissue is referred to as *stress* and the resisting force is referred to as *strain*.[9] When tissues are strained longitudinally, the stress is called *tension*. The stress-strain curve of collagen, a major constituent of tendon (ligament has a similar make-up), is presented in Figure 25–6. At rest, collagen fibers are typically convoluted or crimped; however, when a tension-stress is applied (e.g., the stretching that occurs in crouching before jumping for height), the crimp is straightened in reaction to the strain. During this process, no chemical bonds are broken; thus, when the tension force is released, the crimp returns after the visco*elastic* tendon tissue demonstrates its elasticity and resumes its resting length. If actual tendon lengthening through plastic deformation is the goal, the strain must extend beyond the toe phase (Fig. 25–6) and into the linear phase to strain the bonds between collagen

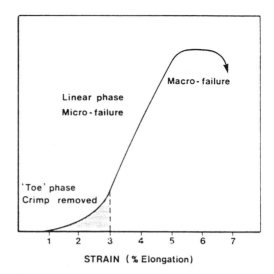

STRAIN (% Elongation)

Fig. 25–6. Stress-strain curve of collagen. With permission from Bogduk N, Twomey LT: Clinical anatomy of the lumbar spine. Melborne: Churchill Livingstone, 1987, p. 53.

fibrils. It is here that the *visco*elastic tendon tissue demonstrates its plasticity. However, if the stress placed on the tissue is too great (e.g., the strain exceeds 4 to 6% of the tendon's length), irreversible damage can

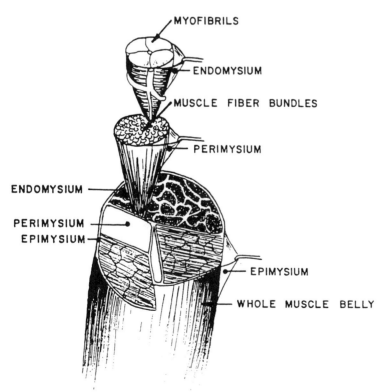

Fig. 25–5. Connective tissue components of skeletal muscle. The tendinous material at the origin and insertion (with the Z-lines of the contractile component, not pictured) is referred to as the series elastic component. The endomysium, perimysium, and epimysium are referred to as the parallel elastic components; they fuse with tendon at the origin and insertion. With permission from Chaffin DB, Andersson GBJ: *Occupational Biomechanics.* 2nd edition. New York: John Wiley & Sons, Inc., 1991, p. 34.

occur. Rupture of the Achilles tendon is an example of such macro-failure.

STRETCHING PROTOCOLS

ROM/flexibility improvement regimens are designed to improve passive and/or active ROM. An example of active ROM is the number of degrees an exerciser is able to raise one leg (knee straight) from the supine position until active end-ROM is reached. An example of passive ROM is having a second party raise the leg. Passive ROM always exceeds active ROM. If the differential between passive and active ROM is too large, the joint can be vulnerable to injury.

Static Stretching

In static stretching, the target musculature is typically lengthened to the point of slight discomfort by increasing the distance between origin and insertion. When this point is reached, the position is held for 10 to 30 seconds, relaxed, and then repeated at least 2 to 3 times per exercise session. Static stretching is generally effective in maintaining ROM. Moreover, it seldom results in injury and/or causes muscle soreness.[10] Although static stretching regimens have been found to be effective in increasing musculotendinous length through plastic deformation,[11] significant improvements have not always been seen.[12] Static stretching appears to have a greater effect on passive than active ROM.

Dynamic/Ballistic

Dynamic stretching protocols were once popular. Although research suggests that they are as effective as static stretching in improving ROM,[10] there is a greater chance of injury, especially if movements become ballistic and exceed end-ROM. (It should be understood that dynamic exercises do not have to have ballistic elements and often never exceed the elastic stretch phase. Therefore each exercise should be judged on the basis of its own merit.) Although ballistic stretching activities have the potential to improve both active and passive ROM through plastic deformation, and are often used in training competitive athletes for sports that have ballistic elements (e.g., jumping, throwing), this type of stretching often causes injury and thus its use is primarily limited to athletic populations.

Proprioceptive Neuromuscular Facilitation

PNF stretching was originally used in clinical settings. However, in recent years this method of improving ROM has received more widespread use. In PNF, the target muscle group is briefly contracted (e.g., 5 to 6 seconds) against resistance *after* the limb is at end-ROM. At one time, PNF protocols recommended *maximal* contraction of the target muscle after end-ROM had been reached. This is one of the possible reasons why muscle soreness and injuries have been reported in the use of PNF.[13] To reduce injury probability, it is recommended that the trainer/partner tell the exerciser to "meet my resistance" and *not* permit a maximal contraction of muscle groups. Then there is an attempt to move the limb beyond this point passively by a partner or with active contraction plus passive assistance. These two PNF techniques are often called Contract Relax (CR) and Contract Relax Agonist Contract (CRAC), respectively.[14] The CRAC technique is more effective in improving active ROM than the CR method.[12]

General Recommendations

For best results, stretching exercises should be performed on a regular basis. If increase in ROM is the goal, a short aerobic warm-up should precede most stretching activity because raising tissue temperature decreases the chance of injury and increases the chance of lengthening the tissue.[11] In addition to reducing the incidence of muscle tearing,[15] it has more recently been advanced that symmetry with respect to flexibility, strength, and balance/proprioception may also be factors that facilitate musculoskeletal function integrity.[16] If the body is viewed as a kinetic or biomechanic chain, it can readily be seen that any "link" out of synch with the same link in the opposite lower extremity obligates joints superior as well as inferior to make compensatory adjustments. This can result in microtrauma to joints and/or exacerbate existing problems.

GUIDELINES IN EVALUATING AND PRESCRIBING STRETCHING ACTIVITIES

Basic Tenets

Unfortunately, there is little evidence to show that certain exercises cause specific microtrauma or damage the musculoskeletal system.[17] The issue often becomes more clouded when well-intentioned writers label many exercises as contraindicated in case someone might do them improperly and/or be inappropriate for a specific subset of the population. Without delineating all aspects of the activity in question, this procedure of exclusion is somewhat analogous to throwing out the baby with the bath water. This can be unfortunate, because often some of these activities are most appropriate and, if performed correctly, are beneficial for at least some exercisers. For example, if one were working with a relatively homogeneous and fit population, as contrasted to a heterogeneous one that included extremity unfit individuals, would it not seem reasonable that some of the exercises used for the former might very well be inappropriate or even contraindicated for the latter? Likewise, if one were working with an elderly population with a greater likelihood of age-related conditions such as osteoporosis, more concern should be given to the body part selected to transmit weight (e.g., the yoga "plough" would be most contraindicated). However, does this mean that the same precautions must be taken when working with younger groups? Age is not the only criterion, an amenorrheic woman in her 20s could have bone mineral density comparable to that of a postmenopausal woman. In the following sections, general guidelines are given on using ROM activities to help ensure that the reader is familiar with some of the nuances of each exercise.

Trunk and Hip Flexion

Testing

The "sit-and-reach" and "fingertips-to-floor" tests have both been used to measure flexibility quantitatively in the sagittal plane. Both tests primarily measure hip-joint flexibility or hamstring length.[18–21] In administering either test, it is essential that the quality of the movement be monitored. One quality point to check is the angle of the sacrum. If the "sit-and-reach" is the measurement, this angle should be 80 or more degrees with the floor (Fig. 25–7). Hamstring length can be specifically checked by administering a straight-leg-raise test (Fig. 25–8). If one is interested in determining lumbosacral mobility in addition to hamstring length, an inclinometer technique is recommended.[22]

Exercise Prescription

Suppleness of the muscles crossing the hip joint is often a goal of a remedial exercise program. However, it is most important to consider characteristics of the individual performing the exercise. If the hamstrings are tight and one performs either the sitting or standing stretch in a bouncing or ballistic manner, the structures of the spine are obligated to absorb these hyperflexion stresses. Over a period

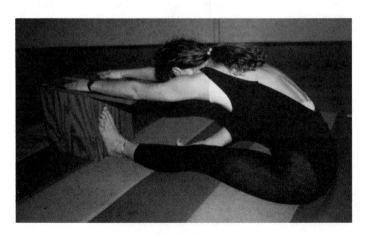

Fig. 25–7. Sit-and-reach test. A book or other rectangular object may be placed adjacent to the sacrum to help determine its angle; a minimum of 80 to 90 degrees is desirable. (The individual depicted is very lithe; her sacral angle approximates 110 degrees.) Superior to the sacrum, the spine should arc smoothly without excessive hyper- or hypomobility.

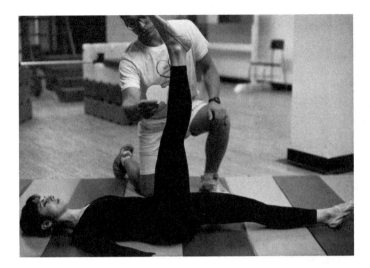

Fig. 25–8. Straight-leg-raise test. In the straight-leg-raise test advocated by Kendall and McCreary,[21] the pelvis is first posteriorly rotated until the low back is snug against the table. One leg is raised by the tester while ensuring that the other one remains stationary. ROM in flexion could be determined with a goniometer, an inclinometer (depicted), or a "home-made" protractor-like device. A minimum of 80 degrees is desirable for this measurement.

of time, this repetitive microtrauma may have a serious consequence.[23] In an attempt to obviate this drawback for the sit-and-reach, Cailliet[24] recommends a "protective hamstring stretch" wherein the leg contralateral to the one being stretched is flexed at the knee. This technique, according to Cailliet, protects the low back from hyperflexion. Although we did not find a significant reduction in lumbosacral flexion following Cailliet's technique,[19] we still believe it is less stressful because of altered pelvic positioning.

Trunk and Hip Extension

Introduction

Although there appears to be a progressive decline in spinal mobility in all planes with aging, this decline has been particularly noted for extension movements in asymptomatic individuals.[25] One explanation offered for the greater diminishment in this ROM than in other spinal ROMs is that extension movements are used less as a person ages.[25,26] Unfortunately, extension of the spine is an issue often ignored or misinterpreted in exercise programs. Although it is acknowledged that ballistic extension movements of the spine (as well as ballistic rotation movements) are totally inappropriate, it is contended that "slow and controlled" extension movements are appropriate for inclusion in exercise programs. However, to be on the safe side, Saal and Saal[27] recommend that *active* back ex-

tension be carried no further than the upper limit of the normal lumbar lordosis seen in standing.

Testing

Figure 25–9 presents a back extension ROM test recommended by Imrie and Barbutto.[28] Even though versions of this test have been in existence for some time, trunk extension is often ignored. For this reason, a scoring protocol based on their guidelines is presented in Table 25–1. It is important to note that this is a *passive* test of spinal extension in that the back musculature is not to be used. Maintenance of spinal ROM is in the best interest of the biomechanics of the spine because it helps the spine contend with the forces encountered in activities of daily living.

A cause of diminished hip-joint extension ROM is tightness in the hip flexors. Although the latter symptomatology may

Table 25–1. Standards for Back Extension Test*

Rating	Back Extension (cm)
Excellent	>30
Good	20–29
Marginal	10–19
Needs work	<9

* Adapted with permission from Imrie D, Barbuto L: *The Back Power Program.* Toronto: Stodarr Publishing Co., 1988.

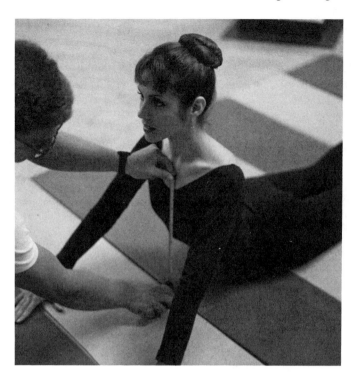

Fig. 25–9. Extension ROM test. While keeping the pelvis in contact with the floor, the subject elevates the chest with arm action; the score is the distance from the suprasternal notch to the floor.

not be as frequently manifested as tightness in the hamstrings, the hip flexors are also "guy wires," which control the attitude of the pelvis and can reduce lumbar ROM in extension. The Thomas test is used to determine if there is hip flexor tightness; it is presented in Figure 25–10.

The Neck

Neck circles and neck hyperextension are often avoided on the grounds that arteries and nerves at the base of the skull may become pinched. However, it has also been argued that neck circles are appropriate *if* they are done slowly and through a normal ROM.[17] What is somewhat ironic is that neck hyperextension exercises (along with neck side bending, flexion, and rotation exercises) appear in a widely accepted therapeutic program designed specifically for individuals with cervical disc and neck problems.[29] If an individual does not use the natural movements which the human body is designed to permit (e.g., *controlled* hyperextension, side bending, and rotation movements of the head), these movement capabilities will diminish with age; to lose

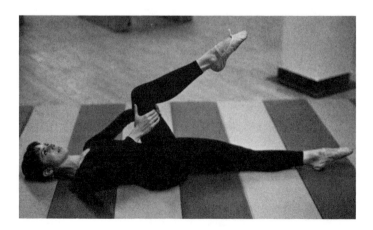

Fig. 25–10. Thomas Test. It is important that the leg be brought to the chest *only* to the point where the lumbar spine is snug against the table. If it is brought farther back, a false sign of short hip flexors might be presented, caused by the attendant posterior rotation of the pelvis. (Plantar flexion at the ankle joints is not necessary.)

range of motion because of disuse is usually unnecessary and undesirable. If intersegmental motion in the neck is limited by a progressive reduction in disc height and/or the condition of arthritis, medical guidance is important before engaging in neck exercises. Often the major distinction that separates appropriate stretching activity from inappropriate stretching activity for the neck is the quality of the movement. Fast and/or ballistic movements of the head are *totally* inappropriate and should never be used in ROM programs.

The yoga plough has been questioned because of the compressive forces it places on the vertebrae. It has also been blamed for causing the postural conditions of forward head and dorsal kyphosis. Although there is a lack of research supporting these contentions, and perhaps it is appropriate for use in some populations,[17] the plough is particularly inappropriate for one who presents with either arthritis of the spine or osteoporosis.[30]

SUMMARY

Although it is unlikely that the performance of almost any exercise will create an immediate problem for any exerciser, poor quality of movement in the performance of a ROM exercise over a period of time can result in repetitive microtraumas. This can have adverse effects on musculoskeletal structures. Stretching exercises that could be interpreted as having a ballistic element should generally be avoided. Although the emphasis in this discussion has been on exercises for the axial skeleton, the same concerns are relevant for movements of the extremities. For example, ballistic horizontal abduction of the upper extremities might be seen by some as an appropriate stretching activity for the pectorales major. However, if the movement exceeds endROM (e.g., this might be more likely if exerciser were holding light dumbbells), softtissue structures of the glenohumeral joint might be damaged. It is also important to understand that some exercises may not be appropriate for an individual because of his or her physical condition and/or age. Exercise leaders should carefully monitor the nuances of any exercise that they teach, the idiosyncrasies of the population to whom they are given, and the quality of the movement of their consumers.

REFERENCES

1. White AA, Panjabi MM: Physical properties and functional biomechanics of the spine. In *Clinical Biomechanics of the Spine.* 2nd edition. Philadelphia: JB Lippincott, 1990.
2. Marshall JL, Johnason N, Wickiewicz TL, et al. Joint looseness: A function of the person and the joint. *Med Sci Sports Exerc, 12:*189, 1980.
3. Mellin G: Correlations of hip mobility with degree of back pain and lumbar spinal mobility in chronic low-back pain patients. *Spine, 13:*668, 1988.
4. Koslow RE: Bilateral flexibility in the upper and lower extremities as related to age and gender. *J Human Movement Studies, 13:*467, 1987.
5. Gracovetsky S, Farfan H: The optimum spine. *Spine, 11:*543, 1986.
6. Nordin M, Frankel VH: Basic biomechanics of the musculoskeletal system. Philadelphia: Lea & Febiger, 1989.
7. Hartley-O'Brien SJ: Six mobilization exercises for active range of hip flexion. *Res Quar Exercise Sport, 51:*625, 1980.
8. Chaffin DB, Anderson GBJ: Occupational Biomechanics. 2nd edition. New York: John Wiley & Sons, Inc., 1991.
9. Bogduk N, Twomey LT: Clinical anatomy of the lumbar spine. Melborne: Churchill Livingstone, 1987.
10. DeVries H: Physiology of exercise for physical education and athletics. Dubuque: William E. Brown, 1980.
11. Safran MR, Seaber AV, Garrett WE: Warm-up and muscular injury prevention an update. *Sports Med, 8:*239, 1989.
12. Etynre BR, Lee JL: Chronic and acute flexibility of men and women using three different stretching techniques. *Res Quart Exer Sport, 59:*222, 1988.
13. Hubley-Kozey CL, Stanish MD: Can stretching prevent athletic injuries? *J Musculoskeletal Med, 1:*25, 1984.
14. Moore, MM, Hutton RS: Electromyographic investigation of muscle stretching techniques. *Med Sci Sports Exer, 12:*322, 1980.
15. Liemohn WP: Factors related to hamstring strains. *J Sports Med Phys Fitness, 18:*71, 1978.
16. Greenwood, PE: Manual medicine-exercise principles in failed low back syndrome. Lecture presented at the American Back Society Fall 1991 Symposium on Back Pain, San Francisco, December, 1991.
17. Lubell A: Potentially dangerous exercises:

Are they harmful to all? *Phys Sports Med, 17:* 187, 1989.

18. Jackson AW, Baker AA: The relationship of the sit and reach test to criterion measures of hamstring and back flexibility in young females. *Research Quarterly for Exercise and Sport, 57:*183, 1986.

19. Liemohn, WP: Lumbosacral posturing and the sit-and-reach. Paper presented at the American Back Society Fall 1991 Symposium on Back Pain, December 13, San Francisco, 1991.

20. Kippers V, Parker AW: Toe-touch test—a measure of its validity. *Phys Ther, 67:*1680, 1987.

21. Kendall FP, McCreary EK: *Muscle Testing and Function.* Baltimore: Williams & Wilkins, 1983.

22. Keeley J, Mayer TG, Cox R, et al.: Quantification of lumbar function—part 5: Reliability of range-of-motion measures in the sagittal plane and an invivo torso rotation measurement technique. *Spine, 11:*31, 1986.

23. Twomey L, Taylor J: Flexion creep deformation and hysteresis in the lumbar vertebral column. *Spine, 7:*116, 1982

24. Cailliet R: Prevention of recurrence of low back pain. In *Low Back Pain Syndrome.* Philadelphia: FA Davis Co, 1988.

25. Einkauf DK, Gohdes ML, Jensen GM, et al.: Changes in spinal mobility with increasing age in women. *Phys Ther, 67:*370, 1987.

26. McKenzie R: Exercises. In *The Lumbar Spine—Mechanical Diagnosis and Therapy.* Upper Hutt, New Zealand: Sinal Publications, 1981, p. 49.

27. Saal JS, Saal JA: Strength training and flexibility. In Conservative Care of Low Back Pain. Edited by White AH and Anderson R. Baltimore: Williams & Wilkins, 1991.

28. Imrie D, Barbuto L: *The Back Power Program.* Toronto: Stoddart Publishing Co., 1988.

29. McKenzie R: *Treat Your Own Neck.* Upper Hutt, New Zealand: Spinal Publications, 1983.

30. Liemohn, W: Exercise and the back. *Rheum Dis Clin North Am, 16:*945, 1990.

Chapter 26

STRENGTH CONSIDERATIONS FOR EXERCISE PRESCRIPTION

Robert J. Moffatt and Nicholas Cucuzzo

MUSCULAR FITNESS

Adequate levels of muscular strength and endurance are typically achieved through systematic programs of weight training. Such programs may be designed for various athletic purposes, for rehabilitation, and for general muscular conditioning. Before discussing either the basic principles of strength training for the development of muscular fitness or the physiology of strength training and muscular endurance, we must first define muscular strength and muscular endurance.

Muscular strength is the force that a muscle group can apply against a given resistance. *Muscular endurance* is defined as the ability of the muscle group to sustain repeated contractions of a given force for an extended length of time. Throughout this section, the word "muscle" refers to a muscle or a muscle group.

ASSESSMENT OF MUSCULAR STRENGTH

Muscular strength is generally measured by one of four methods: (1) tensiometry, (2) dynamometry, (3) one-repetition maximum (1-RM) and a recent approach, (4) computer-assisted force and work output determinations.

A cable tensiometer is easily used, is portable, and records muscular force at nearly all angles in the range of motion at a specific joint during a static or isometric contraction. Batteries of tests for the major muscle groups have been established to be used in evaluations during therapeutic or rehabilitation programs.[1,2] Operating on the compression principle, dynamometers indicate the force required to move a needle a certain distance. The static force applied is then easily determined. The integration of computer microprocessors and mechanical devices now enables nearly in-stantaneous collection of data on muscular forces, acceleration and body part velocities for a wide range of movements in testing, evaluation, and prescription. For a discussion of the traditional 1-RM and muscular endurance assessments, the reader is referred to Chapter 19, Fitness Testing.

When testing individuals for strength by any of these methods, care must be taken to treat all the subjects equally and with well standardized protocols so that proper evaluations can be made among those tested. It is best to select tests of known reliability unless the test administrators are prepared to establish items such as number of trials used, criterion scores, use of the best or average score, and appropriate statistical analysis of the data.

PRINCIPLES OF WEIGHT TRAINING

To develop the muscle effectively, the principles of overload, specificity, and progression need to be designed into the program. Overloading with either standard free weights, pulleys, cams or springs, or stationary bars, or with isokinetic equipment, forces a muscle to perform against workloads greater than it normally encounters. The most rapid gains in strength are attained by exercising the muscle at 80 to 100% of maximum.[3] However, exercise intensities of at least 60% of maximum should be sufficient to develop strength.[1] To develop muscular endurance, muscle groups should be exercised at lower intensities and higher repetitions to the point of fatigue.

For continued muscular development during weight training programs, periodic adjustments to the workload must be made as the muscle becomes stronger. In other words, the resistance against which the muscle trains must continue to overload the muscle. This modification and practical application of the overload principle, referred to as *progressive resistance exercise* (PRE), constitutes the foundation for most of the strength conditioning and weight training programs.

Methods for developing muscular fitness should be selected on the basis of the specific needs of the individual—the principle of specificity. In the early phases of a program, the use of lighter weight or resistance [60% max (or repetition max-RM) and more repetitions (12 to 15) with the avoidance of maximal lifts are considered best for the beginner. This is often a trial-and-error process using several sessions to establish a starting point. Muscular fitness development is not only specific to the muscle group exercised but also to the type of contraction, training intensity and velocity, pattern of movement, and muscle metabolism. The scientific evidence to support the need for movement specific exercises has been reviewed by Sale and MacDougall.[4]

It is essential to consider recovery time when applying classical principles of strength training. Recovery time has been defined as the time allowed for the muscle to partially recover between successive sets of exercise or between training sessions.[5] Insufficient time to recover between contractions can cause a muscle to fatigue. The rate of fatigue and therefore training stress are nearly as much determined by the recovery period as by the load and duration of training.[6] Although research regarding the amount of recovery necessary is sparse, there is general agreement that it is necessary for proper metabolic balance, replenishment of energy stores, and minimizing injury, soreness, and discomfort. Rest periods are essentially determined by the goals of the program.

TRAINING MUSCLES

Numerous methods have been employed to develop muscular strength and endurance. Training procedures are classified according to the type of muscular contraction, isometric, isotonic (concentric and eccentric), or isokinetic (Table 26–1). A comprehensive list of exercises and illustrations are given by Fleck and Kraemer.[5]

Table 26–1. Classification of Muscular Contraction

Type of Contraction	Definition
Isometric or static	No change in muscle length with tension development
Isotonic or dynamic:	
Concentric	The muscle shortens during contraction while it overcomes a constant resistance
Eccentric	The muscle lengthens during contraction while resisting a constant load
Isokinetic	The muscle shortens with maximal tension developed at a constant speed over the full ROM

Isometric Training

Isometric strength has been shown to improve at an average rate of 5% per week with the use of a single 1-second isometric contraction held at two thirds maximum voluntary contraction for 5 days per week.[7] Repeating this contraction 5 to 10 times per day produced greater improvements in isometric strength. Although isometric exercise is effective in providing overload and improving strength, its use may be limited because of the specific nature of the isometric process. Strength gains are specific to the joint angle at which the isometric contraction is performed.[8] To improve strength throughout the range of motion, the exercise needs to be performed at various positions of the joint. Despite its limitations, isometric training does seem to be beneficial in rehabilitation as a countermeasure to strength loss and atrophy associated with limb immobilization. Isometric training may cause increases in intrathoracic pressure and elevations in blood pressure during the static contraction. Therefore, this type of training may be contraindicated for some hypertensive and coronary-prone individuals.

Isotonic Training

Isotonic training consists of movements that contain both concentric and eccentric contractions (see Chap. 3 for definitions) performed against a constant or variable resistance. Delorme and Watkins[9] are credited with the development of a systematic isotonic training program. They determined that strength would increase if resistance were manipulated in three sets of 10 repetitions. The first set began using one half of a 10 RM load (the maximum weight that can be lifted for 10 repetitions). The second set increased the resistance to three fourths of 10 RM followed by the full 10 RM load, which was designed to overload the muscle group being trained.

Research leading to the development of the optimum number of sets, repetitions, and resistance to maximize strength gains and muscular endurance has been summarized by Atha.[6] In general, the stimulus for strength improvement using isotonic training appears to require a three-set program using 5 to 10 RM, 3 to 5 days per week. The weight used for each set should provide sufficient resistance to fatigue the muscle by the last repetition of the set. Work loads greater than 10 RM are more effective when one is attempting to improve muscular endurance.

Isotonic training involves both concentric and eccentric components; however, training programs are usually designed with the concentric component in mind. It has been suggested that, by using eccentric contractions, it may be possible to train at heavier loads and yield greater gains because eccentric contractions use fewer fibers at the same workload.[10] Although eccentric training does not appear to be any more effective than concentric training for strength development, individuals perceive eccentric exercise as easier. Eccentric exercise may also place less strain on the joints involved in the movement.[11] On the other hand, eccentric training produces much more muscle soreness than does concentric training.[12,13]

Isokinetic Training

Isokinetic training involves the use of specialized equipment that permits the muscle to develop maximal tension as it shortens at a constant speed throughout the complete range of motion. The speed of movement is mechanically controlled by the isokinetic exercise device such as the Cybex, Orthotron, and Mini-Gym. The advantage of isokinetic training is the ability to develop strength at different velocities. Isokinetic training is performed at speeds ranging from 24 to 180 degrees per second. This type of training may be especially valuable for athletes who wish to develop strength at speeds that approximate the speeds at which they perform. Studies by Coyle et al.[14] and Lesmes et al.[15] suggest that fast-speed training may be more beneficial than slower-speed training because gains in strength are limited to velocities at or below the velocity of training. Isokinetic training appears to have an advantage over isometric and isotonic methods, partly because of the ability to develop maximum force throughout the full range of motion and develop strength at variable speeds.

The procedures for the development of strength and endurance using isokinetic training are similar to those used for isotonic training. Three sets are performed for each exercise, with 5 to 10 repetitions, 3 to 5 days per week at speeds varying from 24 to 180 degrees per second for strength development. For muscular endurance training, maximum contractions should be performed at 180 degrees per second until exhaustion.

SYSTEMS OF RESISTANCE TRAINING

Most systems of resistance training were designed by Olympic and power lifters and body builders. They are popular because of the increases in muscle size and strength or zealous marketing efforts—not necessarily because they have been scientifically demonstrated to be superior. One system will not work optimally for all individuals and muscle groups. Knowledge of these systems is valuable in manipulating training parameters for attaining optimal gains in strength or muscle hypertrophy. Optimal gains may be attained by varying programs and short- and long-term training parameters appropriately. Following is a brief description of several of the most common resistance training systems currently used. For a comprehensive review and description of the many systems devised to enhance muscular strength and endurance, refer to Fleck and Kraemer.[5]

Single- and Multiple-Set Systems

The performance of each exercise for one set (8 to 12 repetitions) is one of the oldest resistance training programs. Use of this system can lead to significant gains in strength and may be a viable method for those who have little time to dedicate to resistance training.[5] Although effective, Stowers et al.[16] demonstrated that a single set system of one set of 10 repetitions led to significantly less gains in strength than a multiple set system of three sets of 10 reps per set. The multiple set system may be used with any chosen resistance, for any combination of repetitions and sets that are compatible with the preferred intent of the conditioning program. It is recommended that 5 to 6 reps for a minimum of three sets be used for effective increases in strength. Most resistance training programs are a variation of the multiple-set system.[5]

Pyramid (Light to Heavy) System

In this system of weight training, the exerciser performs successive sets of progressive light to heavy resistances while at the same time decreasing the number of repetitions. The Westcott Pyramid Program, as it is commonly known, typically consists of ten repetitions with 55% of the 1 RM weight load/resistance, five repetitions with 75% of the 1 RM weight load, and one repetition with the 95% of the 1 RM weight load.[17]

Circuit Weight Training

Circuit weight training alters the traditional approach to resistance training and has been promoted as a method not only to develop strength but to develop other areas of fitness such as aerobic capacity, body composition, and muscular endurance.[18] This method has been shown to increase muscular strength, especially when low-repetition and high-resistance exercises are included.[18] One of its chief aims is to improve cardiovascular endurance. Increases in maximal oxygen consumption of approximately 4% in men and 8% in women have been reported with 8- to 20-week programs.[18]

Circuit programs are usually devised to enable participants to perform as many repetitions as possible at 40 to 60% of 1 RM for 30 seconds with 15- to 30-second rest periods between exercise stations. Programs typically consist of as few as 6 and up to 15 stations per circuit which, if desired, are repeated two or three times per training session, depending on the specific goals of the program. This system is time-efficient for both the facility, because each piece of equipment is kept in constant use; and for the exerciser, because of its short rest periods.

Super-Set System

Two types of super-set programs have evolved. One alternates the use of groups of antagonistic muscles by using several sets of two exercises for the same body part. An example of this type of super-setting would be: arm curls immediately followed by triceps extensions, or leg extensions immediately followed by leg curls, for three sets. A second form of super-setting uses one set of several different exercises for the same muscle group (e.g., seated and bent-over rowing with lateral pull-downs).

Both forms of super-setting utilize sets of 8 to 12 repetitions with little or no rests between the sets and the exercises. Super-setting is popular among bodybuilders, suggesting the benefits for muscular hypertrophy.

Split Routine System

This system trains various body parts on alternate days to elicit hypertrophy of all muscles in a particular area of the body. A typical routine is training of the chest, shoulders, and back on Monday, Wednesday, and Friday, and the arms, legs, and abdominal muscles on Tuesday, Thursday, and Saturday. Many exercises for the same body part are performed. This splitting of the training system is a time-consuming process because it involves training 6 days per week. The split routine system permits the intensity (resistance) of the training on a muscle group to be maintained at a higher level than would be permissible if the four to six training sessions were combined into two or three long sessions and should realize greater increases in strength.[5]

Plyometrics

Plyometrics is a regimen of training exercise drills involving explosive jumping as a supplement to weight training. The drills are often vertical depth jumping, running or repetitive jumping in place, or single and double leg jumps with and without the use of weight vests or ankle weights.[19] It has been proposed that repetition of such exercises will render suitable neural and muscular training of specific muscles to amplify their power performance.[20] Plyometric exercises are designed with movements to utilize both the inherent stretch-recoil attributes of skeletal muscle and the alteration of a muscle's response by means of the stretch or myotatic reflex. Plyometrics basically overload skeletal muscle by quickly placing the muscle on stretch (eccentric phase) just before the contraction (concentric) phase. The quick stretch or lengthening phase plausibly promotes a more dynamic and powerful maneuver reportedly extending the speed-power advantages of training.[21] The benefits of plyometric training have been well voiced; however, experimentally controlled evaluation of both the benefits and the possible orthopedic risks of such exercises remains to be conducted.[22] To date, further research is needed to validate the position, if one exists, of plyometric training regimens in a total strength-power training program.

COMPARISONS OF WEIGHT TRAINING PROGRAMS

Whatever the training method, when the exercised muscles are overloaded, strength is effectively augmented. A summary of Fleck and Kraemer's comparative review of the acute program variables of resistance training systems[5] suggests that isokinetic training increases both isokinetic strength and isotonic strength and appears to cause less muscle soreness. Isotonic training is superior to isometric training for the development of strength and muscular endurance. Differences between the systems seem to be overwhelmed by the contrasts within them, because the training effects achieved are determined by the selected schedule, i.e., the intensity or the load, frequency, duration, speed, and rests allotted. It is relatively simple to design a number

of distinct programs by rearrangement of system variables. The program should be designed according to the needs of the individual and, in other cases, the competition for which the individual is training. The selection of a training system hinges on the goals of the program, time limitations, and the interaction of goals of the strength training program with those of the overall fitness program. Keeping in mind the need for balance, the entire program for conditioning and fitness is best developed incorporating each component of fitness. Naturally, the focus of the exercise program shifts with the priorities and assessment of the individual.

ADAPTATIONS TO STRENGTH TRAINING PROGRAMS

Various physiologic, morphologic, neural, anthropometric and biochemical alterations occur in muscle tissue in response to a systematic weight training program. Some are modified with training, whereas others are resistant to training regimens. Still others appear to be determined early in life and controlled by genetic factors. Table 26–2 provides a summary of adaptive effects of weight training.

MUSCLE SORENESS AND STIFFNESS

Following a layoff from exercise, one can experience soreness and stiffness in the exercised muscles and joints. A temporary soreness may persist for several hours immediately after unaccustomed exercise, whereas delayed onset muscle soreness (DOMS) may appear 24 to 48 hours later and persist for several days.

The cause of DOMS is uncertain; however, several possible explanations have been proposed. These include a lactic acid build-up in the muscle, muscle spasms and tearing of the muscle and connective tissues.[23–25] Electron microscopy data from Friden, et al.[25] provide strong support for the tissue injury theory in that subjects who reported DOMS revealed microscopic tears in those muscle fibers.

Delayed onset muscle soreness appears to occur most often after intense exercise in muscles unaccustomed to being worked. In addition, eccentric, and, to some extent,

Table 26–2. Summary of Effects of Weight Training on Morphologic, Biochemical, Neural and Anthropometric Factors

	Effect		
	Increase	Decrease	No Change
Morphologic Factors			
—contractile proteins, number and size of myofibrils	X		
—muscle connective tissue	X		
—size of fast-twitch fibers	X		
—number of muscle fiber types			X
—size and strength of ligaments and tendons	X		
Biochemical Factors			
—ATP and CP	X		
—myokinase activity	X		
—mitochondrial density		X	
Neural Factors			
—discharge frequency of motoneurons	X		
—motor unit recruitment	X		
—inhibitions		X	
—motor skill performance	X		
Anthropometrical Factors			
—body weight			X
—lean body weight	X		
—percentage of body fat		X	
—flexibility	X		
—speed and power	X		

isometric muscular contractions also appear to cause the greatest post-exercise discomfort.[26,27]

The Lower Back

Low back pain is generally attributed to abdominal muscle weakness and poor flexibility in the low back-hamstring region. Properly prescribed resistance training can strengthen both the abdominal and lumbar extensor musculature, which support and protect the spine.[28] Proper execution should not be sacrificed when lifting. Harmon et al.[29] report that use of a "weight belt" for heavy near-maximal and competitive lifting significantly reduces intra-abdominal pressure, which may in turn reduce compression forces on vertebral discs. Beginners training at low and moderate loads, or those involved in general conditioning programs, should lift without a belt to recruit and strengthen the deep-lying abdominal muscles, which are utilized to develop proper form and execute good technique. Back problems are best avoided by strengthening the abdominal muscles with proper sit-ups and strengthening the

lower back with appropriate exercises utilizing resistance of light to moderate intensity only in this susceptible area.[5]

MAINTENANCE OF STRENGTH AND ENDURANCE GAINS

Once muscular strength and endurance have developed, they appear relatively easy to maintain. Strength gains were reportedly retained for 6 weeks after stopping an isotonic program.[30] Furthermore, strength was improved by a subsequent 6-week program of training involving 1-RM performed each week.[30] In another study, subjects retained 45% of their strength gains after 1 year.[31] Muscular endurance can also be retained at 70% of training gains after 12 weeks of detraining.[32,33]

REFERENCES

1. McArdle WD, Katch FI, Katch VL: Exercise Physiology. 3rd Ed. Philadelphia, Lea & Febiger, 1991.
2. Clarke DH: Adaptations in strength and muscular endurance resulting from exercise. In *Exercise and Sport Science Reviews*.

Vol. 1. Edited by J. H. Wilmore. New York: Academic Press, 1973.

3. Stone W, Kroll W: *Sports Conditioning and Weight Training.* Boston: Allyn and Bacon, Inc., 1978.

4. Sale D, MacDougall D: *Specificity in Strength Training, a Review for the Coach and Athlete.* Science Periodical on Research and Technology in Sport. Ottawa, The Coaching Association of Canada, March, 1981.

5. Fleck SJ, Kraemer WJ: Designing resistance training programs. Champaign, Illinois: Human Kinetics Books, 1987.

6. Atha J: Strengthening muscle. In *Exercise and Sport Sciences Reviews.* Vol. 9. Edited by D. Miller. Philadelphia: The Franklin Institute Press, 1981.

7. Hettinger T, Muller E: Muskelleistung and Muskeltraining. *Arbeitsphysiologie,* 5:11, 1953.

8. Gardner G: Specificity of strength changes of the exercised and nonexercised limb following isometric training. *Res Quart, 34:*98, 1963.

9. DeLorme T, Watkins A: Techniques of progressive resistance exercise. *Arch Phys Med, 29:*263, 1948.

10. Orlander J, Kiessling K-H, Karlsson J: Low intensity training, inactivity and resumed training in sedentary men. *Acta Physiol Scand, 101:*351, 1977.

11. Johnson B, et al.: A comparison of concentric and eccentric muscle training. *Med Sci Sports Exerc, 8:*355, 1976.

12. Byrnes W: Muscle soreness following resistance exercise with and without eccentric contractions. *Res Quart, 56:*283, 1985.

13. Tulag T: Residual muscular soreness as influenced by concentric, eccentric and static contractions. *Res Quart, 44:*458, 1973.

14. Coyle E, et al.: Specificity of power improvements through slow and fast isokinetic training. *J Appl Physiol, 51:*1437, 1981.

15. Lesme G, Costill D, Coyle E, Fink W: Muscle strength and power changes during maximal isokinetic training. *Med Sci Sports Exerc, 10:*266, 1978.

16. Stowers T, et al.: The short-term effects of three different strength-power training methods. *NSCAJ, 5:*24, 1983.

17. Westcott WL: *Strength Fitness. Physiological Principles and Training Techniques.* Allyn & Bacon, 1982.

18. Gettman L, Pollock M: Circuit weight training: A critical review of its physiological benefits. *Physician Sports Med, 9:*44, 1981.

19. Hatfield FC, Krotee ML. In *Personalized Weight Training for Fitness and Athletics: From Theory to Practice.* 2nd Ed. Kendall Hunt Publisher, 1978.

20. Cho DA: Plyometric exercise. *NSCAJ, 5:*56, 1984.

21. Hakkinen K, et al.: Effect of explosive type strength training on isometric force- and relaxation-time, electromyographic and muscle characteristics of leg extensor muscles. *Acta Physiol Scand, 125:*587, 1985.

22. Boocock MG, et al.: Changes in stature following drop jumping and post-exercise gravity inversion. *Med Sci Spts Exerc, 22:*385, 1990.

23. Tiidus PM, Ianuzzo CD: Effects of intensity and duration of muscular exercise on delayed soreness and serum enzyme activities. *Med Sci Spts Exerc, 15:*461, 1983.

24. Armstrong R: Mechanisms of exercise-induced delayed onset of muscle soreness: A brief review. *Med Sci Sports Exerc, 16:*529, 1984.

25. Friden J, Sjostrom M, Ekblom B: Myofibrillar damage following eccentric exercise in man. *Int J Sports Med, 4:*170, 1983.

26. Talag TS: Residual muscular soreness influenced by concentric, eccentric, and static contractions. *Res Quart, 44:*458, 1973.

27. Trifletti P, et al.: Creatine kinase and muscle soreness after repeated isometric exercise. *Med Sci Sports Exerc, 20:*242, 1988.

28. Pollock ML, et al.: Effect of resistance training on lumbar extension strength. *Am J Sports Med, 17:*624, 1989.

29. Harmon EA, et al.: Effect of a belt on intra-abdominal pressure during weight lifting. *Med Sci Sports Exerc, 21:*186, 1989.

30. Berger R: Comparison of the effect of various weight training loads on health. *Res Quart, 36:*141, 1965.

31. McMorris J, Elkins E: A study of prediction and evaluation of muscular hypertrophy. *Arch Phys Med Rehabil, 35:*420, 1954.

32. Syster B, Stull G: Muscular endurance retention as a function of length of detraining. *Res Quart, 41:*105, 1970.

33. Waldman R, Stull G: Effects of various periods of inactivity on retention of newly acquired levels of muscular endurance. *Res Quart, 40:*393, 1969.

Chapter 27

AEROBIC EXERCISE PROGRAMMING

Deborah Brown Rupp

AEROBIC EXERCISE PROGRAMMING

Fifteen years ago, it was not uncommon to see exercise classes that consisted of calisthenics and stretching, offering little or no cardiovascular workout at all. Today, programming is designed to develop all aspects of fitness components, with an emphasis on cardiovascular conditioning. Additionally, there is a wide range of individuals (in terms of age, health status and fitness levels) pursuing fitness, and therefore a growing need to provide variety and diversity in programming of activities to help motivate individuals in incorporating regular exercise into their lifestyles. Meeting these varying needs has become easier through innovations in technology and creative programming.

Progress in technology, with easier-to-use equipment and creative programming of other activities, makes it essential for fitness instructors to be able to evaluate the technology and new programming ideas to best meet the needs of the various clientele they serve in their setting. Most newer equipment includes computerized readouts, which provide immediate feedback on the time, energy expenditure, and distance covered, and also allow challenges to individuals by varying the workout, some of which allow competition against the computer or other participants on another piece of equipment. Such features certainly serve to motivate individuals in their exercise, but may not always be the optimal training methods. The purpose of this chapter is to evaluate some of the newer modes and approaches to exercise and discuss their advantages and disadvantages (Table 27–1). Fitness instructors should then be able to evaluate the various modes and formats of exercise and determine the most appropriate settings and populations for their use.

Stair Climbing

One of the most popular new machines is the stair climber. The most sophisticated model simulates a flight of stairs revolving around a treadmill. Models most often found in exercise facilities are those referred to as steppers, which use a system of simple hydraulics to vary resistances. These machines offer a low-impact mode of aerobic activity appropriate for most fitness levels. The main concern with using stair climbers is biomechanics. Novices and those with weak quadriceps muscles tend to lean heavily on the hand rails, reducing the total weight on the steps. As the body leans forward, there is also potential for stress on the lower back. Another potential stress area is the knee joint. Biomechanical analysis of stair climbing shows reaction forces in the knee joint to be approximately 3 to 4 times body weight.[1] Because the downward stroke of the pedal on a stair climbing machine is assisted by gravity, one might expect the stress to the knee joint to be comparatively less. More research is needed in the area of stair-stepping biomechanics. In any case, if knee pain is experienced during or after a workout on a climbing machine, the stepping exercise should be discontinued and the knee evaluated. Specific quadriceps and hamstring strengthening exercises should be considered to assist in adding integrity to the knee joint. The tendency to lean forward increases when the resistance is set too high for the fitness level of the individual, and when the participant becomes fatigued. Additionally, if the participant is leaning forward, with significant weight on the arms, the energy expenditure is lower than that displayed on the computer readout. The selected program should, therefore, be appropriate for the fitness level of the individual to avoid alterations in body mechanics and undue fatigue.

Table 27–1. Modes of Exercise

Mode	Advantages	Disadvantages	Population Considerations
Stair climber	Computerized feedback Good cardio workout Wide variety of work levels possible Handrails help balance	Users tend to "lean" on handrails and bend forward from hips Lowest levels may be too demanding for severely deconditioned individuals May aggravate some knee conditions	Caution: Pregnant: OK as long as intensity is within ACOG* guidelines Older: intensity and balance may be of concern Possible mode for overfat and obese
Combined upper body and stepper	Cardio workout uses upper and lower body Provides seat for those who choose to pedal only	Requires some amount of coordination and balance to use hand grips and foot pedals	Same as above
Bench aerobics	Social aspect adds element of fun Can accommodate variety of fitness levels with varying bench heights	People tend to use mode exclusively; potential for overuse injury May aggravate some knee conditions (esp. chondromalacia, arthritis) Beginners may start on bench that is too high	Appeals to variety of fitness levels Older: OK with low bench heights and slower paced movements; participants must be able to maintain balance Pregnant: OK as long as physician approves; she lowers bench height and can see the bench Overfat and obese: OK with intensity modifications
Circuit			
Hand weights/ dumbbells	People often like social aspect Offers variety and fun Combines weighted work with rhythmic aerobic (high impact, low impact, bench, etc.)	Need orientation/education for using dumbbells Increase risk of injuries with use of free weights	With modifications, can be enjoyed by variety of fitness levels
Weight machines	Variety, fun, socialization, greater potential for some strength development	Need orientation to weight equipment Need specialized equipment, which takes up a lot of space	Easy to adapt for special populations especially obese, older, deconditioned and pregnant
Interval	Excellent mode for higher fitness levels Accomplishes more work in given time frame	Higher intensities may increase risk for injury Limited to higher fitness levels unless modifications are given for high intensity bouts	Not appropriate for special populations
Water exercise			
Shallow water	Social aspect, variety, and fun Water helps "hide" body; eases feelings of embarrassment Provides cardio workout and is excellent medium for range-of-motion exercises	Increased risks assumed by instructor and participant	Excellent mode for all fitness levels and special populations Suggested for swimmers and nonswimmers
Deep water	Same as above	Same as above	Recommended for swimmers only (controversial)

* American College of Obstetricians and Gynecologists

An extension of the stair-stepping machines are those that add a climbing action which combines movable hand grips with foot pedals. This action requires a bit of coordination and may be difficult initially, especially in individuals with lower fitness levels. The addition of a seat allows the beginner to sit while using only the foot pedals. Gradually, the participant progresses to the use of moving hand grips while stepping. This piece of equipment may be particularly useful in job-related training (and testing), e.g., police officers or fire fighters. Correct biomechanics are essential for anyone using this equipment to ensure a successful workout and prevention of injuries.

Group Aerobics

Group aerobics have grown in popularity, and most facilities provide classes in high-impact, and low-impact aerobics.

The term high-impact refers to movements that have an unsupported or airborne phase. Examples include running, jogging, jumping jacks, and variations of these moves. It may be easier to achieve higher intensities of exercise using high-impact movements; however, because of the unsupported phase, the impact forces on the joints of the body are greater than the forces resulting from low-impact activities (i.e., walking, low-impact aerobics). This is important to remember when suggesting activities for novice, overweight individuals, and those with a history of bone or joint problems.

Low-impact movements are those in which one foot is in contact with the ground at all times; there is no airborne or unsupported phase to the movement. Low-impact movements reduce the impact forces and thus may be appropriate for a greater proportion of the population than high impact movements. Low-impact activities such as low-impact aerobics and bench-step aerobics can achieve significantly high intensities to satisfy the more highly fit participants, and integration of high- and low-impact activities within a class allows subjects with a variety of fitness levels to participate in the same class.

The term non-impact may not be appropriate to describe movement. If the feet leave the ground and make contact again, there is impact. Clearly, the magnitude of forces can vary greatly; however, use of misleading terms such as non-impact to describe a given program is not appropriate.

It is also important to recognize that the terms impact and intensity are not synonymous. A low-impact activity is not necessarily low-intensity and a high-impact activity is not necessarily high-intensity. Exercise leaders must use their knowledge of levers and range of motion to choreograph moves that elicit the desired intensity of exercise.

Step Aerobics

Bench or step aerobics is a new version that has become very popular. Participants step up and down on a bench that ranges in height from 4 to 12 inches to music that is metered from 120 to about 134 beats·min^{-1}. The routines utilize step patterns that travel up and down off the bench, from one end of the bench to another, and a combination of the two. Bench moves are easily combined with high- and low-impact moves for diversity. Overall, the moves used in step aerobics are less dance and more calisthenic in nature, so there seems to be a broader appeal.

The intensity of exercise of the bench workout can be altered by changing bench height, pace of the music, and use of handheld weights.[2,3] Although research is limited, the few studies that have examined energy expenditure have found that a typical bench routine on an 8-inch bench using 30 lifts per minute (120 beats·min) requires an energy expenditure equivalent to the maximum oxygen uptake of most middle-aged individuals.[3,4] Thus the program for novices or very unfit individuals should begin on a lower bench (4 to 6 inch), incorporate slower cadenced music, and allow the subject to take frequent rests (or march in place) and avoid using the hand weights during the routine. Careful monitoring of heart rate and perceived exertion ensures that these individuals do not exceed their appropriate conditioning intensity.

There are no data on the injury rates or types associated with bench-stepping. Comparison has been made of the vertical impact forces of brisk walking and performing step training on an 8-inch bench. It was reported that the vertical impact forces of a basic step (up, up, down, down) was 1.4 to 1.5 times body weight and similar to the impact of brisk walking.[5] Thus, basic stepping may be considered a low-impact exercise modality. Addition of hand weights may increase the energy cost of the exercise; however, there is a concern that forceful and rapid movement of hand-held weights through a large range of motion may injure the shoulder girdle.

Other guidelines for bench stepping participation include the following:

1. Warm up and stretch the quadriceps, hamstrings, hip flexors, gastocnemius, and Achilles tendon.
2. Step up onto the bench to the center of the platform, contacting the surface with the entire sole of the foot. Use a full body lean when stepping, leaning from the ankle joints and not from the hips. Do not allow the heel to hang over the edge of the step.[9]
3. Step down closely to the bench (not forward off the bench), allowing the heels to contact the floor.[9]
4. Variety and constant changes in lead and support legs are important to avoid excess fatigue and alteration of biomechanics.
5. Step quietly onto the platform; do not jump off the bench.[9]
6. Watch the bench periodically. Inexperienced participants should look at the bench each time they step up.[9]
7. Always face the bench when stepping up or down.
8. Avoid hyperextending the back or locking the knee joints.[9]
9. Master the footwork before adding arm movements.
10. To avoid stress to the shoulder girdle, do not maintain the arms at or above the shoulder level for an extended period. Vary low-, mid-, and high-range arm movements frequently.[9]

Steps 2, 3, 5, 6, 8, and 10 with permission from Francis LL: Step aerobics. *(ACSM), Certified News, 2:* 347, 1992.

Water Exercise

Participation in water exercise has been increasing for several years. Water is an ex-

cellent exercise medium for obese individuals, pregnant women, arthritic patients, and older individuals because of the buoyant forces which decrease weight bearing on the joints. Additionally, many experts believe that the water helps minimize the embarrassment and self-consciousness that some people experience in land-based programs. A wide variety of class formats can be used in the water, including circuit and interval (described below), using a variety of modes, such as swimming, jogging, bench-stepping and other creative adaptations of land exercises. Nonswimmers are typically able to participate in shallow-water classes safely.

Water exercise presents an immediate element of danger not present on land. Thus, minimum standards for instructors include basic CPR, first aid, and completion of the Emergency Water Safety program through the American Red Cross. Qualified lifeguard(s) may be required to be present at any time when there are participants in the water. Non-swimmers should be identified and participate only in shallow-water classes. Their participation in deep-water classes should be discouraged until they can safely propel themselves through the water without the aid of flotation devices.

Adaptation of land exercises to the water takes practice. Instructors must develop an understanding of the characteristics of water and how it affects a given movement. For example, a current is created when all participants jog in the same circular pattern. If the instructor cues the class to change direction, turbulence is created and the jogging is more difficult, increasing the exercise intensity. Practicing the movements and planning the class ensures a safe and effective program. Exercise intensity can be modified by changing the speed of movements and the water depth, and possibly by using accessory devices available for use in water classes.

Accessories such as fins or kickboards are designed to increase resistance to a given movement in the water. The instructor should test the device to assess proper use before using it in the class setting because such devices may place excess stress on joints when used inappropriately in the water. Warnings and precautions should be clearly stated for any device, and any device intended for flotation should be Coast Guard-approved.

Circuit Training

Circuit classes were developed in an effort to achieve gains in strength and muscle endurance in addition to cardiovascular conditioning. A circuit class can be conducted in several ways. One is to set up stations around the perimeter of a room. In this case, participants move from station to station, alternating between a muscular endurance exercise and a cardiovascular activity, or between activities using different muscle groups (i.e., treadmill to bicycle). Ideally, the time spent at each station should be determined by the fitness levels of each participant. However, instructors are faced with the additional considerations of total number of participants and length of the session. A typical one-hour session would alternate 3 minutes on the weighted stations with 5 to 7 minutes on the cardiovascular stations.

A more sophisticated approach includes weight machines that are separated by spring-loaded platforms. As soon as the participants complete a weight bout, they move to the platform and jog in place. The participants are cued to move at predetermined intervals. Work periods in this setting may be shorter than those previously described. Adequate time must be allowed for participants to safely adjust the equipment to the appropriate levels and perform their bout of exercise. The instructor must be certain that all exercises are being executed properly.

Interval Training

Interval training is defined as an exercise session made up of work periods followed by rest periods.[6] Recently, the term has been modified to describe a specific cardiovascular conditioning class format that is similar to Fartlek training or speed-play training in running. Fartlek training is a method of training that varies the pace during a workout, going fast and slow over the entire distance. The cardiovascular portion of the class is constructed of higher-intensity work bouts separated by low- to moderate-intensity bouts. Depending on the fitness level of the participants, the high-intensity movements may include long lever movements, propulsion type moves (sometimes referred to as plyometrics, described subsequently), and faster-paced, high impact moves. The goal is to *average* around the target heart rate *over the entire session*. Interval classes are excellent for the more fit individual who would like to improve performance or simply add variety to the established regimen.

Interval training for individuals such as the very unfit, pregnant women, obese, high-risk, and elderly takes on a very different context. The high-intensity (work interval) bout may be low-level exercise and the low intensity may be a rest (no exercise) bout. This approach is especially important and may be the only way to start individuals with very low fitness with their exercise program. Gradually, the work intervals are increased in duration, with gradual decreases in the rest intervals (or progression of the rest interval becoming a low-intensity exercise interval). Individuals with special needs can participate in high-intensity/moderate intensity interval workouts as long as the high-intensity bouts are modified appropriately to ensure a safe range of participation.

Instructors should plan the class format carefully, choosing moves and combinations that will elicit the desired intensities. Appropriate planning will help to avoid the following common problems with interval classes: (1) intensity stays high throughout the entire conditioning phase; (2) the high-intensity bouts are not appreciably higher than the moderate (or rest) bouts; (3) the moderate bouts are not long enough to allow for adequate recovery. A prolonged warm-up period that includes slow versions of the moves to be used in the high-intensity bout is suggested. A longer active cooldown that includes static stretching is also recommended.

Plyometrics

The term plyometrics has recently come into use in the fitness community. The term is frequently used incorrectly to describe any sort of jumping movements (see Chap. 26). Actually, plyometrics is explosive jump training.[7] This form of training uses the stretch-recoil properties of the muscle to enhance power development in a specific muscle group. The muscle group rapidly lengthens then rapidly shortens. It is the speed element that is believed to contribute to the positive neural and muscular improvements.[8] Plyometric training is most appropriate for use by athletes to improve specific aspects of performance. If these types of moves are to be used in the class setting with individuals of lower fitness levels, extreme caution should be exercised, because anyone unaccustomed to this type of high-intensity, explosive movement may be at greater risk for injury. The instructor should be prepared with alternatives for those who choose to avoid these movements and should monitor the performance of those participants who choose to perform these movements.

SUMMARY

High-technology equipment generally appeals to people of all fitness levels and adds an element of fun to the workouts. Group classes have added equipment such as benches, hand-held weights, and weight machines and have included varied formats such as circuit training and interval work to attract a greater variety of participants. The fitness professional must stay current with trends in the marketplace and be responsive to the needs of various populations to maintain credibility with the public and within the fitness community.

Above all, fitness professionals must be able to appropriately utilize and adapt the technology and new programming methods to their setting and for the populations which they serve.

REFERENCES

1. Nordin M, Frankel VH: *Basic Biomechanics of the Musculoskeletal System.* Philadelphia: Lea & Febiger, 1989.
2. Goss FL, et al.: Energy cost of bench stepping and pumping light handweights in trained subjects. *Res Q Exerc Sport, 60:*369–372, 1989.
3. Olson MS, Williford HN, Blessing DL, Greathouse R: The cardiovascular and metabolic effects of bench stepping exercise in females. *Med Sci Sports Exerc, 23:*1311, 1991.
4. Rupp JC, Johnson BF, Rupp DB, Granata G: Bench step aerobic activity: Effects of bench height and hand held weights. (abst) American College of Sports Medicine Annual Meeting, Dallas, 1992.
5. Johnson BF, Rupp JC, Berry SA, Rupp DA: A comparison of ground reaction forces in bench step aerobics with other aerobic activities (abst). *Int J Sports Med, 13:*1992.
6. Powers SK, Howley ET: *Exercise Physiology: Theory and Application to Fitness and Performance.* Dubuque: William C. Brown, 1990.
7. McArdle WE, Katch FI, Katch VL: *Exercise Physiology: Energy, Nutrition and Human Performance.* Philadelphia: Lea & Febiger, 1991.
8. Chu DA: Plyometric exercise. *NSCA Journal, 5:*56, 1984.
9. Francis LL: Step aerobics. *Certified News (ACSM) 2:*347, 1992

Chapter 28

HOME EXERCISE TRAINING FOR CORONARY PATIENTS

Nancy Houston Miller

In the early 1970s, exercise rehabilitation became commonplace for patients with coronary heart disease. Because little was known about the safety of patients exercising after a coronary event such as a myocardial infarction (MI), it was generally felt that patients performing exercise required medical supervision provided in a group setting. However, the need for medical supervision, including the use of ECG monitoring, has increasingly come into question during the past 20 years. Improved management of patients with ischemic chest pain syndromes and the ability to stratify a patient's prognosis are just two of the advances that have occurred, bringing into question the need for intensive medical supervision of all patients involved in exercise training. In addition, although exercise has a variety of health benefits for patients with coronary heart disease, medically supervised exercise rehabilitation programs reach only about 11 to 15% of the 1,450,000 patients who are eligible for such training following acute MI or coronary revascularization procedures.[1] The majority of such programs exist mainly in hospital settings within major metropolitan areas.

The need for other alternatives to these traditional group-based cardiac rehabilitation programs reflects not only the need to serve larger numbers of patients, but the need for simpler and more cost-effective modes of exercise training. Indeed, of the nearly one million patients who survive a myocardial infarction each year, at least 50 to 60% of them are low risk and could benefit from exercise training without intensive medical supervision.[2] The purpose of this chapter is to describe the methods, results, and benefits of home-based exercise training for patients with coronary heart disease. Although home-based programs can be used to facilitate lifestyle modifica-

tion and education, this chapter focuses on exercise training, including efficacy, patient selection criteria, monitoring and safety, and adherence.

EFFICACY OF HOME EXERCISE TRAINING

DeBusk and colleagues, in the early 1980s, were the first to show the feasibility of home-based exercise training in enhancing the functional capacity of uncomplicated postmyocardial infarction patients.[3] Transtelephonic ECG monitoring was used to enhance the safety of home-based training. The improvement in functional capacity at 6 months post-event among patients exercising in a home environment was similar to that of patients exercising in a medically supervised program within the YMCA. As noted in Table 28–1, others have reported similar findings among patients exercising at home after myocardial infarction or coronary artery surgery.[4-8] Although the number of patients in some of these studies is small, equal improvements in functional capacity are consistently noted in studies comparing home-based training and group-based, medically supervised programs over 12 to 26 weeks.[4-7] Functional capacity increases by approximately 1.5 to 2.0 METS in response to home-based training during the first 3 to 6 months following an MI or coronary artery surgery. No training-induced ventricular tachycardia, ventricular fibrillation, or myocardial infarction have been noted in any of these studies, reflecting appropriate patient selection and adequate safety features employed during home training.

SAFETY OF HOME EXERCISE TRAINING

The advantages of home-based exercise training include greater convenience, cost, and the capacity to train large numbers of

Table 28–1. Home Exercise Training Studies

Study	Type of Patients		Change in Functional Capacity (Pre-Post) METS	Program Duration
DeBusk et al.[3]	M.I.	(n = 40)		8 weeks
	sup	(28)	6.8 ± 1.7 → 10.4 ± 2.2	
	unsup	(12)	7.3 ± 1.1 → 10.3 ± 1.4	
Miller et al.[4]	M.I.	(n = 127)		8–26 weeks
	sup	(66)	6.5 ± 1.4 → 8.5 ± 1.5	
	unsup	(61)	6.0 ± 1.4 → 8.1 ± 1.5	
Thomas et al.[8]	M.I.	(n = 176)		26 weeks
	unsup	(176)	7.0 ± 2.0 → 9.3 ± 2.4	
Stevens et al.[5]	CAS	(n = 204)		12–26 weeks
	sup	(24)	7.5 ± 1.9 → 9.0 ± 1.6	
	unsup	(180)	7.3 ± 1.8 → 8.7 ± 2.1	
Heath et al.[6]	CAS	(n = 45)		12 weeks
	sup	(28)	4.4 ± 1.5 → 8.8 ± 1.7* (p < 0.05)	
	unsup	(17)	4.9 ± 1.5 → 7.6 ± 1.7	
Hands et al.[7]	CAS	(n = 18)		8 weeks
	sup	(10)	6.1 ± 1.1 → 8.1 ± 0.8	
	unsup	(8)	6.3 ± 1.2 → 8.4 ± 0.8	

M.I. = Myocardial Infarction
CAS = Coronary Artery Surgery

patients. The main potential disadvantage of home exercise training is the lack of medical personnel to manage untoward events.

Van Camp found a low rate of training-induced cardiac events among 167 outpatient supervised cardiac rehabilitation programs over a 5-year period in the early 1980s. The incidence of cardiac arrest was 1 per 111,996 patient-hours of exercise and the rate of myocardial infarction was 1 per 293,990 patient-hours of exercise.[9] Combining these rates, an event occurred every 81,101 patient-hours of exercise. No differences in event rates were noted between programs using continuous ECG monitoring and those using intermittent or no telemetry monitoring.

The reported low occurrence of events in supervised programs, compared to an earlier study performed in the 1970s by Haskell,[10] most certainly relates to a number of factors including the ability to identify high-risk patients through methods of risk stratification and the newer technologies that have allowed physicians and others to identify patients at highest risk for cardiac events. Although the event rate in supervised programs is extremely low, the lack of patients involved in home exercise training studies makes it somewhat diffi-

cult to interpret the safety of patients exercising at home. However, it is important to consider that medical therapy including thrombolysis and adjunctive medical therapies (antiplatelet agents, beta-blocking medications) provided soon after the onset of chest pain have decreased mortality after an acute myocardial infarction. Moreover, these medical therapies and revascularization with coronary artery surgery have not only reduced post-MI mortality, but the risk of exercise training in this population. The post-MI and post-coronary artery surgery populations make up an overwhelmingly large proportion of the patients eligible for exercise training.

PATIENT SELECTION

Patient selection criteria appear to be critically important to the safety of both supervised and unsupervised exercise. The American College of Cardiology,[11] American College of Physicians,[12] and American Association of Cardiovascular and Pulmonary Rehabilitation[13] have developed position statements, or guidelines that specify the type and duration of exercise ECG monitoring for coronary patients. The American College of Cardiology[11] recommends ECG monitoring in the following circumstances, all of which reflect a relatively *poor* prognosis:

1. Severely depressed left ventricular function (ejection fraction of less than 30%)
2. Resting complex ventricular arrhythmias (Lown type 4 or 5)
3. Ventricular arrhythmias appearing or increasing with exercise
4. Decrease in systolic blood pressure with exercise
5. Survivors of sudden cardiac death syndrome
6. Patients following an MI complicated by congestive heart failure, cardiogenic shock, and/or serious ventricular arrhythmias
7. Patients with severe coronary heart disease and marked exercise induced ischemia
8. Inability to self-monitor heart rate because of physical or intellectual impairment.

The patients noted above constitute a clinically higher risk group who may benefit from a medically supervised program using ECG monitoring.

The risk of home-based exercise training among moderate-to-low-risk patients is not known with certainty. However, as noted earlier, both coronary artery surgery patients and those with myocardial infarction at low to moderate risk appear to improve substantially with home training without untoward problems. Moreover, undergoing coronary angioplasty or coronary artery surgery significantly improves myocardial functioning, thus decreasing the risks of exercise training. Safety in these low-to-moderate-risk patients appears to relate not only to selection criteria but also to the medical monitoring of patients within such programs.

COMPONENTS OF A HOME EXERCISE PROGRAM

Intake Evaluation

Patients' medical eligibility for home-based exercise reflects their clinical status, including the history and physical examination and the results of a symptom-limited treadmill test. High-risk patients, especially those with marked exercise-induced myocardial ischemia (>2 mm @ HR < 135

or workload < 5 METs), can be considered for coronary revascularization or exercise training in a supervised environment, and low-to-moderate-risk patients may be cleared for home-based exercise training.

In general, as noted in the previous section, patients without significant left ventricular dysfunction or myocardial ischemia are suitable for home training. These patients are capable of initiating home-based exercise training immediately following a symptom-limited treadmill test about 3 weeks after a myocardial infarction or 4 to 5 weeks after coronary artery surgery. Assessment of previous lifestyle habits, including exercise history and other coronary risk factors, as part of the intake evaluation can help to tailor the program to the needs of individual patients. Assessment of psychologic status with methods described in Chapter 36 help to determine the need for appropriate intervention or referral.

Exercise Prescription

Encouraging the patient to choose a favored mode of aerobic exercise facilitates adherence to training. When considering the mode of exercise, however, it is also important that the patient be able to regulate and maintain a heart rate within a given threshold range. Activities that can be alternated from day to day, such as stationary cycling and walking, may further increase adherence to the program. In a recent study, 85% of 176 patients allowed to choose their form of exercise for home-based training carried out walking during the 6-month training period.[8]

The intensity and duration of training in a home environment are similar to those of supervised programs.[4,5] The exercise intensity is usually equivalent to 70 to 85% of the heart rate achieved on symptom-limited treadmill test. Exercise sessions are usually performed 3 to 5 times per week. However, studies in normal middle-aged and older adults indicate that exercise at a lower intensity (60 to 73% of peak treadmill heart rate) may provide cardiovascular benefits similar to those of higher-intensity training.[14] Thus, exercise at a lower intensity for a slightly longer duration may enable a greater number of coronary patients to enjoy the benefits of exercise training.

It is also important that coronary patients exercise below the intensity that produces angina or significant ischemic ST segment depression during treadmill exercise testing. Many patients are taking beta- or calcium channel blockers that lower the peak exercise heart rate and prevent the patient from reaching these ischemic thresholds. Recommendations for home exercise prescriptions based on treadmill test results for patients following acute coronary heart disease are noted in Table 28–2.

Monitoring the Exercise Session

Self-monitoring the intensity of exercise is important for patients involved in home-based programs. Patients should be taught to monitor their heart rates accurately by palpation of the radial or carotid pulse. They should be taught to recognize exercise-induced angina and rhythm disturbances. Patients' skill in monitoring heart rate should be documented by a health care professional.

Another useful self-monitoring technique during exercise is the BORG scale, which rates exercise intensity from 6 (minimal effort) to 20 (maximal effort).[16] Patients can report their level of effort throughout the range of exercise intensities. Patients should be instructed to exercise in the moderate intensity range of 11–14 on the BORG scale. Using this scale to rate the intensity of exercise training sessions helps both patient and health care professional to evaluate the appropriateness of the exercise prescription and any changes in symptoms over time.

Portable heart rate monitors are also useful in regulating exercise intensity. The ExerSentry Monitor emits an audible tone when the heart rate is above or below threshold training heart rate limits. A digital display of heart rate is also provided. Other such monitors include the Polar Accurex, Polar Edge, Heart Speedometer and Elexis Pulse Watch. These inexpensive portable devices allow patients to exercise in comfort and safety. The monitors are especially helpful in regulating exercise intensity during the early phases of home training.

Although it has not been documented that continuous ECG monitoring in a medically supervised program decreases the occurrence of cardiac events, there may be circumstances in which real-time monitoring of ECG at home is desirable. There are now transtelephonic ECG monitoring systems (TEM, Survival Technology) that enable real-time monitoring of cardiac arrhythmias and myocardial ischemia during home-based exercise training sessions. These systems allow intermittent monitoring of individual patients as well as continuous monitoring simultaneously of several patients undertaking exercise at the same time in various home environments. Reimbursement for monitoring with these systems is available in many states. Whether such systems will reduce the risk of untoward events in home programs has not been proven. However, these systems may enable exercise training even among high-risk patients living in rural areas without access to supervised programs.

Monitoring by a health care professional is critically important to the success of home-based training by coronary patients. Regularly scheduled telephone contacts by

Table 28–2. Home Exercise Training Prescriptions

Treadmill Test Response	Recommended Rx
	Heart rate is based on:
No ST dep/angina or <1.5 mm ST dep	70–85% peak TM HR
ST dep >2 mm at HR >135	70–85% of onset of 1.5 mm ST-depression on TM test
ST dep >2 mm at HR <135	High-risk: suggest cardiac catheterization or maximum medical management. Rx just above.
Angina with or without ST depression	70–85% of HR at onset of angina
Other Categories:	
Deconditioned Pts (4–5 MET capacity)	60–75% if peak TM HR
Non-cardiac limitations (PVD, Pulmonary disease, orthopedic problems)	60–85% of peak TM HR
Initiation of beta blocking agents	Standard Rx—decrease range by 10 beats

health care professionals enable discussion of the exercise prescription, any change in the patients' medical status, and problems with adherence to the program. Such contacts also provide the health care professional with the opportunity to give positive feedback regarding lifestyle modification, to solve patients' problems, and to respond to questions. We have found biweekly contacts in the early phase of exercise and monthly contacts at a later phase useful in monitoring the success of home-based exercise training sessions.

Monitoring also includes detection of changes in patients' clinical status that warrant repeat evaluation, including repeat treadmill testing. Annual exercise testing enables exercise prescriptions to be modified or therapy to be altered. If patients develop symptoms during exercise sessions, exercise testing may need to be performed immediately to ascertain a change in the patient's status.

Promoting Adherence

Adherence to an exercise program is often problematic for patients who have recovered from a coronary heart disease event. A drop-out rate of 50% at 6 to 12 months is not uncommon among medically supervised programs.[17] As noted in Chapter 37, the reasons for nonadherence to exercise programs include personal, behavioral, environmental, and programmatic factors. Some of the factors resulting in poor adherence, such as the time and inconvenience of driving to and from a group-based program, are obviated by home-based exercise training. However, group support, which may enhance adherence, is lacking in a home-based exercise program. Consequently, it is critically important to ensure that the patients participating in a home-based exercise program are appropriately instructed and motivated by the health care professional. With proper instruction and the use of behavioral strategies, the rates of adherence to home-based exercise programs among middle-aged older adults may be as high as 75% at one year.[18]

Several factors important to the effectiveness of the exercise prescription may also help to improve adherence. As men-

tioned previously, allowing the patient to choose the mode(s) of exercise, alternating between two activities, and recommending a lower level of activities (60 to 75% of $\dot{V}O_{2max}$) may produce a greater degree of adherence. In a recent study of middle-aged men and women,[14] it was noted that those for whom high-intensity exercise was prescribed actually trained at the low end of the range, whereas those for whom low-intensity exercise was prescribed trained at the high end of the range. Adherence to both high- and low-intensity home-based regimens was similar at 12 months.

Providing proper instructions through the use of written materials or videotapes regarding the exercise program is also essential to the patient's clear understanding of the recommended guidelines. All too often, patients fail to exercise appropriately because of a lack of understanding of how to begin an exercise program. This can be adequately conveyed through combined written and/or videotape materials.

Self-monitoring enhances adherence with calendars or exercise logs. An example of such a form is noted in Chapter 37, Figure 37–3. Exercise logs that allow coronary heart disease patients to record not only the type, intensity, and duration of activity but symptoms of fatigue or angina serve to cue both the patient and health care professional about important changes in the patient's medical status. We have found that a telephone contact initiated by a health care professional one week after receipt of the patient's monthly activity log is an opportune time to discuss the patient's home training program. Telephone and mail prompts may also help to get patients "back on track" if adherence to the exercise logs or program is problematic.

Other methods that may help improve home exercise adherence include the use of contracts between the health care professional and patient, self-administered exercise assessments such as the use of self-tests to measure exercise improvement, encouraging family members or friends to provide social support by exercising at home together, and developing a reward system for regular exercise.

Exercise adherence should also be measured to determine the effects of a home-based program. Self-reported activity sessions measured through activity logs or telephone calls can be calculated as a percentage of those prescribed. In addition, changes in functional capacity as noted through treadmill exercise tests provide some assurance of adherence. Although adherence may be difficult for some patients, employing these methods may help solve this problem and ensure adequate safety for those exercising at home.

In conclusion, home-based exercise training affords a greater opportunity to reach a larger proportion of coronary heart disease patients who can benefit from exercise training. Although lack of direct medical supervision may impose some risk, careful patient selection, developing appropriate exercise prescriptions, and incorporating methods to monitor patients' intensity and adherence by health care professionals may ensure the likelihood that more patients will benefit from rehabilitation.

REFERENCES

1. Leon A, et al.: Scientific evidence of the value of cardiac rehabilitation services with emphasis on patients following myocardial infarction—Section I: Exercise conditioning component. *J Cardiopulm Rehabil, 10:*79, 1990.
2. DeBusk RF, Blomqvist GC, Kouchoukos NI, et al.: Identification and treatment of low-risk patients after acute myocardial infarction and coronary artery graft surgery. *N Engl J Med, 314:*161, 1986.
3. DeBusk RF, Houston N, Haskell W, et al.: Exercise training soon after myocardial infarction. *Am J Cardiol, 44:*1223, 1979.
4. Miller NH, Haskell WL, Berra K, DeBusk RF: Home versus group exercise training for increasing functional capacity after myocardial infarction. *Circulation, 70:*645, 1984.
5. Stevens R, Hanson P: Comparison of supervised and unsupervised exercise training after coronary bypass surgery. *Am J Cardiol, 53:*1524, 1984.
6. Heath GW, Maloney PM, Fure CW: Group exercise versus home exercise in coronary artery bypass graft patients: effects on physical activity habits. *J Cardiopulm Rehabil, 7:*190, 1987.
7. Hands ME, Briffa T, Henderson K, et al.: Functional capacity and left ventricular function: The effect of supervised and unsupervised exercise rehabilitation soon after coronary artery bypass graft surgery. *J Cardiopulm Rehabil, 7:*190, 1987.
8. Thomas RJ, Miller NH, Taylor CB, et al.: Nurse-managed home-based exercise training after acute myocardial infarction: methods and effects on functional capacity. *Circulation, 84:*II-540, 1991.
9. VanCamp SP, Peterson RA: Cardiovascular complications of outpatient cardiac rehabilitation programs. *JAMA, 256:*1160, 1988.
10. Haskell WL: Cardiovascular complications during exercise training of cardiac patients. *Circulation, 57:*920, 1978.
11. American College of Cardiology Task Force: Recommendations of the American College of Cardiology on cardiovascular rehabilitation. *J Am Coll Cardiol, 7:*451, 1986.
12. American College of Physicians: Cardiac rehabilitation services. *Ann Intern Med, 15:* 671, 1988.
13. American Association of Cardiovascular and Pulmonary Rehabilitation: Guidelines for cardiac rehabilitation programs. Champaign, IL, Human Kinetics, 1991.
14. King AC, Haskell WL, Taylor CB, et al.: Group versus home-based exercise training in healthy older men and women. *JAMA, 266:*1535, 1991.
15. DeBusk RF, Stenestrand U, Sheehan MS, Haskell WL: Training effects of long versus short bouts of exercise in healthy subjects. *Am J Cardiol, 65:*1010, 1990.
16. Borg GV, Lindenholm H: Perceived exertion and pulse rate during graded exercise in various age groups. *Acta Med Scand (Suppl), 472:*194, 1967.
17. Oldridge NB: Compliance and dropout in cardiac exercise rehabilitation. *J Cardiopulm Rehabil, 4:*166, 1984.
18. King AC, Taylor CB, Haskell WL: Effects of exercise intensity and format on psychological outcomes in the aging adult. *The Gerontologist, 31:*54, 1991.

Section VI

*SAFETY, INJURIES, AND
EMERGENCY PROCEDURES*

Chapter 29

THE SAFETY OF EXERCISE TESTING AND PARTICIPATION

Paul D. Thompson

The purposes of this chapter are to present the cardiovascular complications that occur during exercise and the pathologic conditions underlying these complications, and to quantify the incidence of exercise-related cardiovascular events. Our ultimate purpose is to enable the exercise leader to recognize potentially dangerous situations and to inform exercise participants of the risks of exercise.

The major cardiovascular complications occurring during exercise are cardiac arrhythmias, myocardial infarction, and sudden cardiac death.[1]

CARDIAC ARRHYTHMIAS

Cardiac arrhythmias are a frequent complication of exercise. The participant and exercise leader are usually unaware of the arrhythmia, except when the individual is exercising in an electrocardiographically (ECG) monitored situation. Some patients do feel palpitations during the arrhythmia, however, or may detect changes in the heart beat when monitoring their pulse. Therefore, the exercise leader should have a general understanding of cardiac arrhythmias during exercise and their significance.

Changes in cardiac control that occur during exercise increase the frequency of cardiac arrhythmias.[1] The decrease in parasympathetic tone and the increase in sympathetic activity with exercise increase cardiac automaticity. Furthermore, exercise may induce myocardial ischemia, which increases cardiac ectopic beats. Cardiac arrhythmias can occur in otherwise healthy people, but are more frequent and more dangerous in patients with heart disease.

Cardiac arrhythmias during exercise may be either supraventricular or ventricular in origin. Supraventricular arrhythmias include paroxysmal atrial tachycardia (PAT), atrial fibrillation, and atrial flutter. These arrhythmias usually produce a rapid ventricular rate of 150 beats per minute or greater. Exercising subjects may complain of a "fluttering" in the chest or use another expression for palpitations. Differentiation from the normal increased heart rate of exercise may be difficult. Whereas the normal exercise heart rate decreases gradually with exercise cessation, the tachycardia of an arrhythmia often persists or suddenly decreases to a much slower rate when the arrhythmia "breaks."

Ventricular arrhythmias during exercise include premature ventricular impulses (PVIs), ventricular tachycardia, and ventricular fibrillation. PVIs occur frequently in the general population and usually are noted as a skipped beat or a pulse drop when subjects monitor their heart rate. As many as 44% of apparently healthy men may demonstrate PVIs during maximal exercise testing.[2] Ventricular tachycardia may be felt only as palpitations, but is often associated with dizziness, weakness, or loss of consciousness. Ventricular tachycardia may precede ventricular fibrillation, which is the probable mediator of most sudden cardiac deaths and requires immediate cardiopulmonary resuscitation.

The exercise leader's response to a subject with a cardiac arrhythmia other than ventricular fibrillation depends on the clinical situation. Arrhythmias causing significant symptoms, such as prolonged palpitations, dizziness, or loss of consciousness, require immediate medical attention. The only exception is in individuals who have an episodic arrhythmia and have been instructed in self-treatment. These patients often have mild PAT. Arrhythmias detected as skipped beats during pulse monitoring but without other symptoms are frequently benign. The subject should discuss the problem with a physician, but it is not of immediate concern, especially in healthy young people. All cardiac arrhythmias are more dangerous in subjects with known cardiac disease and should be brought to the attention of the patient's physician.

EXERCISE-RELATED MYOCARDIAL INFARCTIONS AND SUDDEN DEATH

Myocardial infarctions and sudden cardiac deaths in adults during exercise are usually caused by atheroslerotic coronary artery disease (CAD). This correlation is not surprising in that CAD is the major cause of sudden death in the general adult population.[1] Exercise increases myocardial oxygen demand. CAD limits myocardial oxygen supply with resultant myocardial ischemia. Myocardial ischemia predisposes the myocardium to ventricular arrhythmias, and the final event in most sudden cardiac deaths is almost certainly ventricular fibrillation.[1]

Occasionally, sudden death in adults occurs without pathologic findings of CAD. Muscular contraction of the coronary artery wall or "coronary spasm" may be operative in these instances. A runner in the 1975 Boston Marathon developed ventricular fibrillation and subsequent ECG evidence of a myocardial infarction. He died 2 months later of complications. Autopsy confirmed the myocardial infarction, but the coronary arteries were widely patent.[3] An alternate possibility is that coronary artery thrombosis with subsequent clot lysis may cause exercise-related cardiac events. A 34-year-old participant in the 1982 Montreal Marathon sustained an acute myocardial infarction immediately after the race. Arteriography demonstrated a coronary artery thrombus.[4] Coronary spasm cannot be excluded, even in this instance, however, because coronary spasm can reduce blood flow and may result in clot formation.[5]

CAD is a rare cause of exercise-related sudden death in individuals under 30 years.[6] In this group, various congenital or other abnormalities are associated with exercise-related deaths, including hypertrophic cardiomyopathy, anomalous origin of the coronary arteries, aortic rupture, aortic valve stenosis, cerebrovascular accidents, conducting system abnormalities, and myocarditis.[1] An insufficient amount of information is available to rank-order these diagnoses as to the frequency with which they cause cardiac death.

Hypertrophic cardiomyopathy is a condition in which the left ventricular septum is markedly enlarged and may obstruct blood flow during ventricular contraction. The catecholamine stimulation of exercise increases cardiac contractility and may further compromise left ventricular outflow. Sudden death during exercise with anomalous coronary artery origin most frequently involves the left coronary artery arising from the anterior aortic cusp. Flow in the left coronary artery can be restricted during exercise, leading to myocardial ischemia. Sudden death from aortic rupture received national attention with the death of the Olympic volleyball player, Flo Hyman.[7] Certain very tall individuals have a weakness of connective tissue in the aortic wall produced by an inherited condition called Marfan's syndrome. The increased blood pressure produced by exercise may cause the aorta to rupture. In aortic valve stenosis, the narrowed aortic valve may not permit adequate cardiac output during exercise. Cerebrovascular accidents in young people during exercise are often associated with the rupture of a blood vessel in the brain. Abnormalities of the cardiac conducting system and myocarditis probably cause sudden death by producing ventricular fibrillation.

All of the aforementioned abnormalities are extremely rare, as is sudden death during exertion in young people. Nevertheless, certain warning signs should alert the exercise leader. A history of syncope or chest discomfort during exercise, even in a young person, may be associated with hypertrophic cardiomyopathy, anomalous coronary artery origin, aortic stenosis, or conducting system abnormalities. Sudden death in a close family member aged 50 years or less is also of concern. Professionals supervising sports in which height is an advantage should be aware of the characteristics of Marfan's syndrome: tallness, long fingers and arms, sternal deformity, and nearsightedness. With any of these symptoms or with the characteristics of Marfan's syndrome, the subject should be evaluated by a physician before exercise. Also, because myocarditis may be part of a generalized disease, exercise training should probably be restricted during the febrile period of any illness.

INCIDENCE OF CARDIAC COMPLICATIONS DURING EXERCISE TESTING

In 1969, Rochmis and Blackburn surveyed 130 facilities to determine the risk of exercise testing.[8] Responses were received from the staff of 55% of facilities, yielding a total of 170,000 tests. Eight deaths (0.5 deaths per 10,000 tests) occurred within 1 hour of exercise and an additional eight deaths were attributed to the exercise test over the next 4 days. This rate of one death per 10,000 tests is a convenient figure for estimating the mortality of exercise testing. An additional 3 patients per 10,000 tests were admitted to the hospital for medical treatment. In only 34% of the surveyed test facilities were maximal tests routinely performed.

Stuart and Ellestad mailed questionnaires to 6000 possible exercise test facilities.[9] Professionals from 33% of the institutions replied, for a total of 518,448 tests. Respondents included hospital and office-based facilities. Seventy percent of the respondents used a symptom-limited maximal test. Data showed that only 90.5 deaths, 3.58 myocardial infarctions, and 4.78 arrhythmias requiring intravenous medication or cardioversion occurred per 10,000 tests. The authors did not specify the time after exercise when the cardiac event occurred or the number of patients admitted to the hospital after exercise testing.

Atterhög, Jonsson, and Samuelsson prospectively determined the incidence of cardiac complications in 20 Swedish test facilities in which 50,000 tests were performed during an 18-month period.[10] Only 0.4 deaths, 1.4 myocardial infarctions and 5.2 hospital admissions occurred per 10,000 tests.

In all of the aforementioned studies, the facilities examined conducted exercise testing in the usual clinical situation. Consequently, the risk of such testing is 1 or fewer deaths, 4 or fewer myocardial infarctions, and approximately 5 hospital admissions (including the infarctions) per 10,000 exercise tests—roughly 1 major problem for every 1000 clinical exercise tests. The risk of exercise testing varies with the patient population. Facilities in which the subjects tested are predominantly healthy should experience fewer problems than facilities in which testing primarily involves subjects with severe cardiac disease.[11]

EXERCISE TRAINING IN THE GENERAL POPULATION

Few studies of cardiac complications in the general population have been conducted. Thompson et al. determined the incidence of death during jogging in Rhode Island from 1975 through 1980.[12] Statistics relating to sudden death were collected by the medical examiner, who is required by law to investigate all sudden deaths. The number of Rhode Island men jogging at least twice weekly was determined by using a random-digit telephone survey and population estimates. Results showed only 1 death per year for every 7620 joggers aged 30 through 64 years (95% confidence limits: 1 death per 2,000 to 13,000 joggers). Nevertheless, the hourly death rate during jogging was 7 times that during more sedentary activities (95% confidence limits: 4 to 26 times). The association of exercise with sudden death, therefore, is rare but is probably more than coincidental. If men with known heart disease are excluded and certain assumptions are made, the death rate for healthy men in Rhode Island is only 1 death per year for every 15,200 middle-aged joggers.

Similar results were reported in a case control study of cardiac arrests during vigorous exercise in Seattle.[13] Only 1 episode of cardiac arrest occurred per year during exercise for every 18,000 healthy men. Once again, the death rate during vigorous exercise exceeded that at other times, especially for men unaccustomed to vigorous activity.

We do not know of studies of the general population in which researchers have quantified the risk of myocardial infarction during vigorous exercise. Consequently, the previous estimates of death during exercise underestimate the total risk of cardiac complications. Nevertheless, one can estimate a risk of 1 death per year during exercise for every 15,000 to 20,000 healthy men.

Exercise-related cardiac events are rare in women. Most exercise deaths are due to CAD, and the prevalence of CAD is lower in young and middle-aged women, the group most likely to be physically active. The rarity of cardiovascular events in women has prevented estimates of the incidence of exercise-related deaths in this group. For similar reasons, no incidence figures are available for the occurrence of cerebrovascular accidents, aortic dissection, or other rare exercise complications.

CARDIAC REHABILITATION

Several investigators have examined the incidence of cardiac complications during cardiac rehabilitation.[14] Haskell, in 1978, obtained information from the directors of 30 cardiac rehabilitation programs.[15] The results were based on 13,500 patients and more than 1.6 million hours of exercise. Only 61 major cardiovascular complications, including 50 cardiac arrests, occurred during or soon after exercise, yielding an incidence of only 1 arrest and 1 death per 33,000 hours and 120,000 patient-hours of activity, respectively.

The risks of cardiac rehabilitation were re-evaluated by Van Camp and Peterson in 1986 using data from 167 programs that encompassed 51,000 patients and 2.3 million hours of exertion.[16] There were only 21 cardiac arrests in association with exercise, yielding 1 event per 112,000 hours and 1 death for every 790,000 hours. In addition, 1 myocardial infarction was reported for every 300,000 exercise hours.

The reduction in cardiac arrests between these two studies[15,16] is likely to be caused by multiple factors, including better patient selection, more aggressive management of ischemia, and other factors such as electrocardiographic monitoring.[16] Both studies suggest that the absolute risk of exercise is low even in CAD patients. Both studies also demonstrated the value of prompt cardiopulmonary resuscitation in this group.

Cardiac rehabilitation is currently being used more frequently for patients with severe left ventricular dysfunction and compensated congestive heart failure. The risks and benefits of this practice have recently been reviewed.[17] Some exercise conditioning is beneficial in the patient group to counteract the deconditioning effects of inactivity. On the other hand, patients with importantly decreased left ventricular function are likely to be at increased cardiac risk during exercise training, may fail to benefit from the training regimen, and may even experience deterioration in left ventricular function in association with the exercise program.[17] Consequently, these patients should be carefully observed during rehabilitation for signs and symptoms of deteriorating left ventricular function. Any possible deterioration should prompt reassessment of the value of the exercise program for that patient.

INDICATIONS TO DEFER EXERCISE TESTING

The decision as to whether to perform or to defer an exercise test depends on the clinical situation and the quality and availability of medical assistance. In general, patients with resting blood pressure above 200 mm Hg systolic and 120 mm Hg diastolic should not be tested until the hypertension is controlled. Many facilities stop exercise when systolic and diastolic blood pressure exceed 250 and 120 mm Hg, respectively. Patients with probable or known CAD should undergo exercise testing only when emergency resuscitation equipment and trained personnel are readily available. Similar safeguards are not required for routine testing of healthy subjects, but even in this group, testing should be delayed for otherwise healthy subjects during viral illness. Subjects who report new symptoms suggestive of cardiac disease should undergo exercise testing under supervision. The exercise technicians should also delay exercise testing with any patient or in any situation in which the technician feels uncomfortable because of safety concerns.

INDICATIONS TO LIMIT EXERCISE

Historic evidence of exercise-induced angina, syncope, or cardiac arrhythmias in any participant warrants further evaluation before exercise training. Most fitness leaders know the importance of exercise-induced chest discomfort. Cardiac ischemia may also manifest as jaw, neck, arm, shoulder, or back discomfort or as an uncomfortable shortness of breath. Some middle-aged patients join exercise programs just to "prove" that such symptoms are not evidence of heart disease. It is useful, therefore, to know whether new symptoms have prompted the initiation of an exercise program. Subjects who feel ill or are febrile should be prohibited from training. Similarly, persons returning from a *major* illness should first be evaluated by a physician. The cardiac rehabilitation leader should ensure that the patients have not developed new or progressive symptoms since their last exercise session.

During exercise, significant symptoms, including new or worsening angina, palpitations, dizziness, weakness, unusual and extreme fatigue, or excessive air hunger, should indicate the end of the exercise session for any subject. Subjects who experience such symptoms during exercise should be promptly evaluated by a physician either at the exercise facility or after transport to an emergency room.

SUMMARY

The major cause of important cardiovascular complications during exercise is CAD. Consequently, the risk of exercise complications increases the prevalence of CAD in the exercising population. The risk is extremely small among healthy young adults and nonsmoking women, higher among groups with CAD risk factors, and highest among persons with known disease. The *absolute* risk for cardiac complications in the general population is small. Nevertheless, the exercise leader should be aware of individuals who may be at increased risk and should take appropriate precautions.

ACKNOWLEDGMENT

The author thanks Tess Newton for typing and editing the manuscript.

REFERENCES

1. Thompson PD: Cardiovascular hazards of physical activity. In *Exercise and Sport Sciences Reviews*. Edited by RL Terjung. Philadelphia: Franklin Institute Press, 1982.

2. McHenry PL, Fisch C, Jordan JW, Corya BR: Cardiac arrhythmias observed during maximal exercise testing in clinically normal men. *Am J Cardiol, 29:*331, 1972.

3. Green LH, Cohen SI, Kurland G: Fatal myocardial infarction in marathon racing. *Ann Intern Med, 84:*704, 1976.

4. Chan KL, Davies RA, Chambers RJ: Coronary thrombosis and subsequent lysis after a marathon. *J Am Coll Cardiol, 4:*1322, 1984.

5. Gertz SD, et al.: Endothelial cell damage and thrombus formation after partial arterial constriction: Relevance to the role of coronary artery spasm in the pathogenesis of myocardial infarction. *Circulation, 63:*476, 1981.

6. Ragosta M, Crabtree J, Sturner WQ, Thompson PD: Death during recreational exercise in the State of Rhode Island. *Med Sci Sports Exerc, 16:*339, 1984.

7. Demak R: Marfan syndrome: A silent killer. *Sports Illustrated*, February *17:*30, 1986.

8. Rochmis P, Blackburn H: Exercise tests: A survey of procedures, safety, and litigation experience in approximately 170,000 tests. *JAMA, 217:*1061, 1971.

9. Stuart RJ Jr, Ellestad MH: National survey of exercise stress testing facilities. *Chest, 77:*94, 1980.

10. Atterhög J-H., Jonsson B, Samuelsson R: Exercise testing: A prospective study of complication rates. *Am Heart J, 98:*572, 1979.

11. Young DZ, Lampert S, Graboys TB, Lown B: Safety of maximal exercise testing in patients at high risk for ventricular arrhythmia. *Circulation, 70:*184, 1984.

12. Thompson PD, Funk EJ, Carleton RA, Sturner WQ: Incidence of death during jogging in Rhode Island from 1975 through 1980. *JAMA, 247:*2535, 1982.

13. Siscovick DS, Weiss NS, Fletcher RH, Lasky T: The incidence of primary cardiac arrest during vigorous exercise. *N Engl J Med, 311:*874, 1984.

14. Thompson PD: The cardiovascular risks of cardiac rehabilitation. *J Cardiopul Rehabil, 5:*321, 1985.

15. Haskell WL: Cardiovascular complications during exercise training of cardiac patients. *Circulation, 57:*920, 1978.

16. Van Camp SP, Peterson RA: Cardiovascular complications of outpatient cardiac rehabilitation programs. *JAMA, 256:*1160, 1986.

17. Smith LK: Exercise training in patients with impaired left ventricular function. *Med Sci Sports Exerc, 23:*654, 1991.

Chapter 30

EMERGENCY PLANS AND PROCEDURES FOR AN EXERCISE FACILITY*

William E. Strauss, Diane Panton Lapsley, Terry A. Fortin, Jamil A. Kirdar, and Kevin M. McIntyre

All exercise programs, be they exercise testing, cardiac rehabilitation, or supervised aerobic exercise, should ideally be free of risk. Obviously, however, this is not the case; although the benefits are potentially much greater, the finite risk of a patient developing a problem during exercise does exist. In the following section, we explore this risk and what can be done to reduce it. Many of the guidelines we propose are simple common sense. The central and most important point we stress is the need for an organized, written plan delineating how different levels of patient-related problems are handled *in a particular facility*. Many different types of exercise facilities exist and the health and degree of wellness of the patients or clients, the equipment present, and the expertise of the employees vary considerably. Instead of trying to propose plans and procedures for all, or even many, of these different exercise facilities, we propose certain guidelines that we hope can be models or templates for the exercise technologist, exercise specialist, or program director to use as a stepping stone in modifying the plans to an individual situation. Many references could be cited; we cite a few and include "suggested reading" that may be used as further reference material or as one of many examples we have used to make a point.

RISKS AND BENEFITS OF EXERCISE

The pros and cons of exercise have been controversial for more than 30 years. Results of epidemiologic studies suggest that vigorous exercise is associated with a reduced risk of cardiovascular events and mortality. In addition, a large segment of our population has correctly or incorrectly, over the last decade, become enamored with the overall sense of well-being and health associated with frequent exercise. On the other hand, myocardial ischemia and death have been observed to occur during strenuous exercise. The trade-offs of the risks and benefits of exercise can perhaps be put in perspective by an excellent study performed by Siscovick and colleagues.[1] They examined the exercise habits of a group of previously healthy men who sustained a cardiac arrest and compared them with a random sample of similar men who had not experienced sudden death. The study confirmed that the risk of cardiac arrest did increase transiently during vigorous exercise, although those men who had a high level of habitual exercise had a far lower risk of cardiac arrest during exercise than those with a low level of weekly exercise. Although vigorous physical activity was associated with an increased risk of sudden death, habitual participation in such aerobic activity was associated in an overall reduction in the risk of experiencing sudden death. A far more expanded review of the incidence of complications with exercise is provided in the excellent chapter by Thompson (Chap. 29). Reviewing several studies, Thompson estimated the incidence of death, myocardial infarction (MI) and arrhythmias requiring intravenous medication or cardioversion as being 1 or fewer deaths, 4 or fewer MIs and approximately 5 arrhythmic episodes or admissions per 10,000 exercise tests. The incidence of deaths occurring during unsupervised exercise by a general population was approximately 1 death per year per 7600 joggers, or if men with known heart disease were excluded, one per 15,000 middle-aged joggers. This latter figure was in close agreement with the

* Supported by the Medical Research Service of the US Department of Veterans Affairs.

one episode of cardiac arrest per year per 18,000 healthy men noted by Siscovick in Seattle.[1]

One of the basic premises of this section is that the frequency of cardiac arrest and other serious complications, as well as their ultimate outcome, can be improved. The risk of the development of such events hopefully can be decreased by screening to identify high-risk patients. In addition, the likelihood of surviving those episodes that do occur can be enhanced if trained personnel have developed appropriate plans and procedures ahead of time.

A part of pre-exercise screening involves common sense: patients or clients should be excluded if they have unstable symptoms or major uncontrolled illnesses. In addition, some markers can help to identify the high-risk patient. In a review of their experience with supervised exercise training, Hossack and Hartwig[2] not only provided the data concerning cardiac arrest incidence, but they also delineated clinical findings more likely to be associated with the development of sudden death: myocardial ischemia during exercise and noncompliance with the exercise prescription. Patients with sudden death had more ST depression on the electrocardiogram during pretraining exercise tolerance testing, a reliable manifestation of exercise-induced ischemia. The sudden-death patients not only had more normal exercise capacities pretraining than those individuals who did not experience sudden death, but also they exceeded their prescribed training heart rate range more than twice as frequently. Thus, a high-risk participant may be considered as having continued exercise-related ischemia and a propensity to "push" himself during training.

The need for routine electrocardiographic (ECG) monitoring of all patients during the outpatient exercise rehabilitation programs is controversial, especially because cost is also of major concern.

In a recent survey, 87% of an expert panel of physicians stated that the use of telemetry ECG monitoring is established as essential to the safety and effectiveness of a prescribed regimen of exercise in coronary rehabilitation. There have been no controlled studies comparing the safety of exercise training conducted with on-site medical supervision, with and without continuous ECG monitoring.[3]

Van Camp and Peterson, in a review of 167 programs and assessment of 2 million exercise hours between 1980 and 1984, noted one cardiac arrest per 111,996 patient-hours. Their conclusion was that there was no significant benefit from ECG monitoring; but that the presence of supervision with knowledgeable personnel enhanced survival.[4]

The following list provides the criteria for electrocardiographic monitoring advocated by the American College of Cardiology/American Heart Association Subcommittee on Cardiac Rehabilitation.[5,6] Additional studies examining the safety and efficacy of ECG monitoring in cardiac rehabilitation are necessary if guidelines are to be refined beyond these general recommendations.

1. Severely depressed left ventricular function (ejection fraction below 30%)
2. Resting complex ventricular arrhythmia
3. Ventricular arrhythmias appearing or increasing with exercise
4. Decrease in systolic blood pressure with exercise
5. Survivors of sudden cardiac death
6. Survivors of myocardial infarction complicated by congestive heart failure, cardiogenic shock, and/or serious ventricular arrhythmias
7. Severe coronary artery disease and marked exercise-induced ischemia (ST-segment depression > 2 mm)
8. Inability to self-monitor heart rate because of physical or intellectual impairment.

Despite the ability to screen and to observe high-risk patients more closely, some untoward events continue to happen. In the following sections, we outline guidelines for personnel, equipment, and finally plans or procedures to be put into effect.

CLINICAL KNOWLEDGE REQUIRED OF PERSONNEL IN AN EXERCISE FACILITY

Safe Conduct of an Exercise Program

The conduct of a safe exercise program depends on the knowledge of the personnel and their ability to communicate with the client. Personnel working in the facility must have a degree of competency in the following areas consistent with the program and the particular risk level of the participants involved.

1. Obtain an accurate and complete medical history, and include any physical and emotional limitations.
2. Understand fully the principles of exercise and conditioning, such as frequency, duration, intensity, type of exercise, warm-up and recovery periods.
3. Recognize clinical signs and symptoms and differentiate between normal and abnormal responses to exercise.
4. Understand the physiologic effects of environmental factors as related to heat and cold and humidity on the body, both during and after exercise, and adjust workload up or down as appropriate.
5. Be aware of the pre-exercise habits of the exercise participant as they relate to eating, drinking, clothing, and activity.
6. Know the medication a participant is taking, the patient's compliance with taking this medication, and the effects of the medication.
7. Be able to take vital signs and know what values are appropriate for a particular level of activity.
8. Know how to operate, maintain, and calibrate all equipment.
9. Obtain informed consent from the patient.

Informed Consent

"Consent" implies that the patient or person to be tested (or to participate in an exercise training program) has agreed to be tested, in this case in a form defined by the exercise test protocol to be used. "Informed" consent requires that all of the risks that may be material to the patient's decision to be tested are disclosed and the benefits to be obtained are disclosed. The specific risk of the patient suffering cardiac arrest or myocardial infarction should be disclosed. The patient should be informed of the potential benefit of the procedure to

him or her, especially when the risk may be high and the benefit small.

Informed consent should be viewed more as an exchange of information, or a process rather than a document one may be called upon to sign. The patient should understand, as a result of that process, the specific risks to him and to her of the exercise test. Only when this is achieved can consent be considered "informed." Accordingly, the extent of the legal protection conferred by a patient's signature on an informed consent document when the patient has not been shown to fully understand the risks involved for the potential benefit must be considered to be in question. Certainly, if the patient suffers a complication that he/she had no basis for anticipating, the likelihood of litigation based on the inadequacy of informed consent should be anticipated.

Safe Conduct of the Exercise Session

1. Take vital signs appropriate for the patient's risk level and personal needs (heart rate, blood pressure, rhythm, extremity swelling, respiratory difficulty, unusual weight gain or loss).
2. Elicit information on any symptoms or changes in symptoms since the previous session as well as status of general health before the session.
3. Maintain the patient's adherence to his individual exercise prescription and carefully observe for signals of trouble. Patients often self-deny symptoms.
4. Modify the daily exercise session to meet the patient's present status and refer to the contraindications and reasons for terminating exercise that follow.

Contraindications to Exercise

The importance of being fully aware of the contraindications to exercise cannot be overstated. Table 30–1 is taken from *Guidelines for Exercise Testing and Prescription*,[6] listing both absolute and relative contraindications. The type of facility, level of emergency treatment available, and the benefit or urgency of the test versus the test's safety affect the decision to exercise a person with known relative contraindica-

Table 30–1. Contraindications to Exercise Testing*

Absolute Contraindications
1. A recent significant change in the resting ECG suggesting infarction or other acute cardiac events
2. Recent complicated myocardial infarction
3. Unstable angina
4. Uncontrolled ventricular dysrhythmia
5. Uncontrolled atrial dysrhythmia that compromises cardiac function
6. Third-degree A-V block
7. Acute congestive heart failure
8. Severe aortic stenosis
9. Suspected or known dissecting aneurysm
10. Active or suspected myocarditis or pericarditis
11. Thrombophlebitis or intracardiac thrombi
12. Recent systemic or pulmonary embolus
13. Acute infections
14. Significant emotional distress (psychosis)

Relative Contraindications
1. Resting diastolic blood pressure > 120 mm Hg or resting systolic blood pressure > 200 mm Hg
2. Moderate valvular heart disease
3. Known electrolyte abnormalities (hypokalemia, hypomagnesemia)
4. Fixed-rate pacemaker (rarely used)
5. Frequent or complex ventricular ectopy
6. Ventricular aneurysm
7. Cardiomyopathy, including hypertrophic cardiomyopathy
8. Uncontrolled metabolic disease (e.g. diabetes, thyrotoxicosis, or myxedema)
9. Chronic infectious disease (e.g., mononucleosis, hepatitis, AIDS)
10. Neuromuscular, musculoskeletal, or rheumatoid disorders that are exacerbated by exercise
11. Advanced or complicated pregnancy

---

* With permission from ACSM: *Guidlines for Exercise Testing and Prescription.* 4th edition. Philadelphia: Lea & Febiger, 1991.

Table 30–2. Indications for Stopping an Exercise Test*

1. Progressive angina (stop at 3 + level or earlier on a scale of 1 + to 4 +)†
2. Ventricular tachycardia
3. Any significant drop (20 mm Hg) or systolic blood pressure or a failure of the systolic blood pressure to rise with an increase in exercise load
4. Lightheadedness, confusion, ataxia, pallor, cyanosis, nausea, or signs of severe peripheral circulatory insufficiency
5. > 4 mm horizontal or downsloping ST depression or elevation (in the absence of other indicators of ischemia)
6. Onset of second- or third-degree A-V block
7. Increasing ventricular ectopy, multiform PVCs, or R on T PVCs
8. Excessive rise in blood pressure: systolic pressure > 250 mm Hg; diastolic pressure > 120 mm Hg
9. Chronotropic impairment
10. Sustained supraventricular tachycardia
11. Exercise-induced left bundle branch block
12. Subject requests to stop
13. Failure of monitoring system

---

* With permission from ACSM: *Guidelines for Exercise Testing and Prescription.* Philadelphia: Lea & Febiger, 1991.
† Ibid., Table 4–5, page 73

tant information must be weighed against the safety factor. These termination points are for an exercise test. An exercise session would be stopped earlier in several instances. One would discontinue exercise or reduce the level with the onset of angina and the level of activity would remain below indicators of ischemia (≥ 1 mm ST depression). In these instances, an exercise session may be resumed as symptoms subside. Again, common sense should dictate actions.

Emergency Plan

Not only having an emergency plan but also knowing the plan without having to read it is of utmost importance in any emergency situation. Each facility must have a plan conducive to its particular setting. All personnel must know the plan and review it regularly.

1. Know how to activate the emergency plan (i.e., by wall switch, telephone).
2. Know the location of all necessary

tions. Common sense is essential, especially for an exercise session that can be delayed until problems can be evaluated.

Reasons for Terminating Exercise

The reasons for terminating exercise are also listed in *Guidelines for Exercise Testing and Prescription*[6] and are presented in Table 30–2. As with the contraindications to exercise, these termination points vary with the type of facility and the purpose of the exercise test. The benefit of further impor-

communication equipment (i.e., telephone, including a quarter if necessary; the telephone number to call; warning alarm).

3. Know how to describe the location of the incident, how to get there, and the location of the exits.
4. Know the location of all emergency equipment (i.e., defibrillator, crash cart, and backboard).
5. Know the responsibilities of people assisting with the incident.
6. Be able to provide first-responder assistance.
7. Know how to prepare crash cart and defibrillator for use by those trained to use it (if applicable).
8. Prepare an accurate account of the incident (or drill) and what was done.

Emergency drills in the exercise area, testing labs, locker rooms, and immediate area should be carried out periodically, and as part of each new employee's orientation. This will permit the program director to evaluate the appropriateness of the response of the exercise team members.

Cardiopulmonary Resuscitation

All personnel involved in the exercise program shall be trained in Basic Life Support (BLS) and demonstrate competency in the execution of the skills involved in cardiopulmonary resuscitation (CPR). Consult your local American Heart Association or American Red Cross for further information.

USE OF EQUIPMENT BY PERSONNEL IN AN EXERCISE FACILITY

The safe operation of an exercise facility depends on the condition of the laboratory, the equipment, and the expertise of the staff in its use. Personnel should be competent in the use, care, and instructional techniques for all available equipment within their facility.

Exercise Laboratory

1. The overall floor plan should provide easy access to emergency and monitoring equipment. Locker facilities or separate exercise rooms should be

quickly accessible. Water bubblers or drinking water should be available.
2. Climate control is necessary to maintain a comfortable temperature (72°F or less), ventilation, and humidity for all seasons. The combined effects of temperature, humidity and wind chill must be considered for outdoor activities.
3. Floors should not be slippery. Carpeting or nonslip finishes will reduce the incidence of falls. Areas used for impact activities, e.g., running and aerobics, should be constructed of shock-absorbing materials to prevent injury.
4. Walking or running tracks or lanes should be obstacle-free and have clear traffic patterns. Electrical cords to treadmills or other equipment should be safely tacked down or kept out of traffic patterns.
5. Locker rooms and swimming areas require a dry area suitable for emergency defibrillation. Hand rails in showers and nonslip flooring help prevent falls. Water temperatures in showers should be moderate to prevent post-exercise hypotension.
6. Isolated areas used for exercise and locker-room facilities should have a warning or alarm system for emergency situations.

Exercise Equipment

All exercise equipment must be properly maintained and calibrated to ensure accurate and consistent workloads. The staff should know how to operate and adjust all equipment. They must be capable of providing instruction in the proper use of equipment as well as modifying the techniques to meet the specific demands of any musculoskeletal impairments. Patients should be regularly reinstructed in proper techniques and workloads modified as needed. Not all equipment is appropriate for each patient.

The equipment at any given facility varies, and personnel should be familiar with the manufacturer's safety guidelines and operating instructions, and weight limitations for the models present at the facility. A resistance flywheel should be properly enclosed on any ergometers. General guidelines for common types of equipment follow:

Treadmills—Electrically operated models must be properly grounded and have an easily accessible control panel. Some models have emergency shutoff switches. Patients should be cautioned to stay off belts until the speed is adjusted. Regular maintenance, including calibration and belt inspection, should be performed. Front or side handles should be checked regularly for stability.

Cycle ergometers—Handlebars and seats should be adjustable for proper positioning. Proper calibration of the resistance mechanism is necessary to ensure accurate workloads. Foot straps are not appropriate on all models. Models of combined arm and leg movements and reclined cycles require similar adjustable parts.

Arm ergometers—Free-standing models should be mounted on a stable base when in use. Appropriate resistance, pedal adjustments and seat heights apply.

Rowing machines—Proper instruction will decrease the likelihood of lower back injuries. All moving parts, seats, handgrips, cables, or chains must be regularly maintained.

Weight machines—Cables and chains must be regularly maintained. Proper technique and positioning of seats etc. must be evaluated. It is important to monitor blood pressures during this activity.

Hand weights—A safe storage and spacious usage area is important to protect clients. All weights should be accurately marked and checked for loose ends or fittings.

Swimming pools—Proper supervision and safety equipment is necessary. pH and chlorine levels should be routinely checked. Ladders and railings must be stable. The water temperature should be appropriate for the activity.

Many types of stepping, climbing, and ski machines are available. Proper instruction and maintenance of the machines are the keys to safety. Ascertain the appropriateness of the exercise for the client.

Monitoring Equipment

1. Proper skin preparation and electrode placement are necessary to ensure good contact of electrodes for accurate ECG recording (for more information, see Chap. 1).
2. The ECG monitor should be of the type designed for exercise testing because that allows for easy hookup to electrodes. The choice of hardware models or telemetry units depends on the facility's particular program. Expertise is needed to be able to recognize, analyze, and interpret ECG changes and arrhythmias, both on an oscilloscope and on ECG paper.
3. Quick-look ECGs can be obtained from the paddles of certain monitor-defibrillators. It is imperative that personnel understand fully how to select the proper mode on the defibrillator and where to place the paddles.
4. Blood pressure cuffs should be readily available. Personnel should be trained to take accurate readings while a participant is exercising or at rest (for more information, see Appendix 1).

Emergency Equipment

Emergency equipment includes a crash cart complete with drugs, suctioning apparatus, oxygen, and a defibrillator (Table 30–3 and Table 30–4). Personnel of facilities with such equipment should not be involved with its use unless they are trained in Advanced Cardiac Life Support or some comparable level of training. In an emergency situation, however, having such equipment available and prepared for use when the proper personnel arrive at the scene is of great value. Other equipment that may prove useful in an emergency situation includes an alarm to summon help, a clock to note length of time, and a backboard to provide a firm surface for the victim or to remove someone from a swimming pool.

All emergency equipment must be maintained up to date. It is the responsibility of the personnel who work in the area where the equipment is stored to ensure that it is in working order. Individual policies must be developed to routinely check the expira-

Table 30–3.　Emergency Equipment

Equipment	Maintenance
Defibrillator (portable synchronized)	Check that it is plugged into an electrical outlet (recharge battery)
	Test the delivery of energy output is adequate by turning on set energy level, charge and discharge (to be done exactly according to specific manufacturer's instruction)
	Check that accessory equipment is available (i.e., electrode paste, patient cable with electrodes)
Oxygen tanks	Check level of fullness
	Check for tubing present
Airways (oral and endotracheal tubes)	Present and clean (oral) or sterile (endotracheal tube)
Laryngoscope and intubation equipment	Present and in working order (i.e., laryngoscope light works)
Ambu bag	Present and clean (keep inside plastic bag) with tubing attached
Syringes and needles	Present, sterile
Intravenous tubing and solutions	Present, sterile
Intravenous stand (to hang solutions on)	Present
Adhesive tape	Present
Blood drawing tubes and equipment (i.e., for blood chemistry, blood gas)	Present
Suction apparatus and supplies (tubing, gloves, etc.)	Present
	Works when switched on
	Gloves, suction tubing are sterile

tion dates of emergency drugs. This can be easily accomplished by keeping the drugs in a locked cart with a date on the lock showing when the earliest expiration date of any drug will be. Thus there is no need to break the lock to handle individual drugs unless they are needed for an emergency, and this ensures that all drugs are valid and have not reached this date of expiration. Oxygen tanks should be checked for fullness by checking the gauge. Defibrillators are usually checked by turning them on, setting a particular energy level (recommended by the manufacturer) and discharging the energy out of the paddles without removing the paddles from their position on the defibrillator. This ensures that the defibrillator will emit an accurate amount of electrical energy if required to do so, and avoid any mishaps which may occur (i.e.: the defibrillator battery charge runs out because the unit was inadvertently left unplugged) from neglecting the equipment. Other equipment, such as intravenous catheters, needles, solutions, tubing, endotracheal intubation tubes, and laryngoscope, should be kept in the same locked cart with the drugs to ensure availability when needed.

Electrical defibrillation of the heart is obtained by the passage of enough electrical current through the heart to cause depolarization of the heart muscle. This is accomplished with the use of an external device—a portable or direct current defibrillator. The electrical energy is selected (i.e., 200, 300, or 360 joules), paddles (greased with paste to avoid burning the skin) placed on the victim's chest, and buttons pushed to deliver the energy selected from the defibrillator to the victim (making sure no one else is touching the victim at the time the electrical energy is being delivered). According to the AHA, electrical defibrillation is currently the most effective method of terminating ventricular fibrillation (a lethal cardiac arrhythmia) and early use is recommended when a cardiac arrest occurs.[7]

Oxygen is necessary to improve tissue oxygenation. Thus, when a person is complaining of chest pain or shortness of breath or is in cardiac arrest, supplemental oxygen is beneficial. Oxygen can be stored in a cylinder which contains a pressure gauge (telling you how much oxygen remains in the tank) and flow meter (letting you adjust the amount of oxygen to be

Table 30–4. Emergency Drugs (American Heart Association Classification of Drugs Most Commonly Used in a Life-threatening Emergency)

Drug	Mechanism of Action
1. Drugs to correct hypoxemia and metabolic acidosis:	
Oxygen	Increases alveolar oxygen tension
	Improves tissue oxygenation
Sodium bicarbonate	Reacts with hydrogen ions to form water and carbon dioxide to buffer metabolic acidosis. Not recommended in an arrest situation until after 10 minutes of CPR, defibrillation, oxygen and drugs are tried and metabolic acidosis is present
2. Drugs to increase heart rate:	
Atropine	Exerts a parasympatholytic action (i.e., blocks the vagus nerve) that allows sympathetic stimulation to predominate, thereby increasing the rate of sinus node discharge and enhancing atrioventricular node conduction
Isoproterenol	Increases heart rate and vasodilates coronary and peripheral arteries by means of beta-adrenergic stimulation
3. Drugs to correct ventricular dysrhythmias:	
Lidocaine	A Class IB agent that blocks the fast sodium Purkinje fibers, thereby raising the fibrillation threshold, and suppressing ventricular ectopy
Bretylium	A Class III agent that lengthens repolarization and increases refractoriness of the cardiac muscle cell, which raises the fibrillation threshold
Procainamide	A Class IA agent that exerts a direct electrophysiologic effect on the heart to lengthen repolarization, thus suppressing ventricular as well as supraventricular arrhythmias
4. Drugs to raise blood pressure and cardiac output:	
Epinephrine	A sympathomimetic amine with both alpha and beta-adrenergic effects, which contribute to the restoration of spontaneous cardiac activity and increase in perfusion pressure during external chest compression. During a cardiac arrest, epinephrine should be given after oxygen, defibrillation, and CPR
Norepinephrine	An alpha receptor stimulant which produces vasoconstriction and raises blood pressure
Dopamine	A catecholamine with dose-dependent cardiovascular effects. At low doses ($0.5–2$ μg/kg/min), renal and mesenteric vasodilation occurs. At doses of $2–10$ μg/kg/min an increase in myocardial contractility (beta stimulation) occurs as well as some increase in systemic vasoconstriction (alpha stimulation). High doses (over 10 μg/kg/min) cause peripheral vasocontriction because of alpha stimulation
Dobutamine	A synthetic sympathomimetic amine that, at low doses, acts directly on cardiac B_1 receptors (thus increasing myocardial contactility). Higher doses produce B_2 and alpha receptor stimulation, producing peripheral vasoconstriction
5. Miscellaneous	
Nitroglycerine	A smooth muscle relaxant that primarily dilates veins, thus decreasing venous return to the heart. It also produces some arterial vasodilation, thus decreasing systemic vascular resistance. It decreases myocardial oxygen demand and reduces myocardial ischemia. It is available for sublingual, oral, topical, or IV use
Sodium nitroprusside	A potent peripheral vasodilator used to treat hypertension and heart failure by reducing peripheral arterial resistance and increasing venous capacitance
Furosemide	A potent diuretic that inhibits reabsorption of sodium and chloride in the ascending loop of Henle. This results in a marked increased excretion of electrolytes and water
Morphine sulfate	Has both an analgesic and a sympatholytic effect. It is effective in treating ischemic chest pain in patients with acute myocardial infarction as well as patients with acute pulmonary edema
Digoxin	Improves the availability of calcium to myocardial contractile elements (a positive inotropic effect); thus increases cardiac output in heart failure. There is also an increase in the AV nodal refractory period through an increase in vagal tone and sympathetic withdrawal and moderate vasoconstriction of arterial and venous smooth muscle. It is available for IV and oral administration

given). Connecting tubing from the oxygen tank and an administration unit (i.e., nasal cannula, face mask or bag-valve device) must also be available.

To prevent airway obstruction and improve oxygen administration, equipment such as an oral airway (a device placed in the mouth that, when in proper position, prevents the tongue from occluding the trachea) or an endotracheal tube (a larger tube passed directly into the trachea using a laryngoscope to aid correct placement of the endotracheal tube) may be used. Intubation equipment must be used by properly trained personnel only. This equipment is a part of advanced life support for a cardiac/respiratory arrest victim. An Ambu bag (bag-valve-mask hand respiratory) device consists of a self-inflating bag and non-rebreathing valve. These devices can be used with a mask over the victim's nose and mouth, or attached to an endotracheal tube to ventilate a victim. Supplemental oxygen can be delivered to the victim by the Ambu bag to the oxygen tank with connecting tubing and turning the oxygen up to 15 L/min of oxygen flow.

Because many cardiac arrest victims may vomit or have a large amount of respiratory secretions, suction equipment is necessary on any emergency cart. A suction apparatus attached to the emergency cart will provide suction as well as connecting tubing and suction catheters to clear secretions from the victim's mouth or trachea.

Equipment to start an intravenous line (catheters, tubing and solution) are necessary to enable trained personnel to start an intravenous line and administer drugs intravenously.

Table 30–3 provides a list of emergency equipment and the minimum standards to maintain to ensure that this equipment is in proper working order.

Emergency drugs serve as effective adjuncts to chest compression, artificial ventilation, and cardioversion during advanced cardiac life support. Classification and mechanism of action of drugs most commonly used in a life-threatening emergency are presented in Table 30–4. It is beyond the scope of this chapter to give a detailed description of all drugs used in cardiac arrest situations, and we recommend other sources for those who want a more detailed description (i.e.: dosage, interactions, etc.) of these drugs.[7,8]

EMERGENCY ACTION PLANS

Having a "plan" in case of an emergency situation is necessary. In this section, emergencies are divided into life-threatening, potentially life-threatening, and nonemergency situations. Remember also that the exercise sessions may be held in a variety of settings, from "Basic" (i.e., an area that has only the basic equipment of a clock and nearby telephone) to "Intermediate" (i.e., a facility that may also have an emergency defibrillator and possibly a "start up" kit containing a few essential drugs, intravenous lines, an oxygen tank, and a mask hand ventilator) to "High" level, which has all necessary emergency equipment available.

Guidelines for each level of emergency are presented within the particular setting of the exercise program. These guidelines are intended for use as models that each staff should modify to fit individual needs. Remember, having a basic plan of action for your individual facility and following this plan is most important when an emergency arises.

Throughout this section, we discuss the roles of the first, second, and third rescuers. Certainly, instances occur when only a single rescuer or more than three rescuers are involved. For a single rescuer only in a life-threatening emergency (CPR being performed), the rescuer follows the AHA guideline that states "Activate the EMS system first" before performing CPR. The sequence of BLS is: assessment, EMS activation, and the ABC's of CPR. In all instances, the first rescuer stays with the victim, calls for help, and performs CPR, if necessary. The second rescuer activates the emergency medical system (EMS) for the facility, waits for the emergency team to direct him or her to the scene, or returns to the scene and provides assistance. The third (or more) rescuer provides assistance at the scene or waits at a common location to direct the emergency team to the scene.

The level of education and training in emergency care of persons involved with exercise programs varies greatly. No one should do any more than one is trained to

Table 30–5. Possible Medical Emergencies

Problem	First Aid Procedure
Heat cramps	Replace lost fluid. Increase sodium and potassium through excessive sweating
Heat exhaustion and heat stroke	Move victim to a shaded area, have victim lie down with feet elevated above the level of the heart
	Remove excess clothing
	Cool victim with sips of cool fluid; sprinkle water on him or her and fan area; rub ice pack over major vessels in armpits, groin, and neck areas
	Victim should seek immediate medical attention and be given IV fluids as soon as possible
Fainting	Leave the victim lying down. Turn on his or her side if vomiting occurs
	Maintain an open airway
	Loosen any tight clothing
	Take blood pressure and pulse if possible
	Seek medical attention because it is a potentially life-threatening situation and cause of fainting must be determined
Hypoglycemia (symptoms include diaphoresis, pallor, tremor, tachycardia, palpitations, visual disturbances, mental confusion, weakness, lightheadedness, fatigue, headache, memory loss, seizure, or coma)	May become life-threatening—seek medical attention to treat cause
	Oral glucose solutions to give include Kool-aid with sugar, Coke, orange soda, ginger ale, Tang, orange juice, apple juice. If patient is able to ingest solids, gelatin sweetened with sugar, milk chocolate, or a banana may be given
Hyperglycemia (symptoms include dehydration, hypotension and reflex tachycardia, osmotic diuresis, impaired consciousness, nausea, vomiting, abdominal pain, hyperventilation, odor of acetone on breath)	May be life-threatening if it leads to diabetic ketoacidosis
	Seek immediate medical attention
	Rehydrate with intravenous normal saline
	Correct electrolyte loss (K^+)
	Correct acid/base disturbance (sodium bicarbonate)
	Insulin
Sprains/strains	No weight-bearing on affected extremity
	Loosen shoes, apply a pillow or blanket type splint around extremity
	Elevate the extremity
	Apply bag of crushed ice on the affected area
	Seek medical attention if pain or swelling persist
Simple/compound fractures	Immobilize the extremity
	Splint the extremity to prevent further injury to bone or soft tissue. Use anything at hand as a splint
	Do not attempt to reduce any dislocation in the field unless there is danger of losing life or limb
	Seek immediate medical attention
	Protect the victim from further injury
Bronchospasm	Maintain open airway
	Give bronchodilators via nebulizer if prescribed for patient
	Give oxygen by nasal cannula if available
Hypotension/shock	Lie the victim down with feet elevated
	Maintain open airway
	Monitor vital signs (pulse, blood pressure)
	Call for immediate advanced life support measures because this is a life-threatening emergency that requires intensive monitoring of vital signs, administration of intravenous fluids and drugs to maintain adequate tissue perfusion while evaluation is done as to the cause (i.e., hypovolemia, cardiogenic, septic, etc.)
	Give fluids by mouth only if medical attention is delayed and the victim is conscious without nausea or vomiting
Bleeding	Apply direct pressure over the site to stop the bleeding
Lacerations	Protect the wound from contamination and infection
Incisions	May need to seek medical attention; victim may need stitches, tetanus shot
Puncture wounds	
Abrasions	If bleeding is severe; in addition to direct pressure, elevate the injured part of the body, and if an artery is severed, apply direct pressure over the main artery to the affected limb and seek immediate medical attention
Contusions	

do. All recommendations state that all personnel involved with exercise training should be certified in BLS. Common sense is a must for any nonemergency or potential life-threatening emergency situation. Any additional skills (i.e., pulse or blood pressure taking, reading monitors, and administering first aid) are, of course, helpful to any situation. When called upon to "assist a physician," your assistance will be of greater value if you:

1. Know the exact time and nature of the emergency.
2. Know all the pertinent information leading up to the emergency situation to be able to provide a history.
3. Have any available data at hand for review (e.g., vital signs or ECG strip).
4. Are able to administer BLS.
5. Are familiar with the contents of an emergency cart/box to give to the physician.

6. Are familiar with the operation of all emergency equipment to set up for use by the physician (i.e., ECG machine or defibrillator).

Table 30–5 is a list of possible medical emergencies that may occur during an exercise test or training session. Basic first aid procedures to aid the victim before the arrival of an emergency medical team are also given. Obviously, the exercise must be stopped immediately once an event occurs, and the victim should seek medical attention even if the event is of minor consequence (i.e., the victim "feels faint" but does not lose consciousness) at the time. It is not possible to predict the severity of any of the various problems which might arise with any one individual. Also, the likelihood of encountering problems rises when the participant is older and has a pre-existing medical condition. Common sense should prevail in any situation. More in-

Table 30–6. Plan for Nonemergency Situations

Level: Basic	Intermediate	High
At a YMCA pool or park without emergency equipment	At a gym or other outside facility with basic equipment plus defibrillator and possibly a small "start-up" kit with drugs	Hospital or hospital-adjunct with all the equipment of intermediate level plus a "code cart" containing emergency drugs; equipment for intravenous drug administration, intubation, drawing arterial blood gas samples, and suctioning. Victim may be inpatient or outpatient

First Rescuer
1. Instruct victim to stop activity
2. Remain with victim until symptoms subside
  a. If symptoms worsen, follow steps for Table 30–2
  b. If symptoms do not subside, bring victim to the ER/MD office for evaluation
3. Advise victim to seek medical advice before future activity
Second Rescuer
1. Assist rescuer #1, drive victim to ER/MD office if necessary
	First Rescuer
	Same as Basic level #1–3
	Add:
	4. Take vital signs
	5. Monitor and record rhythm
	6. Bring record of vital signs and strip to ER/MD office if symptoms do not subside and visit is necessary
	Second Rescuer
	Same as Basic level #1
	Add:
	2. Bring B/P Cuff, monitor to site
	3. Assist with taking and monitoring vital signs
		First Rescuer
		Inpatient Facility
		Same as Intermediate level #1–5
		Add:
		6. Call for RN if on ward for RN or MD if in clinic to evaluate
		7. Notify primary MD
		8. Document in record
		9. Request new consult from MD to resume exercise if more than 3 consecutive exercise sessions are interrupted for same complaint
		Second Rescuer
		Same as Intermediate level #1–3

Table 30–7.   Plan for Potentially Life-Threatening Situation

Level: Basic	Intermediate	High
At a YMCA pool or park without emergency equipment	At a gym or other outside facility with basic equipment plus defibrillator and possibly a small "start-up" kit with drugs	Hospital or hospital-adjunct with all the equipment of intermediate level plus a "code cart" containing emergency drugs; equipment for intravenous drug administration, intubation, drawing arterial blood gas samples, and suctioning. Victim may be inpatient or outpatient

First Rescuer
1. Establish responsiveness
   a. Responsive:
   Instruct victim to sit
   Call for help
   Direct rescuer #2 to call EMS
   Stay with victim until EMS team arrives
   Note time of incident
   Apply pressure to any bleeding if necessary
   Keep victim comfortable
   Note if victim takes any medication (i.e., TNG)
   Take pulse
   b. Unresponsive:
   Place victim supine
   Open airway
   Call for help
   Check respiration. If absent, go to Life-Threatening section
   Maintain open airway
   Check pulse. If absent to to Table 30–8
   Direct rescuer #2 to call EMS
   Stay with victim, continue to monitor respiration and pulse
2. Other considerations
   a. If bleeding, compress area to decrease/stop bleeding
   b. Suspected neck fracture: open airway with a jaw-thrust maneuver. Do not hyperextend the neck
   c. If seizing: prevent injury by removing harmful objects
   Place something under the head (if possible). Turn victim on side once seizure activity stops to help drain secretions

Second Rescuer
1. Call EMS
2. Wait to direct emergency team to scene or
3. Return to scene to assist

Third Rescuer
1. Direct emergency team to scene or
2. Assist rescuer #1

First Rescuer
Same as Basic level #1 and 2
Add:
3. Apply monitor to victim and record rhythm. Monitor continuously
4. Take vital signs every 1–5 minutes
5. Document vital signs and rhythm. Note time, and victim complaints

Second Rescuer
Same as Basic level #1–3
4. Bring all emergency equipment and
   a. Place victim on monitor
   b. Run strip
   c. Take vital signs

Third Rescuer
Same as Basic level #1 and 2

First Rescuer
Same as Intermediate level #1–5
Also may adapt/add:
1. Call RN on ward
2. Call RN/MD if off ward
3. Document in patient record
Out-patient program:
1. Request rescuer #2 to call ER
2. Bring to ER if in same building
3. Notify primary MD as soon as possible

Second Rescuer
Same as Intermediate level #1–4

Third Rescuer
Same as Intermediate level #1 and 2

depth discussions of many of these problems may be found in Chapters 13 and 31.

In summary, the aforementioned guidelines are meant to be models for the many and varied types of exercise facilities and personnel so that they may develop appropriate and specific plans for their individual needs. Outlined examples of emergency plans follow in Tables 30–6 through 30–8; however, of paramount importance

Table 30–8. Plan for Life-Threatening Situation

Level:	Basic	Intermediate	High
	At a YMCA pool or park without emergency equipment	At a gym or other outside facility with basic equipment plus defibrillator and possibly a small "start-up" kit with drugs	Hospital or hospital-adjunct with all the equipment of intermediate level plus a "code cart" containing emergency drugs; equipment for intravenous drug administration, intubation, drawing arterial blood gas samples, and suctioning. Victim may be inpatient or outpatient

First Rescuer
1. Position victim (pull from pool if necessary) and place supine, determine unresponsiveness
2. Call for help (911 or local EMS number)
3. Open airway; look, listen, and feel for air
4. Give 2 ventilations if no respirations
5. Check pulse (carotid artery)
6. Administer 15:2 compression/ventilation ratio if no pulse
7. Continue ventilation if no respiration

Second Rescuer
1. Locate nearest phone and call EMS
2. Return to scene and help with 2-man CPR, or
3. Remain at designated area and direct emergency team to location

Third Rescuer
1. Assist with 2-man CPR or
2. Help direct emergency team to site
3. Help clear area

First Rescuer
Step #1–7 for Basic level
Second Rescuer
Step #1–3 of Basic level.
Add:
4. Return to scene, bringing defibrillator: take "quick look" at rhythm. Document rhythm [you are not to defibrillate a victim unless certified to do so (i.e., ACLS)], and this activity is part of your clinical privileges for the facility in which the work is being completed
5. Place monitor leads on patient and monitor rhythm during CPR
6. Bring emergency drug kit if available
   a. Open oxygen equipment and use Ambu bag with oxygen at 10 L if trained to do so
   b. Open drug kit and prepare intravenous line and drug administration. (These steps must only be done by trained, licensed professionals)
   c. Keep equipment at scene for use by emergency personnel

Third Rescuer
Same as Basic level

First Rescuer
In-patient program:
Step #1–7 of Basic level
Out-patient program:
Step #1–7 of Basic level
Second Rescuer
In-patient program:
Step #1–6 of Intermediate level
Out-patient program:
Step #1–6 of Intermediate level
Third Rescuer
In-patient program:
Step #1–3 of Basic level
Out-patient program:
Step #1–3 of Basic level

is that each facility have its own structured emergency plan developed in parallel as exercise programs are developed. These written and specific plans must be prepared *in advance* and then included in the orientation and training for all personnel.

EXAMPLES OF EMERGENCY PLANS

Nonemergency Situation

The victim complains of angina or not feeling well, has nausea/vomiting, fever, dizziness or shortness of breath during exercise, and exhibits a drop or excessive rise in blood pressure (B/P) during exercise or an excessive rise or a fall in pulse with exercise.

Potentially Life-Threatening Situation

This can be any event in which the victim suddenly loses consciousness (respirations and pulse present), such as seizure activity, an accident with large blood loss, or chest pressure and pain with activity or angina symptoms that are unrelieved by 3 nitroglycerin tablets (TNG). This type of situation may lead to a life-threatening emergency if action is not taken immediately.

Life-Threatening Situation

This is any event accompanied by unresponsiveness or absence of respiration and/or pulse.

REFERENCES

1. Siscovick DS, Weiss NS, Fletcher RH, Lasky T: The incidence of primary cardiac arrest during vigorous exercise. *N Engl J Med, 311:* 974, 1984.
2. Hossack KF, Hartwig R: Cardiac arrest during cardiac rehabilitation. Identification of high risk patients. *Am J Cardiol, 49:*915, 1982.
3. Diagnostic and Therapeutic Technology Assessment (DATTA): Coronary rehabilitation services. *JAMA, 258:*1959, 1987.
4. Van Camp SP, Peterson RA: Cardiovascular complications of outpatient cardiac rehabilitation programs. *JAMA, 256:*1160, 1986.
5. American College of Cardiology Position Report on Cardiac Rehabilitation. *J Am Coll Cardiol, 7:*451, 1986.
6. *Guidelines for Exercise Testing and Prescription* (4th edition). Philadelphia: Lea & Febiger, 1991.
7. *Textbook of Advanced Cardiac Life Support.* Dallas, TX, American Heart Association, 1987.
8. Lapsley D: Drug therapy for sudden cardiac death. In *Sudden Cardiac Death. Theory and Practice.* Edited by P. Owen. Chapter 9. Gaithersburg, Maryland. Aspen Publication, 1991, pp. 183–191.

SUGGESTED READING

1. Ellestad MH, Blomqvist CG, Naughton JP: Standards for adult exercise testing laboratories. *Circulation, 59:*421A, 1979.
2. Standards and guidelines for cardiopulmonary resuscitation (CPR) and Emergency Cardiac Care (ECC). *JAMA, 268:*2135, 2298, 1992.
3. Alexander J, Holder AR, Wolfson S: Legal implications of exercise testing. *J Cardiovasc Med, 3:*1137, 1978.

Chapter 31

EXERCISE-RELATED MUSCULOSKELETAL INJURIES: RISKS, PREVENTION, AND CARE

Bruce H. Jones, Katy L. Reynolds, Paul B. Rock, and
Michael P. Moore

Musculoskeletal injuries are an inherent risk of vigorous physical activity and exercise. In the exercise testing and prescription setting, there is naturally a tremendous concern about hazards to the health of patients and fitness program participants. This concern frequently focuses on myocardial disease; however, the most common risk of exercise is that of musculoskeletal injuries. This chapter discusses the injuries associated with physical activity and exercise, including the incidence of and risks for their occurrence, strategies to prevent them, and the initial identification and the primary care of such injuries.

INCIDENCE OF INJURY

The incidence of injuries associated with exercise varies depending on the type and amount of activity. For many activities, the risks are not known. The activity for which the best data exist is running. The results of several studies suggest that, in any given year, 40 to 50% of competitive runners will experience an injury and 10 to 20% of these runners will seek medical care for their injuries. The incidence of injury for noncompetitive runners and joggers is about half that of competitors. Injury incidence for similarly vigorous weight-bearing activities such as high-impact aerobics is probably similar to that for running. Among middle-aged adults engaged in less intense fitness activities, the annual rates of exercise-related injury are about 10%, with half of these requiring medical care. The incidence of exercise-induced injury associated with non-weight-bearing activities such as swimming and cycling is lower than for weight-bearing activities. In bicycling, however, there are other more serious hazards such as falls and collisions, which must be considered. Although good data are not available for many common exercise activi-

ties, it is clear from the information that does exist that higher injury rates can be expected to be a associated with almost any vigorous exercise.

RISK FACTORS FOR INJURY

Although hypotheses about the causes of exercise-related injuries are abundant, little scientific data clearly identify risk factors for specific activities other than running. To scientifically determine whether a particular activity or environmental feature (extrinsic factor) or individual characteristic (intrinsic factor) is a risk factor, the incidence of injury in the suspected high risk group must be compared to the risks of those in the low risk or "normal" population who are not exposed to the condition or do not exhibit the characteristic. These comparisons are quantified as relative risks or rate ratios (i.e., the incidence of injuries in the risk group divided by the incidence of injury in the low-risk or nonrisk group). Information on injured individuals without comparison to normal or low-risk individuals is not sufficient to determine what factors are "truly" associated with increased risk of injury. Consideration of the actual risks associated with different extrinsic and intrinsic factors is the best foundation for development of preventive strategies.

Commonly cited risk factors for weight bearing, exercise-related injuries are listed in Table 31–1. These are categorized as either extrinsic or intrinsic factors. Extrinsic factors are variables outside the individual and to which he or she might be exposed, such as training parameters, terrain features, other environmental conditions, equipment, and so forth. Intrinsic factors are inherent characteristics of the individual, such as physical fitness, body composition, gender, and age.

Table 31–1. Risk Factors for Musculoskeletal Injuries Associated with Weight-bearing Exercise and Activity

Extrinsic Factors
  Training Parameters (excessive or rapid increase)
    Intensity
    Frequency
    Duration
  Environmental Conditions (extremes)
    Terrain (hilly vs flat)
    Surfaces (too hard, too soft, irregular)
    Weather (hot or cold)
    Other
  Equipment (appropriate for activity)
Intrinsic Factors
  Physical Fitness (low levels)
    Low endurance (cardiovascular and muscle)
    Strength (low and/or imbalances)
    Flexibility (too high or low, imbalances)
    Body composition (overweight, too lean)
  Anatomic abnormalities
    High arches
    Bowed legs
    Leg length discrepancies
    Others
  Gender
  Age
    Young
    Old
  Past Injury
  Musculoskeletal disease
    Osteoporosis
    Arthritis

Extrinsic Risk Factors

Training

The most important risk factor for exercise-related injuries is training activity. The parameters of training, frequency, duration, and intensity all influence the likelihood of injuries. For running, it is well documented that greater frequency and longer duration of training are associated with higher risks of injury. For example, the improvement in aerobic capacity ($\dot{V}O_{2max}$) in novice runners or joggers does not increase as rapidly as the risks of injury when training is escalated above 3 days per week or more than 30 minutes per day, respectively (see Table 31–2). Among runners who compete in road races, those who run more miles per week sustain more injuries (see Table 31–3). Although this is not well documented, higher intensity of training can also be expected to increase the risks of injury. Fortunately, training parameters such as frequency, duration, and intensity are easily modified to reduce the risks of injury.

Type of Exercise

Type of activity also affects the risks of injury. Overuse injuries, such as stress fractures and Achilles tendinitis, are extremely common with running, high-impact aerobics, and other strenuous weight-bearing activities. For activities in which speed is a factor, the overall injury rates may be lower, but more serious; acute and traumatic injuries, such as fractures and concussions, are more likely to occur. Individual factors such as dexterity, balance, and skill are important considerations in determining risks for certain activities such as cycling and skiing. In assessing the risks of a prescribed exercise activity, the exercise specialist must consider the type and severity of potential injury associated with a specific activity and the fitness and skill re-

Table 31–2. Effects of Training Frequency and Duration on Incidence (%) of Injury and Improvement in $\dot{V}O_{2max}$ among Previously Sedentary Men*

Effect of Frequency (30 Min/Session for 20 Weeks)			Effect of Duration (3 Days/Week for 20 Weeks)		
Days/Wk	Injuries	$\dot{V}O_{2max}$ % increase	Mins/Day	Injuries	$\dot{V}O_{2max}$ % increase
1	0%	8.3%	15	22%	8.6%
3	12%	12.9%	30	24%	16.1%
5	39%	17.4%	45	54%	16.9%

* Adapted from Pollock ML et al.: Effects of frequency and duration of training on attrition and incidence of injury. *Med Sci Sports,* 9:31, 1977.

Table 31–3. Yearly Incidence (%) of Training Injuries* among Men and Women by Average Number of Miles Run per Week†

| Gender | Measure | Miles Run per Week | | | | | |
		0–9	10–19	20–29	30–39	40–49	50+
Men	n	70	191	183	93	25	31
	Incidence	21.4%	29.3%	36.1%	40.9%	52.0%	71.0%
Women	n	89	221	158	72	14	21
	Incidence	29.2%	32.1%	41.1%	52.8%	35.7%	57.0%

* Injuries = injurious events that caused a runner to decrease his or her training, to take medicine for the injury, or to see a physician.
† Adapted with permission from Koplan JP, Powell KE, Sikes RK, et al.: An epidemiologic study of the benefits and risks of running. *JAMA, 248*:3118, 1982.

quired for safe performance of that activity. If an individual's relative lack of fitness or skill causes increased risk, a different type of exercise should be recommended.

Environmental Conditions

It has been speculated that certain characteristics of the environment where exercise takes place affect the risks of injury, but there are few data to document the effects. For instance, running on hilly terrain probably places more biomechanical stress on the musculoskeletal system than training on flat terrain. Likewise, it seems reasonable to assume that surfaces with different characteristics of shock absorbency, such as roads, sidewalks, dirt tracks, trails, or grass, will affect the risks of injury for running. However, there may be trade-offs in the choice of surfaces. For instance, running on softer, more shock-absorbent, but irregular surfaces such as trails or grass may reduce the risk of overuse injuries but increase the risk of acute traumatic injuries such as ankle sprains. For sports such as tennis, surfaces with high amounts of friction may enhance some aspects of performance but also contribute to higher risk of injury. Other external environmental factors such as temperature, precipitation, and visibility, may be important risk factors to consider in choosing an exercise activity for a particular day, season, or location. Most choices involve compromises that must be weighed in the context of other extrinsic and intrinsic factors.

Equipment

Exercise equipment is another factor which undoubtedly affects the risks of injury. Unfortunately, even for common equipment such as running shoes, although there is much circumstantial evidence and a lot of opinion about associated injury, little reliable experimental or epidemiologic data exists to indicate which characteristics of shoes actually offer the wearer protection. Although reliable data are not available, it is difficult to believe that today's carefully designed athletic shoes do not offer greater protection against injuries. The age and state of repair of shoes is another consideration. Old or worn footwear may be the functional equivalent of having an anatomic defect causing hyperpronation or supination and resulting in injuries.

Equipment for activities other than running may be an important factor in the causation or prevention of injuries. Choices such as racquets of different sizes, weights, and materials for tennis or bicycles of different types, and dimensions for cycling and so forth may not only affect the performance of the activity, but also change the risk of injury.

Intrinsic Risk Factors

Physical Fitness

Level of physical fitness is one of the more important intrinsic risk factors associated with exercise-related injuries. Physical fitness has at least five health-related com-

Table 31–4. **Incidence (%) of Training-Related Injuries by Endurance Level (Quartiles) as Measured by Mile Run Times among Male and Female Army Trainees during 8 Weeks of Basic Training***

Gender	Measure	Quartiles of Mile Run Times			
		Q1 Fast	Q2	Q3	Q4 Slow
Men†	n	21	20	19	19
	Incidence	14.3%	10.0%	26.3%	42.0%
Women‡	n	36	36	35	33
	Incidence	36.1%	33.3%	57.1%	60.6%

* Adapted with permission from Jones BH, Bovee MW, Knapik JJ: *Associations among Body Composition, Physical Fitness, and Injury in Men and Women Army Trainees.* Chap. 9. Body Composition and Physical Performance. Marriott, B. (Ed.). Washington DC: National Academy Press, 1992, pp 141–173

† Median mile run time for men 7.0 min (Range: 5.9 to 11.5 min, upper cutpoints for Q1 and Q3 = 6.4 and 7.7 min, respectively); p-value for trend in risks = 0.02.

‡ Median mile run time for women = 9.8 min (Range: 6.0 to 16.3 min, upper cutpoints for Q1 and Q3 = 9.0 and 10.4 min, respectively); p-value for trend in risk = 0.03.

ponents, including cardiorespiratory endurance, muscle endurance, strength, flexibility, and body composition. The degree to which each of these components contributes to risk of muscle or skeletal injury depends on the type of physical activity. For instance, low levels of aerobic fitness (see Table 31–4) and low muscle endurance are risk factors for injury during Army Basic Training, which contains large amounts of running and marching. In general, individuals of lower-than-average fitness appear to be more likely to experience exercise-related injuries. This may be because less fit exercise participants experience higher relative levels of physiologic and biomechanical stress at any given level of activity.

Some components of physical fitness, such as flexibility, exhibit a complex relationship with injury. For example, Army trainees with both the most and least hamstring and low back flexibility are at greater risk of physical training injuries than their more average peers (Table 31–5). It may be that individuals who are inflexible sustain more muscle and tendon strains, whereas those who are highly flexible experience more sprains and dislocations of joints.

Body Composition

Body composition is another potential risk factor for musculoskeletal injury, exhibiting a complex association with injury.

Table 31–5. **Incidence (%) of Training-Related Injuries among Male Army Infantry Trainees during 12 Weeks of Infantry Basic Training by Level of Flexibility (Quintiles) as Measured by a Toe-Touching Test***

Quintile of Flexibility†	Q1 Low	2	3	4	Q5 High
n per quintile	61	60	60	60	62
Incidence of injury‡	49.2%	38.3%	20.0%	33.3%	43.6%

* Adapted with permission from Jones BH, Cowan DN, Tomlinson JP, Robinson JR, Polly DW, Frykman PN: Epidemiology of injuries associated with physical training among young men in the Army. Med Sci Sports Exerc. In press, 1993.

† Median flexibility = 1.7 inches beyond toes (range: −9.4 inches to +11.2 inches beyond toes; upper cut points for Q1 to Q4: −0.8 inches, 0.6 inches, 2.9 inches and 5.5 inches, respectively).

‡ p-value for chi-square Q1 vs Q3 = 0.001, p-value for chi-square Q5 versus Q3 = 0.005.

Higher percents of body fat are thought to increase risks of exercise-related injuries because higher relative amounts of fat to muscle mass place overweight individuals under greater physiologic and biomechanical stress during weight-bearing activities. It is also likely that some individuals may be too lean and at risk of injury from that condition. Hypothetically, individuals who possess little muscle mass relative to their total body mass may also be under greater physiologic stress during weight-bearing exercise.

Gender

Gender-related factors influence the risks associated with exercise. In general, however, much of the apparent differences in injury risks between men and women may be the result of differences in levels of physical fitness. On the average, women have lower aerobic capacity, less muscle strength, and higher percents of body fat than men of the same age and stature, which increases their risk for injury. Consistent with this supposition, recent Army data indicate that, although the overall injury rates are higher for women during basic training, the rates are the same for men and women exhibiting similar physical fitness levels and doing the same activities.

Age

Age also influences the risks of injury during exercise. Both younger and older individuals appear to have increased risk. Young children may be vulnerable because of musculoskeletal immaturity and high energy and nutrient requirements for growth. Adolescents may be particularly susceptible to injury during growth spurts when skeletal size increases disproportionately to muscle mass. Older individuals are thought to be more injury-prone because endurance, strength, and flexibility decline with age. Interestingly, however, a number of recent studies of runners and exercising adults have failed to show higher rates of injuries among older individuals. This failure probably results at least partly from the fact that older individuals modulate their risks of injury by decreasing the frequency, duration, and intensity of their exercise activities. Because older individuals have been shown to experience a training effect and other benefits of exercise similar to younger individuals, older age should not be viewed as a contraindication for exercise, but careful attention should be paid to modifying risk factors that can be altered.

Anatomic Variants

Anatomic factors such as leg length discrepancies, bowed legs, flat feet, and high arches are reputed to be associated with higher risks of injuries during weight-bearing activities. The existence and magnitude of these associations, however, are not well documented. Presumably, individuals may develop compensatory adaptations. The presence of an anatomic abnormality should not be viewed as a contraindication to exercise unless persistent injuries result from training activities.

Past Injuries

Past injuries are a well documented risk factor for current exercise-related injuries. The reasons for this are probably multifactorial and may involve imbalances in strength and flexibility resulting from past injuries which predispose the injured area to reinjury and/or other body parts to new injuries. In this regard, it should be remembered that it may take months or years to re-establish near-normal strength and flexibility after a serious injury. Also, serious injuries limit activity, causing a decrease in physical fitness, which predisposes to further injury.

Musculoskeletal Diseases

Several chronic musculoskeletal conditions may pose a risk for exercise-related injuries. These include osteoporosis and arthritis. Osteoporosis results from loss of bone mineral content which leads to porosity and loss of structural strength of bone. Osteoporosis is common among postmenopausal women, but occurs with higher frequency among elderly men as well. Some young women, especially those who engage in routine vigorous physical training or do not eat an adequate diet, may develop osteoporosis. Among such young women, osteoporosis may be associated with menstrual irregularity or absence of menstrual periods. Osteoporotic individuals are more likely to develop stress fractures and even pathologic fractures, so weight-bearing exercise should be prescribed cautiously and in moderation for those at risk of this condition.

Two very common forms of arthritis may have an impact on risk of injury and physical performance. Osteoarthritis is associated with the destruction of the cartilage of joints; rheumatoid arthritis is characterized by inflammation of the lining of joints. These diseases do not preclude individuals from exercising and are not caused by exercise. Studies suggest that aerobic exercise may actually improve the functional status and joint mobility of arthritic patients. However, it may be necessary to prescribe non-weight-bearing exercise (e.g., biking or swimming) because high-impact weight-bearing activities such as running may exacerbate the inflammation of arthritic joints. Individuals whose functional activities are impaired as a result of arthritis should seek medical advice before initiating an exercise routine.

PREVENTIVE STRATEGIES

The key to preventing injuries is reduction or elimination of risk factors. Few strategies for preventing exercise-related injuries by altering risk factors have actually been tested; however, circumstantial evidence and common sense suggest numerous measures that could help to minimize injuries and enhance fitness and performance simultaneously. These measures include gradual progression of training for improvement of physical fitness levels, individualization of exercise activities, warm-up, cool-down, stretching, and use of appropriate equipment. A key factor in preventing injuries is physical fitness. A sensible program for improving physical fitness should be a part of all strategies for preventing injury, because individuals who exhibit lower-than-average levels of physical fitness are more likely to sustain injuries. Some groups deserve special consideration because of the likelihood that their fitness levels are low. These groups include sedentary individuals, overweight men and women, young children, the elderly, and those recovering from injuries. Finally, it is

important to monitor exercise participants for warning signs of impending injury so that activity can be modified to prevent the injury from occurring.

Progression and Individualization of Exercise

Probably the most common mistake made by those who engage in vigorous exercise is progressing training too quickly. Although it is necessary to overload the cardiorespiratory and musculoskeletal systems to make improvements in physical fitness, if the overload is too great, the body systems break down rather than building up. To ensure the enhancement of fitness and prevention of injury, increases in training should progress gradually.

Optimally, a physical fitness program should be balanced to develop all fitness components (endurance, strength, flexibility, etc.), even though it may focus more on one component than another. If fitness is to be improved and injuries prevented, programs must, to some extent, be tailored to the individual. For instance, those who are overweight, elderly, or recovering from lower extremity injuries may need to be guided to low-intensity weight-bearing activities such as walking or to non-weight-bearing activities such as swimming or biking to improve fitness and decrease risk of injury. Overweight individuals may also need to diet in addition to exercising. As the fitness and experience of individuals increase, the duration, intensity and frequency of exercise may be progressively increased.

Warm-up

A structured warm-up prepares the body for more vigorous activity and may reduce the risk of injury. At rest, muscles receive only 15 to 20% of the blood pumped from the heart, but during vigorous exercise, they may receive as much as 75% of the body's blood flow. Adequate warm-up allows a gradual redistribution of blood flow to the muscles. The increased blood flow to exercising muscle has a literal warming effect, which increases the elasticity of connective tissue and other muscle components and decreases muscle viscosity. These changes should theoretically reduce the incidence of injuries to muscles, tendons and ligaments. To be optimally effective, warm-up should last 15 to 20 minutes, gradually progressing to target activity levels and involving large muscle groups.

Cool-down

An appropriate cool-down period is recommended to allow the body to gradually return to the resting state. Reduction of physical activity to 50 to 70% of maximum allows washout and metabolism of the by-products of strenuous exercise such as lactate. Further reductions in activity level to 25 to 50% allow the circulatory system to return to resting levels, which should prevent venous pooling in the legs which reduces the likelihood of postexercise syncope. It is suggested that cool-down should last 10 to 15 minutes and involve the same large muscle masses as the exercise activity. Whether cooling down gradually actually reduces the risk of injury has not been demonstrated.

Stretching

Stretching exercises increase or maintain the range of motion of joints and theoretically reduce the risk of injury to tight muscles and joints with constricted range. Static or nonballistic stretching is recommended. The stretch position of an exercise should supposedly be held from 10 seconds to 60 seconds. Forceful bouncing motions (ballistic stretching) are discouraged because they may actually cause injury. The types of stretching needed vary according to which muscle groups and joints are subjected to stress by a given activity. A sports medicine or physical training textbook should be consulted for the specific stretching exercises for particular activities or sports. Stretching should be done after muscles are warmed up and may be incorporated in both the warm-up and cool-down routine.

Protective Equipment

Protective equipment is another important consideration in the prevention of injuries. The most important item of equipment for weight-bearing activities is a good shoe, because the foot may strike the ground with an impact of 2 to 3 times body weight as frequently as 1000 times per mile in running. Appropriate shoes offering maximum protection for a particular activity or sport should be chosen. The shoe should provide adequate shock absorbency, heel counter height and stability, forefoot flexibility, and durability for the activity. For instance, a running shoe is designed for forward motion with the right amount of shock absorbency for the impact of running and appropriate lateral stability. It does not have the right amount of lateral support, traction, and durability for sports such as tennis or an exercise such as aerobics, which require more lateral support. Footwear should be well maintained and replaced or resoled when excessive wear is apparent.

Other protective devices to modify footwear may be considered for special circumstances. Individuals who hyperpronate or supinate may require a prescription for orthotics if they experience injuries associated with physical training or activity. Individuals with discrepancies in leg length also may require appropriately manufactured orthotics or lifts to compensate for this deformity.

Other specifically designed protective equipment may be necessary for a variety of activities and sports. Vulnerable body parts such as the head and eyes need special protection. Helmets are essential for activities such as bicycling, in which speed and the frequency of collisions contribute to the likelihood of serious head injuries. For racquet sports and games played with small balls or similar objects, goggles or other appropriate eye protection should be worn. Individuals should educate themselves and consult local experts regarding appropriate equipment and protective devices before beginning a new or potentially hazardous exercise activity. Exercise training professionals should be well acquainted with the specific risks for injury and protective equipment for the activities they prescribe or supervise.

Monitoring Warning Signs of Injury

Finally, to prevent serious injury and prolonged recovery periods, both exercise participants and those supervising them should monitor for signs of early or impending injury. Fatigue or lack of enthusiasm are indicators that exercise intensity or frequency are too great or that rest and recovery are inadequate. The remedy for these symptoms is decreased intensity and frequency of activity, and in some instances a period of complete rest before resumption.

Pain is another important warning sign. It indicates that a body part or organ system has been overstressed or actually injured. Pain that develops precipitously or that gradually but consistently increases with successive activity should be heeded, and training should be curtailed until the pain improves or abates. Discomfort accompanied by changes in function (limping gait, etc.) also indicates excessive physiologic or biomechanical stress. Individuals with recent severe injuries, degenerative conditions, or history of problems secondary to an anatomic malalignment should pay particular attention to these warning signs. If adequate alterations of training are not made in response to warning signs, injuries will result.

EXERCISE-RELATED INJURIES

Exercise-induced injuries can be broadly classified as either acute traumatic or "overuse" injuries (Tables 31–6 and 31–7). Acute traumatic injuries result when ligaments, bones, or muscle-tendon units are subjected to an abrupt force which exceeds their stress-strain threshold or yield point. Forces which exceed that yield point cause

mechanical deformation of the structure, resulting in failure and injury. Acute injuries most often result from a single violent event such as twisting an ankle in a pothole or breaking a bone in a collision between two soccer players.

In contrast, overuse injuries result from small repetitive overload forces on the structural (bones, ligaments, and tendons) and force-generating (muscles) elements of the body. With weight-bearing activities such as running, microtraumatic events that slightly exceed the body's ability to repair itself accumulate stride after stride, mile after mile. Eventually, the accumulation of these slight insults results in a noticeable injury. Because it is necessary to overload not only the cardiovascular but also the musculoskeletal system to achieve a training effect these injuries are bound to occur to some extent with any exercise program. The majority of overuse injuries to the musculoskeletal system are soft tissue injuries.

Traumatic Injuries

The two most common traumatic injuries encountered in the exercise setting are sprains (ligament) and strains (muscle).

Sprains

Injuries to ligaments are termed "sprains." Ligaments are fibrous connective tissues that connect bones or cartilage providing support and strength to joints. Sprains are classified into three categories—first, second, and third degree—depending on the severity of ligamentous

Table 31–6. Summary of Common Exercise Induced Acute (Traumatic) Injuries

Type	Location	Signs/Symptoms	Treatment
Sprain	Ligament	Pain, swelling, joint instability, Grades 1–3	RICE** Grade 3 (surgery)*
Strain	Muscle	Pain, swelling, tightness Loss of function, Grades 1–3	RICE** Grade 3 (surgery)*
Fracture	Bone	Pain, swelling, instability	Immobilize, Transport to ER
Dislocation	Separation of joint	Pain, swelling, instability	Immobilize, Transport to ER
Blisters and other wounds	Skin	Pain, swelling, bleeding, infection	Wound care, Sterile dressing

* Reconstructive surgery may be required
** RICE = Rest, Ice, Compression, Elevation

Table 31–7.   Summary of Common Exercise Induced Chronic (Overuse) Injuries

Type	Location	Signs/Symptoms	Treatment
Bursitis	Bony prominence	Pain, swelling, warmth, limitation of motion	RICE* Anti-inflammatory**
Tendinitis	Tendon	Pain, swelling, limitation of motion	RICE* Anti-inflammatory**
Patellar-femoral syndrome	Bone, tendon, cartilage, ligament	Pain, grating, instability	RICE* Anti-inflammatory**
Sprain	Ligament	Same as acute but milder	RICE* Anti-inflammatory**
Strain	Muscle, muscle-tendon	Same as acute but milder	RICE* Anti-inflammatory**
Stress fracture	Bone	Persistent pain, x-ray/bone scan	RICE* Anti-inflammatory**
Low back injury	Vertebrae, disc, ligament, muscle	Pain, limitation of motion, neurological symptoms	RICE* Anti-inflammatory**
Shin splints	Bone, tendon, fascia	Pain, swelling	RICE* Anti-inflammatory**
Metatarsalgia	Bone, joint, nerve	Pain, swelling	RICE* Anti-inflammatory**

* RICE = Rest, Ice, Compression, Elevation
** Anti-inflammatory: ASA, NSAID

tearing. First-degree sprains result from minimal tearing of the ligament and are characterized by microfailure of collagen fibers within the ligament. There is no associated joint instability, and only mild pain and swelling. Second degree sprains are more severe, with partial tearing of the ligament and possibly the joint capsule. They may be associated with varying degrees of joint instability, although instability may not be apparent if there is associated muscle spasm. There is substantial damage to the collagen fiber and considerable loss of strength of the ligament with second degree sprains. These injuries are characterized by severe pain and marked swelling. A second-degree sprain that is inadequately treated may result in further injury or complete tearing of the ligament. Third-degree sprains result from a complete tear of the ligament. These injuries are characterized by severe pain at the time of injury and obvious joint instability. Injuries of this severity often require surgical reconstruction and stabilization and should have prompt evaluation by an orthopedic surgeon.

Strains

Strains are commonly referred to as "muscle pulls" and generally result from stretch-ing or tearing of muscle. They are also classified as first-, second- or third-degree strains by the severity of muscle damage and the resulting loss of function. First-degree strains produce only mild signs and symptoms with minimal local pain, which is increased with passive stretch or vigorous contraction of the injured muscle. Often only a sensation of muscle tightness with activity is present with mild strains. Second-degree strain is a more severe injury, with partial tearing of the injured muscle. There is substantial pain and considerable loss of function. With second-degree strains there may be varying degrees of hemorrhage and discoloration from bruising. Third-degree muscle strains cause marked muscle disruption and possible avulsion of the muscle-tendon unit. These injuries may require surgical intervention and should be promptly evaluated by an orthopedic surgeon.

Muscle strains are common injuries, particularly in the lower extremity, where the hamstring and quadriceps musculature and the calf muscles are the groups most commonly injured. They may also occur in the upper extremities and back. Most strains of the lower extremity are mild to moderate in severity but may require up to three weeks for recovery. More severe muscle strains may require several months to heal. Muscle strains often recur, particularly if there has been inadequate rehabilitation, because the inelastic scar tissue that forms at the site of injury impairs flexibility. For this reason, it is felt that both flexibility and strength of the injured muscle should be restored to near normal before returning to previous levels of activity.

Fractures and Dislocations

More serious, but less frequent acute injuries include fractures (broken bones) and dislocations (separation of joints). These injuries usually result in severe pain, swelling, and weakness. Also, fractures can be associated directly with open wounds (compound fracture), making infection virtually certain. Suspected fractures should be immobilized (splinted) to prevent further separation of bone fragments and damage to blood vessels and nerves. Dislocated joints should also be immobilized. Following immobilization, individuals with these injuries should be transported immediately to an appropriate medical facility for evaluation and treatment.

Skin Wounds and Blisters

Blisters and open skin wounds (i.e., abrasions, lacerations, punctures) are common acute injuries that can become readily infected if not properly treated. Blisters are friction injuries related to shearing forces between the skin and equipment. The hands and feet are especially vulnerable. Keeping the blister top intact with some type of sterile dressing has been shown to promote faster healing and reduce infection rates. If the blister is painful and must be punctured, the procedure should be done with sterile precautions. To drain blisters, several punctures should be made if the age of the blister is less than 24 hours. However, a single puncture is recommended for older blisters. Keeping the acute wound clean and covered is extremely important and a physician should be consulted for any signs of infection.

Unfortunately, there has not been any clear-cut evidence of effective preventive measures that reduce risk of blistering. Anecdotal reports and common sense suggest strategies that include keeping the skin dry with socks that wick away moisture and using drying agents (i.e., antiperspirants). Ensuring good shoe fit should also help prevent foot blisters.

Open wounds can occur in any type of sport. Whether it be a ruptured blister, abrasion or a laceration, special care must be taken to keep the lesion covered to prevent infection and indirect transfer of blood-borne pathogens (i.e., Hepatitis B, HIV, etc.). Large deep wounds or significant bleeding indicate the need for medical evaluation and treatment.

Overuse Injuries

Overuse injuries can affect most of the musculoskeletal elements of the limbs including the bursae (bursitis), tendons (tendinitis and tenosynovitis), muscle (strains), ligaments (sprains), and bones (stress fractures).

Bursitis

"Bursitis" refers to the presence of inflammation of a fluid-filled sac called a "bursa." A bursa normally functions to reduce friction between adjacent tissues and is located where muscle or tendon pass over a body prominence.

The key symptoms of bursitis are pain and limitation of motion. Signs of bursitis include point tenderness over the bursa, swelling, and limited motion. Occasionally the skin over an inflamed bursa appears red (erythematous) and warm. The majority of bursitis results from acute and/or chronic mechanical irritations or trauma; although acute septic bursitis requiring antibiotic therapy also occurs. Treatment of nonseptic bursitis consists of rest, ice application, and anti-inflammatory medication.

Tendinitis

Tendinitis refers to acute or chronic painful inflammation of a tendon. It results from repetitive stress of forceful muscle contractions, which leads to overload of the tendon and "mechanical fatigue" with micro-tears in the tendon itself. Excessively violent force may cause a complete tear or rupture of the tendon an acute injury which requires surgical correction. Overload of tendons is greater with eccentric (lengthening) muscle contractions such as occur running downhill or lowering a weight than with concentric contractions (shortening). Force overload is believed to be a major etiologic factor in the development of such conditions as Achilles tendinitis, tennis elbow (lateral epicondylitis), rotator cuff tendinitis, and jumper's knee (patellar tendinitis).

Tendinitis may be classified by the presence or absence of activity-related pain and its severity. In the initial stage, the primary complaint is pain. Repeated stress results in progressive inflammation, which is characterized by mild pain before activity, which generally improves with exercise and frequently reappears following activity. This stage is characterized by varying degrees of point tenderness of the tendon at the site of injury and pain with passive stretching. Progressive inflammation results in continuous activity pain, which heralds more serious pathology of the tendon. If adequate rest for recovery is not allowed, pain frequently prohibits the individual from participation in exercise or sports. This degree of inflammation is characterized by swelling, point tenderness and considerable pain to stretch of the tendon. Treatment consists of rest, ice massage of the tendon, and anti-inflammatory medication. The goal of treatment is pain-free activity and restored flexibility and strength.

Patellofemoral Syndrome

One of the most common overuse injuries encountered in exercise programs is knee pain. The most common cause of overuse knee pain is the patellofemoral pain syndrome. This syndrome is particularly common among individuals participating in running programs, and frequently is referred to as "runner's knee." The term "chondromalacia" is often inappropriately used to describe overuse knee pain. Chondromalacia literally means "soft cartilage" and specifically describes the pathology and appearance of deteriorating cartilage.

The cause of patellofemoral syndrome is complex, but is felt to be caused by abnormal patellofemoral (thigh-knee) mechanics. Multiple biomechanical factors have been described as predisposing to this injury. Among the most common are femoral anteversion, "squinting" patella, shallow femoral groove, and excessive Q-angle. The amount of exercise may be of greater importance, however. The syndrome is often associated with abrupt increases in training mileage and/or intensity of running. Also, hill running is often cited as an exacerbatory factor. The lay term "runner's knee" for patellofemoral syndrome is testament to the role of exercise in its development.

The primary symptom of patellofemoral syndrome is pain that increases with activity and localizes to the region below or around the patella. Running downhill, ascending or descending stairs, and prolonged sitting with the knee flexed typically intensify the symptoms. Frequently, the individual complains of instability or "giving way" of the knee. A sensation of grating behind the kneecap and pain on compression of the kneecap are other symptoms reported in this syndrome. Treatment for this syndrome consists of rest, ice, and anti-inflammatory medications.

Sprains and Strains

Although many sprains and strains are acute injuries, they may also result from or be aggravated by overuse and therefore can be classified as chronic injuries. Whatever the cause, the symptoms are the same as for acute traumatic sprains and strains, except that symptoms are generally milder. The treatment of these overuse injuries is the same as for the acute injuries.

Stress Fractures

Most stress fractures from overuse occur to the lower extremities, especially in the tibia of the leg and metatarsals of the foot. They occur in two successive stages in response to repetitive overloading of bones during activities such as running, walking, or marching. The first stage is a normal physiologic response called "remodeling," in which the body attempts to strengthen stressed bone by removal of old bone and the laying down of new bone. If excessive, this response is called a "stress reaction." The response can be documented with bone scans and x rays. If the stress continues, the repair process may actually weaken the bone by removing more bone than is laid down. The weakened bone is more susceptible to mechanical failure, and the second stage occurs when the weakened bone fractures. Because of the potentially serious consequences of stress reactions of bone, any individual with aching bone pain associated with exercise which does not abate in a few days or worsens should be evaluated by an appropriate medical practitioner.

Low Back Injuries

It is beyond the scope of this chapter to discuss back injuries in great detail. However, low back pain is such a common symptom of injury either associated with or exacerbated by exercise that a few generalities about the causes, treatment, and prevention of back injuries merit mention.

Low back pain as a result of musculoskeletal injury may be a symptom of damage to the bony structural elements of the spine (vertebrae), to the shock-absorbing discs between vertebrae, to the ligaments connecting vertebrae, or to the supportive musculature of the back and abdomen. The possible injuries include traumatic and stress fractures of the vertebra, ruptured discs, torn or sprained ligaments, and muscle strains or spasms. Unless neurologic symptoms accompany the low back pain, it may be difficult to differentiate between serious causes of discomfort, such as a ruptured disc, and less serious causes, such as muscle strains. If symptoms of neurologic involvement, such as pain radiating into the buttocks or down one or both legs, numbness or tingling of the legs, or weakness occur, a physician should be consulted. Chronic back pain of unknown origin or severe pain are additional reasons to consult a physician.

The most common causes of low back pain are sprains or strains of the soft tissues connecting and supporting elements of the vertebral column. Initial treatment for these consists of rest, ice application, and pain-relieving and anti-inflammatory medication like aspirin. A few days of complete bed rest may also be beneficial, but longer periods of bed rest may be counterproductive.

Flexibility and strengthening exercises are frequently prescribed for both rehabilitation and prevention of recurrent low back injuries. No one set of exercises has proven efficacy, however, and there is some debate concerning what specific exercises should be done. The best strategy for preventing strains and sprains of the back is a general overall conditioning program that includes nonballistic stretching of the back muscles, hamstrings, and hip muscles, and exercises specifically to strengthen not only the back but the abdomen as well. Exercises that involve excessive flexion or rotational motions of the low back should be avoided especially by older individuals.

Other Common Overuse Syndromes

Shin splints and metatarsalgia are common descriptive terms frequently used to describe symptom complexes that may have several underlying causes. "Shin splints" (i.e., shin soreness) is a vague term for overuse injuries involving the lower leg. These injuries are more accurately defined by anatomy, specific site of pain, and cause of injury. Key sites of pain are proximal lateral tibia and the distal medial tibial border of the lower leg. This injury complex may involve inflammation of musculotendinous units attached to the tibia or stresses on the periosteal or bony tissues.

Metatarsalgia is another vague term used to describe painful overuse injuries of the foot. The usual symptom is forefoot pain during weight-bearing activity. Tenderness is usually detected on the sole of the foot under the second or third metatarsal head. This condition usually results from chronic foot strain caused by significant changes in the intensity of weight-bearing activity (e.g., running, marching). Other conditions that can present with metatarsal pain include stress fractures, neuromas, and arthritis. These conditions should be considered if forefoot pain does not respond to conservative measures, and the appropriate medical evaluation should be obtained.

Excessive running is frequently associated with the occurrence of these overuse syndromes and injuries. However, rapid changes in intensity, frequency or duration of any exercise activity (i.e., excessive walking, marching, swimming, biking etc.) can result in these conditions. Pain occurring at the beginning of exercise, and disappearing during activity and then returning in the cool down phase suggests inflammation of soft tissue. Pain that persists during exercise and improving with rest suggests bone injury. Immediate care is essentially the same for all overuse conditions—rest, ice, compression, elevation, and anti-inflammatory medication.

It should be kept in mind that numerous infrequent but serious conditions may also masquerade with the same symptoms and signs as overuse syndromes. These conditions include pathologic fractures, compartment syndromes, and tumors. Symptoms that persist despite conservative measures warrant further investigation.

INFLAMMATION

A basic understanding of inflammation is essential to ensure the proper treatment of musculoskeletal injuries because it is associated with most injuries. Inflammation is the result of a complex series of physiologic reactions to injury. There are three main categories of factors involved in the inflammatory process: (1) vasoactive compounds, (2) chemotactic factors, and (3) degradative agents. During the initial injury phase, vasoactive substances (i.e., prostaglandins, etc.) are released by injured tissues, leading to vasodilation and increased permeability of capillaries in the injured area. This results in leakage of plasma and often bleeding, which cause swelling and edema. Swelling causes tissue hypoxia and continued release of chemical mediators. White blood cells are attracted to the site by these mediators. The white cells function to clean up debris from the injury, but their digestive enzymes (lysozymes) may leak into the area damaging healthy tissues. They also release still more mediators. Although inflammation is an important part of the healing process, it may contribute to a self-perpetuating cycle of chronic inflammation unless appropriate interventions are initiated.

The end result of the inflammatory process is the classic signs and symptoms of musculoskeletal inflammation—swelling, redness, loss of function, warmth and pain. These signs and symptoms vary according to the severity of the injury and whether it is acute or chronic in nature. Excessive and persistent swelling caused by inflammation impairs the healing response and lengthens recovery time. Swelling and bleeding also cause pain by mechanical stimulation of free nerve endings. In an attempt to splint (protect) the injured area, secondary muscle spasm may occur, which further aggravates the pain from other causes. Consequently, one of the major goals of initial treatment of musculoskeletal injuries is to minimize swelling and edema, which helps to decrease other associated symptoms.

BASIC PRINCIPLES OF CARE FOR EXERCISE-RELATED INJURIES

The objectives of initial treatment of exercise-related injuries are to decrease pain, limit swelling and excessive inflammation that might retard healing, and prevent further injury. In acute injuries, these objectives may be accomplished by a combination of rest, ice application, compression, and elevation of the injured part. The acronym "RICE" (R-rest, I-ice, C-compression, E-elevation) is used to refer to this treatment protocol. Chronic injuries may require additional treatment modalities, including physical therapy. Anti-inflammatory medication may be helpful for both chronic and acute injuries.

Rest

For both acute and chronic conditions, the initial rest period should be at least 1 to 2 days until the inflammatory response has diminished. Severe injuries may require more rest (several days to weeks) to prevent further injury and ensure healing. For some cases of mild acute or mild chronic conditions, rest may be relative, requiring only a decrease in the intensity, duration, and frequency of exercise. In most cases, normal exercise may be resumed when pain-free activity is possible.

Joint immobilization using casts or splints is an extreme method of enforcing the rest that may be necessary to heal some injuries. These treatments carry their own risk, however, and require medical supervision. Although immobilization may be beneficial, prolonged immobilization may result in muscle wasting, weakness, joint stiffness, and decreased cardiovascular fitness.

Ice (Cryotherapy)

Ice or other cold modality is applied to reduce swelling, bleeding, inflammation, and pain. Cold causes local constriction of blood vessels, which limits bleeding and escape of fluid into the area. It also decreases pain by a direct effect on nerves. Decreased pain and nerve conduction velocity minimize muscle spasm.

Cold therapy is especially helpful, even crucial, in the first 24 to 72 hours following acute injuries. It is also helpful in limiting the inflammatory process in chronic injuries, particularly when daily activities routinely reactivate the inflammatory process. Common methods for applying cold include ice packs, ice baths, ice towels, ice massage, gel packs, chemical packs, and vapocoolant sprays. The type, duration, and frequency of application of cold should be specifically tailored for each injury. The time and depth of cooling of the subcutaneous tissue and underlying muscle are dependent on the size and depth of the injury. Frequency of applications is based on amount of pain and muscle spasm.

Ice can be applied in the form of an ice pack, ice towel, or ice bath. Placing ice in plastic bags is probably the simplest way to apply cold. Crushed or chipped ice in plastic bags wrapped with an elastic bandage will conform to the contour of the injured part better than ice cubes. Application should be for only 20 to 30 minutes at a time; otherwise reflex vascular dilation may result in increased swelling and bleeding. Acutely, cold can be applied each hour for the first several hours. Later, it can be applied twice a day if pain and spasm are diminished. Some injuries, especially those to the hands or feet, may be immersed in a cold water bath made by adding ice to cold water until a temperature of 13 to 18°C (55 to 65°F) is reached.

For chronic injuries, ice massage with chunks of ice or ice frozen in paper cups is an effective means to apply cold locally. Slow circular strokes are used for a duration of 10 to 20 minutes to cool the underlying tissue. Brief applications may be sufficient for tendinitis, bursitis, and sprains.

Ice massage two or three times per day combined with range-of-motion exercises can be effective in treating these chronic injuries.

Gel packs also conform well to injured areas when wrapped with an elastic pressure bandage, but they lose their cooling properties rapidly. Also, they can cause frostbite if special precautions are not taken to insulate the packs from the skin.

Chemical cold packs contain a mixture of chemicals that must be activated to produce a cooling effect. These packs are expensive and are not reusable. Also, they can cause "burns" and may leak. They are no more effective than other means, but may be more convenient in certain circumstances. Vapocoolant sprays provide a circumscribed anesthetic effect. They should not be used for deeper tissue cooling. Improper use can lead to frostnip and frostbite.

Also, caution should be exercised because cold therapy can be harmful. Contraindications for cold therapy include individuals with a history of peripheral circulatory problems or cold hypersensitivity such as Raynaud's syndrome.

Compression

Compression helps to reduce swelling and bleeding. Compression is achieved by the use of elastic wraps and sleeves. Compression and ice may be applied simultaneously by wrapping an ice pack within an elastic bandage over the injured area. Care should be taken to avoid cutting off the circulation with excessive compression.

Elevation

Elevation of the injured part decreases blood flow and excessive pressure in the injured area. It allows gravity to assist drainage and thus decrease swelling. For elevation to be most effective, the injured extremity should be raised above the level of the heart and placed on a comfortable padded surface.

Heat

Heat is a commonly used treatment to relieve pain and muscle spasm, increase blood flow, and reduce stiffness. Because it increases blood flow, heat should not be applied until 2 to 3 days after an acute injury because it may increase leakage and swelling. Furthermore, heat should not be applied when swelling and bleeding persist because it may aggravate some inflammatory conditions. Heat is contraindicated in patients with impaired sensation, skin circulation, or thermal regulation.

Warm whirlpool or immersion baths are effective for relaxation and facilitation of range-of-motion of deeper tissues. Immersion is usually limited to 20 or 30 minutes, and care must be taken not to immerse too long because of the risk of dangerous elevation of body core temperature.

Anti-inflammatory Medication

Anti-inflammatory drugs, such as aspirin, inhibit key steps in the inflammation process. Anti-inflammatory medications are useful adjuncts for the treatment of acute and chronic exercise related-injuries. However, their use is not indicated within the first few days of injury because initially the inflammatory response promotes healing. These medications are most beneficial for relief of chronic inflammatory conditions like tendinitis and bursitis, and they are also good pain relievers. Common anti-inflammatories include aspirin, ibuprofen, indomethacin, and a number of other nonsteroidal drugs. Most of these anti-inflammatory medications have side effects, including heartburn (gastritis) and bleeding of the gastrointestinal tract. As a consequence, the medications should always be taken with meals or snacks unless specifically indicated otherwise. Also, patients should be aware that these medications can mask symptoms of injury.

Acetaminophen (Tylenol) is not an anti-inflammatory medication but is a good pain reliever. Therefore, it is useful for pain relief but not for reduction of inflammation.

CONCLUSION

Most training injuries result from excessive intensity, duration, or frequency of activity for the existing intrinsic condition of the participant or the extrinsic environ-mental conditions. Training routines should be based on an assessment of the individual's physical fitness level and potential risk factors. The majority of exercise-related injuries can be prevented by the use of good judgment and moderation. Periodic re-evaluation of training should be conducted, especially if warning signs of injury such as pain, fatigue or markedly decreased performance occur. If preventive measures and common sense fail to prevent injury, the training should be stopped, prompt treatment should be instituted. Finally, professional medical attention should be sought whenever the severity of injury merits it or if complaints persist after rest and first aid measures.

BIBLIOGRAPHY

Articles

American College of Sports Medicine: Position statement on the recommended quantity and quality of exercise for developing and maintaining fitness in healthy adults. *Med Sci Sports Exer, 22:*265, 1992.

Halvorson GA: Therapeutic heat and cold for athletic injuries. *Phys Sports Med, 18:*87, 1990.

Koplan JP, et al.: An epidemiologic study of the benefits and risks of running. *JAMA, 248:* 3118, 1982.

Koplan JP, Siscovick C, Goldbaum GM: The risks of exercise: A public health view of injuries and hazards. *Public Health Rep, 100:*189, 1985.

McKeag DB, Dolan C: Overuse syndromes of the lower extremity. *Phys Sports Med, 17:* 108, 1989.

Myburgh KH, Grobler N, Noakes TD: Factors associated with shin soreness in athletes. *Phys Sports Med, 16:*129, 1988.

Powell KE, Kohl HW, Caspersen CJ, Blair SN: An epidemiologic perspective on the causes of running injuries. *Phys Sports Med, 14:* 100, 1986.

Ramsey ML: Managing friction blisters of the feet. *Phys Sports Med, 20:*117, 1992.

Books

Dirix A, Knuttgen HG, Tittel K (eds.): The Encyclopedia of Sports Medicine: The Olympic Book of Sports Medicine. Boston: Blackwell Scientific Publications, Vol 1, 1988.

Pollock ML, Wilmore JH, Fox SM: Exercise in

Health and Disease. Philadelphia: WB Saunders, 1984.

Schneider RC, Kennedy JC, Plant ML (eds.): Sports Injuries: Mechanisms, Prevention, and Treatment. Baltimore: Williams and Wilkins, 1985.

Shepard RJ, Astrand P-O (eds.): Endurance in Sport. London: Blackwell Scientific Publications, 1992.

Torg JS, Walsh RP, Shepard RJ: Current Therapy in Sports Medicine. 2nd ed. Toronto: BC Decker Inc., 1990.

Section VII

HUMAN DEVELOPMENT AND AGING

Chapter 32

PHYSIOLOGIC CHANGES OVER THE YEARS

Roy J. Shephard

In considering physiologic changes over the years, it is useful to subdivide the overall population into three broad age categories (Table 32–1). There is first the phase of growth and development. Information on the toddler and pre-school child is limited, but there is a growing amount of data on the preadolescent and adolescent. Next follows the well documented phase of maturity, the young adult phase. Finally, there is the phase in which most physiologic functions show an age-related deterioration, accelerating through early and later middle age into the three subcategories of old age. Calendar age provides general guidance as to an individual's place on this continuum, but both during growth and development and in later life, individuals sometimes show wide discrepancies between their calendar and biologic ages.

Normal age-related changes in cardiovascular function and peak oxygen transport, skeletal muscles, bones, joints and overall body composition are first considered. Orthopedic problems in relation to age are then examined. Finally, this discussion includes the effects of chronic exercise and pathologic conditions such as hypertension and obesity.

NORMAL PHYSIOLOGIC CHANGES WITH AGE

Cardiovascular Function

Age-related changes in resting and maximal heart rate are important when prescribing exercise, conducting a maximal effort test, and attempting to predict cardiovascular performance from the heart rate observed during submaximal exercise.

The school-age child (and probably the preschool child) have what has been described as a "hypokinetic circulation," with a small stroke volume and peak cardiac output in relation to size.[1] The hemoglobin level (and thus the oxygen carriage per unit volume of blood) is also lower than in an adult. Partly because of these disparities and partly because of a high resting metabolism and some anxiety exhibited during evaluation, the resting heart rate of the young child is often high (typically 80 beats per minute and sometimes as high as 100 beats per minute). Hypokinesis apparently disappears with a combination of growth and more vigorous training at the time of the adolescent growth spurt.[2] At puberty, boys also show an increase of hemoglobin concentration to about 14.5 g/dL, with a peak of 16.5 g/dL in the postadolescent period. Girls parallel the changes seen in the boys through to puberty, but thereafter their hemoglobin remains relatively constant at 14.0 to 14.5 g/dL. Because of these changes, the resting heart rate decreases in both sexes, typically dropping to values of 65 to 70 beats per minute in the adolescent and postadolescent. The resting heart rate of a young adult depends greatly on the individual's physical condition. In sedentary subjects, resting values of 65 to 70 beats per minute remain usual, but in top-level endurance competitors with a large stroke volume, resting heart rates as low as 26 beats per minute have been described. Usually, some loss of physical condition occurs with further aging, and the resting heart rate may thus increase by a small amount over the span of adult life.

The maximal heart rate is usually quoted as 220 minus age in years, with the implication that this formula is applicable to subjects of all ages. It is difficult to motivate toddlers and young schoolchildren to the sustained effort needed when determining maximal heart rate. Some authors have seen peak values of 210 to 215 beats per minute in young schoolchildren, but a figure of 195 to 200 beats per minute is a more usual finding. A maximum of 195

Table 32–1.   Phases of Growth and Aging

Phase One: Growth and development
  Toddler and preschool (<5 years)
  Preadolescent (5 to 11 years)
  Adolescent (12 to 14 years)
Phase Two: Maturity
  Postadolescent (15 to 19 years)
  Young adult (20 to 30 years)
Phase Three: Aging
  Early middle age (30 to 45 years)
  Late middle age (45 to 65 years)
  Young elderly (65 to 75 years)
  Middle elderly (75 to 85 years)
  Very old (>85 years)

beats per minute is typical of the sedentary young adult, but values may be 5 to 10 beats per minute lower in an endurance athlete, particularly if the test is not performed on a sport-specific ergometer.[3] The peak heart rate declines progressively throughout middle age, the main reason apparently being an increase in the "stiffness" of the ventricular walls, and thus a slowing of ventricular filling. By age 65 years, the estimate of peak heart rate derived from the classical formula (155 beats per minute) still seems appropriate for an endurance athlete,[4] but is too low for a sedentary person. Particularly during treadmill exercise, the true maximum of a well-motivated sedentary individual seems at least 170 beats per minute.[5] It is difficult to motivate the middle-old and very old to all-out effort, but a further reduction of maximum heart rates apparently occurs in these age groups. One study found respective average values of 144 and 135 beats per minute for active men and women aged 70 to 79 years.[4] Weisfeldt et al.[6] have argued that the older person can compensate for the declining maximal heart rate by an increase of maximal stroke volume, at the expense of some increase of end-diastolic volume. However, such compensation seems limited to a small group of the healthy elderly who have been screened thoroughly for coronary vascular disease. More usually,[7] the circulatory limitation imposed by the decrease of peak heart rate is compounded by a decrease of stroke volume as maximal effort is approached, because the aging coronary circulation is no longer able to meet peak cardiac oxygen demands.

Exercise prescription commonly assumes a linear relationship between heart rate and oxygen consumption. Such a relationship has been demonstrated in children and young adults, at least when they are using the large muscles of the body to perform exercise at an intensity between 50 and 100% of maximal oxygen intake (for example, from heart rates of 128 to 195 beats per minute in young men, and from 135 to 198 beats per minute in young women). However, the tendency to a decline of stroke volume as maximum effort is approached[7] distorts the linear relationship of heart rate to oxygen consumption in an older person, and to sustain oxygen delivery to the working muscles, the heart rate must come closer to its maximal value at any given oxygen consumption. The situation in an ever-increasing proportion of middle-aged and elderly individuals is further complicated by the administration of beta-blocking drugs, which greatly restrict the increase of heart rate with oxygen consumption. These drugs are prescribed to treat hypertension and various arrhythmias, and for the prophylaxis of arrhythmias in postcoronary patients.

Maximal Oxygen Intake

The most appropriate method of expressing maximal oxygen intake ($\dot{V}_{O_2max}$) has had extensive discussion. It may simply be reported as an absolute value (L per minute or mmol per minute), but to compare individuals of differing body size, it is common to attempt a standardization of results (for example, by expressing data per unit of body mass, mL/kg/min). Notice that a low relative $\dot{V}_{O_2max}$ may reflect either a poor oxygen transport or an excessive accumulation of body fat. A body mass adjustment has logic for many types of aerobic exercise, because the energy cost is also roughly proportional to body mass. However, units relative to body mass are inappropriate for weight-supported activities (for example, the child on a bicycle, the young adult in a rowing skiff, or the senior citizen exercising on a chair or in a swimming pool).

Methods of size standardization have understandably had greatest discussion in children. Theoretic arguments have been advanced for adopting a relationship to height^2,[8] although experimental data vary as height$^{2.5-3.0}$,[9] the dimensional equivalent of body mass. If a height^2 standardization is adopted, functional capacity appears to remain relatively constant through childhood and adolescence, but if data are expressed relative to body mass, there is an apparent loss of function beginning at about 12 years of age, a finding that has led physical educators to demand more rigorous and/or more frequent school programs of physical education.[10] In young and middle-aged adults, mass standardization generally provides a satisfactory basis for comparing subjects, although very muscular individuals (such as large football players) often achieve low relative scores. In the old and very old, any form of height standardization is progressively complicated by decreases of stature caused by (1) kyphosis; (2) compression of intervertebral discs; and (3) sometimes frank intervertebral collapse. Mass standardization is more satisfactory for the elderly, although such scores may also be increased somewhat by a loss of bone and lean tissue, without any improvement of cardiovascular condition.

The essential principle of $\dot{V}O_{2max}$ measurement is to choose a form of activity that involves the majority of the body muscles and can be continued to exhaustion without peripheral muscular fatigue. Motivation is important to obtaining a true maximal effort at all ages. The ideal measuring device for the toddler and the preschool child is an adaptation of a toy such as a pedal car. From age 6 or 7 years through to old age, however, the $\dot{V}O_{2max}$ of the average person is best determined by progressive uphill treadmill exercise, running, or walking, depending on physical condition.[8,11,12] The endurance athlete should be assessed using a combination of treadmill testing and measurements made on a sport-specific ergometer.[13] The well-trained competitor is able to match or even exceed the treadmill value while performing his or her chosen sport. The young child is liable to stumble while running on the treadmill belt, and a safety harness is thus desirable when testing the youngest age groups. Beyond age of 50 or 60 years, subjects may again experience problems on the treadmill, caused by unstable knee

joints. In such circumstances, walking becomes a preferable form of exercise to running and the subject may then be allowed to rest the hands lightly on the supporting rail (although, if this approach is adopted, it is important to measure the oxygen consumption rather than estimate it from the speed of walking and the treadmill slope). The cycle ergometer has some superficial attraction as a means of evaluating a person with unstable knees, although in practice many elderly people have difficulty in riding a cycle ergometer, and their performance is often limited by quadriceps weakness (rather than cardiac function, as intended).

Field laboratories sometimes estimate the oxygen consumption from the rate of working (for example, the power output on a cycle ergometer, or the product of body mass, step height, and stepping rate), as when using the "work" scale of the Åstrand nomogram.[8] A resting metabolism of 3.5 mL/kg/min is generally assumed, along with a constant net mechanical efficiency of exercise (for example, 23% on a cycle ergometer, or 16% during the repeated ascent and descent of a stepping bench). Unfortunately, efficiency is not constant. The energy cost of an unfamiliar task (such as uphill running on a laboratory treadmill) decreases progressively as the task is repeated. Young children tend to perform most types of exercise in a mechanically inefficient way through a combination of natural exuberance and an incomplete development of motor skills. Performance becomes more consistent and closer to the assumed mechanical efficiency through young adult life and middle age, but deteriorates in the elderly; thus, the net mechanical efficiency of cycle ergometry drops from an average of 23% at age 25 years to 21.5% at an age of 65 years, with the probability of a further decrease in the middle-old and very-old, due to (1) weakness of postural muscles, (2) loss of coordination, (3) stiffness and deterioration of joints, and (4) lack of recent practice of the required skills.

Age-related variations in mechanical efficiency are an equally important source of error when attempting to estimate physical condition from physical performances such as the time required to run 1.6 km.[13]

If $\dot{V}_{O_{2max}}$ is expressed relative to body mass, the value for a fit male subject remains fairly constant from school entry to early adult life, at about 50 mL/kg/min. In young men selected and trained for top-level endurance sports, figures of 80 to 85 mL/kg/min are possible. In contrast, the peak oxygen transport of sedentary and somewhat obese young men can be 40 mL/kg/min or lower. The aging of function in adult years has been studied in both small longitudinal samples[14,15] and larger cross-sectional populations.[4] With either approach, there are difficulties in distinguishing the inherent rate of aging from changes in patterns of physical activity that are related to either aging or experimental involvement. Typically, sedentary subjects show a loss of 5 mL/kg/min per decade from age 25 to 65 years. In cross-sectional samples of continuing athletes that have been matched for habitual activity, the rate of loss of function does not seem greatly reduced, although the active person has a 5 to 10 mL/kg/min larger aerobic power than a sedentary peer at any given age.[7] After age 65, the rate of functional loss is thought to accelerate, although the subjects who have been studied in this age range are few and highly selected, and it becomes increasingly difficult to assure constancy of physical activity patterns when making comparisons.

In theory, there is no apparent reason why the relative $\dot{V}_{O_{2max}}$ value of a preadolescent girl should not match that of a boy, although in practice (probably because of social conditioning to a less active lifestyle), figures of 40 to 45 mL/kg/min are usually observed in female subjects. The relative aerobic power of the female subject as an adolescent and a young adult is further restricted relative to that of the male subject because of a higher percentage of body fat and a lower hemoglobin level. From adolescence through to about age 35, values for sedentary female subjects are typically in the range 35 to 40 mL/kg/min, and it is unusual to find values greater than 60 to 65 mL/kg/min even in top endurance competitors. A steady decline begins around age 35. Values for sedentary women decrease to about 25 mL/kg/min at age 65, with an accelerating loss of function thereafter.[4,16]

Skeletal Muscles

The relative proportions of slow- and fast-twitch fibers are largely determined at birth (although vigorous endurance training can cause some interconversion, particularly of fast glycolytic to fast oxidative and glycolytic fibers). The total number of muscle fibers is also fixed at an early age, although considerable enlargement of muscles remains possible by fiber splitting and hypertrophy of existing fibers.

As with $\dot{V}_{O_{2max}}$, there is considerable discussion of methods of standardizing muscle strength data for interindividual differences of body size. Some authors have argued on theoretic grounds that muscle force should be related to the square of stature,[8] or to the cross-section of the active limb; however, observations on the growing child[9] show that the development of muscle strength is more closely related to the third power of height, or the dimensionally equivalent variable of body mass. Because muscle force must often be used to displace body mass, standardization per kg of body mass is both convenient and functionally meaningful. In male subjects, rapid hypertrophy of muscle occurs coincident with or immediately subsequent to the adolescent growth spurt.[17] In contrast, girls do not show any disproportionate development of their muscles at puberty. Thus, although the strength of an active young girl is similar to that seen in a boy of similar age, the postadolescent female has only about 60% of the strength of her male counterpart.[18,19] The discrepancy by gender in maximal force is greater for the arms than for the legs. About one half of the difference seems attributable to the shorter stature and thus the smaller muscle dimensions of adult women. Of the residual difference, one part probably reflects a lesser secretion of androgens in the female subject and another part is an expression of socially-conditioned sex differences in patterns of habitual activity. Both sexes reach maximal levels of muscle tissue quantity and strength in their early twenties. A plateau of strength is generally maintained until 40 to 45 years of age, followed thereafter by an accelerating loss of lean tissue and an associated decrease in strength.[17] At all ages, women seem somewhat more vulnerable to loss of lean tissue than men, and with any tendency to anorexia, muscle atrophy may begin even in adolescence or early adult life. The aging of both sexes apparently leads to a selective loss of type II fibers, with a corresponding loss of contractile speed.[20,21] By age 65, a typical muscle group shows a 20% loss of maximal force. Again, it is unclear how much of this functional loss is an inevitable consequence of aging and how much is a reflection of a decrease in habitual activity with advancing years. Some recent reports have shown a substantial restoration of both strength and lean tissue when nonagenerians have undertaken appropriate muscle-strengthening programs.[22]

The anaerobic power, as measured by a staircase sprint (Margaria test) or 5 seconds of appropriately loaded all-out cycle ergometer exercise (Bar-Or Test), develops in parallel with the mass of muscle in children, adolescents, and young adults.[23] Typical values for the young school child are under 6 W/kg, and in older children scores are still at least 20% less than in adolescents and young adults; the latter age groups have staircase sprint scores of 11 to 18 W/kg in males and 9 to 11 W/kg in females, whereas their corresponding figures for the Wingate test are 8 to 11 W/kg in males and 8 to 10 W/kg in females. The anaerobic power deteriorates in later middle age as the loss of lean tissue and the selective atrophy of type II muscle fibers become of practical significance. In both sexes, scores on the staircase sprint show a 45 to 60% decrease between 25 and 65 years of age, although a part of this loss may reflect decreased habitual activity, decreased coordination of muscular contraction, decreased motivation, decreased efficiency of movement, and, in the case of the staircase sprint, a fear of stumbling.[24]

As gauged by peak blood lactate levels, the anaerobic capacity in a child of either sex is 8 to 9 mmol/L.[24] This value is lower than the maximum developed in a young adult. Some authors have attributed the difference in tolerance of anaerobic effort to a deficiency of glycolytic enzymes such as phosphofructokinase in the muscles of the growing child. A second important consideration is a smaller ratio of muscle mass to total blood volume, and there may also

be difficulties of motivation or coordination in a very young child. The peak anaerobic capacity increases at adolescence, allowing a blood lactate of 10 to 12 mmol/L. This figure is also typical of the sedentary young or middle-aged adult who performs a single bout of all-out effort,[12] although middle-distance runners and competitors in team games such as ice hockey can realize values of 14 to 18 mmol/L. By age 65, the peak blood lactate concentrations of the average person have decreased to 8 or 9 mmol/L, even if good motivation is shown during testing;[16] the main reason why anaerobic capacity declines in older adults seems a reduced ratio of active muscle volume to blood volume.

The 30-second Wingate cycle ergometer test of anaerobic capacity reflects similar trends to the peak blood lactate figures.[24] In young children of both sexes, the Wingate test anaerobic capacity is about 170 joules (J)/kg. In adolescent boys, the value rises to 213 J/kg, but in pubertal girls the increase is much more modest, to 177 J/kg. Both sexes then maintain a plateau of anaerobic capcity through about age 35, and thereafter there is an accelerating loss of function.

Bones

In the child, the epiphyses are not yet united with the shafts because the long bones are still growing. Two practical problems result. The first is a traction epiphysitis that may develop through overuse, for example, at the medial epicondyle of the humerus (baseball thrower's elbow), less commonly at the upper epiphyseal plate of the humerus (baseball shoulder), at the tibial tubercle (in young jumpers) and at the distal radial epiphysis in young gymnasts.[26] Second, fractures developed during contact sports may pass through the epiphyseal plate, leading to a disruption in normal growth.[27]

The dangers of osteoporosis are gaining increasing recognition.[28] Amenorrheic young women (who are often ballet dancers, gymnasts, or endurance runners) with inadequate energy and mineral intake may already be at some risk of bone demineralization from early adolescence. Unless deliberate measures are taken to strengthen the bones, their calcium content diminishes progressively throughout adult life. In women, the process commonly begins between ages 20 and 30, and the rate of loss of calcium is particularly rapid in the 5 years immediately succeeding the menopause. Calcium loss generally commences about 10 years later in men than in women, and tends to progress less rapidly. Nevertheless, by the age of retirement, both sexes have lost sufficient calcium to increase the vulnerability to fractures, and this hazard becomes progressively more marked in the middle-old and very old. Calcium loss can be checked, if not reversed, by a program of progressive weight-bearing exercise.[29]

Degeneration of and damage to the articular cartilages causes a progressive increase in the incidence of osteoarthritis with aging. By age 50 to 60, radiographs of the spine show characteristic lesions in 70 to 80% of subjects, although only a small proportion of individuals (15 to 20%) complain of specific symptoms.[30] It is unclear how far overuse and sport-related injuries contribute to this problem. Studies of middle-aged and older joggers[31,32] suggest that they are not at any increased risk of osteoarthritis of the knees, and subjects with back pain may respond favorably to a moderate increase of physical activity.[33] Nevertheless, it is important to remember that the middle-old and very old can obtain adequate endurance exercise from walking, and this imposes only one third to one sixth of the impact stress on the joints associated with jogging.[31,32] If degenerative changes in the knee, hip, or spine are severely limiting standard forms of endurance exercise, water-supported exercises provide a useful alternative.[34]

Joints

Problems of flexibility do not normally impose any limitations on the desired activity patterns of the child and young adult. However, a progressive loss of function begins in young adulthood from a combination of factors that include muscle shortening caused by disuse, age-associated deterioration of joint structures (including both ankylosis of fibrocartilaginous joints and osteoarthritis), and (particularly in the middle-old to very old) a progressive degeneration of the collagen molecules that provide the structural basis of tendons. Cross-linkage between individual collagen fibers not only reduces flexibility, but also increases the risk of injury if excessive force is applied.[35] The extent of the functional loss has been studied most fully for flexion of the hips and spine, as measured by the Dillon sit-and-reach test. About a 20% decrease in the range of movement on this test occurs between the ages of 25 and 65.[36] The rate of deterioration probably accelerates beyond age 65, although detailed population data are lacking.

An important fact to note is that the relationship between flexibility and function is not linear, but rather shows important discontinuities when the range of movement is no longer adequate to allow the performance of specific tasks such as climbing into or out of a bathtub. Likewise, if a small increase in the range of movement can be developed by an appropriate training regimen, a large gain in the quality of life may result.

Body Composition

Although many simple methods for the analysis of body composition have assumed a two-compartment model (fat and lean tissue), in reality the overall body density depends on the relative amounts and the respective densities of at least four body components (fat, bone, muscle and visceral tissues).[37]

In young children, the proportion of body fat is fairly small (10 to 15% of total body mass), although, probably mainly for cultural reasons, even prepubertal girls carry slightly more fat than boys of similar age. In boys, some increase in the percentage of body fat usually occurs with the decreasing habitual activity of adolescence; a figure of 15 to 20% fat is thus typical by age 20 to 30. In girls, the pubertal decrease of physical activity is often more marked, and the effects of this change are supplemented by an accumulation of fat in the breasts and around the hips, so that a figure of 20 to 25% body fat is typical from adolescence through to young adult life. In both sexes, 5 to 10 kg of fat usually accumulate in early middle age, so that the percentage may rise to 20 to 25% in men and 25 to 30% in women at this stage of life. A further build-up of adipose tissue after the menopause takes many older women to 30 to 35% fat.

There is a general parallel between age-related changes in muscle mass[37] and the course of muscle strength, as discussed above. Boys show a large increase of muscle protein during and immediately after puberty, and both sexes progressively lose muscle tissue after age 40 to 45. Because bone is very dense, the loss of calcium has a substantial effect upon total body mass.[37] In men, bone mass has decreased by about 10% at age 65, and by 20% at 80. In women, the loss is greater, amounting to about 20% by 65 and 30% by age 80.

These various alterations of body composition complicate the assessment process. A gain of body mass over the course of adult life (in the absence of specific training) generally reflects an accumulation of fat, but any loss of mass may be attributable to fat, muscle, bone, or some combination of all three. The relationship between skin fold readings and body density changes with age, in part because the skin's contribution to the double fold of tissue (4 mm in a young adult) becomes smaller with aging, and partly because the density of the lean tissue compartment decreases with bone demineralization.[37] Even underwater weighing, widely regarded as the "gold standard" of body composition determinations, has only limited validity, because the two compartment models that most authors have used to interpret hydrostatic data fail to accommodate interindividual differences in the density of lean tissue.[37]

Attempts to assess a person's lean body mass from determinations of his or her percentage of body fat and body mass are even less satisfactory. More direct estimates of lean tissue based upon body water, [40]K, or tissue impedance are complicated by age-related changes in the water and mineral content of the cells. Neutron activation and whole body counter technology can provide accurate assessments of body protein and bone calcium levels, but such procedures are expensive and are still available only in major hospitals.[38] Other techniques now becoming available include ultrasound, computerized tomography (CT), dual photon absorptiometry, magnetic resonance imaging (MRI) and infrared interactance.[37,39]

ORTHOPEDIC PROBLEMS

Orthopedic problems can arise from excessive exercise at any age. In the child athlete, the most frequent cause of difficulty is inflammation of the epiphyseal regions through repeated overloading of the tendon, for example, the medial epicondylar lesion noted with repeated throwing of "curved" balls by a little-league baseball player, the lesion of the tibial tubercle seen with excessive repetition of running and jumping, and the distal radial epiphysitis encountered in overambitious young gymnasts. Lesions can usually be avoided by moderating the intensity of training and competition until closure of the epiphyses is complete through appropriate age classification of participants. Any children reporting symptoms around the epiphyses should also be examined carefully for this problem.[26,27]

In middle age, many exercise programs have an alarming toll of injuries, particularly among recent recruits. From 30 to 50% of Masters competitors are injured each year,[40] and as many as 50% of sedentary recruits to exercise programs can develop incapacitating musculoskeletal injuries over the first 6 months of conditioning, because of such factors as inadequate warm-up, poorly developed muscle strength, sudden violent movements, and over-rapid progression of the exercise prescription. Surprisingly, such injuries do not always have a negative impact on subsequent intentions to exercise; perhaps for some subjects the excitement associated with a risk of injury is (at least subconsciously) a desired aspect of exercise. This way of thinking naturally complicates the task of prevention.[41]

The incidence of muscular tears can reputedly be reduced by a preliminary phase of gentle stretching of the limbs and an adequate warm-up period (at least 5 minutes of exercise) at a moderate pace. In middle-aged and older individuals, the latter precaution also helps to reduce the frequency of cardiac arrhythmias during the early phases of exercise.[42]

Swelling of the knees and an exacerbation of previous back injuries are common complications of jogging, particularly when the exercise is performed on a hard or uneven surface. Even mild symptoms are an indication for moderation of the prescription. Physical activity should leave the individual no more than pleasantly tired the following day. The likelihood of problems can be reduced by the use of well-cushioned shoes, a strengthening of the knee and back muscles, and a reduction of body mass. If symptoms persist or worsen, the only alternative may be to adopt some form of weight-supported exercise, such as swimming, cycling, or aqua-fitness classes.

Tendo-Achilles injuries and "shin splints" are also common early complications of increased physical activity. A hard or uneven running surface and inadequately cushioned shoes are again a factor in such injuries. The tendo Achilles can be damaged by allowing the heel to drop too far, and problems thus arise if the shoe that is worn has an inadequate heel. Shin splints and other orthopedic problems of the ankle and foot commonly reflect inappropriate angulation of the knee and ankle joints, and can thus be countered by simple orthotic devices.[42,43]

Currently, an increasing number of middle-aged and older individuals are preparing for marathon and even longer races. Plainly, a minimum training distance is an essential component of preparation for such events, but a ceiling of perhaps 70 to 80 km per week (40 to 50 miles per week) should also be set. If athletes exceed such a limit, the potential of normal, recuperative processes is surpassed, and injuries (including stress fractures of bones such as the metatarsals[44]) become increasingly frequent. In one series of Master's track and field competitors, we found that 50% had sustained injuries over the past year, and in one third of the injured group, the lesion had been sufficiently severe to interrupt training for 1 month or more. Long-distance runners frequently take vitamin C in the belief that it will protect them against injury or speed their recovery. However, we find that this makes no difference in either the incidence of injuries or the duration of disability.[45]

As a person reaches later middle age and old age, there is an increasing likelihood of knee and back problems from osteoarthritis. The prime cause of osteoarthritis is an injury to hyaline cartilage at the articular surface. Few studies of former athletes have been undertaken. Trauma experienced during contact sports such as ice hockey at an earlier age is almost certainly a significant etiologic factor, yet there is a surprising divergence between extent of symptoms and radiographic appearances.[30] An important determinant of residual function is the conservation of muscle and ligamentous strength about an arthritic joint by a combination of passive and active movements, plus isometric contractions of the principal muscles. If the knee can no longer be fully extended and has thus become unstable, a cane can be provided. However, the use of such an aid limits activity, and encourages an unnatural gait. A cane should thus be regarded as a temporary expedient to keep the person active while the quadriceps muscles are being strengthened. Aspirin can also be given to relieve pain, and in the event that the limitation of movement at a hip or knee joint is already extensive, an artificial joint can be considered.

Painful corns and calluses develop frequently on the feet of the middle-old and very old. Although they can be treated quite simply by a trained podiatrist, if ignored, they can also lead to abnormal movement patterns and a worsening of condition at deteriorating joints.

Lastly, demineralization of bones leaves the middle-old and very old person vulnerable to fractures of the long bones, hips, and pelvis.[27] The risk of falls increases with obesity, a deterioration of equilibrium, poor eyesight, reduced leg lift, and a tendency to develop postural hypotension.[47] Clearly, contact sports should be avoided after early middle age, and as the bones become weaker, it is also important to avoid activities that have a high risk of falls or collisions with stationary objects.

CHRONIC EXERCISE

The response to chronic exercise depends upon the intensity, frequency, and duration of training relative to the initial physical condition of the subject. Young children have difficulty in sustaining interest over long bouts of physical conditioning, and a nominal hour of required school gymnastics is too readily dissipated in changing, showering, and theoretical instruction. In the studies of Goode et al.[48] the minimum time needed to elicit a training response was only 6 minutes per session, provided that the student was brought to at least 80% of maximal oxygen intake five times per week.

In adults, high intensities of effort are needed to increase the condition of an athlete, but the training regimen for an average sedentary person is usually held below the anaerobic threshold to reduce the likelihood of injuries and the discouragement of excessive fatigue. A Position Statement from the American College of Sports Medicine[49] recommended that an endurance training program involve a large muscle mass 3 to 5 days per week at 50 to 85% of the individual's maximal oxygen intake. The choice of initial intensity depends on the person's condition. The recommended duration of an individual session ranges from 20 to 60 minutes per session, longer times being required if it is necessary to adopt a low intensity regimen. The ACSM further suggests that such activity be supplemented on at least 2 days per week by strength training (one set of 8 to 12 repetitions of 8 to 10 exercises to condition the major muscle groups).

The extent of the training response in middle age and old age depends greatly on the individual's motivation. Authors have described sedentary subjects in their 40s and 50s who have largely restored both the strength and the aerobic power that they enjoyed in their early 20s, but such individuals are exceptional. At age 65, an effective program more usually induces the same *percentage* gain that would be seen in a sedentary young adult who undertook rigorous training. The absolute response of the elderly is thus about half of that observed in a young adult.[16] Some of the middle-old and very old lack the initial condition necessary to commence continuous 30-minute sessions of endurance exercise at an appropriate fraction of their maximal oxygen intake. In such individuals, the pre-scription can initially be split into two or more bouts per day.

HYPERTENSION

As many as 20% of Canadian adults have been told at some time by their physicians that their blood pressure was too high.[50] Often this reflects a temporary elevation of the blood pressure associated with the anxiety-provoking circumstances of a medical consultation,[51] rather than clinically significant hypertension.

The systemic blood pressure at rest normally shows a small but steady rise from early adulthood through age 65, with a minimal increase thereafter. This is because an unchanged stroke volume is pumped into an increasingly rigid arterial system. The main cause of high blood pressure in old age is "benign essential hypertension." The separation of the normal from the abnormal is arbitrary, however, and a small rise in the systolic reading may be no more than an exaggeration of the normal aging process.

During a single bout of vigorous exercise, the well-trained individual generally develops a somewhat higher systolic pressure than that of a sedentary person, probably because of a larger increase in stroke volume. There is also some evidence that a large rise of pressure during exercise is a warning that the individual concerned is at increased risk of developing hypertension.[52] Evidence is now abundant that a regular training program reduces the resting systolic and diastolic blood pressures of hypertensive patients by about 10 mm Hg.[52] Such a reduction of pressures has therapeutic importance; indeed, on a population basis, regular exercise compares favorably with most available drugs, while lacking many of their unpleasant side effects. The training response is somewhat less consistent in normotensives, and no reduction of pressures may be expected if the initial readings are less than 125/85 mm Hg.

OBESITY

Physical activity plays an important role in prevention and treatment of moderate obesity at all ages, although the value of exercise in the correction of massive obesity is less clearly established. The body fat of the moderately obese person typically accumulates as the result of a small imbalance between food intake and energy expenditure, continued over many years. Studies of preschool children, school-age children, and adults all show that moderately obese individuals are less active than their sedentary peers[53] although because the obese spend more energy to move about, it is less clearly established that they have a lower daily energy expenditure than their thinner counterparts. An increase of physical activity necessarily has preventive value, unless there is a compensatory increase of food intake. In terms of treatment, exercise prescription is positive advice, in contrast to the usually restrictive tone of a dietary recommendation, although the exerciser must be prepared to persist with the recommended program for months rather than weeks. The mood-elevating tendency of moderate exercise may counter the dysphoria encountered with dietary restriction; it also lessens the protein loss associated with a simple restriction of energy intake, and in the moderately obese person it can achieve a substantial loss of fat without a need for specific dieting. Finally, because the fat is lost progressively over a period of some months, a new and more active lifestyle is established that helps to avoid the all-too-common recidivism associated with rapid and drastic dieting.

If the obesity is severe, adolescents and adults are frequently embarassed to exercise in the presence of the opposite sex. The initial exercise tolerance of the grossly obese may also be quite limited, and over-enthusiastic demands on the part of an instructor can lead the program participant to a sense of failure, with poor compliance and a further deterioration of body image. Walking or weight-supported exercise is initially more practical than jogging or calisthenics for the severely obese. A low body density and good insulation make swimming one of the more agreeable forms of exercise for such subjects. A substantial daily energy expenditure is needed to realize fat loss, and sometimes the required expenditure is best attained by two or three relatively brief sessions rather than one protracted bout of exercise. Such a schedule not only reduces the liability to fatigue, but also avoids an excessive rise of core temperature; heat elimination is necessarily made more difficult by the insulation of a thick layer of subcutaneous fat. The energy cost of most tasks is augmented by the heavy limbs and the large overall body mass. The normal assumptions of 23% mechanical efficiency on a cycle ergometer or 16% efficiency on a step test are incorrect in an obese person, and an appropriate allowance must be made for the increased cost of movement when prescribing exercise.

Finally, the very obese are often lacking in agility, and tend to fall heavily. Older obese individuals with some osteoporosis are thus at increased risk of bone injury, and this should be considered when recommending an appropriate exercise program.

REFERENCES

1. Bar-Or O, Shephard RJ, Allen CL: Cardiac output of 10–13 year old boys and girls during submaximal exercise. *J Appl Physiol, 30:*219, 1971.
2. Raven PB, Drinkwater BL, Horvath SM: Cardiovascular responses of young female track athletes during exercise. *Med Sci Sports, 4:*205, 1972.
3. Dal Monte A, Faina M, Menchinelli C: Sport-specific equipment. In *Sports and Human Endurance.* Edited by RJ Shephard and PO Åstrand. Oxford: Blackwell Scientific Publications, 1992.
4. Kavanagh T, Shephard RJ: Can regular sports participation slow the aging process? Data on Masters athletes. *Phys Sports Med 18:*94, 1990.
5. Londeree BR, Moeschberger ML: Effect of age and other factors on maximal heart rate. *Res Q, 53:*297, 1982.
6. Weisfeldt ML, Gerstenblith G, Lakatta EG: Alterations in circulatory function. In *Principles of Geriatric Medicine,* Edited by R Andres, EL Bierman, and WR Hazzard. New York: McGraw-Hill, 1985.
7. Shephard RJ: The aging of cardiovascular function. In *Academy Papers. Physical Activity and Aging.* Edited by WW Spirduso and HM Eckert. Champaign, IL: Human Kinetics Publishers, 1988.
8. Åstrand PO, Rodahl K: *Textbook of Work Physiology.* 3rd Ed. New York: McGraw-Hill, 1986.

9. Shephard RJ, et al.: On the basis of data standardization in pre-pubescent children. In *Kinanthropometry II*. Edited by M Ostyn, J Borms and J Simons. Basel: Karger, 1980.

10. Bailey DA: Exercise, fitness and physical education for the growing child. In *Proceedings of National Conference on Fitness and Health*. Edited by WAR Orban. Ottawa: Health and Welfare, Canada, 1974.

11. Cumming GR: Body size and the assessment of physical performance. In *Physical Fitness Assessment. Principles, Practice and Applications*. Edited by H Lavallée and RJ Shephard. Springfield, IL: Charles C Thomas, 1978.

12. Shephard RJ: Maximal oxygen intake. In *Sports and Human Endurance*. Edited by RJ Shephard and PO Åstrand. Oxford: Blackwell Scientific Publications, 1992.

13. Pate RB, Shephard RJ: Characteristics of physical fitness in youth. In *Youth, Exercise and Sport*. Edited by C Gisolfi and DR Lamb. Indianapolis: Benchmark Press, 1989.

14. Kasch FW, Wallace JP, Van Camp SP, et al.: A longitudinal study of cardiovascular stability in active men aged 45 to 65 years. *Phys Sports Med, 16(1):*117, 1988.

15. Åstrand PO: Exercise physiology for the mature athlete. In *Sports Medicine for the Mature Athlete*. Indianapolis: Benchmark Press, 1986.

16. Shephard RJ: *Physical Activity and Aging*. 2nd Ed. London: Croom Helm, 1987.

17. Mirwald RL, Bailey DA: *Maximal Aerobic Power. A Longitudinal Analysis*. London, Ontario: Sports Dynamics, 1986.

18. Celentano EJ, Nottrodt JW: Analysing physically demanding jobs: The Canadian Forces approach. In *Proceedings of the 1984 Conference on Occupational Ergonomics*. Edited by DA Attwood and C McCann. Toronto: Human Factors Association of Canada, 1984.

19. Shephard RJ, Vandewalle H, Bouhlel E, Monod H: Sex differences of physical working capacity in normoxia and hypoxia. *Ergonomics, 31:*1177, 1988.

20. Davies CTM, White MJ: Contractile properties of elderly human triceps surae. *Gerontology, 29:*19, 1983.

21. Aoyagi Y, Shephard RJ: Aging and muscle function. *Sports Med, 14:*376, 1992.

22. Fiatarone MA, Marks EC, Ryan ND, et al.: High-intensity strength training in nonagenarians. Effects on skeletal muscle. *JAMA, 263:*3029, 1990.

23. Bar-Or O: *Pediatric Sports Medicine*. New York: Springer, 1983.

24. Bouchard C, Taylor AW, Dulac S: Testing maximal anaerobic power and capacity. In *Physiological testing of the elite athlete*. Edited by JD MacDougall, HA Wenger, HJ Green. Ottawa: Canadian Association of Sport Sciences, 1982.

25. Shephard RJ: *Physical activity and growth*. Chicago: Year Book Publishers, 1982.

26. Roy S, Caine D, Singer KM: Stress changes of the distal radial epiphysis in young gymnasts: A report of 21 cases and a review of the literature. *Am J Sports Med, 13:*301, 1985.

27. Roy S, Irvin R: *Sports Medicine. Prevention, Evaluation, Management and Rehabilitation*. Englewood Cliffs, NJ: Prentice Hall, 1983.

28. Smith E: Bone changes with aging and exercise. In *Physical Activity, Aging and Sports*. Edited by R Harris, S Harris. Albany, NY: Center for Studies on Aging, 1989.

29. Chow R, Harrison JE, Notarius C: Effect of two randomized exercise programmes on bone mass of healthy post-menopausal women. *Br Med J, 295:*1441, 1987.

30. Hult L: Cervical, dorsal and lumbar spinal syndromes. *Acta Orthop (Suppl.), 17:*7, 1954.

31. Lane NE, Bloch DA, Jones HH, et al.: Long distance running, bone density and osteoarthritis. *JAMA, 255:*1147, 1986.

32. Panush RS, Brown DG: Exercise and arthritis. *Sports Med, 4:*54, 1987.

33. Nachemson AL: Exercise, fitness and back pain. In *Exercise, Fitness and Health. A Consensus of Current Knowledge*. Edited by C Bouchard, RJ Shephard, T Stephens, JR Sutton, BD McPherson. Champaign, IL: Human Kinetics Publishers, 1990.

34. Shephard RJ: Physical activity for the senior: A role for pool exercises? *CAHPER J, 50(6):*2, 1985.

35. Hall DA: Metabolic and structural aspects of aging. In *Textbook of Geriatric Medicine and Gerontology*. 2nd Ed. Edited by JC Brocklehurst. Edinburgh: Churchill-Livingstone, 1978.

36. Fitness and Amateur Sport. *Fitness and Lifestyle in Canada*. Ottawa: Fitness and Amateur Sport, 1983.

37. Shephard RJ: *Body Composition in Biological Anthropology*. London: Cambridge University Press, 1991.

38. Mernagh JR, et al.: Composition of lean tissue in healthy volunteers for nutritional studies in health and disease. *Nutr Res, 6:*499, 1986.

39. Brodie D: Techniques of measurement of body composition. *Sports Med, 5:*11, 74, 1988.

40. Kavanagh T, Lindley LJ, Shephard RJ,

Campbell R: Health and socio-demographic characteristics of the Masters competitor. *Ann Sports Med, 4:*55, 1988.

41. Shephard RJ, Godin G, Valois P: Exercise-induced injury and current exercise behaviour. *Clin Sports Med, 1:*197, 1990.

42. Barnard RJ, MacAlpin RN, Kattus AA, Buckberg GD: Ischemic response to sudden strenuous exercise in healthy men. *Circulation, 48:*936, 1973.

43. Nigg BM: Biomechanics, load analysis and sports injuries in the lower extremities. *Sports Med, 2:*367, 1985.

44. Shephard RJ, Taunton J: *Foot and Ankle in Sport and Exercise.* Basel: Karger, 1987.

45. Clement DB: Stress fractures of the foot and ankle. In *Foot and Ankle in Sport and Exercise.* Edited by RJ Shephard and J Taunton. Basel: Karger, 1987.

46. Kavanagh T, Shephard RJ: The effects of continued training on the aging process. *Ann NY Acad Sci, 301:*656, 1977.

47. Overstall PW: Falls. In *Principles and Practice of Geriatric Medicine.* Edited by MSJ Pathy. Chichester, John Wiley, 1985.

48. Goode RC, Virgin A, Duffin J, et al.: Effects of a short period of physical activity on adolescent boys and girls. *Can J Appl Sport Sci, 1:*241, 1976.

49. American College of Sports Medicine. Position Stand. The recommended quantity and quality of exercise for developing and maintaining cardiorespiratory and muscular fitness in healthy adults. *Med Sci Sports Exerc, 22:*265, 1990.

50. Shephard RJ, Cox M, Simper K: An analysis of Par-Q responses in an office population. *Can J Publ Health, 72:*37, 1981.

51. Young MA, Rowlands DB, Stallard TJ, et al.: Effect of environment on blood pressure: Home versus hospital. *Br Med J, 286:*1235, 1983.

52. Tipton CM: Exercise training, and hypertension: An update. *Exerc Sport Sci Rev, 19:*447, 1991.

53. Bray G: *Exercise and obesity.* In Exercise, Fitness and Health. Edited by C Bouchard, RJ Shephard, T Stephens, J Sutton and B McPherson. Champaign, IL: Human Kinetics, 1990.

Chapter 33

EXERCISE PRESCRIPTION FOR CHILDREN

Linda D. Zwiren

PHYSIOLOGIC ASPECTS

Unless otherwise indicated, this chapter refers to prepubescent children. It should be noted that data on prepubescents are limited by the fact that many experimental procedures are not appropriate for use with children.[1] In addition, most studies have used chronologic age to classify subjects as prepubescent. Because age of maturation is variable, it is unclear whether subjects were truly prepubescent when classified solely by chronologic age.

Major differences in physiologic responses to exercise exist between children and adults. These differences and the implications for exercise are presented in Table 33–1. Apart from low economy of locomotion and limitations of exercising in climatic extremes, no apparent underlying *physiologic* factor has been identified that would make children less suitable than adults for prolonged, continuous activities. The American Academy of Pediatrics (AAP), in reference to endurance, recommends that "if children enjoy the activity and are asymptomatic there is no reason to preclude them from training for or participating in such events."[2]

Although children can perform exercise over a wide variety of intensities and durations, they *spontaneously* prefer short-term intermittent activities with a high recreational component and variety rather than monotonous, prolonged activities. In accordance with their physiologic profile and from a psychologic viewpoint, children seem best suited to repeated activities that last a few seconds, interspersed with short rest periods. The least suitable forms of exercise for children, from a physiologic viewpoint, are highly intense activities lasting 10 to 90 seconds.[3]

PRECAUTIONS FOR EXERCISING IN CLIMATIC EXTREMES

Because children have a higher metabolic level at a given submaximal walking or running speed, children produce excessive body heat. This higher metabolic load in addition to a poor sweating capacity, large surface-to-mass ratio, and immature cardiovascular system (Table 33–1), causes children to have shorter tolerance for exercising in hot climates and greater susceptibility to heat stress.[3] The AAP recommends: "Clothing should be light weight, limited to one layer of absorbent material to facilitate evaporation of sweat and to expose as much skin as possible. Sweat-saturated garments should be replaced by dry ones. Rubberized sweat suits should never be used to produce loss of weight."[4]

Children have low tolerance to extreme heat or extreme cold; they thermoregulate as effectively as adults, however, when exercising in neutral or moderately warm climates.[1] The AAP emphasizes "that heat-related disorders are particularly pronounced in races that exceed 30 minutes in duration."[2] Activities lasting 30 minutes or more should be reduced whenever relative humidity and air temperature are above critical levels (Table 33–2).[4]

ACCLIMATIZATION

Children tend to lag behind adults in the *rate* of physiologic acclimatization and, therefore, should be involved in a longer and more gradual program. The AAP recommends ". . . that intensity and duration of exercise should be restrained initially and then gradually increased over a period of 10 to 14 days to accomplish acclimatization to the effects of heat."[4] Children can

Table 33–1. Physiological Characteristics of the Exercising Child*

Function	Comparison to Adults	Implications for Exercise Prescription
Metabolic:		
Aerobic		
$\dot{V}O_{2max}$ (L·min^{-1})	Lower function of body mass	
$\dot{V}O_{2max}$ (ml·kg^{-1}·min^{-1})	Similar	Can perform endurance tasks reasonably well
Submaximal oxygen demand (economy)	Cycling: similar (18–30% mechanical efficiency); walking and running: higher metabolic cost	Greater fatigability in prolonged high-intensity tasks (running and walking); greater heat production in children at a given speed of walking or running
Anaerobic		
Glycogen stores	Lower concentration and rate of utilization of muscle glycogen	
Phosphofructokinase (PFK concentration)	Glycolysis limited because of low level of PFK	Ability of children to perform *intense* anaerobic tasks that last 10 to 90 seconds is distinctly lower than that of adults
LA$_{max}$	Lower maximal blood lactate levels	
Phosphagen stores	Stores and breakdown of ATP and CP are the same	Same ability to deal metabolically with very brief intense exercise
Oxygen transient	Faster reaching of steady state than adults. Shorter half-time of oxygen increase in children	Children reach metabolic steady state faster. Children contract a lower oxygen deficit. Faster recovery. Children, therefore, are well suited to intermittent activities
LA$_{submax}$	Lower at a given percent of $\dot{V}O_{2max}$	May be reason why children perceive a given workload as easier
HR at lactate threshold	Higher	
Cardiovascular:		
Maximal cardiac output ($\dot{Q}_{max}$)	Lower because of size difference	Immature cardiovascular system means child is limited in bringing internal heat to surface for dissipation when exercising intensely in the heat
$\dot{Q}$ at a given $\dot{V}O_2$	Somewhat lower	
Maximal stroke volume (SV$_{max}$)	Lower due to size and heart volume difference	
SV at a given $\dot{V}O_2$	Lower	
Maximal heart rate (HR$_{max}$)	Higher	Up to maturity HR$_{max}$ is between 195 and 215 beats/min
HR at submax work	At given power output and at relative metabolic load, child has higher HR	Higher HR compensates for lower SV
Oxygen-carrying capacity	Blood volume, hemoglobin concentration, and total hemoglobin are lower in children	
O_2 content in arterial and venous blood (C_aO_2-C_vO_2)	Somewhat higher	Potential deficiency of peripheral blood supply during maximal exertion in hot climates

Table 33–1. (*Continued*)

Function	Comparison to Adults	Implications for Exercise Prescription
Blood flow to active muscle	Higher	
Systolic and diastolic pressures	Lower maximal and submaximal	No known beneficial or detrimental effects on working capacity of child
Pulmonary Response:		
Maximal minute ventilation $\dot{V}_{Emax}$ ($L \cdot min^{-1}$)	Smaller	Early fatigability in tasks that require large respiratory minute volumes
$\dot{V}_{E2max}$ ($mL \cdot kg^{-1} \cdot min^{-1}$)	Same as adolescents and young adults	
$\dot{V}_{Esubmax}$; ventilatory equivalent	$\dot{V}_E$ at any given $\dot{V}_{O_2}$ is higher in children	Less efficient ventilation would mean a greater oxygen cost of ventilation. May explain the relatively higher metabolic cost of submaximal exercise
Respiratory frequency and tidal volume	Marked by higher rate (tachypnea) and shallow breathing response	Children's physiologic dead space is smaller than that of adults; therefore, alveolar ventilation is still adequate for gas exchange
Perception (RPE: rating of perceived exertion):	Exercising at a given physiologic strain is perceived to be easier by children	Implications for initial phase of heat acclimatization
Thermoregulatory:		
Surface area (SA)	Per unit mass is approximately 36% greater in children (percentage is variable, depends on size of child, i.e., SA per mass may be higher in younger children and lower in older ones)	Greater rate of heat exchange between skin and environment. In climatic extremes, children are at increased risk of stress
Sweating rate	Lower absolute amount and per unit of SA. Greater increase in core temperature required to start sweating	Greater risk of heat-related illness on hot, humid days because of reduced capacity to evaporate sweat. Lower tolerance time in extreme heat
Acclimatization to heat	Slower physiologically; faster subjectively	Children require longer and more gradual program of acclimatization; special attention during early stages of acclimatization
Body cooling in water	Faster cooling due to higher SA per heat, producing unit mass; lower thickness of subcutaneous fat	Potential hypothermia
Body core heating during dehydration	Greater	Prolonged activity: hydrate well before and enforce fluid intake during activity

* Adapted with permission from Bar-Or O: Exercise in childhood. In *Current Therapy in Sport Medicine, 1985–1986*. Edited by RP Walsh and RJ Shephard. Toronto: CV Mosby, 1985, with information from related references[1,3,6,11,28,29]

Table 33-2. Weather Guide for Prevention of Heat Illness*

Air Temperature (°F)	Danger Zone (% Relative Humidity)	Critical Zone (% Relative Humidity)
70	80	100
75	70	100
80	50	80
85	40	68
90	30	55
95	20	40
100	10	30

* With permission from Haymes EM, Wells CL: *Environment and Human Performance.* Champaign, IL: Human Kinetics, 1986.

acclimate, to some extent, when they exercise in *neutral* environments, and when they *rest* in hot climates; however, they acclimatize *subjectively* faster than adults. Therefore, children, especially at the early stages of acclimatization, may *feel* capable of performing physical exercise in the heat, despite a marked physiologic heat stress.[5]

FLUID REPLACEMENT

During continuous activity of more than 30 minutes' duration, fluid replacement should be 100 to 150 mL every 15 to 30 minutes, even when the child is not thirsty.[1,4] Bar-Or recommends that replacement fluids for children should not exceed 5 mEq/L Na$^+$ (0.3 g/L NaCl), 4 mEq/LK$^+$ (0.28 g/L KCl), and 25 g/L sugar. Haymes and Wells suggest that a child weighing 40 kg should ingest 150 mL of cold tap water every 30 minutes during activity.[6]

OVERUSE INJURY

The most common musculoskeletal problems in young runners are those that result from repeated mechanical stress over a long period of time (overuse injuries). The recent increases in overuse injuries in children have been attributed to the increase in children who compete and train intensely because such injuries are *not* seen in free play.[7] Children may be more anatomically susceptible to overuse injuries than adults because of the presence of growth tissue. Risk factors include:

- Abrupt change in intensity, duration, or frequency of training (intensity should not be increased more than 10% per week)
- Musculotendinous imbalance in strength and flexibility
- Anatomic malalignment of lower extremities
- Poor footwear and running surface

EXERCISE PRESCRIPTION

Although positive scientific verification is still lacking, the recommended guidelines for exercising adults, in terms of frequency, duration, and intensity, can be used for older children.[1,8,9] Some controversy remains, however, as to whether the use of adult guidelines for younger children will increase the level of maximal oxygen intake ($\dot{V}O_{2max}$) beyond the level associated with growth.[3,8-11] It has been suggested that the intensity of exercise based on the adult guidelines to improve $\dot{V}O_{2max}$ may be appropriate for pubescent and postpubescent children but unacceptable for younger children.[12,13] Because evidence exists that health benefits in the adult are related to activity level, perhaps the best prescription for prepubescent children involves keeping them active, with less concern for increasing $\dot{V}O_{2max}$. When the goal of an exercise prescription is to improve health status, the emphasis should be on increasing energy expenditure through regular physical activity, with minimal concern for the intensity of the exercise. Recommended activities are those that require moving of the whole body mass (e.g., walking, running, cycling, cross-country skiing, swimming), which are performed at an intensity lower than that recommended for increasing maximal aerobic capacity but of longer duration and greater frequency.[13]

The increase of light to moderate activity in which a child engages is not only important for reducing risk factors for chronic diseases but is also a major component of multidisciplinary programs for obese children.[13,14] Because obesity in children has been identified as the risk factor that has the greatest impact on reduction of adult coronary heart disease,[15] increasing energy expenditure in this group of children would be beneficial from a public health perspective. It must be cautioned, however, that one cannot use adult-based equations to predict $\dot{V}O_2$ (and, therefore, energy expenditure) for walking and running in children. ". . . even when corrected for body mass, the $\dot{V}O_2$ of walking or running is higher than that of adolescents or adults. Thus, adult-based equations that predict the $\dot{V}O_2$ from walking and running speeds and slopes underestimate the actual metabolic cost when used with children."[14]

Children with an illness or disability with resultant hypoactivity may require a specific exercise prescription (Table 33–3). A specific prescription may also be advised for children identified as having two or more risk factors for coronary artery disease.

STRENGTH TRAINING

Strength training (also known as resistance or weight training) was not recommended for prepubescent children by the American Academy of Pediatrics (AAP) in 1983.[15] These 1983 recommendations were based on results of relatively few studies that stated that prepubescent children could not gain in strength with resistance training because of lack of circulating androgens.[13] Recent studies, however, have shown that strength gains can be realized, with minimal risk of injury, in both boys and girls with proper weight training programs.[15]

Strength is a measure of the greatest force that can be produced by a group of muscles. *Muscle endurance* is the ability to contract repeatedly (or to maintain a contraction) without fatigue, and *muscle power* is the speed at which muscle force can be generated.[13] Strength training is the use of a variety of methods, including free weights, weight machines, and/or one's body weight, to increase muscular strength, endurance, and/or power.[16] Usually strength training involves doing a series of repetitions against some resistance. The more repetitions (and, therefore, the lower the resistance), the more likely training effect will improve muscle endurance; fewer repetitions with higher resistance will maximize strength gains.[13] Weight training is usually engaged in to increase fitness, to enhance performance in a sport, or to prevent injury. On the other hand, weight *lifting* or power lifting, are competitive sports in which maximal weight is lifted in a single attempt.[16] Body building is a competitive sport in which the participants use various resistance methods to develop muscle size, symmetry, and definition.[16]

Because the most recent ACSM guidelines for adults include recommendations for muscular strength and training as well as for cardiovascular training, and because some recent studies have indicated that children lack upper-arm strength, recommendations for children are included here.[17,18] The AAP recommends that strength training programs for prepubescents should be conducted by well-trained adults. Children should avoid the practices of weightlifting, power lifting, and body building as well as the use of maximal amounts of weight in strength training programs until they have reached Tanner stage 5 level of developmental maturity. Appropriate weight training programs for children should focus on a higher number of repetitions and low resistance, in which muscle balance, flexibility, and proper technique are emphasized.[13,18] Several excellent sources are available for developing such programs.[13,18–20]

GRADED EXERCISE TESTS

Rationale for Exercise Testing

The various reasons for using exercise testing in pediatric diagnosis are listed in Table 33–4. Application of graded exercise testing (GXT) to specific diseases or problems is beyond the scope of this monograph, and we refer the reader to other references for more detailed information.[1,21–24] In many cases, the GXT is used most successfully as an affirmation to the child and parents that exercise can be performed at high intensity with no ill effects.

Ergometers

The same types of ergometers can be used with children and adults, although preferably children, especially those younger than 7 years, should be tested on a treadmill. Premature local muscle fatigue and the inability to maintain a specific cadence prevent many children from reach-

Table 33-3.   Exercise Prescription in the Management of Specific Pediatric Diseases*

Disease	Purposes of Program	Recommended Activities
Anorexia nervosa	Means for behavioral modification; educate regarding lean mass versus fat	Various; emphasize those with low energy demand
Bronchial asthma	Conditioning; possible reduction of exercise-induced bronchospasm; instill confidence	Aquatic, intermittent, long warm-up
Cerebral palsy	Increase maximal aerobic power, range of motion, and ambulation; control of body mass	Depends on residual ability
Cystic fibrosis	Improve mucus clearance, training of respiratory muscles	Jogging, swimming
Diabetes mellitus	Help in metabolic control; control of body mass	Various; attempt equal daily energy output
Hemophilia	Prevent muscle atrophy, contractures, and possible bleeding in joints	Swimming, cycling; avoid contact sports
Mental retardation	Socialization; increase self-esteem; prevent detraining	Recreational, intermittent, large variety
Muscular dystrophies	Increase muscle strength and endurance; prevent contractures; prolong ambulatory phase	Swimming, calisthenics, wheelchair sports
Neurocirculatory disease	Increase effort tolerance; improve orthostatic response	Various; emphasize endurance-type activities
Obesity	Reduction of body mass and fat; conditioning; socialization and improved self-esteem	High in calorie uptake but feasible to child; emphasize swimming
Rheumatoid arthritis	Prevent contractures and muscle atrophy; increase daily function	Swimming, calisthenics, cycling, sailing
Spina bifida	Strengthen upper body; control of body mass and fat; increase maximal aerobic power	Arm-shoulder resistance training, wheelchair sports (including endurance)

* With permission from Bar-Or O: Exercise in childhood. In *Current Therapy in Sport Medicine, 1985–1986.* Edited by RP Walsh and RJ Shephard. Toronto: C.V. Mosby, 1985.

ing maximal values on the cycle ergometer. Cardiorespiratory measurements must be directly assessed on the treadmill. Prediction of maximal values from submaximal $\dot{V}O_2$ are not applicable with children because the efficiency of a child's gait is so variable.[3]

If a cycle ergometer is used, an electronically braked cycle ergometer is preferred, because power output is not dependent on a given pedal rate. On mechanically braked ergometers, pedal rates of 50 to 60 rev min^{-1} are recommended.[1] If children aged 8 or 9 years or younger are to be

tested, special pediatric models should be used or existing cycle ergometers should be modified. The handlebars should be lengthened, the seat height must be adjusted so that the angle of the knee joint at the extension is 15°, and the pedal crank length should be reduced (13 cm for age 6; 15 cm for age 8 to 10 years).[1] In addition, because smaller resistance increments may be needed, resistance unit indicators on the cycle ergometer should be in 5W gradations. Testing of children with diseases that involve the legs may require the use of arm ergometers.

Table 33–4. Rationale for Exercise Testing in Pediatric Diagnosis

Measure physical working capacity
1. Assess function—establish whether a child's daily activities are within the child's physiologic functioning level
2. Identify deficiency in specific fitness component—muscular endurance and strength may limit daily performance rather than aerobic capacity (e.g., in muscular dystrophy)
3. Establish a baseline before the onset of an intervention program
4. Assess the effectiveness of an exercise prescription
5. Chart the course of a progressive disease (e.g., cystic fibrosis, Duchenne muscular dystrophy)

Exercise as a provocation test
1. Amplify pathophysiologic changes
2. Trigger changes otherwise not seen in the resting child

Exercise as an adjunct diagnostic test
1. Noninvasive exercise test can be used for screening to determine the need for an invasive test
2. Assessing the severity of dysrhythmias
3. Assessing the functional success of surgical correction
4. Assessing the adequacy of drug regimens at varying exercise intensities

Assessment and differentiation of symptoms: chest pains (asthma from myocardial infraction), breathlessness (bronchioconstriction from low physical capacity), coughing, easy fatigability

Instill confidence in child and parent

Motivation or compliance in intervention program

* Adapted with permission from Bar-Or O: Exercise in pediatric assessment and diagnosis. *Scand J Sport Sci* 7:35, 1985.

PROTOCOL

Various exercise protocols are available for children who are symptomatic.[1,21–25] Some protocols are similar to those used with adults. In some instances, protocols are modified so that the initial power output and subsequent incremental increases are lowered. The specific protocol selected depends on the specific question(s) to be answered, measurements to be obtained, whether submaximal and/or maximal data are needed, and the abilities and limitations of the patient. A GXT is not required when evaluating asymptomatic children.

SUPERVISORY PERSONNEL

During GXT, a technician and/or nurse should be present, and a physician should be available within 30 to 60 seconds. For the following conditions, a physician should be actively involved in the testing:[1,27]

- Serious rhythm disorders
- Aortic stenosis with anticipated gradients over 50 mm Hg
- Myocardial disease
- Cyanotic heart disease
- Advanced pulmonary vascular disease
- Ventricular dysrhythmia with heart disease
- Coronary arterial disease

CONTRAINDICATIONS

In addition to the contraindications listed in the *Guidelines*, the contraindications for testing pediatric patients follow:

1. Asthmatic child who is dyspneic at rest or whose 1-second forced expiratory volume (FEV_1) or peak expiratory flow is less than 60% of predicted value
2. Acute renal disease
3. Hepatitis
4. Insulin-dependent diabetic who did not take prescribed quantity of insulin or who is ketoacidotic[1]

CRITERIA FOR TERMINATION OF TEST

Criteria for stopping an exercise are similar to those for adults included in the *Guidelines*.[17]

Attainment of Maximal Values

Maximal Oxygen Uptake ($\dot{V}O_{2max}$)

The evidence of a plateau is less common in children than in adults. Data on intraindividual variation in $\dot{V}O_{2max}$ indicate, however, that acceptable data can be obtained even if criteria for identifying a plateau in $\dot{V}O_{2max}$ are not always satisfied.[1,10] Strategies and procedures have been suggested for increasing the likelihood of achieving a physiological $\dot{V}O_{2max}$ in younger children.[26]

Maximal Heart Rate

Children with peripheral musculature that is weak or atrophied (e.g., as in muscular dystrophy or cerebral palsy) are not able to generate enough power to reach maximal heart rates associated with other children their age (Table 33–1). In addition, children with congenital heart block (and a number of other congenital heart defects), anorexic children, and children receiving beta-blocker therapy also may have reduced maximal heart rates.[1,27]

REFERENCES

1. Bar-Or O: *Pediatric Sports Medicine for the Practitioner: From Physiologic Principles to Clinical Applications.* New York: Springer, 1983.
2. American Academy of Pediatrics: Risks in running for children. *Pediatrics, 86:*799, 1990.
3. Bar-Or O: Exercise in childhood. In *Current Therapy in Sport Medicine*, 1985–1986. Edited by RP Walsh and RJ Shephard. Toronto: C.V. Mosby, 1985.
4. American Academy of Pediatrics: Climatic heat stress and the exercising child. *Phys Sport Med, 11:*155, 1983.
5. Inbar O: Exercise in the heat. In *Current Therapy in Sport Medicine*, 1985–1986. Edited by RP Walsh and RJ Shephard. Toronto: C.V. Mosby, 1985.
6. Haymes EM, Wells CL: *Environment and Human Performance*, Champaign, IL: Human Kinetics, 1986.
7. Micheli L: Pediatric and adolescent sport injuries: Recent trends. *Exerc Sport Sci Rev, 14:*359, 1986.
8. Rowland TW: Aerobic response to endurance training in pre-pubescent children: A critical analysis. *Med Sci Sport Exerc, 17:*493, 1985.
9. Sady SP: Cardiorespiratory exercise in children. In *Clinics in Sports Medicine.* Vol. 5. Edited by F Katch and PF Freedson. Philadelphia: WB Saunders, 1986.
10. Krahenbuhl GS, Skinner JS, Kohrt WM: Developmental aspects of maximal aerobic power in children. *Exerc Sport Sci Rev, 13:*503, 1985.
11. Wells CL: The effects of physical activity on cardiorespiratory fitness in children. In *American Academy of Physical Education Papers*, No. 19. Edited by GA Stull and HM Eckert. Champaign, IL: Human Kinetics, 1986.
12. Cureton KJ: Commentary on "Children and fitness: A Public health perspective." *Res Quart Exer Sports, 58:*315, 1987.
13. Rowland TW: *Exercise and Children's Health.* Champaign, IL: Human Kinetics Books, 1990.
14. Bar-Or O: Discussion: Growth, exercise, fitness, and later outcomes. In *Exercise, Fitness, and Health: A consensus of Current Knowledge.* Edited by C Bouchard, RJ Shephard, T Stephens, JR Sutton, BD McPherson. Champaign, IL: Human Kinetics, 1990.
15. Zwiren LD: Exercise in children and youth. In *Exercise and the Heart in Health and Cardiac Disease.* Edited by RJ Shepard, H Miller. New York, NY: Marcel Dekker, 1992.
16. American Academy of Pediatrics: Committee on Sports Medicine: Strength, training, weight and power lifting, and body building by children and adolescents. *Pediatrics, 86:*801, 1990.
17. American College of Sports Medicine: *Guidelines for Exercise Testing and Prescription.* 4th Ed. Philadelphia: Lea & Febiger, 1991.
18. Freedson PS, Ward A, Rippe JM: Resistance training for youth. In *Advances in Sports Medicine and Fitness, Vol 3.* Edited by WA Grana, JA Lombardo, BJ Sharkey, JA Stone. Chicago: Yearbook Medical Publishers, 1990.
19. Webb DR: Strength training in children and adolescents. *Pediatr Clin North Am, 37:* 1187, 1990.
20. Anderson B, Burke ER: Scientific, medical, and practical aspects of stretching. *Clin Sports Med 10(1):*63–86, 1991.
21. American Heart Association Council on Cardiovascular Disease in the Young: Standards for exercise testing in the pediatric age group. *Circulation, 66:*1377A–1397A, 1982.
22. Driscoll DJ: Diagnostic use of exercise testing in pediatric cardiology: The non-evasive approach. In *Advances in Pediatric Sport Sciences Vol 3.* Edited by O Bar-Or. Champaign, IL: Human Kinetics, 1989.
23. Golden JC, Janz KF, Clarke WR, Mahoney LT: New protocol for submaximal and peak exercise values for children and adolescents. *Pediatr Exer Sci, 3:*129, 1991.
24. Cummings GR, Langsford S: Comparison of nine exercise tests used in pediatric cardiology. In *Children and Exercise.* Edited by RA Binkhorst, HCG Kemper, WHM Saris. Champaign, IL: Human Kinetics, 1985.
25. Godfrey S: *Exercise Testing in Children. Applications in Health and Disease.* Philadelphia: WB Saunders, 1974.
26. Hester D, Hunter G, Shulevak, Dunaway D: Conducting maximum treadmill tests

with young children—procedures and strategies. *JOPERD, 61:*23, 1990.

27. Cumming GR: Exercise tests in pediatric cardiology. In *Current Therapy in Sport Medicine* 1985–1986. Edited by RP Walsh and RJ Shephard. Toronto: CV Mosby, 1985.

28. Bar-Or O: The child athlete and thermoregulation. In *Exercise in Sport Biology.* Edited by P Komi. Champaign, IL: Human Kinetics, 1982.

29. Inbar O, Bar-Or O: Anaerobic characteristics in male children and adolescents. *Med Sci Sport Exerc, 18:*264, 1986.

BIBLIOGRAPHY

Bar-Or O: Importance of differences between children and exercise and adults for exercise testing and exercise prescription. In *Exercise testing and exercise prescription for special cases. Theoretical basis and clinical application.* Edited by J Skinner. Philadelphia: Lea & Febiger, 1987.

Bar-Or O: Exercise in pediatric assessment and diagnosis. *Scand J Sport Sci, 7:*35, 1985.

Freed MD: Recreational and sports recommendations for the child with heart disease. *Pediatr Clin North Am 31:*1307, 1984.

Chapter 34

EXERCISE PROGRAMMING FOR THE OLDER ADULT
Gregory W. Heath

Older individuals who engage in regular vigorous physical activity have an increased physical working capacity,[1] decreased body fat,[2] increased lean body tissue,[2] increased bone density,[3] and lower rates of coronary artery disease (CAD),[4] hypertension,[5] and cancer.[6] Increased physical activity is also associated with greater longevity.[7] The benefits of regular physical activity and exercise can also assist older adults in enhancing their quality of life, improving their capacity for work and recreation, and altering their rate of decline in functional status.[8]

When designing and prescribing exercise programs for older adults, several physiologic, anatomic, and psychologic characteristics should be considered to ensure a safe, effective, and enjoyable exercise experience.

CHARACTERISTICS THAT AFFECT PHYSICAL ACTIVITY IN OLDER ADULTS

Cardiovascular System

Aging is associated with changes in the cardiovascular system.[9] Resting heart rate shows little or no change with increasing age; however, maximal exercise heart rate shows a decline.[10] Functional and structural changes take place that affect the myocardium. One such change is a reduction in resting cardiac output, which results partly from a fall in resting stroke volume in the face of myocardial hypertrophy.[11]

When comparing older and younger individuals, we note that submaximal exercise leads to similar increases in stroke volume and cardiac output.[11] At maximal exercise intensities, however, older individuals have cardiac outputs that are 20 to 30% lower than those of younger individuals.[11]

Elasticity of the major blood vessels declines with aging. Higher resting and exer-

cise blood pressure determinations result.[9] The increase in blood pressure, both at rest and on exercise, often peaks at age 65 to 70 years, with little or no further change beyond this age level.

Maximal oxygen uptake ($\dot{V}O_{2max}$) shows a steady decline with age.[12] The level of physical activity, however, dramatically influences this change. The decline in $\dot{V}O_{2max}$ that can be attributed to aging per se is primarily caused by changes in the myocardium that are related to maximal cardiac output expressed as the product of maximal stroke volume and maximal heart rate. A decrease in myocardial sensitivity to catecholamines and the effect of prolonged diastole that occurs with age appear to be the most likely explanations for the decline seen in heart rate.[13] Peripheral vascular changes and the ability of the skeletal muscle to extract oxygen are minimally involved in this decline; however, loss of skeletal muscle mass that occurs with aging results in a decrease in oxygen extraction and also has an impact on the $\dot{V}O_{2max}$.[14] In consideration of the above mentioned cardiovascular characteristics, many older adults who are just beginning a regular program of physical activity will have low initial levels of cardiorespiratory fitness. Therefore, the initial exercise prescription will need to be tailored more specifically and the progression of activity will need to be slower than in younger adults.

Coronary artery disease (CAD) is a major threat to cardiovascular health in the elderly.[15] This disease, with its underlying process of atherosclerosis, is the most prevalent chronic disease found in older individuals. Many of the limitations within the cardiovascular system that appear to be associated with aging are often a result of CAD and its complications. Atherosclerosis can also affect the arteries of the brain, kidney, and peripheral vascular system. Numerous contraindications for exercise in older people with CAD and other heart disease exist (Table 34–1). Modification of the exercise prescription can usually be made to accommodate most of the relative contraindications for exercise. The effects of disease should be understood in light of the physiology of aging and the desired effects of regular physical activity.

Older individuals can obtain cardiovas-

Table 34–1. Contraindications to Physical Activity for Older Adults*

Absolute Contraindications
  Severe CAD—unstable angina pectoris and acute myocardial infarction
  Decompensated congestive heart failure
  Uncontrolled ventricular arrhythmias
  Uncontrolled atrial arrhythmias (compromising cardiac function)
  Severe valvular heart disease including aortic, pulmonic, and mitral stenosis
  Uncontrolled systemic hypertension (e.g., > 200/105)
  Pulmonary hypertension
  Acute myocarditis
  Recent pulmonary embolism or deep vein thrombosis
Relative Contradictions
  CAD
  Congestive heart failure
  Significant valvular heart disease
  Cardiac arrhythmias including ventricular and atrial arrhythmias and complete heart block
  Hypertension
  Fixed-rate, permanent pacemaker
  Cyanotic congenital heart disease
  Congenital anomalies of coronary arteries
  Cardiomyopathy including hypertrophic cardiomyopathy and dilated cardiomyopathy
  Marfan's syndrome
  Peripheral vascular disease
  Severe obstructive or restrictive lung disease
  Electrolyte abnormalities, especially hypokalemia
  Uncontrolled metabolic diseases (e.g., diabetes, thyrotoxicosis, myxedema)
  Any serious systemic disorder (e.g., mononucleosis, hepatitis)
  Neuromuscular or musculoskeletal disorders that would make exercise difficult
  Marked (gross) obesity
  Anemia
  Idiopathic long-QT syndrome

* Adapted with permission from Van Camp SP, Boyer JL: Exercise guidelines for the elderly. *Phys Sports Med,* 17:83, 1989.

cular endurance benefits from regular endurance exercise training that are similar to those benefits observed in younger adults.[15] The level of $\dot{V}O_{2max}$ can increase in sedentary older persons with regular endurance activity. Lower heart rate, blood pressure, and blood lactate levels at submaximal exercise can be demonstrated with regular endurance exercise.[15]

Respiratory System

Changes in the lung and respiratory system occur with aging. The residual volume increases 30 to 50%; the vital capacity decreases 40 to 50% by age 70.[16] Therefore, as individuals age, there is a greater dependency on increased respiratory frequency rather than increased tidal volume during exercise. This dependency increases the overall work in breathing.[16]

Respiratory function does not limit exercise capacity unless function is significantly impaired, as with chronic obstructive pulmonary disease (e.g., emphysema, chronic bronchitis). The ventilatory changes that are seen with aging do not interfere with the ability of the individual to manifest significant improvements in $\dot{V}O_{2max}$ after training.

Nervous System

Significant changes occur in the central and peripheral nervous system with age. Reaction times become slower and the velocity of nerve conduction slows by 10 to 15% by age 70.[17] More specifically, sensory defects increase in incidence with increasing age. Mechanical and neurologic changes occur in the older individual's auditory system.[18] These changes are responsible for impaired auditory activity and decreased sound discrimination.

The visual system also undergoes significant change with increasing age.[18] The lens undergoes a yellowing and, in some cases, lens opacity occurs (cataracts). The number of rods and cones is usually reduced. The iris loses the ability to open as wide as in younger individuals. These changes are responsible for the common complaint of impaired night vision in the elderly as well as the general need for better visual conditions, such as improved lighting.

Regular lifetime physical activity appears

to delay the slowing of reaction times with aging;[17] however, results of studies in which scientists examined these variables in response to regular exercise in previously sedentary older individuals are inconclusive. Although few researchers have documented positive or negative effects of regular exercise on neurologic function, some investigators report the possibly decreased level of anxiety in older regular exercisers and the consistent finding of an increased sense of well-being in older participants with regular exercise.[19,20]

Musculoskeletal System

A 20% decline in muscle strength usually occurs by age 65. This decline in strength is attributed not only to advancing age but also to the effects of disuse.[21]

A progressive loss in bone mass occurs with aging.[3] This loss is particularly evident in women, but also occurs in men. Women over 35 lose bone mass at a rate of 1% per year.[3] Men begin to sustain bone loss at about age 55 and usually lose 10 to 15% by age 70.[3] Bone loss can be exacerbated in the elderly by an inadequate dietary calcium intake, diabetes mellitus, lack of supplemental estrogen and progestin in postmenopausal women, renal impairment, or immobility.[3] Bone loss with resultant loss of bone strength predisposes many older individuals to fractures, particularly of the hip, vertebrae, and forearm.[22] These are a significant cause of morbidity and mortality (hip) in the elderly.[22]

Older adults can have significant limitations in flexibility. Changes that occur with aging have not been well documented; however, investigators have found the major cause of declining flexibility is the lack of movement with joints that are not usually used in daily activities. The aging joint is generally less flexible and mobile.[23] Connective tissue changes in muscles, ligaments, joint capsules, and tendons appear responsible for most of the loss of flexibility and mobility.[24]

Regular strength training in older individuals has demonstrated increased strength with a mild to moderate muscle hypertrophy.[21,25] Regular weight-bearing exercise can cause an increase in bone density in middle-aged and older women.[22]

Men who exercise regularly have reportedly higher bone densities than their sedentary counterparts.[3]

Exercise programming for the elderly emphasizing flexibility activities has brought about significant improvement to joint range of motion, including the neck, shoulder, wrist, back, hip, knee, and ankle.[23]

Other Systems

Renal function declines approximately 30 to 50% between the ages of 30 and 70. Along with the decline in kidney function is a decrease in acid-base control, glucose tolerance, and drug clearance.[26]

A general reduction in total cellular water occurs with aging, with a decline of 10 to 50% in total body water.[26] This change predisposes the older individual to a more rapid dehydration when confronted with a hot environment, burns, or diarrhea. Evaporative water losses and perspiration need to be considered when older adults exercise. The added stress of a hot and humid environment can be assessed in older adults by noting the increase in heart rate at any given rate of physical activity. This failure of thermoregulation in older adults is often exacerbated by such common medications as beta-blocking agents.[27]

Metabolism

Basal metabolic rate gradually decreases with age, as does $\dot{V}o_{2max}$.[28] Sedentary men have been shown to have decreases in their $\dot{V}o_{2max}$ of 9% per decade, with regularly active men showing only a 5% per decade decline.[29] Glucose tolerance is diminished with increasing age, accompanied by an increasing likelihood of developing noninsulin-dependent diabetes mellitus.[30] Lean body mass decreases, whereas body fat increases.[2]

Regular physical activity can increase $\dot{V}o_{2max}$, increase lean body mass, and decrease body fat.[2] Alterations in glucose and lipid metabolism have also been demonstrated in older individuals who engage in regular endurance activities, with some researchers reporting apparently improved glycemic control in diabetic persons.[31]

The pharmacologic needs of older adults warrant consideration. Certain medicines for diseases that commonly affect the elderly influence an individual's response to exercise (e.g., beta-blockers). Vigorous exercise affects the action of some medicines (e.g., decreased insulin requirement, increased sensitivity to dehydration from diuretics).

Psychosocial Elements

In American society, retirement often marks the end of the productive period of life. Certain attitudes have led the majority of society to relegate the older adult to a sedentary lifestyle. Regular physical activity can be an effective tool in maintaining functional ability and promoting an enhanced sense of well-being in older adults.[32]

EXERCISE PROGRAMMING

Medical History and Clearance

Exercise programming for the elderly may be offered on three different levels: (1) A program-based level that consists primarily of supervised exercise training; (2) exercise counseling and exercise prescription followed by a self-monitored exercise program; and (3) community-based exercise programming which is self-directed and self-monitored.

Within supervised exercise programs and programs offering exercise counseling and prescription, participants should complete a brief medical history and risk factor questionnaire (Table 34–2).[28]

From the questionnaire, important information regarding potential limitations and restrictions for the individual participant's activity program can be made. Exercise leaders do well to require their senior participants to have had a recent (within the last 6 months) physical examination with a physician before beginning a program of moderate exercise. Participants should be encouraged to consult a physician if they have any questions regarding their medical status.

After an appropriate medical history is gathered, potential participants should undergo a preprogram evaluation in which flexibility, endurance capacity (aerobic), and strength are assessed. The primary purpose of the preprogram evaluation is

Table 34–2. Medical History and Clearance: Essential Elements

Medical History
  Cardiovascular disease
  Degenerative joint disease
  Hypertension
  Back syndrome
  Obstructive or restrictive lung disease
  Hypothyroidism
  Diabetes mellitus
  Dizziness, ataxia
Risk Factors
  Familial history of CAD
  Cigarette smoking
  Physical inactivity
  Obesity
  Hypertension (blood pressure > 140/90)
  Elevated blood lipids (cholesterol ≥ 240 mg/dL
    and/or low density lipoprotein cholesterol ≥
    130 mg/dL)
Medications
  Beta blockers
  Calcium channel blockers
  Antihypertensives
  Nonsteroidal anti-inflammatory drugs
  Analgesics
  Bronchodilators
  Thyroid replacement
  Hypoglycemic

to document baseline measures of flexibility, cardiorespiratory endurance, and strength. These baseline measures not only assist the exercise leader in prescribing an appropriate physical activity level, but also provide feedback to participants regarding progress when the evaluation is repeated periodically. The evaluation measures need not be sophisticated. Flexibility may be assessed with sit-and-reach assessments, both on the floor and in a chair.[33]

The use of a goniometer is helpful in determining limitations in joint flexibility and mobility. Observation of gait and movement from a seated to a standing position provides insight into sensory impairment, impaired equilibrium, or orthostatic hypertension. Strength testing may take the form of simple grip strength testing combined with modified push-up and sit-up performance. Cardiorespiratory endurance capacity may be assessed by appropriate field tests, such as a walking speed test for 12 minutes or the chair-step test.[33] Submaximal bicycle testing with pulse palpation and blood pressure measurements may also be employed. The previously mentioned cardiorespiratory tests are intended to be functional evaluations that are at submaximal levels and in appropriately screened individuals are relatively safe and effective while providing data for exercise prescription and physical activity education.

Potential participants with documented CHD, diabetes mellitus, or known risk factors for these diseases should be recommended for diagnostic exercise tolerance testing as well as functional assessment. The testing and evaluation should be directed by a physician. Typical methods of exercise tolerance testing include graded treadmill exercise testing with continuous electrocardiographic (ECG) monitoring and simultaneous measurement of heart rate and blood pressure. Exercise tolerance testing often involves a symptom-limited testing protocol through which an estimation of Vo_{2max} can be made. Several appropriate treadmill testing protocols are currently in use. The modified Balke and modified Bruce protocols, in which the speed and grade are initially at less than 2.5 METS with gradual increases in workload of 1 to 2 METS every 2 to 3 min, are examples of appropriate testing protocols.[33]

An alternative to treadmill testing is bicycle ergometry. The principles of ECG, heart rate, and blood pressure monitoring are the same. The most common reason for using the bike is selected medical contraindications for the use of the treadmill, including the presence of osteoarthritis or an artificial limb, as well as an unstable gait or severe obesity. The use of the bike has one major disadvantage in symptom-limited testing—the common experience of localized muscle fatigue in the legs. This result sometimes interferes with the participant's ability to achieve sufficiently high heart rates to be of diagnostic value.

When developing a community-based, self-directed program, medical clearance is left to the judgment of the individual participant. An active physical activity promotion campaign in the community seeks to educate the senior population regarding precautions and recommendations for moderate and vigorous physical activity. These messages should provide steps for seniors to follow before beginning a regular moderate to vigorous physical activity program. These steps should include:

1. Awareness of pre-existing medical problems (i.e., CHD, arthritis, osteoporosis, or diabetes mellitus).
2. Consultation before starting a program with a physician or other appropriate health professional if any of the above mentioned problems are suspected.
3. Appropriate mode of activity and tips on different types of activities.
4. Principles of training intensity and general guidelines as to rating of perceived exertion (RPE) and training heart rate (THR).
5. Progression of activity and principles of starting slowly and gradually increasing activity time and intensity.
6. Principles of monitoring symptoms of excessive fatigue.
7. Making exercise fun and enjoyable.

GENERAL EXERCISE PRESCRIPTION GUIDELINES[33,34]

Mode of Activity

Many older individuals who wish to participate in regular exercise programming have significant limitations. Degenerative joint disease, including osteoarthritis, is common in this age group. The mode of exercise must be appropriately modified to accommodate these participants. Emphasis on minimal or nonweight-bearing activities such as cycling, swimming, and chair and floor exercises may be the most appropriate. For participants with difficulty in joint mobility of the knees and hips, movement down and up from the floor may be initially contraindicated. Generally, most seniors are able to engage in moderate walking activities. Individualization of the mode of activity is important, including variation of activity as well as adjustments for participant bias and preference. Prescribing calisthenics for individuals suffering from degenerative joint changes should be done with care. Modified stretching and strengthening exercises should be employed where indicated. Guidelines for prescribing activities for selected chronic conditions are listed in Table 34–3.

Table 34–3. Modification of the Exercise Prescription: Selected Aging-Related Conditions

Condition	Recommended Modification
Degenerative joint disease	Nonweight-bearing activities such as stationary cycling, water exercises, and chair exercises
	Emphasis placed on interval activity. Low-resistance-low-repetition strength training
Coronary artery disease (CAD)	Physician oversight. Symptom-limited activities. Moderate-level endurance activities preferred (i.e., walking, slow cycling), although at physician's discretion more vigorous activities can be prescribed
	Low-resistance, higher-repetition strength training (see Chap. 16)
Diabetes mellitus	Daily, moderate endurance activities
	Low-resistance, higher-repetition strength training. Flexibility exercises. Monitoring of symptoms and caloric intake. In the presence of obesity, nonweight-bearing exercises may be indicated
Dizziness, ataxia	Chair exercises may be preferred. Low-resistance, low-repetition strength training. Moderate flexibility activities with minimal movement from supine or prone to standing positions
Back syndrome	Moderate endurance activities (i.e., walking, cycling, chair exercises)
	Modified flexibility exercises; low-resistance, low-repetition strength training; modified abdominal strengthening activities; water activities
Osteoporosis	Weight-bearing activities with intermittent bouts of activity spaced throughout the day. Low-resistance, low-repetition strength training, chair-level flexibility activities
Chronic obstructive lung disease	Moderate level endurance using an interval or intermittent approach to exercise bouts. Low-resistance, low-repetition strength training; modified flexibility and stretching exercises
Orthostatic hypotension	Minimize movements from standing to supine and supine to standing
	Sustained moderate endurance activities with short rest intervals. Emphasize activities that minimize the changing of body positions
Hypertension	Emphasize dynamic large-muscle endurance activities; minimize isometric work and focus on low-resistance, low-repetition isotonic strength training

Frequency

Emphasis on more frequent activity (5 to 7 days per week) should be made with seniors. This recommended increase in frequency has physiologic relevance for the maintenance of endurance capacity as well as flexibility. In addition, the greater frequency may enhance compliance and lead to a greater probability of the subject assimilating physical activity into the daily routine.

Duration

An appropriate goal for most seniors is 20 to 40 minutes of endurance activity per session. However, because of physiologic and pathophysiologic limitations, shorter exercise sessions of 10 to 15 minutes repeated 2 or 3 times throughout the day may be necessary for some seniors. In addition, because of aging-related limitations, the intensity of activity may have to be de-

creased, justifying an increase in duration approaching one hour to derive optimal benefits for older adults.

Intensity

Because of the general medical and physiologic limitations often seen in older individuals, the intensity of activity is of critical importance. For participants who have a history of CAD or are at high risk for CAD, the exercise prescription should be based on the results of a recent ECG (within 3 months) monitored exercise evaluation. An appropriate target heart rate based on the formula of Karvonen can be calculated, as well as an appropriate MET level, both of which are adjusted for symptoms and/or ECG changes noted in the exercise test. Usually young-old ($\leq$ 75 years) individuals can have peak work capacities of 7 METs or greater whereas the old-old ($>$ 75 years) participants usually have peak levels that do not exceed 4 METs. Unfortunately, the medical status and physical activity status of participants can vary considerably, so that generalization of workloads often becomes difficult. When an individual's work capacity has been assessed, the use of MET levels in calculating an appropriate intensity is useful. Use of the principles of RPE have proven helpful in regulating intensity in exercising older individuals. Usually a level of 12 to 15 on a 6 to 20 scale is adequate for most conditioning activities. When participants are well oriented to this method, it becomes a useful self-monitoring mechanism for regulating intensity of exercise.

Progression of Activity

A gradual approach to increasing activity levels is most appropriate. With initiation of exercise, a 4-to-6-week period is usually necessary for seniors to progress from a moderate to vigorous conditioning level. Another 4 to 6 weeks are often necessary to achieve an appropriate maintenance level. Individual variability in fitness and adaptation to the exercise usually dictate the appropriate progression of activity.

LEADING AN EXERCISE PROGRAM FOR OLDER PARTICIPANTS[35]

Planning

Community-based exercise programs require adequate research before implementation. Focus groups with seniors are an appropriate approach to assessing the physical activity needs of older individuals. Facilities and environmental settings can then be adequately planned.

Types of supervised programming should be well researched. Seniors should have adequate input regarding the types of activities for the program; community surveys of senior groups can provide invaluable information regarding the perceived exercise needs of the population. Interviews with local and regional senior organizations can be another source of important information for program planning. Information gathered from local governmental agencies often provides data on demographics and senior programs and resource lists that aid in identifying key resources and contacts for program support and further information.

The promotion of the exercise programming should be focused, often with differing messages aimed at particular target groups. This step is important in exercise program leadership to ensure that an adequate subset of the senior community is involved in physical activity programming, whether supervised or self-directed.

Facilities

When selecting facilities for supervised exercise programming, consider the previously mentioned limitations of older individuals. A facility with adequate lighting and ventilation is important. Ideally, a facility should limit background noise as much as possible because of the greater prevalence of hearing impairment in the elderly. A resilient surface is necessary, and well-cushioned mats for floor exercise are important.

Programming

The program should offer a good variety of activities that are designed not only for conditioning effects, but also for fun and enjoyment.

Well-trained and amiable personnel are critical. Many programs succeed without the best of facilities or equipment because of personnel who are empathetic, knowledgeable, and fun. Knowledge of the community and its resources is important in the promotion of programming. Selection of sites for programming should be convenient and easily accessible.

Emergency Skills

All staff involved in supervised programming should be certified in cardiopulmonary resuscitation and knowledgeable about basic first aid. Familiarity with the major medical disorders of the elderly (i.e., CAD, diabetes, arthritis, hypoglycemia) ensures a safer environment for exercise.

Participants who are in supervised programming or for whom exercise counseling and prescription are provided should have a basic knowledge of their medical and pharmaceutical regimens and how these might influence their response to exercise.

An appropriate emergency plan is essential in supervised programs. A file card for each participant with important emergency phone numbers as well as the name and phone number of his or her physician should be readily available.

A pattern of referral for medical consultation should also be provided in the event that participants are without a primary physician and are in need of medical evaluation and treatment.

SUMMARY

If the above considerations are taken into account, effective and safe physical activity programs can be developed for the increasing numbers of older adults in this country. In light of its disproportionately high levels of illness, disability, and health care utilization, the elderly population remains an important target for physical activity intervention.

REFERENCES

1. Bortz WM: Disuse and Aging. *JAMA, 248:* 1203, 1982.
2. Sidney KH, Shephard RJ, Harrison JE: Endurance training and body composition of the elderly. *Am J Clin Nutr, 30:*326, 1977.
3. Smith DM, Khairi MRA, Norton J, et al.: Age and activity effects on rate of bone mineral loss. *J Clin Invest, 58:*716, 1976.
4. Paffenbarger RS, Hyde RT, Wing AL: Physical activity as an index of heart attack risk in college alumni. *Am J Epidemiol, 108:* 161, 1978.
5. Tipton CH: Exercise, training and hypertension. *Exerc Sport Sci Rev, 12:*245, 1984.
6. Lee I-M, Paffenbarger RS, Hsieh C-C: Physical activity and risk of developing colorectal cancer among college alumni. *J Natl Cancer Inst, 33:*1324, 1991.
7. Paffenbarger RS Jr, Hyde RT, Wing AL, Hsieh CC: Physical activity, all-cause mortality, and longevity of college alumni. *N Engl J Med, 314:*605, 1986.
8. Frontera WR, Evans WJ: Exercise performance and endurance training in the elderly. *Top Geriatr Rehabil, 2:*33, 1986.
9. Schulman SP, Gerstenblith G: Cardiovascular changes with aging: The response to exercise. *J Cardiopulm Rehab, 9:*12, 1989.
10. Fleg JL: Alterations in cardiovascular structure and function with advancing age. *Am J Cardiol, 57:*33c, 1986.
11. Rodeheffer RJ, Gerstenblith G, Berker LC,

et al.: Exercise cardiac output is maintained with advancing age in healthy human subjects. Cardiac dilatation and increased stroke volume compensate for diminished heart rate. *Circulation, 69:*203, 1984.
12. Buskirk ER, Hodgson JL: Age and aerobic power: The rate of change in men and women. *Fed Proc, 46:*1824, 1987.
13. Weisfeldt ML, Gerstenblith G, Lakatta EG: Alterations in circulatory function. In *Principles of Geriatric Medicine.* Edited by R Andres, EL Bierman, WR Hazzard. New York: McGraw Hill, pp. 249–279, 1985.
14. Fleg JL, Lakatta EG: Role of muscle loss in the age associated reduction in $\dot{V}O_{2max}$. *J Appl Physiol, 65:*1147, 1988.
15. Van Camp SP, Boyer JL: Cardiovascular aspects of aging. *Phys Sports Med, 17:*121, 1989.
16. DeVries HA, Adams GM: Comparison of exercise responses in old and young men, II. Ventilatory mechanics. *J Gerontol, 27:* 344, 1972.
17. Spirduso WW: Reaction and movement time as a function of age and physical activity. *J Gerontol, 30:*435, 1975.
18. Smith EL: Special considerations in developing exercise programs for the older adult. In *Behavioral Health: a handbook of health enhancement and disease prevention.* Edited by JD Matarazzo, SM Weiss, JA Herd, NE Miller, SM Weiss. New York: John Wiley & Sons, 1984.
19. Barry AJ, Page JF, Steinmetz JR, et al.: Effects of physical conditioning on older individuals: motor performance and cognitive function. *J Gerontol, 21:*192, 1966.
20. Sidney KH, Shephard RJ: Attitudes towards health and physical activity in the elderly: effects of a physical training program. *Med Sci Sports Exerc, 8:*246, 1977.
21. Moritani T: Training adaptations in the muscles of older men. In *Exercise and Aging: The Scientific Basis.* Edited by EL Smith and RC Serfass. Hillside, NJ: Enslow Publishers, 1981.
22. Chow R, Harrison JE, Notarius C: Effects of two randomized exercise programmes on bone mass of healthy post-menopausal women. *Br Med J, 295:*1441, 1987.
23. Adrian MJ: Flexibility in the aging adult. In *Exercise and Aging: The Scientific Basis.* Edited by EL Smith and RC Serfass. Hillside, NJ: Enslow Publishing, pp. 45–58, 1981.
24. Munns K: Effects of exercise on the range of joint motion. In *Exercise and Aging: The Scientific Basis.* Edited by Smith EL and Serfass RC. Hillside, NJ: Enslow Publishers, 1981.
25. Frontera WR, Meredith CN, O'Reilly KP, et al.: Strength conditioning in older men:

Skeletal muscle hypertrophy and improved function. *J Appl Physiol, 64:*1038, 1988.

26. Rowe JW, Shock NW, Defronzo RA: The influence of age on the renal response to water deprivation in man. *Nephron, 17:*270, 1976.

27. Gordon NF, Myburgh DP, Schwellnus MP, Van Rensburg JP. Effect of B-blockade on exercise core temperature in coronary artery disease patients. *Med Sci Sports Exerc, 19:*591, 1987.

28. Fitzgerald PL: Exercise for the elderly. *Med Clin North Am, 69:*189, 1985.

29. Heath GW, Hagberg JM, Ehsani AA, et al.: A physiological comparison of young and older endurance athletes. *J Appl Physiol, 51:* 634, 1981.

30. Meyers DA, Goldberg AP, Bleecker ML, et al.: Relationship of obesity and physical fitness to cardiopulmonary and metabolic function in healthy older men. *J Gerontol, 46:*M57, 1991.

31. Seals DR, Hagberg JM, Hurley BF, et al.: Effects of endurance training on glucose tolerance and plasma lipid levels in older men and women. *JAMA, 252:*645, 1984.

32. Emery CF, Pinder SL, Blumenthal JA: Psychological effects of exercise among elderly cardiac patients. *J Cardiopulm Rehab, 9:*46, 1989.

33. Smith EL, Gilligan C: Physical activity prescription for the older adult *Phys Sports Med, 11:*91, 1983.

34. Shephard RJ. The scientific basis of exercise prescribing for the very old. *J Am Geriat Soc, 38:*62, 1990.

35. Smith EL, Stoedefalke KG, Gilligan C: *Aging and Exercise: Freedom through fitness.* Biogerontology Laboratory, Department of Preventive Medicine, University of Wisconsin, Madison, Wisconsin, 1980.

Section VIII

HUMAN BEHAVIOR/PSYCHOLOGY

Chapter 35

PRINCIPLES OF HEALTH BEHAVIOR CHANGE

C. Barr Taylor and Nancy Houston Miller

Helping people begin and maintain changes in health behavior is a challenge for the most experienced counselor. Nevertheless, behavioral scientists have identified some strategies that, if systematically applied, are useful in helping an individual begin and sustain health behavior change. We describe one model for such change that includes some practical approaches. This is derived from social learning theory, a comprehensive analysis of human functioning in which human behavior is assumed to be developed and maintained on the basis of three interacting systems: behavioral, cognitive, and environmental.[1,2] Social learning theory emphasizes the human capacity for self-directed behavior change. Willingness to change is related to self-efficacy (self-confidence), which is influenced by four main factors: persuasion from an authority, observation of others, successful performance of the behavior, and physiologic feedback. Social learning theory is a useful model to help in the understanding of why people change; behavioral therapy provides the methods and strategies for effecting and maintaining behavior change. Many excellent and detailed discussions of behavior change programs are available.[3-6]

Other theoretical models have added useful ideas for conceptualizing behavior change. Fishbein and Ajzen[7] emphasize the importance of expectations and attitudes as precursors to behavior. The Health Belief Model also places emphasis on the role of beliefs in determining health care behavior.[8] In this model, the important variables influencing behavior include the patient's readiness to make a change, the perceived benefit of the change, cues to action, and modifying factors such as knowledge and socioeconomic background. Prochaska and DiClimente[9] have described how behavior change occurs through a series of changes, beginning with precontemplation, leading to contemplation, then actual behavior change and maintenance of that change. Finally, comprehensive models of behavior change, involving systems and even community factors, have been developed that may provide helpful ideas for designing more effective programs.[10,11]

In this chapter, the person helping another person make a health behavior change—a physician, nurse, exercise specialist, fitness instructor, or health educator—is the *instructor*; the person making the changes is the *participant*.

HEALTH BEHAVIOR CHANGE MODEL

Health behavior change can be conceptualized as occurring in stages, arbitrarily divided into the antecedent, adoption, and maintenance phases (Figure 35–1). Antecedents refer to all existing conditions that can help initiate, hinder, or support change. Observing the benefits that a friend receives from exercising may serve as an antecedent or stimulus for motivating a person to begin an exercise program. Adoption refers to the early phases at the start of a behavior change program. Maintenance applies to later phases when the participant is already undergoing behavior change.

Antecedents

People sometimes decide to change for reasons that even they do not understand or that are beyond their control. A chance encounter with a friend who has made important changes and looks better for it; an illness; a caustic remark from a coworker; and clothes, once loose, that become tight-fitting, are all events that may push a per-

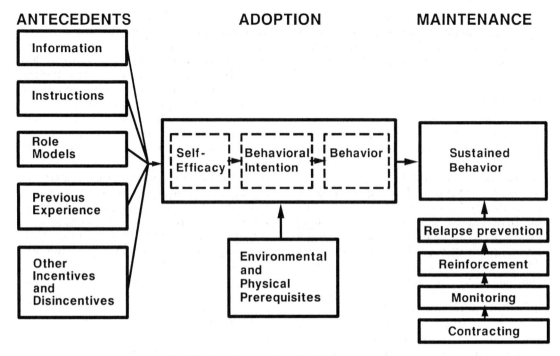

Fig. 35–1. Stages of health behavior change.

son to adopt a health behavior change. Such chance occurrences, life experiences, and opportunities are often critical factors in instigating change. Nevertheless, social learning theory predicts that certain antecedents to behavior change can be identified that are useful in increasing a person's intention to change. We prefer to use the phrase "intention to change" rather than motivation, the customary term describing a person's willingness to change, because motivation implies dichotomy (the individual will or will not change), whereas intention implies a continuous psychologic state. If you ask a person to rate his or her intention on a scale from 0 to 10 in which 0 indicates no intention to change and 10 indicates certainty, people with little intention are not likely to change, whereas those with higher "scores" of intentions are more likely to change. For example, in a study evaluating an intervention to help postmyocardial infarction patients stop smoking, the participants were asked about their intentions to quit smoking while in the hospital. At 12-month follow-up, 33% of those who said that they had little or no intention to quit, and 76% of those who had definitely said they would quit had done so.[12]

Intentions frequently change and can be influenced by the factors listed in Figure 35–1.

Information

Intention to change often begins with information. Information should be presented in simple and clear ways, with the use of language or writing that is understandable to the audience. Keep in mind that 30 to 40% of the American public reads at a 7th grade level or lower. Information is most effective when combined with instructions on how to make the changes. Although pamphlets, self-help books, and handouts are often used to communicate health information, most people read only 10 to 15% of such material, unless they are extremely interested in the topic or are held accountable for it. Some audiences that would seem to benefit most from information tend to ignore it: for instance, smokers tend to ignore messages describing the risks of smoking, nonexercisers know less about the benefits of physical activity than exercisers, and less educated groups may not read lengthy or complicated materials. Any knowledge critical for behavior change should be tested by the instructor at the beginning of the program so that the client's myths or misperceptions can be corrected early on.

Instructions

Persuasion from a person of authority, e.g., instructions to change a particular behavior, is a powerful source of behavior change. Health care professionals are considered the most credible source of information by the public. Persuasion from an authoritative figure should occur in a kind but firm manner. People reluctant to make health behavior changes listen for ambivalence in a health professional's message. They are not, for example, likely to follow this message: "Smoking is bad for your health; you should think about stopping." They are more likely to be affected by: "You must stop smoking." Instructions should be clear, achievable, and accompanied by the necessary information about how to bring about changes. In addition, they should be reinforced by reminders and feedback. Participants should be asked to repeat the critical information.

Models

Role models, whether family, friends, or other credible sources (e.g., health professionals), can facilitate change by allowing the participant to see how other individuals make changes, react to those changes, generalize those changes to different types of situations (e.g., how people practice food changes at home, in restaurants, and in grocery stores), and cope with difficult situations to maintain their healthy habits. People undergoing health behavior change can benefit from being asked by their instructors to think of persons whom they know or admire who have made changes like the ones they want to make. Videotapes or films demonstrating how individuals have made changes and the effect of these changes can be effective in increasing intention to change.

Previous Experience

Previous experience is a major factor in determining whether we begin a new health behavior. We are more likely to take an aspirin for a headache, for instance, if it was helpful in the past. Previous experience also leads to many superstitious health traps. If we happen to take an extra vitamin C tablet at a time when a cold seemed to resolve more rapidly than usual, we are likely to take an extra dose of vitamin C the next time we get a cold, whether or not it is really helpful. The level of our confidence to try a new behavior is largely determined by our previous experience. In helping a person change a health care behavior, have him or her review previous success or failure with it. If he or she started exercise, for instance, but then quit, an important step is to determine why he or she quit last time and what can be done differently if the same problem occurs. As another example, participants might fail to adopt a new diet because they feel unable to prepare the meals they are expected to prepare. People often need to develop new skills to be and feel more effective before change can occur. Developing new skills leads to increased confidence and increased intention to change.

Other Incentives and Disincentives

Other incentives and disincentives are also important antecedents for health behavior change. Incentives should be built into the program and should outweigh the disincentives. Clients should be encouraged to answer the question, "How can I make sure that I benefit from this program?" Some of the benefits may be obvious, e.g., exercising to feel and look better; other benefits may not be as obvious, e.g., exercising to prevent disease. Reducing the disincentives anticipated with beginning a health program are equally important. Many people begin exercising at an inconvenient time, in a place that does not appeal to them, and with an activity they do not enjoy. Such disincentives almost ensure that the program will be short-lived. Careful attention to these antecedents can influence a person's intention to adopt behavior change. With sufficient information, compelling instructions, appropriate models for change, positive physiologic feedback, increased confidence to change, and maximized incentives and minimized disincentives, a person is more likely to adopt a health behavior change. An examination of the antecedents for change answers the questions: What does the participant need to know about the reasons for and methods of bringing about the desired change? What instructions has the participant been given from significant people in his or her life about the importance of making these changes? What are existing and potential models for change? What has been the participant's success with making this and comparable changes in the past? How confident does the participant feel that he or she can make the changes this time? What can be done to increase the participant's confidence? What are the potential incentives and disincentives for change?

Adoption

When to intervene or to encourage a person to adopt a new behavior is more art than science, and is facilitated by carefully listening to participants' needs and interests. Continued, gentle reminders are often useful, even for a chronic smoker who has refused to quit many times in the past. Simply asking a person if he or she is ready to try a new behavior (e.g., increase level of exercise, alter diet) may be sufficient to instigate the process of behavior change. Crises—medical or personal—also present an incentive, and often an opportunity, for change. On the other side, at times the instructor needs to back off and not push a person beyond his or her willingness to change. Questions like, "Are you ready to try (some behavior change)?" or "Do you want to consider (some behavior change)?" may help the instructor decide to encourage further change.

Goal-setting is an important part of the adoption phase. Some programs ask participants to list their goals and to identify the areas where they may need or want extra help. Numerous studies have demonstrated that the more flexible, individually tailored, and achievable the goals are, the better the ensuing adherence. Goals should be specific rather than global, and short-term, although linked to longer-term goals. A useful way to determine if a goal is likely to be achieved is to ask a person how confi-

dent he or she is (on a scale anchored from 0 = no confidence to 100% = entirely certain) of being able to attain the goal within the given time frame. Participants who report that they are 70% or more confident that they can achieve a goal are likely to be able to do so. Again, in setting goals, it is important to ensure that the participant's needs, goals, and preferences are included in setting the goals.

Once a person intends to make a behavior change and has high confidence that he or she will be able to succeed with the change, the adoption of the health change is often precipitated by "cues to action." For instance, many people begin a health care program on the basis of their symptoms or how they are feeling. Such physiologic and emotional feedback both cues people to change and is critical in influencing whether a program is sustained. Smoking relapse often occurs in the first few days after quitting because tobacco withdrawal symptoms may overwhelm intentions to stop. Poorly conditioned people may stop exercising in the first days of a new exercise program because of unpleasant feelings of being out of breath.

Certain environmental and physical prerequisites are often necessary for health behavior change and should be discussed with participants. Such prerequisites for exercising include such things as clothing, equipment, access to facilities, necessary written materials, and a release from a physician if appropriate.

The early stages of change are often the most difficult. Replacing one activity, even a self-destructive one, with another involves many subtle and important shifts in people's lives. Cigarette smokers often say they feel as though they have lost a good friend when they stop. The instructor should be particularly available and supportive at such times.

Maintenance

Once a behavior is adopted, different factors determine whether it is maintained. Behaviors generally are maintained if they are satisfying (reinforcing) or if not doing them causes more discomfort than doing them. Four strategies have proven useful in enhancing maintenance: (1) the activity is monitored and feedback of change occurs (monitoring); (2) the activity is made as satisfying as possible (reinforcement); (3) relapse or interruptions are anticipated (see Relapse Prevention); and (4) commitment is formalized (see Contracts).

Monitoring

Self-report, diary, physiologic, or other types of monitoring are useful to sustain behavior change and to help instructors determine the progress made by their participants. Monitoring forms can be used by instructors for review and problem solving. In addition, monitoring through the use of self-report forms and diaries provides the participant with important feedback that may increase the likelihood that the behavior is maintained.

Many monitoring forms have been developed. In general, they should be simple and convenient to use. Chapter 38 provides an example of a simple exercise monitoring form.

Reinforcement

Positive reinforcement is a powerful factor in sustaining behavior change. Many environmental stimuli are natural reinforcers, for example, food, water, sexual activity, and warmth. Other activities are social or symbolic reinforcers, such as attention, praise, money, and diamonds. When considering reinforcers, it is necessary to bear in mind that reinforcers are idiosyncratic; that is, what is reinforcing to one person may not be reinforcing to another person. An obvious example would be attempting to reinforce jogging behavior with cigarettes in a nonsmoker. Several excellent references are available concerning how to use reinforcement for health behavior change.[13-14]

Relapse Prevention

Various techniques are used to help participants avoid slips (lapses) that may lead to relapse or to prepare for interruptions or other events that may cause discontinuation of a program. The relapse prevention model is derived from studies of alcoholics and smokers trying to quit. Marlatt and colleagues[15] observed that even one cigarette may lead to total relapse, and that preparation for the situations in which the cigarette urges are strongest (e.g., while drinking or experiencing stress) could help to prevent this relapse. The model can be applied to other behaviors, such as exercise. For instance, to help exercisers continue with their program, the Stanford Cardiac Rehabilitation Program staff encourages people to monitor their exercise; to identify clear relapse danger signals, such as an actual or anticipated reduction in exercise frequency; and to develop strategies to deal with these potential relapses.[12] When beginning an exercise program, participants are encouraged to write down what they will do when illness, injury, or changes in work schedule interrupt their exercise program. They might ask a jogging partner for a telephone call to remind them to exercise as soon as they return from a vacation, leave a money "deposit" with a friend that is refundable when they have started exercise again after an illness, or ask the instructor to call them periodically to determine if they are exercising.

Contracts

Written contracts are also extremely useful to maintain change and to help people continue with a program. Instructors should not have participants write contracts that are unrealistic or unlikely to be achieved.

Behavior change is dynamic, and goals need to be updated and revised. If the goal has not been achieved, it may be important to undertake some "problem solving" with the participant. With problem solving, the participant identifies a list of possible solutions to help him or her achieve the goal, develops a plan for implementing these solutions, tries them out, evaluates the results, and repeats the process if the initial solutions have not been successful.

Developing a Program

A program consists of the antecedent, adoption, and maintenance phases of behavioral change, how the interventions associated with this phase are sequenced and integrated, and the interaction between the instructor and the client. An example of the components integrated into the Stanford exercise studies of moderate exercise is detailed in Table 35–1.[16]

Table 35–1.　Elements of Exercise Program Design

Antecedents and Adoption
　Written description of benefits of exercise
　Assessment of expectations; review of expectations to make them realistic
　Assessment of confidence; skills training to enhance confidence
　Videotape instruction on how to warm up and keep heart rate within guidelines
　Physical examination, treadmill, weight, and skinfold assessment
　Experimentation to identify most enjoyable locations
Maintenance
　Monitoring
　　Weekly diaries of exercise duration and intensity
　　Heart rate monitor with auditory feedback
　Reinforcement
　　Social: Biweekly phone calls from staff; group meetings
　　Monetary: None built into program
　　Physical: Three- and six-month treadmill test and weight assessment
　　Symbolic: T-shirts
　　Accomplishment: Monitoring of confidence, psychologic variables
　Contracts
　　None built into program
　Relapse prevention
　　Participant develops own plans for coping with interruptions of exercise

Organization

Implementing a behavior change program requires time. Programs need to ensure that such time is available for both the instructor and the participants. Some programs include a session before exercise devoted to aspects of education and behavior change. This time can be spent in presenting new information, reviewing how people have done with the goals they have set, sharing solutions for problems, etc. It is also important that programs include time for the instructors to formally review with peers and administrators the behavioral aspects of the program. Such sessions can be spent evaluating educational material, reviewing progress of clients, problem-solving, and designing new aspects of the intervention.

The components listed in Table 35–1 can be readily organized into a step-by-step approach. The first step is to ask the participant to consider making a change. Often people intend to adopt a behavior, but sometimes an important step is to recommend additional changes, for instance, to advise and help an exerciser to stop smoking. Suggesting such changes can be difficult, but few people resent a thoughtful attempt to help them improve their health. The second step, and perhaps most important part of asking a participant to consider making a change, is to provide information, instructions, and models; to review past experiences; to build confidence to change; and reduce disincentives and increase incentives to change. The third step is to request a commitment that is specific in time and place as to when the new behavior will occur. The fourth step is to develop with the participant a way to monitor progress with the new behavior and to determine when and how their progress will be reviewed. Early in the adoption phase, the participant should be trained in relapse prevention, if possible. Problem-solving should be used as necessary to help overcome difficulties. Such problem-solving can occur with the group as a whole, at either the beginning or the end of an exercise session, or by telephone or in a face-to-face counseling session.

Instructor Qualities

Different instructors achieve different outcomes, even when the same program is used. Instructors seem to be more effective if participants feel that the instructor is competent and likes, understands, and is interested in them. This relationship translates into a bond between the instructor and the participant that makes the program effective. Role-playing of typical participant situations with peers and receiving feedback is a particularly good way for instructors to develop interpersonal skills.

Overpersistence with a participant unwilling to change is a problem for some instructors. Instructors who take too much responsibility for the action of another person are particularly likely to be overpersistent. Unfortunately, overpersistent instructors often begin to resent the participant's inaction, feel chronic frustration, or devote too much time to that person. To avoid these problems of overpersistence, instructors must have or develop guidelines as to when a program or request for change is discontinued. In one YMCA program, participants meet with the nurse-coordinator to review reasons for their noncompliance, to solve problems, and to set measurable compliance goals. A second meeting is scheduled if the client continues to be noncompliant. If the client fails after the second meeting, a termination meeting is scheduled to drop the participant from the program. During the termination meeting, the nurse-coordinator explains that this program is not appropriate for that person, and that in light of the dangers of noncompliance both to the participant and to persons who might be influenced by noncompliance (e.g., overexerting), the participant should not continue in the program.

Social learning theory is the basis for a model for understanding behavior change; behavior therapy helps to develop many effective change procedures. Information, instructions, models, increasing a person's confidence in performing the exercise program, and maximizing incentives and minimizing disincentives can increase intentions to change and lead to actual adoption of exercise. Once it is adopted, maintenance can be improved by monitoring and feedback, reinforcement, relapse prevention, and the use of contracts.

REFERENCES

1. Bandura A: Self-efficacy: Toward a unifying theory of behavioral change. *Psychol Rev, 84:*191, 1977.
2. Bandura A: *Social Learning Theory.* Englewood Cliffs, NJ: Prentice-Hall, 1977.
3. Agras WS, Kazdin AE, Wilson CT: Behavior therapy: *Toward an Applied Clinical Science.* San Francisco: WH Freeman, 1979.
4. Melamed BC, Siegel LJ: *Behavioral Medicine: Practical Applications in Health Care.* New York: Springer, 1980.
5. Watson DL, Tharp RC: *Self-directed Behavior Change.* Monterey: Brooks/Cole, 1981.
6. Blumenthal JA, McKee DC: *Applications in Behavioral Medicine and Health Psychology: A Clinician's Source Book.* Sarasota, Florida: Professional Resource Exchange, 1987.
7. Fishbein M, Ajzen I: *Belief, Attitudes, Intention and Behavior.* Reading, MA: Addison-Wesley, 1975.
8. Becker MH, Maiman LA: Sociobehavioral determinants of compliance with health and medical care recommendations. *Medical Care, 13:*10, 1975.
9. Prochaska JO, DiClimente CC: Stage process of self-change of smoking: Toward an integrative model of change. *J Consult Clin Psychol, 51:*390, 1983.
10. Winett RA, King AC, Altman D: *Psychology and Public Health: An Integrative Approach.* New York: Pergamon, 1989.
11. Green LW, Kreuter MW: *Health Promotion and Planning: An Education and Environmental Approach.* Mayfield: Mountain View, 1991.
12. Taylor CB, Houston-Miller N, Killen JD, DeBusk RF: Smoking cessation after acute myocardial infarction: Effects of a nurse-managed intervention. *Ann Intern Med 113:* 118, 1990.
13. Goldfried M, Davison CC: *Clinical Behavior Therapy.* New York: Holt, Rinehart and Winston, 1976.
14. Cautela JR, Kastenbaum RA: Reinforcement survey schedule for use in therapy, training, and research. *Psychol Rep, 29:*115, 1967.
15. Marlatt GA, Gordon JR (eds): *Relapse Prevention: Maintenance Strategies in the Treatment of Addiction.* New York: Guilford Press, 1985.
16. Gossard D, et al.: Effects of low and high intensity home exercise training on functional capacity in healthy middle-aged men. *Am J Cardiol, 57:*446, 1986.

Chapter 36

BASIC PSYCHOLOGIC PRINCIPLES RELATED TO GROUP EXERCISE PROGRAMS

C. Barr Taylor and Nancy Houston Miller

When conducting exercise programs, personnel encounter a variety of psychologic issues and problems. Therefore, these professionals should be familiar with basic psychologic principles and ideas to manage their clients and groups most effectively. The following discussion is a brief overview of some of the psychologic principles that affect exercise participants. The topic areas reflect those areas of concern frequently encountered by exercise instructors, and address the learning objectives in *ACSM's Guidelines for Exercise Testing and Prescription (4th Ed.)*.

CRISIS MANAGEMENT/FAILURE TO COPE

A crisis is a period of life, usually brief, when demands from an event exceed the ability and resources to cope, leading to distress.[1] People in crisis feel hopeless and extremely anxious and tense. Other common feelings are fear, anger, guilt, embarrassment, and shame. The high level of anxiety often impedes thinking and impairs coping.

The most common crises are situational: premature delivery, status and role change, rape, physical illness, physical abuse, divorce, or loss of a loved one. Maturation, however, may also precipitate crises as a new stage in life requires new coping responses. People in crises should not be considered mentally ill, yet their distress should be taken seriously. Crisis management follows four broad steps:

1. *Psychosocial assessment of the individual in crisis.* Always determine if individual is capable of suicide or assault to other persons.
2. *Development of a plan.* Usually involves referral to an expert in crisis management.
3. *Implementation of the plan.* Involves drawing on the person's personal, social, and material resources.
4. *Follow-up.* Continued support and reinforcement of patient's actions (when appropriate) are important.

The exercise instructor is involved with the first two steps, and needs to continue to ascertain the status of the participants during the final two steps.

Psychosocial Assessment

The purpose of assessment is to determine the origin of the problem, the risk of suicide or assault, and if the participant is able to take care of himself or herself. The key risk factors for suicidality can be seen in Table 36–1.[2] Prediction of suicide is difficult, but the possibility should be entertained when the participant exhibits any of the features listed in Table 36–1. If the instructor in any way suspects that a participant is depressed or upset, or for other reasons is suicidal, the instructor needs to ask the participant if he or she is suicidal. Participants with physical illness who feel helpless and hopeless are at particularly high risk of suicide. Any suggestion that suicide is a possibility should be followed up to determine the seriousness of the intent. A common belief is that asking about suicide may plant the idea; the opposite is true. An open discussion about suicidal feeling is helpful in and of itself and can set the stage for referral. Participants who are suicidal or dangerous and unable to take care of themselves should be referred for immediate professional help. Suicide crisis centers and community mental health centers exist in all large communities and have capable staff members who can provide advice and recommendations as to how and where to refer a person. Participants can also be taken to hospital emergency rooms. Make

Table 36–1.   Risk Factors For Suicide

1. Previous suicide attempt
2. Overt or indirect suicide talk or threats
3. Depressed mood
4. Significant recent loss, e.g., spouse, job
5. Unexpected change in behavior or attitude
6. Being elderly, male, isolated with chronic illness
7. Sense of hopelessness, helplessness, loneliness, exhaustion, "unbearable" psychologic pain
8. Alcohol or drug abuse or intoxication
9. Failing health, particularly if previously independent

sure that the participant has an immediate place to go and a way to get there. Suicidal participants should not take themselves for help. They should be accompanied by police, mental health staff, family, or friends to the place of referral.

Most crises, however, do not lead to or are accompanied by emergency situations. Further assessment includes answering questions like these: To what extent has the crisis disrupted normal life patterns? Is the individual able to hold a job? Can the person handle the responsibility of daily living? Has the crisis disrupted the lives of others? Has the crisis distorted the individual's perception of reality? Is the usual support system present, absent, or exhausted? What are the available resources?

The exercise instructor may occasionally encounter a potentially violent patient or client. Anyone can become violent, but certain groups are at particular risk, e.g., young males; urban, violent cultural subgroups; alcohol or drug users or abusers. Individual predictors include: a past history of violence, active use of alcohol, physical abuse as a child, or some form of brain injury. All threats of violence must be taken seriously. The exercise instructor must be willing to seek help from police as necessary for his or her protection and the protection of other participants.

Management Plan

Development and implementation of a crisis management plan is not appropriate for most exercise instructors; however, follow-up contact is appropriate. People in crisis appreciate the concern of other persons and often can benefit substantially from such concern.

COMMUNICATION SKILLS

Certain basic interviewing skills are useful for obtaining information and for establishing a positive relationship with an individual.[3,4] In acquiring information from patients and in problem solving and making recommendations for change, the use of facilitative or neutral communication skills is important, i.e., skills that encourage the participant to speak openly and to avoid disruptive communication behaviors. Definitions of some facilitative communication behaviors are provided in Table 36–2.

Confronting the individual is sometimes necessary. Confrontation involves directing attention to something that the client may not be aware of or is reluctant to admit. Confrontation should address only observable facts and not make inferences about the patient's motives or specific emotional state. For example, a postmyocardial infarction participant who is intoxicated at the time of an exercise session and is disruptive may need to be confronted about the behavior. An example of an overly aggressive confrontation follows:

> *Exercise instructor:* You have been drinking. You had better not drink before you come here.

Table 36–2.   Facilitative Communication Behaviors

Noncommittal Acknowledgment (Verbal and Nonverbal)
  Brief expressions that communicate understanding, acceptance, and empathy, such as: "Oh," "I see," "Mm-hmmm," head nodding, focused posture
Door Openers
  Invitations to expand or continue the expressions of thoughts and feelings (without specifying the content), such as "Could I hear more?" "Please go on," "I don't quite understand," "Please pursue that," and (use some of the last words the patient said)
Content Paraphrase
  Rephrase the factual portion of the message and send it back to check your accuracy in understanding.

A more appropriate confrontation might be:

> *Exercise instructor:* You seem to be acting funny today. Have you been drinking?
> *Participant:* Nah.
> *Exercise instructor:* I can smell alcohol on your breath. When did you last have something to drink?
> *Participant:* Oh, a couple of beers about an hour ago.
> *Exercise instructor:* I can't allow people to exercise here if they have been drinking. Will you make sure you have not been drinking before you come next time?

Most of us are uncomfortable with direct confrontation, but it is often necessary as well as useful.

PSYCHOPATHOLOGY

The Diagnostic and Statistical Manual of the American Psychiatric Association—Revised lists over 100 diagnostic categories.[5] Only the few general problems the exercise leader is likely to encounter, however, are discussed in this section.

Depression

Depression affects 5 to 10% of adults at one time or another.[5,6] In addition to feeling "down", depression is often accompanied by somatic symptoms (Table 36–3).

Table 36–3.   Symptoms of Depression

Emotional features
   Depressed mood, feeling blue
   Irritability, anxiety
   Loss of interest
   Withdrawal from others
   Preoccupation with death
Cognitive features
   Feeling worthless or guilty
   Hopeless, in despair
   Poor concentration
   Indecisive
   Suicidal feelings
Vegetative features
   Fatigue, lack of energy
   Trouble sleeping
   Loss of appetite
   Weight loss or gain
   Lack of interest in sex
   Depressed look

Depressed patients may exhibit psychomotor retardation, easy crying, and a sad face. Depressed patients often feel helpless and hopeless and exhibit self-reproach. Most importantly, from an assessment standpoint, depression is frequently accompanied by suicidal feelings. Suicidal feelings in depressed patients should be assessed directly, and such patients should be referred for care, following the aforementioned guidelines for emergency crises.

Hospitalization for psychiatric care is sometimes necessary, but more often depressed patients recover with outpatient professional help, medication, and the passage of time. The symptomatology of depression makes exercising difficult, but exercise appears to be beneficial in removing many of the symptoms of depression.[7]

Patients hospitalized for myocardial infarctions often feel depressed, a feeling that usually resolves after they return home. Moderate or worse depression, which persists 2 to 3 weeks after return home and resumption of usual activities, requires further evaluation. Such patients should be considered for referral to local mental health professionals, or their primary care physician, for further assessment and treatment.

Anxiety Disorders

Anxiety affects everyone at one time or another. Severe anxiety, however, can lead to avoidance and restriction of life's activities, and can be associated with severe depression and terrifying panic attacks. Acute anxiety can often be resolved with reassurance or brief periods of psychotherapy.

Chronic anxiety is usually secondary to depression, but may represent a primary anxiety disorder. The three most prevalent primary anxiety disorders are generalized anxiety disorder and panic disorder with and without agoraphobia. Generalized anxiety disorder is characterized by excessive worry and signs of motor tension (e.g., trembling, muscle tension, restlessness), autonomic hyperactivity (e.g., sweating, dry mouth, and frequent urination), vigilance, and scanning (e.g., feeling keyed up or on edge all the time). Panic disorder is characterized by recurrent panic attacks, which are discrete periods of apprehension or fear accompanied by such symptoms as dyspnea, palpitations, choking, chest pain or discomfort, sweating, dizziness, and fear of going crazy and/or doing something uncontrolled. The first panic attack occurs usually in the early 20s and comes "out of the blue." Many panic disorder patients develop severe phobic avoidance (agoraphobia). Such patients are not likely to be able to participate in an exercise class or program, but doing so is of great benefit. Chronic anxiety can occur secondary to psychiatric problems besides depression, such as alcoholism, drug abuse, and schizophrenia. It can also be caused by medical problems, most commonly hyperthyroidism, hypoglycemia, and temporal lobe epilepsy.[8]

Some patients with anxiety may report unpleasant symptoms with exercise. Use of a treadmill can help reassure anxious patients that exercise is safe and can help the exercise instructor identify any contraindications to exercise.[9] Furthermore, exercise may help reduce symptoms in patients with severe anxiety disorders.[10]

Alcohol and Drug Abuse

Drug and alcohol abuse are very common. When the instructor suspects alcohol abuse, e.g., the patient smells of alcohol, reports blackout periods, and seems preoccupied with alcohol, the instructor may need to confront the participant about alcohol use. Four questions, referred to as the CAGE Questionnaire for Alcoholism,[10] can be used to screen for alcoholism:

1. Have you ever tried to cut down on your drinking?
2. Are you annoyed when people ask you about your drinking?
3. Do you ever feel guilty about your drinking?
4. Do you ever take a morning "eye-opener"?

A "yes" response to any of these questions increases the suspicion that the participant may have alcoholism. Participants who are suspected of using alcohol before an exercise session should be confronted in the manner discussed above.

Patients who appear to be abusing alcohol may benefit from referral to a treatment program. For information on where to find treatment for alcohol and other drug problems, the best place to look is in the telephone book's Yellow Pages under "Alcoholism Information" or "Drug Abuse and Addiction Information." Usually there is a listing of the nearest Council on Alcoholism (or Council on Alcohol and Drug Abuse). These Councils provide information over the phone on the availability of the nearest alcohol treatment programs. Alcoholics Anonymous (AA) or Narcotics Anonymous (NA) may also be listed. Both offer immeasurable help in enabling people to cope with problems with alcohol and other drugs. You can also contact the National Clearinghouse for Alcohol and Drug Information (1-800-729-6686) to find the number of local or state alcohol treatment resources.

Bulimia Nervosa

Bulimia nervosa is characterized by recurrent episodes of binge eating (rapid consumption of a large amount of food over a short period of time); feeling a lack of control over eating during the binges; self-induced vomiting, use of laxatives or diuretics; strict dieting or fasting, or vigorous exercise to prevent weight gain; and persistent overconcern with body shape and weight.[5] The food consumed during a binge is usually high in calories, tastes sweet, and is easy to swallow. Binges usually occur secretly, and the food is gobbled down rapidly with little chewing. A binge usually ends because of abdominal discomfort, sleep, social interruption, extreme guilt or induced vomiting. A study of college freshmen indicated that 4.5% of the women and 0.4% of the men had a history of bulimia. It is more common among exercisers than nonexercisers. Bulimic patients often feel very guilty about their vomiting or laxative and/or diuretic abuse and are likely to suffer from some depression. Frequent vomiting can lead to dental erosion. Electrolyte imbalance and dehydration can occur, and can lead to serious physical complications. Cognitive/behavioral psychologic interventions have proven effective in helping bulimic patients reduce their symptoms, and such patients should be encouraged to seek treatment.[11,12] Many mental health professionals specialize in treating eating disorders. The National As-

Table 36–4. Clinical Picture of Anorexia Nervosa

Loss of more than 25% premorbid body weight
Distorted body image
Fears of weight gain or of loss of eating control
Adolescent and young adult women primarily affected
Perfectionist behavior
Refusal to maintain normal body weight
No known physical illness to account for weight loss

sociation of Anorexia Nervosa and Associated Disorders (708-831-3438) can be contacted to identify referral sources in your area.

Anorexia Nervosa

Anorexia nervosa is a rare, potentially life-threatening eating disorder; the clinical picture of this condition is listed in Table 36–4.[12,13] Most anorectic patients exercise to excess. If anorexia is suspected, a weight and dietary history should be obtained, and if possible the percentage of body fat should be measured.

Anorectic patients are best helped by professionals specializing in eating disorders, but the exercise specialist can play an important role in their care by confronting the patient as to the seriousness of the disorder and by insisting that the patient seek help. Once the patient has begun therapy, the exercise instructor can help the patient design a normal eating and activity pattern emphasizing health and proper nutrition, not weight, and in general providing psychological support.

GROUP DYNAMICS

Because many exercise programs are conducted in groups, an understanding not only of how to handle individual problems but also of the effects of certain behaviors on the group is important. Several good references are available concerning group dynamics.[14]

Within any group are chronic complainers, comedians, disruptive individuals, noncompliers, and participants who overexert themselves. If not addressed early in the program, such individuals can dominate group time and make extraordinary demands on staff members.

When dealing with behaviors that may cause significant reactions by both the staff and the group, important points to assess are: (1) how you are feeling about the patient; (2) what the patient is doing or saying; and (3) what the dynamics of the interaction itself are, especially in terms of how to manage the situation from the start to avoid problems that ultimately influence the entire group.

Chronic Complainers

Typical initial reactions of the chronic complainer are feelings of avoidance, impatience, and anger. Anger is especially common if the patient continually criticizes people or things that you admire. In managing such an individual, first determine whether the patient is simply looking for a sympathetic ear and is really not complaining, or whether this problem is constant. Accordingly, appropriate steps to follow are:

1. Listen attentively
2. Acknowledge what the patient has said and how the patient must feel about the situation
3. Do not agree with the patient; this implies acceptance
4. Set limits regarding staff time
5. Agree upon how the situation should be stopped

Disrupters/Comedians

Disrupters and comedians have many of the same characteristics and may be handled somewhat the same in a group setting. The disrupter may cause feelings of impatience, frustration, and anger, whereas initial reactions to the comedian may be mild. If, however, the comedian's humor becomes disruptive, your reaction may be the same as that to the disrupter. In addition, the comedian's senseless humor may lead to avoidance of this person because of a lack of wanting to listen to this type of behavior. The disrupter and the comedian often feel insecure or unappreciated, or need attention. Although staff members may need to spend more time with these individuals to ascertain their needs, the added time may help to resolve the problems. If continued disruptive behavior occurs, however, limits must be set, with goals for changing the behavior. If the disruptive behavior persists, dropping the patient from the group warrants consideration to avoid unpleasant reactions that may develop from other group members.

Noncompliers

The noncompliant participant in a group exercise program is at risk when exercising haphazardly, and detracts from the sense of cohesion necessary to ensure positive group dynamics. The leader of a group exercise session should keep in mind the following points when handling noncompliance:

1. Assess the intention of the patient's behavior
2. Determine the barriers to attendance
3. Provide positive reinforcement
4. Seek solutions to the lack of attendance
5. Set incremental, realistic goals
6. Choose methods to enhance compliance, such as contracting, self-rewards, and telephone prompts
7. Monitor change in behavior
8. Consider dropping the participant from the program if person is unwilling to cooperate

Overexerters

Instructors often find a participant in an exercise program who is unwilling to listen to instructions about target heart rates and the necessity for maintaining them. This person tends to exhibit characteristics of the type A personality (competitive attitude, underlying hostility, and time urgency). The overexerciser foolishly undertakes bursts of exercise at high heart rates, and may disrupt the class with behavior similar to that of the disrupter. Because maintenance of heart rate is critical to the safety of any program, this person must be addressed immediately upon ascertaining the negative behavior. By using the following steps, the instructor can counteract the behavior and ensure increased safety for the participant.

1. Identify for the participant the type of behavior exhibited and the effects regarding safety (participant is often unaware and has not listened)
2. Reinforce for the participant the fact that this type of behavior is unacceptable
3. Set limits regarding the consequences of continued negative behavior
4. Positively reinforce the participant when he or she is exercising appropriately
5. Consider dropping the participant if unwillingness to comply with instructions persists

This brief overview of some psychologic issues relevant to exercise programs is only a starting point. Exercise instructors should identify mental health professionals in their communities with whom they can consult as well as to whom they can refer clients in need of care.

REFERENCES

1. Hoff LA: *People in Crisis.* 2nd Ed. Menlo Park: Addison-Wesley, 1984.
2. Tomb DA: *Psychiatry for the House Officer,* 3rd Ed. Baltimore: Williams & Wilkins, 1988.
3. Enelow AF, Swisher SN: *Interviewing and Patient Care.* New York: Oxford, 1979.
4. Froelich RE, Bishop EM: *Medical Interviewing: A Programmed Text.* St. Louis: CV Mosby, 1969.
5. American Psychiatric Association: *Diagnostic and Statistical Manual of Mental Disorders* (Third Edition, Revised). Washington, DC: American Psychiatry Association, 1987.
6. Rush AF, Altshuler EZ (eds): *Depression: Basic Mechanisms, Biology and Treatments.* New York: Guilford, 1986.
7. Taylor CB, Sallis JF, Needle R: The relation of physical activity and exercise to mental health. *Public Health Rep, 100:*195, 1985.
8. Taylor CB, Arnow B: *The Nature and Treatment of Anxiety Disorders.* New York: The Free Press, 1988.
9. Taylor CB, et al.: Treadmill exercise test and ambulatory measures in patients with panic attacks. *Am J Cardiol, 60,*48J, 1987.
10. Ewing JA: Detecting alcoholism: The CAGE Questionnaire. *JAMA, 252:*1905, 1984.

11. Agras WS: *Eating Disorders: Management of Obesity, Bulimia, and Anorexia Nervosa.* New York: Pergamon, 1987.

12. Garfinkel PE, Garner DM: *Anorexia Nervosa: A Multidimensional Perspective.* New York: Brunner/Mazel, 1982.

13. Harris RT: Bulimarexia and related serious eating disorders with medical complications. *Ann Intern Med, 99:*800, 1983.

14. Yalom ID: *The Theory and Practice of Group Psychotherapy.* 3rd Ed. New York: Basic Books, 1985.

Chapter 37

EXERCISE ADHERENCE AND MAINTENANCE

Abby C. King and John E. Martin

EXTENT OF THE PROBLEM

Over the past few decades, we have witnessed an explosion of interest by the American public and health professionals alike in physical activity as a means for achieving a variety of goals in areas related to health, functioning, and quality of life. Despite this increased interest, as well as the belief by most adults that they would benefit personally from additional physical activity, available evidence indicates that two thirds or more of American do not exercise regularly (i.e., weekly) and 25% or more do not exercise at all. Population segments that are notably under-represented among the ranks of those engaging in regular exercise include older individuals (particularly women); the less educated; smokers, and overweight individuals. For the 10% or less of sedentary adults likely to begin a regular exercise program within a year, and those already participating in group or individual exercise, approximately one half can be expected to drop out within 3 to 6 months. For individuals enrolled in secondary prevention programs, a 50% dropout by 12 months is typical.

Such statistics indicate that helping many individuals to stay regularly involved in a physical activity program is a challenge requiring creativity and patience on the part of the health professional. In addition, finding ways to encourage the extremely sedentary to adopt a more active lifestyle represents an increasingly important public health goal. Health professionals can be helped in their efforts by taking advantage of the current public enthusiasm for becoming more active as well as the growing wealth of findings suggesting the types of strategies that can be effective in enhancing physical activity participation.

REASONS FOR THE ADHERENCE PROBLEM

A belief that has grown in popularity is that, in at least some ways, physical activity may be a unique health behavior, governed by factors that differ somewhat from other health behaviors.[1-3] Certainly the demand for regularity in performing physical activity to continue to reap health benefits throughout life calls for innovative methods of studying the *process* of making regular exercise a habit. A related observation receiving increasing attention is that the factors influencing initial adoption and early participation in exercise may differ from those affecting subsequent maintenance. Such observations call for the application of *stages of change* models to better identify strategies that will work best for individuals at different stages and levels of exercise participation, e.g., persons contemplating joining an exercise program, those in the early stage of exercise adoption, and those committed to maintaining their program across the long-term. Although our understanding of the factors influencing this process generally remains in its infancy,[4] a number of potentially important variables have been identified that have received a growing amount of scientific support. These factors are discussed subsequently.

Current Knowledge

Although no one theory allows investigators to explain fully why individuals become or stay active, researchers have been aided in their efforts to understand such health behaviors by placing them in the context of a *social learning/social cognitive model* of health behavior change. This social cognitive approach, broadly defined, views

443

such behaviors as being initiated and maintained through a complex interaction of personal, behavioral, and environmental factors and conditions. Put another way, an individual's past experiences with physical activity, how they view physical activity in general and different forms of activity in particular, the extent of their current activity-related knowledge, skills, and beliefs, and how the surrounding environment either helps or hinders their efforts to increase physical activity levels, all play a role in influencing how active the individual currently is and will remain.

Personal Factors

In addition to *demographic* and *health* factors, such as age, educational attainment, body weight, and smoking status, variables influencing initial participation in regular physical activity include *past experiences* with physical activity; an individual's *perceptions of health status* as well as exercise ability and skills; *self-efficacy* beliefs, defined as the level of confidence in one's ability to successfully perform a specific physical activity regimen; perceptions related to *access to exercise facilities, lack of time, and exercise intensity;* and an understanding of how increased physical activity will *personally benefit* the individual, in both the short term and the long term. In addition, a person's rating of *self-motivation* may be related to continued participation in an exercise regimen. Importantly, when "self-motivation" is defined as the ability to find rewards for behavior independent of external rewards available for that behavior, it is something that conceivably can be *learned* by the individual. This concept is preferable to definitions of motivation that place the blame for nonadherence on internal processes related to "personality" and similar constructs. These latter definitions, aside from being unfair to the individual by ignoring extrapersonal influences on behavior (e.g., the environment), do not provide the health professional with a firm direction for intervention.

Although many of the above-mentioned factors are associated to some extent with *initial participation* in physical activity, relatively few appear to influence substantially how long an individual maintains an exer-

cise regimen. Among those that do are smoking status, body weight, self-efficacy levels, and perceived lack of time.

Behavioral Factors

Behavioral factors include the actual *skills* an individual possesses to carry out physical activity to maximize exercise-related benefits while minimizing injury, boredom, and other impediments to maintenance. Such skills include the knowledge and use of behavioral and psychological strategies that help the individual to negotiate the barriers and pitfalls that inevitably interfere with being active on a regular basis.

An example of a useful behavioral skill involves knowing how to plan ahead by identifying and preparing for periods when disruption to an exercise program is likely (e.g., during holidays). This type of strategy is known as *relapse prevention.*[5] Another potentially effective strategy involves the implementation of a *decision balance-sheet* whereby the individual carefully evaluates and weighs the expected or experienced benefits and costs of participating in an activity program.

Environmental and Program Factors

Environmental and program-based factors can influence initial participation as well as longer-term adherence, including *family influences* and support, with individuals who report their spouses to be neutral or unsupportive of their physical activity more likely to drop out; *proximity and access to facilities,* for persons preferring facility-based activities; *weather; regimen flexibility;* the *convenience* of the activity (either real or perceived); immediate *cues and prompts* in the environment promoting physical activity (e.g., reminders to exercise); and the *immediate consequences* of the activity for the individual.

The type of exercise being offered (e.g., swimming, aerobic dance), as well as the intensity, frequency, and duration of the proposed regimen can influence subsequent participation levels. The format in which the activity is offered (e.g., class; home-based, with or without partners) can also have an important effect on both initial participation rates and longer-term adherence. Although the majority of exercise programs in the U.S. are offered in a class or group format, evidence indicates that the American public generally prefers programs offered outside of a formal group, with important benefits to long-term adherence occurring with adequately structured home-based regimens.[6]

Immediate consequences, including observance of physical activity-related benefits and the enjoyability of the activity itself, are other program-related factors that are likely to have a strong impact on subsequent adherence. Conversely, the sedentary person persists in this unhealthy state principally because it is immediately reinforcing, with attempts to become physically active likely having resulted in immediate aversive consequences. Thus, it is the task of the health professional to ensure that initial attempts to exercise are painless, enjoyable, and highly reinforcing (see later discussion). Although time constraints are typically noted as a major reason for inactivity, regular exercisers complain as much about time-related difficulties as persons who are not regularly active. Thus, perceived available time may reflect in large part the priority the individual places on being physically active rather than actual time limitations per se.

Several points must be made concerning the identification of the factors influencing physical activity adoption and adherence. First, as mentioned previously, the factors that most strongly influence initial adoption are most likely to be different from those that affect how well activity is maintained once it is started.[7] Second, the currently noted variables clearly constitute only part of all the relevant factors in affecting activity levels, many of which have yet to be identified. Because of the complex interrelationships among these variables, many individuals may have difficulty in reporting why they are having trouble starting or maintaining an exercise program unless they actually *monitor* their activities. Third, some factors that have been identified as predictive of inactivity (e.g., smoking status, being overweight) indicate that individuals who can reap the most health benefits from regular physical activity, in terms of reducing health risks, are those who are currently least likely to adopt or

maintain an activity program. Finally, the variety of factors implicated indicates the importance of developing programs and strategies that fit the needs and preferences of different population groups. This matching or *"tailoring"* approach can be contrasted with the more typical method of trying to get individuals to "fit into" ongoing, already existing programs. By tailoring physical activity approaches to fit population or individual needs more closely, health professionals may be able to decrease the dropout rate during the initial "critical period" (i.e., the first 3 to 6 months), when reduced participation or dropping out typically occurs.

CHANGING PHYSICAL ACTIVITY PATTERNS

Increasing Adoption and Early Adherence

Adoption of increased physical activity patterns can be enhanced through paying particular attention to factors in each of the aforementioned personal, behavioral, environmental, and program-related spheres.

Personal and Behavioral Factors

In terms of personal factors, previous experiences with physical activity should be explored, along with any unreasonable beliefs and misconceptions the person may harbor toward exercise (e.g., "no pain, no gain," or that older individuals should not be active, because they need to "conserve their energy"). For example, many would-be exercisers believe that exercise is an inherently painful and aversive process; these individuals not only must be told but also must be shown that this statement is untrue. The utility of more moderate activities of daily living (e.g., brisk walking) is often unknown to many sedentary individuals, and may for many persons be more appealing than more structured, vigorous activity regimens. Behaviorally, many sedentary individuals can benefit from specific instruction (accompanied by actual rehearsal and feedback) on appropriate ways of performing specific activities (e.g., jogging, striding, cycling, and warmup exercises) to obtain health-related benefits while avoiding injury.

In addition to development of activity-related attitudes, knowledge, and skills, a physical activity program should be made *personally relevant* for the individual, in terms of both the type of activity or activities chosen and the goals of the program. For instance, if stress reduction is a motivating factor for an individual, activities that can be helpful in reducing stress (i.e., not overly competitive, noisy, or demanding) should be targeted. Examples of such activities include brisk walking, jogging, or bicycling programs conducted outdoors in pleasant surroundings, which could allow the individual time to "get away from it all."

Additional useful measures include structuring appropriate *expectations* concerning physical activity and what it can and cannot do as early as possible, stressing the varied benefits for the individual of making the change, as well as exploring any perceived *barriers* to increasing physical activity (e.g., unreasonable expectations; fear of embarrassment, failure, or boredom). A simple questionnaire regarding expectations for the individual can provide the health professional with early clues as to where such expectations may lie.

Environmental and Program-Related Factors

Numerous environmental and program-related variables can enhance initial adoption and early adherence to physical activity.

Convenience. Three convenience factors are important to the successful initiation and maintenance of an exercise program. First, researchers have clearly demonstrated that the greater the effort required to prepare for physical activity, such as a long drive to and from an exercise facility, the greater the potential for dropout (up to twice the dropout and one half the initial participation rates for inconvenient facilities). Facilities should be within easy access to the individual. Alternatively, encouraging methods of being physically active in or around the home (the place where many people prefer to exercise) can make convenience less of a potential deterrent to adherence. Care is needed to ensure that the person is encouraged to participate in an exercise program (i.e., joining a spa or health club) that is close to the home or

workplace or located conveniently between these two settings if at all possible.

The second important convenience factor is time. If the program being offered utilizes a class structure, offering several time options can be helpful. For some members of groups with extreme time constraints, such as working mothers, discussing alternatives to a class format is often necessary. Alternatively, some health programs and establishments, as well as worksite settings, now offer child care services.

The third convenience factor concerns the exercise mode itself. If the exercise selected requires special, costly, or time-consuming preparation, such as skiing or possibly swimming, the level of exercise adherence can be expected to be potentially lower. Thus, the selection of the exercise type or mode, the location of facility, and the time of day can be of critical importance in the early stages of acquisition of the exercise habit. Each choice should therefore be evaluated carefully by both the participant and the health professional before embarking on any systematic program.

Behavior Shaping. For sedentary persons, the major objective is to establish a physical activity habit through allowing the individual *success* in accomplishing activity goals while decreasing opportunities for failure. Therefore, the initial activity prescription should be one that, although less rigorous than the health professional might prefer, is easy to do given the person's current preferences, motivation, skills, and present life circumstances. For some individuals, this shaping may translate into an initial increase simply in activities of daily living (e.g., walking more at work and at home; taking stairs). For other persons, the initial prescription may involve structured endurance activities twice a week, with a concomitant increase in routine activities until the person is ready to move on to a more vigorous activity schedule.

The key consideration in all exercise programs and prescriptions should be the *gradual shaping* of successive approximations of the ultimate exercise and/or fitness goal. When this important behavior-shaping principle is violated, such as starting exercisers at too high an intensity, frequency, or duration, adherence is almost always negatively affected. For example, when beginning exercisers are exposed to exercise intensities greater than 85% of aerobic capacity, exercise frequencies equal to or greater than 5 days per week, and/or exercise sessions of more than 45 minutes in duration, the rates of injuries and dropout significantly increase, affecting as many as one half of participants.

Thus, the exercise regimen should be *easy* and *gradually incremented,* ensuring success at each stage. Most importantly, health professionals and beginning exercisers should focus primarily on shaping and maintaining the *exercise habit* for about the first 6 to 12 weeks, rather than on rapid establishment of the optimal regimen for desired benefits. It is important to keep in mind that any benefits of even the most successful physical training program are lost completely unless the exercise habit foundation is solidly established. This approach of first establishing behavioral control of the exercise habit implies that health professionals should encourage early participants to "just show up" (e.g., "No matter how little you may feel like doing or are able to do . . . remember, we are working on reinforcing the habit of exercising; the benefits will definitely come, and stay, if you can master this first 'habit step'").

Several methods might be considered for use to properly shape exercise and avoid overextending persons during the early stages of a program. Exercisers should be encouraged to maintain an intensity level at which they can still comfortably talk without breathing or sweating heavily. This level can be easily monitored by the participant as well as the health professional. Exercising with other participants and talking throughout the session is an excellent method for controlling intensity levels. However, group instructors should be aware that simply telling those having difficulty in keeping up to "take it easy," when the instructor himself or herself and most of the class are working at the higher intensity level, is often an ineffective strategy for helping individuals maintain the lower intensity levels. A more effective strategy is to provide the class with an additional role model who demonstrates the lower-intensity alternative alongside the instructor.

Heart rate is also a good physiologic index of intensity: exercisers can monitor pulse rates during the exercise (this assessment can also be done by using portable heart rate monitors with preset alarms). The Borg Scale, or rating of perceived exertion (RPE), is excellent for tracking the perception of exercise intensity (in many ways just as important as the actual physical work output).[8] In practice, these measures can be used together. For example, in more sedentary and unfit participants, an RPE no higher than 12 and a heart rate of less than 70% of maximum would be recommended for optimal enjoyment and lifetime habit establishment, whether the form of exercise is routine activities such as walking or programmed endurance training. Figure 37–1 provides an example of individual monitoring of heart rate within an "effective comfort zone" of 60 to 75% of maximum, representing an optimal training intensity for both motivation and physical benefit.

Enjoyability. It is critical that the individual in some way enjoy or reap some immediate benefits from an activity if the activity is to be continued. The physical discomfort that often accompanies the early stages of increased activity must in some way be minimized or offset by positive factors if the person is to be kept from dropping out. Ways of enhancing enjoyability include the tailoring of the type(s) of activity, the actual exercise regimen, and the format of the regimen (group or alone; class or home-based) to individual preferences. For instance, does the person prefer a group aerobics class with music, or would a walking/jogging program augmented with a portable stereo cassette player fit better with the person's work schedule and personal preferences? As noted previously, discomfort can be minimized by gradually shaping the regimen from mild (e.g., RPE below 13) to more challenging. Again, the individual can monitor whether the regimen is too demanding by focusing on ease of breathing and talking during the activity. Individuals can also be taught distraction techniques, when relevant, to help them refocus their attention away from what are for some persons aversive aspects of activity (e.g., increased exertion and sweating). One method of assessing enjoy-

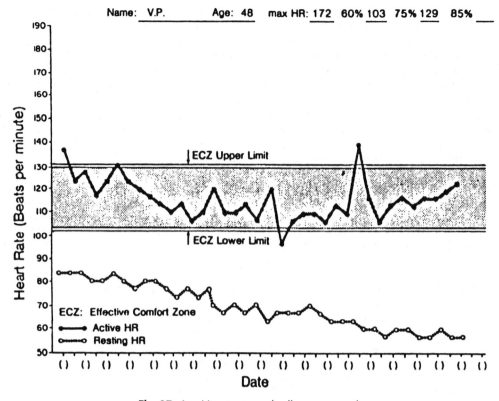

Name: V.P.   Age: 48   max HR: 172 60% 103 75% 129 85% ___

ECZ Upper Limit

ECZ Lower Limit

ECZ: Effective Comfort Zone
●——● Active HR
○——○ Resting HR

Heart Rate (Beats per minute)

Date

Fig. 37–1. Heart rate and adherence graph.

ability of the exercise session is to ask participants to note their levels of enjoyment on self-monitoring records that reflect a range of values from "very unenjoyable" to "very enjoyable" (e.g., 1 to 5 scale). If two or more sessions are in the "unenjoyable" range, the exercise regimen might best be modified or varied, perhaps with more reinforcement provided.

External Rewards and Incentives. As noted previously, the initial steps involved in becoming more physically active are found by many persons to be anything but rewarding. Often it is not until several months into a regular physical activity program that participants begin to report experiencing positive benefits from physical activity on a regular basis. In fact, the longer the period of inactivity and the more unfit the individual (e.g., obese smoker), the longer the period is likely to be before any physical activity becomes intrinsically reinforcing (i.e., feels good). Therefore, beginners need external rewards early in their program to help to encourage and motivate them. For our highly unfit overweight smokers, "beginner" status might extend to 6 months or 1 year, and special external incentive may need to be programmed throughout that time period. For other, more fit persons, this "beginner" phase may need to occur for only a short time.

One extremely valuable form of reward is *social support*. Social support has proven to be a powerful motivator for many people. Social support can be delivered in many forms, including through a class instructor, exercise partners, and family members who encourage increased activity regardless of whether they themselves actually participate, as well as through telephone contacts and letter prompts from a caring health professional. *Praise* is a critical component of social support. To be most effective, this vocal encouragement should be both immediate (during or very shortly after the exercise) and specific. For example: "Your effort level is great . . . you'll be able to keep that pace for some time!"; "Great going, your attendance has been perfect over the past month!" The praise of exercise therapists, family members, and fellow participants should occur consistently and frequently during the early stages of acquisition of the exercise habit. Families of neophyte exercisers might also be encouraged to exercise with them, or at least accompany them whenever possible to enhance this support. When the support from significant others is active and ongoing, exercisers are two to three times more likely than those with little or no family support to persist in their physical activity program. Therapists, family members, and "helpers" alike should be cautioned, however, against even the best-intentioned nagging or employment of other aversive procedures (e.g., inviting guilt for failure to exercise) designed to induce the recalcitrant person to exercise. These counterproductive actions almost inevitably increase the punishing characteristics of the exercise, further upsetting the delicate balance between motivation to exercise and remaining pleasantly inactive.

The use of social support can also be extended and formalized using written *contracts* between the individual and a significant person in the environment. Contracts are written, signed agreements that help to specify the person's activity-related *goals* in a public format (Fig. 37–2). They typically specify short-term, concrete goals and the types of positive consequences that will occur on reaching the goals. The contract should have some flexibility in daily goal-setting, so that the person is not faced with rigid daily goals that are difficult or impossible to meet, thereby providing frequent failure experiences (see following section). Thus, in the earlier stages of the program, an appropriate goal might be related to attendance rather than performance within the session. These contracts often work best if developed in tandem with an interested person or "helper" in the person's environment. Such contracts can help to increase an individual's personal responsibility and commitment to the program. An alternative to the value-exchange contract is the written agreement, through which the participant agrees in writing to perform certain behaviors. Although not as effective as the formal contract, the agreement can be useful for persons who refuse to go so far as to sign a contract.

The use of appropriate and consistent

Two-Week Contract:

Plan to Increase Amount of Brisk Walking

My Responsibilities:
    1. To focus on increasing my brisk walking while at work, especially during my lunch hour.
    2. To reward myself on each day that I reach 2½ miles on my pedometer with thirty minutes (or more) of reading for my own enjoyment.
    3. To record my data in my exercise journal at 10:00 each night.

My Helper's Responsibilities:
    1. To prompt me during work to do my activity.
    2. In return, I will prompt him concerning a behavior of his choice, as desired.

This contract will be evaluated in two weeks, on *(date)*.

Signed:

_____
_____ (helper)
_____ (health provider)

_____
(date)
_____
(date)
_____
(date)

Fig. 37–2. Sample contract.

exercise *models* in the person's environment (i.e., other individuals the person can observe exercising) can also motivate people to begin and continue to exercise. These models should be as similar as possible to the targeted individuals (some programs use successful graduates as future participant-assistants) for maximal effectiveness. Furthermore, whenever possible, the health professional or therapist should set an appropriate example by exercising along with the program participants.

Another type of incentive occurs in the form of *feedback* to the person concerning how he or she is doing on what the person deems as relevant or important dimensions. Such feedback can be delivered by another person or it can be generated by the individual through the use of self-recorded monitoring sheets, an activity diary (see Fig. 37–3), and/or a graph showing progress in one or more variables (e.g., see Fig. 38–1, plotted heart rates, and attendance/adherence across time). Computer-generated feedback letters currently show promise as an efficient, systematic method for providing personalized feedback to participants on a regular basis. When used in conjunction with *goals* that are reasonable, personally relevant, and short-term, feedback can be a powerful motivating factor.

Behavioral Success. A key factor in adherence is recognizing that continued adherence is typically a consequence of *behavioral success*, rather than the education or instruction that constitutes the early portions of most programs. In other words, often the feelings of success and accomplishment that accompany actually *doing* an activity on a regular basis are what shape our beliefs and attitudes about continuing

Name _____ Social Security #: _____ Exercise Goal _____
Date _____

	Sun.	Mon.	Tues.	Wed.	Thurs.	Fri.	Sat.
Activity Type:							
Total Time:							
Distance:							
Heart Rate Before exercise:							
During exercise:							
After exercise:							
Enjoyment 1. very enjoyable 2. somewhat enjoyable 3. neutral 4. somewhat enjoyable 5. very enjoyable	1 2 3 4 5	1 2 3 4 5	1 2 3 4 5	1 2 3 4 5	1 2 3 4 5	1 2 3 4 5	1 2 3 4 5
Where did you exercise?							
With whom did you exercise?							

Fig. 37–3. Activity record.

the activity rather than vice versa. This fact helps to explain why many individuals, despite being knowledgeable concerning physical exercise, are not currently active. Health professionals can help this process by pointing out to individuals the changes and gains they have made, no matter how modest. Participants should be "shaped," so that they engage in the exercise no matter how they feel (barring illness or injury) or what their attitude. Eventually, this regular and successful participation will produce appropriate feelings of mastery, if not enjoyment, as well as positive attitudes toward their own exercise program—a process that enhances the probability of sticking with the exercise program over the long run.

Self-management. Success in behavior change correlates with building in, early on, training in *self-management strategies* and an understanding of the importance of taking *personal responsibility* for physical activity. Individuals must recognize the importance of taking charge of their physical activity as a lifelong goal rather than as something that occurs only so long as their 12-week class or program lasts. Such programs are a *vehicle* for establishing the lifelong habit, and are not the sole means by which physical activity should be defined. Early in all programs, persons should be taught methods of being able to prompt and successfully engage in activity in various settings and under various circumstances, e.g., specific instruction on how to set the occasion for exercise (e.g., carry exercise clothes in car, or lay them by the bed; spend time with exercise "buffs"; park car and walk) and what to do if an exercise class or episode is missed or a relapse has occurred (e.g., admit responsibility for the "slip"; develop a restart plan, call exercise "buddy," arrange reinforcement, simplify or change regimen).

ENHANCING MAINTENANCE

In addition to sedentary individuals who have difficulty in starting a physical activity program, some individuals spend much of their time *restarting* exercise programs that they terminated for various reasons. Often they stopped the program completely after an inevitable "break" in the activity sched-ule because of illness or injury, travel, holidays, inclement weather, or increased demands at work. Therefore, a useful step is to prepare individuals, both psychologically and behaviorally, for breaks or "slips" in their activity that can lead to a full-blown relapse and a return to their previous sedentary ways.[7] Persons should first be warned that such breaks are inevitable and do not indicate that the person is hopelessly lazy or a failure. Having individuals identify their own types of "high-risk situations" that lead to inactivity, as well as devising strategies to prepare them for "slips" ahead of time, can be profitable.

Recommended Strategies

Useful plans include identifying types of alternative activities (e.g., brisk walking), planning to exercise as soon as possible after the break in the schedule, arranging to exercise with someone else, and resetting goals to an easier level to avoid discouragement.

Other methods that can be used for enhancing maintenance are described in the following paragraphs.

Reminders of Benefits

Provision of continued evidence of relevant personal benefits from regular exercise (in the physical, social, and psychological arenas) is important. The professional staff should ask individuals on a regular basis what types of benefits and positive consequences they are reaping from their current physical activity program. For some persons at particular risk for dropping out, such questioning might be posed frequently (e.g., one or more times a month). If an individual cannot define positive aspects of the exercise or can provide a list of negative aspects that is twice as long, that participant is at serious risk of dropping out and should be targeted for increased attention.

Generalization Training

Directors of exercise programs or classes should try to avoid halting the program abruptly, especially if no generalization training has been conducted. To ensure continued adherence, the exercise habit must be generalized or re-established in the new (e.g., home) environment before programmed sessions are discontinued in the old setting. This generalization might be accomplished in one of several ways, including requiring unsupervised home exercise sessions from the beginning or at an early stage of the program; including family or significant others in exercise sessions for a period before cessation of the more formal program; and adding additional exercises before "graduation" that are more easily maintained in the home environment. Ideally, responsibility for session supervision, reinforcement, and feedback characteristics should be gradually transferred from the instructor to the participants themselves as the change date approaches, to approximate more closely the conditions the exerciser is likely to experience in the new (maintenance) setting.

Reassessment of Goals

Reassessment of goals provides the opportunity to verify that they are still relevant, realistic, and motivating. Again, goals that are too long-term or are vague do not provide enough motivation to maintain the individual through trying or rough periods. During the early stages of an exercise program (i.e., the first 3 to 6 months), goals should be adjusted frequently if necessary (i.e., once every 2 weeks) to keep the person on course.

Social Support

The continued use of social support in as many forms as possible is valuable. If the format of the exercise is a class situation or group headed by an exercise leader, the leader should take responsibility for calling participants on the telephone when they miss two classes in a row (one class, if the person has been targeted as someone at high risk for dropping out). The purpose of the telephone call is not to scold or in any way make these individuals feel guilty for not attending. Rather, it should be used to let these persons know that they were missed and that other participants noticed and care about them. Other individuals in the class can assume this type of responsibility as well (a "buddy system"). If the exercise program is conducted outside of a formal class or group, the health profes-

sional can continue support in the form of periodic telephone calls, letters, and newsletters. Family members, co-workers, and friends of the person should continue to encourage and support their exercise efforts as well.

Relevant Rewards

When used for exercise behavior and achievements in conjunction with the person's activity goals, rewards should change periodically to maintain their motivating impact. Rewards may include "points" that are accumulated as the person continues to exercise and that can be totaled to obtain a large reward (e.g., a new exercise outfit, dinner out, a small trip), or small rewards in such areas as "time off" (to read or engage in other enjoyable activities).

Feedback

Self-monitoring and other forms of *feedback* are useful for noting progress and enhancing motivation. For some individuals, this feedback may take the additional form of professional or self-administered exercise or fitness *assessments*. Such fitness assessments can involve setting up a standardized exercise "course" in the person's immediate environment so that the individual can easily measure current fitness levels against past performance. Frequently, such assessments involve seeing how fast a person can complete a specific distance, or noting his or her exercise heart rate during the completion of a specific amount of work undertaken over a specified amount of time.

Contracts

As noted previously, contracts should be updated and changed frequently, if warranted, and should include specific goals, rewards, and helpers. Contracts that are too easy do not provide the challenge needed to motivate many individuals. In contrast, contracts that are too difficult lead to frustration and discouragement (as well as injury, in some cases).

Avoidance of Boredom

Individuals should be encouraged to monitor the amount of enjoyment they derive from their activity, and to take responsibility for making it more enjoyable, if it is not currently meeting their needs. The health professional should work collaboratively with the individual to achieve this goal (e.g., through implementation of new activities, environments, goals, and partners). With the wide variety of aerobic activities from which to choose, and the diversity of settings currently available in which to conduct such activities, the "I'm bored" response should not be allowed for long. For some individuals, boredom may be licked by coaching them in an exercise regimen that involves a variety of activities. For other participants, one activity conducted in varied settings and formats may be more appropriate or preferable. Some form of enjoyable competition (e.g., fun runs or walkathons) may also stimulate exercise maintenance.

Importance of Routine Activities

For many individuals, particularly as they age, an increase in activities of daily living can provide a useful "backdrop" of activity that can keep them loose and "peppy," even during times when they are not engaged in more vigorous activity. It is important for participants to understand that the health benefits obtained from an active lifestyle can be more effectively realized if they become more active in a variety of ways, both within and outside of formal programs.

Helping individuals to begin and maintain increased levels of physical activity can undoubtedly be a challenge to even the most enterprising health professional. Such a task requires continued creativity and flexibility in developing and modifying programs to meet the changing needs of participants. Health professionals can be helped in their efforts by remembering the guidelines to changing and maintaining behavior that behavioral scientists have found to be particularly useful. A summary of some of the more general guidelines follows:

1. Behavior (including physical activity) is strongly influenced by its immediate consequences for the individual.

2. To increase the likelihood that a behavior will occur, increase the immediately rewarding aspects of the behavior, and decrease the negative or punishing aspects.

3. Rewards, used to reinforce behavior change and to motivate future behavior, are in the "eye of the beholder." Let the individual choose rewards that are personally motivating.

4. Set appropriate activity-related goals, and modify these goals as necessary. Encourage individual tailoring of and flexibility in exercise goal-setting, emphasizing adherence/attendance at first rather than performance per se.

5. Provide relevant feedback whenever possible. Encourage (teach) exercisers to plot their progress (e.g., heart rate, distance covered, exercise duration) on graphs for visual motivation purposes.

6. Gradually "shape" an initially difficult behavior; have individuals start with less demanding activity goals to help "ease" them into the habit of being physically active.

7. Structure appropriate expectations in the *early* stages of the program.

8. Prepare participants for inevitable lapses or breaks in their exercise regimen by encouraging them to "plan ahead", and to put unexpected breaks in their regimens into perspective.

9. Whenever possible, offer people choices as a means of better tailoring exercise programs to fit individual needs and preferences.

10. Encourage public expressions of commitment to the exercise program through the use of written contracts, decision balance sheets, and other strategies.

11. Teach participants how to use environmental or social prompts and reminders to "set the stage" for regular exercise adherence. Examples include writing session times into a daily schedule book and encouraging individuals to keep their exercise apparel in a prominent place.

12. Foster self-management of the exercise regimen as much as possible.

13. Utilize as many types of social support as is feasible; when relevant, adequately prepare individuals ahead of time for changes in instructors to minimize disruptions to the exercise class or group.
14. Use the exercise program as an opportunity to model and promote an overall healthy life-style.

In addition, health professionals should keep in mind the usefulness of a *public health perspective* in attacking exercise adoption and adherence problems with their clients. This perspective emphasizes the importance of inspiring as many individuals as possible in a community to engage in *some* physical activity, rather than a relatively small number doing a large amount. Although use of the traditional prescription of "3 times per week, for at least 30 minutes at a time at an aerobic heart rate" is certainly a useful general goal, for many individuals in our society this goal is currently unreachable. Alternatively, striving to motivate the very sedentary among us to increase their general activity levels through more moderate, convenient activities of daily living can be a worthwhile endeavor that should not be ignored. Health professionals must remain open to the various options available in enhancing physical activity levels in their clients, particularly on a community-wide, cost-efficient basis.

ACKNOWLEDGMENTS

Preparation of this chapter was supported in part by US Public Health Service grant #AG-00440 from the National Institute on Aging, Bethesda, Md, awarded to Dr. King.

REFERENCES

1. Dishman RK: Compliance/adherence in health-related exercise. *Health Psychol, 1:*237, 1982.
2. Oldridge NB: Compliance with exercise rehabilitation. In *Exercise and Public Health.* RK Dishman (Ed.). Champaign, IL: Human Kinetics Publishers, 1988, pp. 283–304.
3. Martin JE, Dubbert PM: Exercise adherence. *Exerc Sport Sci Rev, 13:*137, 1985.
4. Marcus BH, Takowski W, Rossi JS: Assessing motivational readiness and decision-making for exercise. *Health Psychol,* in press.
5. King AC, Frederiksen LW: Low-cost strategies for increasing exercise behavior: The effects of relapse preparation training and social supports. *Behav Modif, 4:*3, 1984.
6. King AC, Haskell WL, Taylor CB, et al.: Group- vs home-based exercise training in healthy older men and women: A community-based clinical trial. *JAMA, 266:*1535, 1991.
7. Sallis JF, Haskell WL, Fortmann SP, et al.: Predictors of adoption and maintenance of physical activity in a community sample. *Prev Med, 15:*331, 1986.
8. Borg GV: Perceived exertion as an indicator of somatic stress. *Scand J Rehabil Med, 2:*92, 1970.

Chapter 38

WEIGHT MANAGEMENT
Kelly D. Brownell and Carlos M. Grilo

Obesity is a serious, prevalent, and growing public health problem. Excess weight is associated with increased risk of coronary heart disease, type II diabetes, hypertension, and other illnesses. Despite the known seriousness of obesity, increased public concern, and record rates of dieting, obesity remains a common problem. Thirty-four million Americans are believed to be obese, and this figure may be increasing.

This discussion of weight management applies to people of all categories—the millions of overweight persons along with the millions who are at or close to "ideal" weight but struggle to maintain desirable body size. Although some of this discussion is relevant to the casualties of the ubiquitous pressure to be thin (individuals with anorexia nervosa and bulimia nervosa), the special characteristics of those populations are beyond the scope of this chapter.

DEFINITION

Obesity is a surplus of adipose tissue containing fat stored in triglyceride form, resulting from excess energy intake relative to energy expenditure. The point at which excess fat constitutes obesity is somewhat arbitrary.

Overweight is defined as deviation in body weight from some standard or "ideal" weight related to height. The most frequently used standard was published in 1959 by the Metropolitan Life Insurance Company. Although newer Metropolitan Life tables were published in 1983, and others, such as the U.S. Department of Agriculture, have released tables, the 1959 Metropolitan tables still represent the best body weight health standard. Most research adopts the figure of 20% above the ideal weight as the definition of overweight. Although the precise point at which increasing weight exceeds the

threshold for good health is unclear, the 20% figure was adopted at the NIH Consensus Conference on the Health Risks of Obesity in 1985.

Overweight does not always reflect obesity (e.g., athletes can weigh more than the "ideal" weight, yet be quite lean). The various weight for height measures [e.g., % overweight, weight/height, and body mass index (weight/height squared)] tend to correlate at approximately 0.7 with body fat measured directly. Figure 38-1A shows a nomogram for body mass index and recommendations for assessment and intervention.

An important new development has occurred with the study of body fat distribution. Fat distributed in the abdomen, called upper-body or android-type obesity (because it occurs most often in men), is associated with greater morbidity and mortality than is body fat distributed below the waist, called lower-body or gynoid obesity. The simple ratio of waist-to-hip circumference is a stronger predictor of cardiovascular risk than is body weight, body fat, or body mass index. Figure 38-1B shows a nomogram for assessment of this ratio and associated risk.

THE PSYCHOLOGY AND PHYSIOLOGY OF BODY WEIGHT REGULATION

The public and many health professionals believe that excess weight reflects lack of willpower, poor self-concept, and deep-seated psychological problems. This is incorrect. Excess weight results from a complex interaction of cultural, genetic, physiologic, and psychologic factors. Even when studies show psychologic distress in overweight persons (these results are noted in a minority of studies), the distress could be the consequence rather than the cause of their condition.

Body Mass Index (BMI) Nomogram

Place a straightedge across the scales for weight and height.
The BMI is the number in the middle scale where the straightedge crosses it.

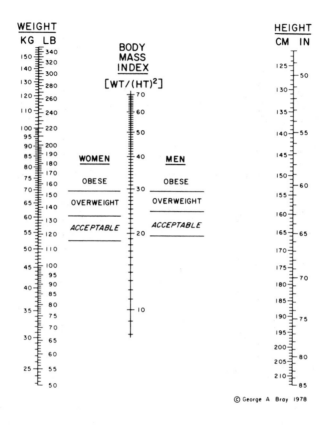

© George A Bray 1978

Adult Intervention Guidelines		
BMI kg/m²		
19–34 years	≥35 years	
<25	≤27	Normal; refer to waist-to-hip ratio
25–27	—	Intervention indicated if there is a family history or presence of heart disease, type II diabetes, hypercholesterolemia, or hypertension.
≥27	≥27	Intervention indicated even in the absence of another risk factor

A

Fig. 38–1. Nomograms for A. body mass index (BMI) and B. waist-to-hip ratio (WHR). Also shown are recommendations for adult interventions based on BMI and classification of health risk based on WHR. BMI nomogram reprinted with permission from Bray GA: Definitions, measurements, and classification

Waist-to-Hip Ratio (WHR) Nomogram

Place a straightedge across the scales for waist and hip circumferences.
The WHR is the number in the middle scale where the straightedge crosses it.

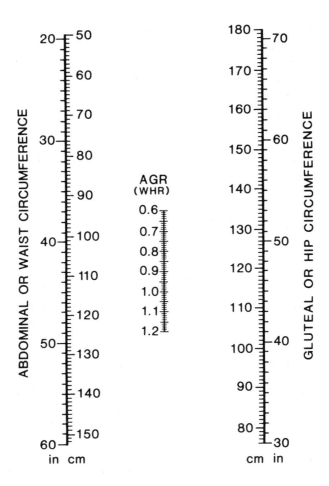

Waist Circumference. Measure the circumference below the xiphoid process of the sternum and above the iliac crest at the level of the umbilicus. If the abdomen is very large, the measure may be taken with the patient supine on the examining table.

Hip Circumference. Measure the maximum circumference around the hips over the buttocks.

Risk Classification	
Group	**At Risk WHR Values**
Men	>1.0
Women	>0.8

B

of the syndrome of obesity. *Int J Obesity,* 2:99, 1978. WHR nomogram reprinted with permission from Bray GA, Gray DS: Obesity: Part I—Pathogenesis. *West J Med, 149:*429, 1988.

Much of the interest in physiologic factors has focused on the concept of a body weight "set point." The set point theory proposes a "natural weight" for each individual, i.e., the weight the body seeks to protect against pressures to be too heavy or too thin. If some people have a set point above the ideal, they are destined to fight their physiology to lose weight. The concept of set point is appealing because it leads to a search for factors that regulate body weight. Whether a set point exists is a matter of considerable debate. In working with overweight individuals, one must walk a fine line between acknowledging the importance of biology and painting a pessimistic picture of the body resisting all attempts at weight change.

Recent research has shown that body weight is under substantial genetic control. Moreover, the pattern of body fat distribution (e.g., upper or lower body) also appears to be genetically influenced. Studies have also found that resting metabolic rate (RMR), which accounts for roughly 70% of daily expenditure and can vary considerably across individuals, is also influenced by genetics.

These findings, however, do not suggest that it is fruitless to diet. What they do suggest is that individuals should adopt more "reasonable" goals and should avoid wholesale pursuit of aesthetic or even health ideals. The professional should also explain to overweight people that they *inherit only a tendency towards obesity and that the extent of its expression can be influenced by diet and exercise.*

IMPORTANCE OF EXERCISE IN WEIGHT CONTROL

Several lines of evidence demonstrate the importance of exercise in weight control. First, overweight persons are rarely among the ranks of the physically active. However, inactivity could be either the cause or consequence of weight problems. Second is the finding that people in weight loss programs who maintain their loss are most likely to exercise. The most convincing evidence, however, comes from studies in which dieters are randomly assigned to groups that do or do not receive an exercise program to accompany dietary change. Only a few such studies exist, but they point to a consistent conclusion—that exercise facilitates long-term weight loss. Thus, available data suggest that weight control programs ought to include exercise.

Exercise has been prescribed as a component of weight control programs for years, but only as a formality. Professionals held little hope for compliance because they knew how daunting the prospect of exercise could be to someone with the physical burden of excess weight. Compelling reasons exist, however, to emphasize physical activity.

1. *Exercise expends energy.* Exercise does use calories, but some dieters make the mistake of believing they can burn enough calories from low-level activity to permit increased food intake. The cumulative effects of exercise over long periods of time can be substantial, so even modest levels of activity can be beneficial. The caloric expenditure of various physical activities can be found in a book by McArdle, Katch, and Katch (see Recommended Readings).

2. *Exercise may suppress appetite.* This issue has been studied more in animals than in humans, but exercise may help to suppress appetite in some persons. Other individuals may increase intake enough to offset the increased expenditure, so the effects of exercise on appetite are either neutral or positive for the dieter. Some people find it helpful to schedule exercise at times when they typically overeat.

3. *Exercise can counteract the ill effects of obesity.* Exercise can have positive effects on blood pressure, serum cholesterol levels, body composition, and cardiorespiratory function. Obese persons are at increased risk for abnormalities in each of these areas. Exercise can provide these benefits independent of weight loss.

4. *Exercise can improve psychologic functioning.* Changes in anxiety, depression, general mood, and self-concept are noted in people who maintain an exercise program. In someone attempting to lose weight, the psychologic changes can enhance dietary compliance. Exercise may have this

effect by increasing a general sense of personal control.

5. *Exercise may minimize loss of lean body mass.* As much as 25% of the weight lost by dieting alone can be lean body mass (LBM). Overweight people typically have increased LBM as well as fat, but the loss of LBM during dieting is considered potentially dangerous if the body depletes protein reserves in essential areas of the body. The percentage of LBM lost decreases when exercise is combined with diet. Researchers have not studied formally what seems intuitively correct—that strength training protects LBM more than endurance activities. Because endurance activities are more likely to be part of most exercise prescriptions, this potential for accelerating or decelerating loss of LBM is an important area for further research.

6. *Exercise may counter the metabolic decline produced by dieting.* Calorie restriction produces a rapid reduction in resting metabolic rate (RMR). The decline can be as much as 20%, and because RMR accounts for 60 to 70% of total energy expenditure, such a decline is noteworthy. This RMR reduction may account, in part, for the "plateau" reached by many dieters when weight loss slows or stops, even when calorie intake remains stable. Exercise is known to increase the RMR, but the magnitude and duration of the increase are controversial. How the type, frequency, intensity, and duration of the exercise can be altered to offset the metabolic decline produced by dieting is not clear.

Professionals should be aware of these benefits of exercise and can be enthusiastic about exercise as one aspect of weight control. Describing the benefits to dieters can provide an added incentive to become more physically active.

Exercise Adherence

As is the case with dieting, compliance with exercise is a major challenge. In addition to providing education regarding the importance of exercise for weight control, the professional might enhance compliance in several ways.

1. *Emphasize the Psychologic Benefits.* The psychologic benefits of exercise can be substantial. Exercise, in addition to expending energy and improving health, can enhance self-esteem, provide motivation, decrease anxiety, and buffer individuals against stress (a common trigger for overeating). The professional can do much to enhance adherence by stressing to individuals that each time they do some form of physical activity, it represents a positive step. Motivationally, it is important to keep track of such "successes" (e.g., parking and walking to the mall), which may contribute to the feeling of greater *personal control.*

2. *Be Sensitive to the Excess Weight.* When inactive people state what prevents them from exercising, they usually say they are too busy. This "barrier to exercise" can often be overcome by creative scheduling and by alerting people to the many benefits of exercise. The "busy schedule" reason, however, often masks other, more important barriers. One such barrier is the excess weight itself. Becoming active can be difficult, tiring, and painful when the body carries an extra load. People must be instructed to set reasonable exercise goals and to expect some time to elapse before they can do high levels of activity.

   Another obstacle to exercise involves the negative associations that plague many people, particularly persons who have been overweight since childhood. They are likely to be self-conscious and embarrassed about their bodies because they have been teased, have been picked last for teams, and have suffered from poor performance at sports. When the mere prospect of exercise evokes such negative feelings, care is necessary to prescribe levels of activity consistent with abilities and fitness level, and to work with individuals to select activities they enjoy.

3. *Avoid an Exercise Threshold.* When professionals encourage individuals

to exercise, a common question is, "How much should I do?" Too often the response is well-meaning, but is automatic and perhaps counterproductive. Individuals are told of the famous, three-part equation involving *frequency, intensity,* and *duration.* A typical prescription from this equation is that exercise should be done 3 times per week at 70% maximum heart rate for at least 15 minutes each time. This equation is born from extensive research showing that such exercise is necessary to improve cardiorespiratory conditioning. This goal is important but is not the only goal of exercise.

Use of this equation implies an exercise "threshold," i.e., that exercise must be done at specific levels to have any value. If an activity meets or exceeds the levels dictated by the equation, an individual is thought to have exercised "enough," having incurred some physiologic benefit. If the effort falls below this level, people often assume they have not profited. This threshold may be a useful incentive for some individuals but represents a deterrent to others.

Recent research has found that modest physical activity and modest weight loss can both have significant health benefits. Relatively low levels of activity are associated with decreased mortality. Modest exercise also predicts weight loss. Moreover, surprisingly small weight losses can normalize blood pressure among some obese hypertensive subjects, and improve control among obese Type II diabetics.

Professionals should make a specific point about exercise—*any exercise is better than no exercise.* When a person asks if walking one block is "enough," tell them it is far better than being inactive. Moreover, it should be underscored that such an effort represents a positive commitment to oneself. *Consistency may be more important than the type or amount of exercise.*

4. *Select the "Right" Exercise.* The selection of a realistic and appropriate exercise program is a key predictor of

adherence. People are more likely to continue activities that they find enjoyable. Two questions can be asked as a starting point: *Is it fun?* and *Will you do it regularly?* The professional can then assist the person in choosing activities that will match their lifestyle and schedule.

For obese individuals, the choice of low-impact activities is particularly important. For many people, obese or lean, regular walking represents a potentially rewarding option. Beginning "moderate" intensity programs should be preceded by a consultation with a physician. (See ACSM Guidelines for Exercise Stress Testing.)

A COMPREHENSIVE APPROACH TO WEIGHT CONTROL

Weight problems are not easily remedied by simple advice for people to "eat less and exercise more." Important elements of programs should have a broad base with consideration of at least three factors: nutrition, exercise, and behavior change, with the assumption that each area is done well. This breadth of focus is not easy because most professionals are expert in only one area.

There exists a staggering range of options for weight control programs. Commercial groups, self-help groups, professional counseling, and various other approaches are successful for some people. Therefore, *educated referrals are an important aspect of work with overweight persons.* Unfortunately, we must rely on clinical judgment for making such referrals, because research has not yet provided clear guidelines.

Figure 38-2 provides a conceptual scheme showing a recommended three-stage process proposed by Brownell and Wadden for selecting a treatment for an individual. This comprehensive approach represents the integration of three approaches (i.e., classification, stepped care, and matching individuals to treatment) to the selection of treatment. The classification approach employs overweight level to determine treatment. The stepped-care approach prescribes the least intensive interventions first (e.g., self-help programs) followed by more intensive treatments

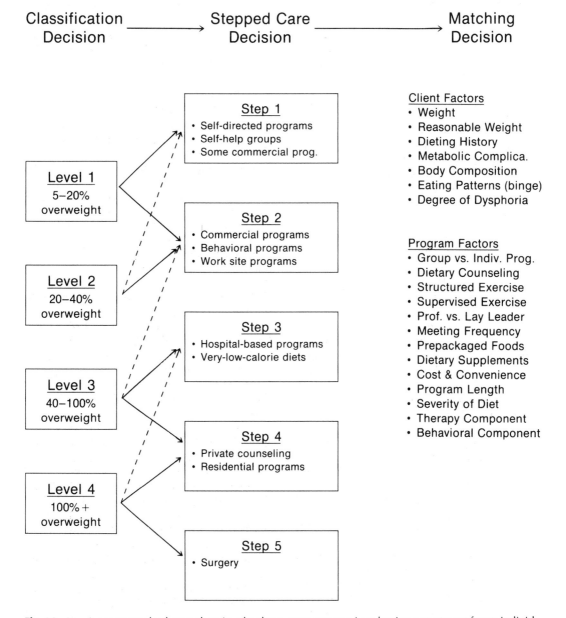

Classification Decision ⟶ Stepped Care Decision ⟶ Matching Decision

Step 1
• Self-directed programs
• Self-help groups
• Some commercial prog.

Step 2
• Commercial programs
• Behavioral programs
• Work site programs

Step 3
• Hospital-based programs
• Very-low-calorie diets

Step 4
• Private counseling
• Residential programs

Step 5
• Surgery

Level 1
5–20%
overweight

Level 2
20–40%
overweight

Level 3
40–100%
overweight

Level 4
100% +
overweight

Client Factors
• Weight
• Reasonable Weight
• Dieting History
• Metabolic Complica.
• Body Composition
• Eating Patterns (binge)
• Degree of Dysphoria

Program Factors
• Group vs. Indiv. Prog.
• Dietary Counseling
• Structured Exercise
• Supervised Exercise
• Prof. vs. Lay Leader
• Meeting Frequency
• Prepackaged Foods
• Dietary Supplements
• Cost & Convenience
• Program Length
• Severity of Diet
• Therapy Component
• Behavioral Component

Fig. 38–2. A conceptual scheme showing the three-stage process in selecting a treatment for an individual. The first step, the Classification Decision, divides individuals according to percent overweight into four levels. This level indicates which of the five steps would be reasonable in the second stage, the Stepped Care Decision. This indicates that the least intensive, costly, and risky approach will be used from among alternative treatments. The third stage, the Matching Decision, is used to make the final selection of a program, and is based on a combination of client and program variables. The dashed lines with arrows between the Classification and Stepped Care stages show the lowest level of treatment that may be beneficial, but more intensive treatment is usually necessary for people at the specified weight level. Reprinted with permission from Brownell KD, Wadden TA: The heterogeneity of obesity: Fitting treatments to individuals. *Behavior Therapy, 22*:153, 1991.

(e.g., hospital-based) for those who have failed at lower levels. Individual matching involves matching individuals to treatment based on consideration of personal needs and program characteristics (e.g., a dieter with significant distress might be evaluated for counseling).

Components of Effective Treatment

As noted above, nutrition, exercise, and behavior change represent the three key elements of weight control programs. An overview of important components follows. Several available manuals and books for weight control are cited in the reference section of this chapter.

Behavior Modification

Lifestyle and behavior change are the cornerstones of effective treatment. Behavioral interventions are critical to ensure such changes, and focus on much more than just eating and exercise habits. They involve teaching individuals the relationship between *antecedents* (i.e., events, thoughts, and feelings leading up to eating), *behaviors* (i.e., eating, binging, etc), and *consequences* (i.e., events, thoughts, and feelings that follow eating and can determine subsequent problematic eating). In addition, individuals can be taught specific *coping skills* to change eating and exercise. Teaching dieters coping skills to overcome difficult situations and prevent negative reactions is perhaps one of the most important treatment interventions.

Exercise

Exercise is a key component of weight control for the reasons discussed above. We recommend that *consistency* be the focus of exercise programs for weight control rather than the type or amount of exercise. Consistency, adherence, and enjoyment are the goals.

Nutrition

Adequate nutrition and a decreased calorie intake relative to expenditure (negative energy balance) are the general goals of dietary interventions. Nutrition is discussed in detail in Chapter 39. There are two primary methods for monitoring caloric intake. One is to count calories. The individual is instructed to eat a specific number of servings from basic food groups, but to do so with total calorie intake not exceeding a defined level. The second method involves the exchange plan developed by the American Dietetic Association and the American Diabetic Association. Individuals are taught to eat a specific number of "exchanges" within food groups. Exchanges represent amounts of different foods within a group that are equivalent in nutrition and calories. In our experience, both approaches are acceptable, so personal preferences of the client and professional can be used to select one over the other.

Negative Energy Balance. The first question often asked is *How many calories?* Although numerous methods exist to arrive at such a figure, we recommend the following general approach. Begin with 1500 kcal/day for men and 1200 kcal/day for women. Modify caloric consumption from this starting point depending on the needs of the individual. Calorie intakes below 1000 kcal/day should be medically monitored. We generally recommend setting a weekly goal of a 1 to 2 lb weight loss. Determination of the caloric intake necessary to produce a 1 to 2 lb loss per week can be difficult. Many complex factors influence metabolic needs. For example, people have been told for years that if they reduce their calorie intake by 500 per day (3500/week), they will lose 1 pound each week. This calculation is valid only when intakes and expenditures are averaged across many people. There is considerable variability. Moreover, there is also variability within individuals over time. Thus, keeping a dietary record over time may aid in the adjustment of intake to help establish specific calorie goals.

Adequate Nutrition. Nutrition needs to be considered carefully when choosing an approach to weight reduction. Inadequate nutrition during weight reduction can have serious medical consequences. Hypocaloric diets must be nutritionally adequate with particular attention to protein, vitamin, and mineral intake. Moreover, diet composition may influence various mechanisms relevant to weight control such as diuresis, appetite, and satiety. Specific nutritional considerations are discussed in Chapter 39 and in referenced texts.

Very-Low-Calorie-Diets. A particularly aggressive approach to weight loss, very-low-calorie diets (VLCD), has become popular in recent years. These involve fasting supplemented by either a powdered supplement or small amounts of lean meat, fish, or fowl. Calorie levels vary from 400 to 800 kcal/day, and programs vary considerably in the quality of behavioral and nutritional intervention that accompanies the diet. These diets are typically reserved for individuals 40% or more over ideal weight and are to be undertaken only under medical supervision. They are appealing because the weight loss is so rapid (2 to 3 lbs/wk for women and 3 to 5 lbs/wk for men), and because the dieter does not have to make choices about foods. The issue, of course, is long-term maintenance. The first studies with follow-up periods of 1 year found good maintenance of weight loss if a VLCD was combined with a high-quality behavioral program. Recent results of 3- to 5-year follow-ups show nearly total weight regain.

We believe it is premature to abandon use of these diets, but individuals must be cautioned about the probability of relapse. In the meantime, research needs to examine methods for sustaining the impressive losses produced by these diets.

Cognitive Change

People's thoughts and attitudes about themselves, nutrition, and exercise play key roles in weight maintenance. It is important to help people become *actively* aware of their thoughts. People often have *"automatic"* thoughts, which are over-learned responses to particular situations. These thoughts influence how we feel and can have a profound impact on dietary compliance. Examples are self-deprecating thoughts following dietary violations, adoption of unreasonable goals, and all-or-none thinking (e.g., foods are legal or illegal, being on or off a diet). Teaching awareness of thoughts and ways to substitute more objective thoughts can be help-

ful. The professional can also help individuals *focus on progress* (not shortcomings) and look for *problems in behaviors and situations* (not characterologic defects).

Social Support

The social environment influences our health behaviors. Social support represents a potential resource for dietary change. It is our experience, however, that some individuals benefit from social support whereas others do not. Some individuals prefer to lose and maintain weight loss privately, whereas others benefit from social support. It is helpful for professionals to examine this issue with individuals, and with those who would profit from support, to teach them methods for eliciting and sustaining the support.

Relapse Prevention

Keeping weight off represents the greatest challenge that dieters face. Many people who lose weight are unable to maintain the loss. Many individuals "successfully" lose weight numerous times only to regain it. This problem (i.e., relapse) has negative psychologic and medical consequences. Recent research has found that individuals whose body weight fluctuates repeatedly over time (e.g., weight loss and weight regain cycles) may have increased risk for coronary heart disease compared to individuals with stable body weights.

Figure 38-3 shows a schematic model of the process of relapse. We view relapse as a process, not an outcome. Dieters, regardless of their motivation, commitment, or level of success, inevitably experience temptations and, almost universally, have episodes of overeating. How a dieter *copes* with such situations may determine whether that isolated event (i.e., temptation or lapse) escalates into repeated overeating (relapse), leads to abandonment of the diet (collapse), or, ideally, leads to increased confidence and continued maintenance. Relapse prevention techniques have been developed to identify potential *high-risk* dieting situations and develop *coping skills* to overcome those situations. In cases in which lapses do occur, individuals must be taught to avoid negative reactions and

The Process of Lapse and Relapse

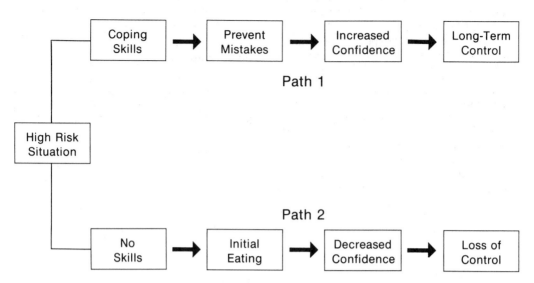

Fig. 38-3. Schematic diagram of the process of lapse and relapse. Dieters inevitably encounter "high-risk" dieting situations in which dietary control is challenged. Two general paths are possible. The lack of coping skills or the inability to successfully apply coping during high-risk situations may result in overeating, which decreases confidence. Lack of coping skills, coupled with decreased confidence, increases the probability of continued loss of dietary control. Alternatively, the application of coping skills during a high-risk situation may help the dieter to overcome the temptation, which increases confidence. Coping skills coupled with increased confidence increase the probability of continued dietary control. Reprinted with permission from Brownell KD, Rodin J: *Weight Maintenance Survival Guide.* Dallas: American Health Publishing Co., 1990. Adapted originally from Marlatt GA, Gordon JR (eds): *Relapse Prevention: Maintenance Strategies in the Treatment of Addictive Behaviors.* New York: Guilford Press, 1985.

to react instead with an attempt to learn from the lapse, solve problems for future events, and renew commitment to the program.

SUMMARY

Obesity is a significant health problem in our society. Complex physiologic, genetic, cultural, and psychologic factors contribute to the problem, so it should not be automatically attributed to weak will power or personal deficits. Exercise is an important predictor of success at weight reduction, so increased physical activity is one of the key aims in working with people who wish to reduce weight. Compliance is jeopardized, however, if the special physical and psychologic burdens of being overweight are not considered. Regardless of the level of intervention, a comprehensive program involving nutrition, behavior, cognitions, and

social support, in addition to exercise, appears to hold the greatest promise for long-term results. The frequency of relapse and its potential psychologic and medical consequences highlight the need for aggressive relapse prevention work. Consistency and lifestyle change are the key goals.

RECOMMENDED READINGS

1. Bouchard C, et al: Genetic effect in resting and exercise metabolic rates. *Metabolism, 38:* 364, 1989.
2. Bray GA: Nutrient balance and obesity: An appropriate control of food intake in humans. *Med Clin North Am, 73:*29, 1989.
3. Brownell KD: *The LEARN Program for Weight Control.* Dallas: American Health Publishing Co., 1990.
4. Brownell KD, Foreyt JF (eds): *Handbook of Eating Disorders: Physiology, Psychology, and Treatment of Obesity, Anorexia, and Bulimia.* New York: Basic Books, 1986.

5. Brownell KD, Wadden TA: Etiology and treatment of obesity: Towards understanding a serious, prevalent, and refractory disorder. *J Consult Clin Psychol, 60:*505, 1992.

6. Dishman RK (ed): *Exercise Adherence: Its Impact on Public Health.* Champaign, Illinois: Human Kinetics Books, 1988.

7. Grilo CM, Shiffman S, Wing RR: Relapse crises and coping among dieters. *J Consult Clin Psychol, 57:*488, 1989.

8. Marlatt GA, Gordon JR (eds): *Relapse Prevention: Maintenance Strategies in Addictive Behavior Change.* New York: Guilford, 1985.

9. McArdle WD, Katch FI, Katch VL: *Exercise Physiology: Energy, Nutrition, and Human Performance (3rd Edition).* Philadelphia: Lea & Febiger, 1991.

10. Stunkard AJ, Harris JR, Pedersen NL, McClearn GE: A separated twin study of the body mass index. *N Engl J Med, 322:*1483, 1990.

11. Wadden TA, Van Itallie TB, Blackburn GL: Responsible and irresponsible use of very-low-calorie-diets in the treatment of obesity. *JAMA, 263:*83, 1990.

Chapter 39

NUTRITION

Suzanne Nelson Steen and Kelly D. Brownell

An adequate and balanced diet is essential for optimal functioning. What we eat influences our work, play, psychologic status, and health. Considering the abundance of food in industrialized societies, the continued existence of nutrient deficiencies is surprising. The more significant problem, however, is that of *overnutrition*. The excessive consumption of calories, fat, cholesterol, and sodium has been linked to cardiovascular disease, certain forms of cancer, obesity, and other diseases.

Changing an individual's diet is not always easy. Food preferences are strongly ingrained and are influenced by family and culture. Ethnic groups who migrate to another culture are likely to change language, customs, and even religious practices before changing food preferences. Food acquires symbolic meaning when mothers feed children, families assemble for meals, holidays are celebrated, and so forth. Hectic lifestyles also influence food choices. The fast food that is an easy solution to a busy schedule tends to be high in fat, sodium, and calories. What, then, constitutes a healthy diet, and how can health professionals encourage positive changes?

BASIC FOODS AND FUNCTIONS

More than 50 known nutrients are needed by the body. These nutrients are divided into six classes: fat, carbohydrate, protein, vitamins, minerals, and water. This section discusses each of the basic nutrients, including their functions and food sources.

Fats and Cholesterol

Fat is stored in large quantities in adipose tissue and represents a large potential energy store. One gram of fat supplies 9 kcal, which is slightly more than the 7 kcal supplied by alcohol and more than twice the energy of carbohydrate or protein. In addition to providing energy, dietary fats transport the fat-soluble vitamins A, D, E, and K and protect and insulate vital organs.

Fats found in the body are classified as simple fats, compound fats, and derived fats, and are referred to as triglycerides, phospholipids, and cholesterol, respectively. Triglycerides, which are composed of three fatty acids and a glycerol molecule, represent more than 90% of the fat stored in the body. Dietary fats are categorized as either saturated or unsaturated (including polyunsaturated and monounsaturated) depending upon their chemical structures.

As shown in Table 39–1, saturated fats come primarily from animal products and are solid at room temperature. Vegetable sources of saturated fat include coconut oil, palm oil, and cocoa butter. These fats are widely used in commercially prepared foods (crackers, cookies, and pastries), and can easily become a significant source of fat in the diet. Unsaturated fats (Table 39–1) are liquid at room temperature and are vegetable oils.

Essential Fatty Acids

Linoleic acid is an essential fatty acid (EFA). It cannot be synthesized by the body and must be supplied by the diet. Arachidonic acid is also an EFA, but the body can produce it from linoleic acid. These EFAs are required for proper growth and healthy skin. Deficiency results in poor growth, dermatitis, lowered resistance to infection, and poor reproductive capacity. All of the EFAs can be obtained by consuming one tablespoon of oil per day (12 g or 108 kcal of fat).

Omega-3 Fatty Acid

Eicopentaenoic acid (EPA) and omega-3 fatty acid are names for this important fish

Table 39–1.   The Effects of Various Fats on Blood Lipids

Type	Sources	Effects on Blood Lipids
Saturated Fat	beef, veal, pork butter, lard cheese, cream, milk chocolate coconut oil cocoa butter hydrogenated vegetable oils lard palm oil shortenings	increases total cholesterol level increases LDL cholesterol level increases HDL cholesterol level
Polyunsaturated Fats (Vegetable Oils)	corn oil safflower oil sesame oil soft margarine soybean oil sunflower oil	decreases total cholesterol level decreases LDL cholesterol level decreases HDL cholesterol level
Monounsaturated Fats	avocados canola oil olive oil peanut oil	decreases total cholesterol level decreases LDL cholesterol level HDL level remains unchanged
Omega-3 Fatty Acids (Fish Oils)	mackerel salmon sardines shellfish trout tuna	decreases total cholesterol level decreases LDL cholesterol level increases HDL cholesterol level

oil that appears to have many health benefits. It has been shown to decrease serum triglycerides, total cholesterol, and blood pressure, and to increase the proportion of HDL cholesterol to total cholesterol. Mollusks and crustaceans contain significant amounts of cholesterol; however, the presence of omega-3 fatty acids appears to offset its effects. Three meals per week containing fish and shellfish with high levels of EPA are recommended.

Overall Fat Intake

Recommendations for dietary fat include reducing the percentage of total calories from fat to no more than 30%, and reducing the percentage of calories from saturated fat to 10%. Table 39–2 provides the American Heart Association goals and eating plan tips for reducing the risk of coronary heart disease.

The food industry has addressed the need for reduced fat intake by producing fat substitutes, which mimic the taste and feel of fat in the mouth. Milk and egg proteins and various carbohydrates have been modified to resemble fat. The resulting products are similar to sugar substitutes in that they provide taste with fewer or no calories. The hope is that these substitutes will aid in weight control and in improving general health. Nutritionists are concerned, however, that people may compensate for the calorie reduction by eating less healthy foods, or may substitute foods containing artificial fats and sugars for more nutrient- and fiber-rich foods such as fruits, vegetables, and grains. The only fat substitute currently on the market is Simplesse, which contains 1 to 2 kcal/g.

Cholesterol (cho) is a waxy, fat-like substance essential to all animal life. It is contained in all cells of the body and hormones (testosterone, estrogen, and steroid hormones), and is unique to animals—it is not found in plants or plant products. The body can use saturated fat to produce sufficient cholesterol; it does not need to be obtained through the diet. When too much saturated fat is consumed, the body produces excess cholesterol. Therefore, although it is important to monitor cholesterol intake, saturated fats, not dietary

Table 39–2.   American Heart Association Eating Plan

Goals of the American Heart Association Eating Plan

Reducing your "controllable" risk factors—those you can change—may prevent a heart attack in the future.

The best way to help lower your blood cholesterol level (a major risk factor for heart attack) is to eat less saturated fatty acids and cholesterol, and control your weight.

The eating plan is based on these AHA dietary guidelines:

- Total fat intake should be less than 30 percent of calories.
- Saturated fatty acid intake should be less than 10 percent of calories.
- Polyunsaturated fatty acid intake should be no more than 10 percent of calories.
- Monounsaturated fatty acids make up the rest of total fat intake, about 10 to 15 percent of total calories.
- Cholesterol intake should be no more than 300 milligrams per day.
- Sodium intake should be no more than 3000 milligrams (3 grams) per day.

Eating Plan Tips

To control the amount and kind of fat, saturated fatty acids, and dietary cholesterol you eat:

- Eat no more than 6 ounces (cooked) per day of lean meat, fish and skinless poultry.
- Try main dishes featuring pasta, rice, beans and/or vegetables. Or create "low-meat" dishes by mixing these foods with small amounts of lean meat, poultry or fish.
- The approximately 5 to 8 teaspoon servings of fats and oils per day may be used for cooking and baking, and in salad dressings and spreads.
- Use cooking methods that require little or no fat—boil, broil, bake, roast, poach, steam, saute, stir-fry or microwave.
- Trim off the fat you can see before cooking meat and poultry. Drain off all fat after browning. Chill soups and stews after cooking so you can remove the hardened fat from the top.
- The 3 to 4 egg yolks per week included in your eating plan may be used alone or in cooking and baking (including store-bought products).
- Limit your use of organ meats such as liver, brains, chitterlings, kidney, heart, gizzard, sweetbreads and pork maws.
- Choose skim or 1% fat milk and nonfat or low-fat yogurt and cheeses.

To round out the rest of your eating plan:

- Eat 5 or more servings of fruits or vegetables per day.
- Eat 6 or more servings of breads, cereals or grains per day.

---

* Modified from the American Heart Association Diet: An Eating Plan for Healthy Americans. 7272 National Center, Greenville Ave, Dallas, Texas 75231

cholesterol, have the greatest impact on total blood cholesterol levels. Cholesterol levels are also affected by heredity. The National Cholesterol Education Program considers a blood cholesterol level of less than 200 mg/dL desirable; 200 to 239 md/dL is considered borderline high; and levels of 240 mg/dL or greater are considered high.

Lipoproteins are produced by the liver and intestinal mucosa to transport insoluble fats such as cholesterol and triglycerides through the bloodstream. Low-density lipoproteins (LDL) are principally cholesterol. The cholesterol transported by LDL may be deposited on the arterial walls, contributing to atherosclerosis. Very low-density lipoproteins (VLDL) are a major carrier of triglycerides in the blood. The smallest group of lipoproteins, the high-density lipoproteins (HDL), however, appear to play a protective role by carrying cholesterol away from the arterial walls to the liver for catabolism and excretion, and by interfering with the binding of LDL to cell membranes. Therefore, high levels of HDL (greater than 45 mg/dL for men, greater than 55 mg/dL for women), low levels of LDL (less than 130 mg/dL), low total cholesterol (less than 200 mg/dL), and low total cholesterol/HDL cholesterol ratio (less than 4.9 for men, less than 4.4 for women) carry the lowest risk of cardiovascular disease. As shown in Table 39–1, the kind of fat consumed has an impact on these blood lipid levels. Exercise has also been shown to favorably increase HDL levels.

CARBOHYDRATES AND FIBER

Two types of carbohydrates, simple and complex, are consumed in the diet. Simple carbohydrates include glucose, fructose, sucrose (table sugar), and galactose (milk sugar), and can be found in foods such as candy, cake, soda, and jelly. Complex carbohydrates are made from chains of simple sugars, and include foods such as pasta, bread, cereal, rice, fruits, and vegetables. During the digestive process, simple and complex carbohydrates are broken down into glucose, which then circulates in the blood.

The typical diet contains more than the recommended amount of simple sugars and too few complex carbohydrates. These foods supply "empty calories" and few useful nutrients. Complex carbohydrates contain B-vitamins, minerals, fiber, and protein, which contribute to a balanced diet. The recommendation for the current U.S. diet is that 58% of daily calories come from carbohydrate; 48% from complex carbohydrates, and only 10% from simple sugars.

Dietary fiber is the nondigestible portion of carbohydrate. It is found only in plant foods; the best sources are foods high in complex carbohydrates. Fiber may play a role in the prevention and treatment of diabetes, cardiovascular disease, and hemorrhoids. It may also benefit dieters by creating a feeling of fullness without a high level of calories.

There are two types of fiber: water-soluble and water-insoluble. Water-soluble fiber is contained in pectin and gum; food sources are citrus fruits and apples. Soluble fiber may help lower cholesterol levels, thereby protecting against atherosclerosis and heart disease. Insoluble fiber absorbs water in the large intestine and produces soft stools that pass quickly through the intestinal tract. It is theorized that insoluble fiber thereby protects against colon cancer by reducing the amount of time that potential carcinogens can be absorbed through the intestinal tract. Insoluble fiber may also help prevent irritable bowel syndrome and diverticulosis. It is contained in whole-grain products, particularly bran.

Recommended fiber intake is 25 to 50 g/day, compared with the current average intake of 10 to 20 g/day. Intake should be increased gradually, however, as sudden increases can cause diarrhea, gas, and bloating. Cooked legumes provide approximately 9 grams per 1/2 cup; corn and peas have 5 grams per 1/2 cup; and bran cereal with raisins has 4 grams per 1.3 oz. By substituting whole foods for processed ones, fiber intake can also be increased (Table 39–3).

Protein

Proteins are composed of amino acids and are found in both plant and animal products. Eight (9 in children) of the 20 amino acids found in proteins are essential; i.e., they cannot be synthesized by the body

Table 39–3.   Fiber in Whole and Processed Foods

Instead of:	Use:	Change in Fiber Content:
Apple juice (0.4 g)	Fresh apple (3.5 g)	+875%
Orange juice (0.5 g)	Fresh orange (2.6 g)	+520%
Polished rice (0.2 g)	Brown rice (1 g)	+500%
Pasta (1.1 g)	Whole wheat pasta (4 g)	+360%
White bread (0.4 g)	Whole wheat bread (1.4 g)	+350%
Potato, no skin (1.4 g)	Potato with skin (2.5 g)	+180%

and must be supplied in the diet. Proteins from animal sources generally contain all the essential amino acids and are considered "complete." Protein from plant sources is "incomplete" in that one or more of the essential amino acids are missing. Vegetarians must be careful to complement their sources of protein to ensure consumption of all essential amino acids. Table 39–4 shows examples of complementary proteins.

Approximately 12% of total calories should come from protein. The RDA for protein is based on body weight, with increased amounts required during times of growth, certain disease states, pregnancy, and lactation. For the average man, the recommended intake is 0.8 g/kg body weight. This requirement can be met with 8 oz of meat or poultry.

Vitamins

Vitamins are essential for life and cannot be manufactured by the body. They are therefore required in the diet, but in very small amounts. The *fat-soluble* vitamins, A,

D, E, and K, are stored in the fat tissues of the body. *Water-soluble* vitamins are not stored in the body, so it is important to consume adequate amounts daily. They include C, thiamine, riboflavin, B_6, niacin, folacin, B_{12}, biotin, and pantothenic acid.

Vitamins have numerous functions. The majority facilitate metabolic reactions where energy is released from carbohydrate, fat, and protein; others are needed for blood clotting (vitamin K) and visual processes (vitamin A). Table 39–5 summarizes the primary functions and dietary sources. Table 39–6 gives the RDAs.

Americans spend $500 million annually on vitamins, which reflects the unfounded belief that vitamins can cure and prevent disease, increase energy level, improve athletic performance, enhance sexual potency, and reduce stress. Some vitamin producers market general-purpose multivitamins as meeting the special needs of active people, individuals with stressful lifestyles, and so forth, and health-food establishments promote "natural vitamins." The vitamin hysteria has also been promoted in books by nutrition "experts" who claim expertise in sports nutrition, wellness, or other areas. Miraculous benefits are often promised, including a longer life.

Vitamins have not been shown to prevent or cure any illness (including the common cold) except when specific deficiencies exist. Some vitamins aid in energy metabolism, but do not themselves provide energy, because they contain no calories. Essentially, no difference exists between a vitamin synthesized in a laboratory and a "natural" vitamin from plants or animals. Overuse of vitamins is not advisable. Taking too many vitamins may pose serious health hazards and can be expensive. Megadoses of fat-soluble vitamins can lead to hypervitaminosis and potential liver and

Table 39–4.   Complementing Proteins to Make Complete Proteins
For best results, foods should be eaten at the same meal or within 2–3 hours of each other

Legumes and grains	Dairy products and grains
Lentil soup & wheat bread	Low-fat yogurt and a peanut-butter sandwich
Barley soup w/navy beans	
Baked beans & brown rice	Macaroni & cheese
Split pea soup & rye bread	**Legumes and nuts & seeds**
	Raisin nut sunflower seed snack

Table 39–5. Vitamins

Vitamin	Main Function	Good Sources
A	Maintenance of skin, bone growth, vision, and teeth	Eggs, cheese, margarine, milk, carrots, broccoli, squash, and spinach
D	Bone growth and maintenance of bones	Milk, egg yolk, tuna, and salmon
E	Prevents oxidation of polyunsaturated fats	Vegetable oils, whole-grain cereal, bread, dried beans, and green leafy vegetables
K	Blood clotting	Cabbage, green leafy vegetables, and milk
Thiamine (B_1)	Energy-releasing reactions	Pork, ham, oysters, breads, cereals, pasta, and green peas
Riboflavin (B_2)	Energy-releasing reactions	Milk, meat, cereals, pasta, mushrooms, and dark green vegetables
Niacin	Energy-releasing reactions	Poultry, meat, tuna, cereal, pasta, bread, nuts, and legumes
Pyridoxine (B_6)	Metabolism of fats and proteins and formation of red blood cells	Cereals, bread, spinach, avocados, green beans, and bananas
Cobalamin (B_{12})	Formation of red blood cells and functioning of nervous system	Meat, fish, eggs, and milk
Folacin	Assists in forming proteins and in formation of red blood cells	Dark-green leafy vegetables, wheat germ
Pantothenic acid	Metabolism of proteins, carbohydrates, and fats, formation of hormones	Bread, cereals, nuts, eggs, and dark green vegetables
Biotin	Formation of fatty acids and energy-releasing reactions	Egg yolk, leafy green vegetables, and egg yolk
C	Bones, teeth, blood vessels, and collagen	Citrus fruits, tomato, strawberries, melon, green pepper, and potato

kidney damage. Complications have also been reported from large doses ("pharmacologic" levels of 10 times or more of the RDA) of vitamin C, niacin, and vitamin B_6. Vitamin supplements should not be used to make up for poor dietary habits. Supplementation is advised, however, during certain phases of the life cycle, such as infancy, pregnancy, and lactation.

Minerals

Minerals exist in the body in minute amounts, but are vital. Fifteen minerals have been identified, but dietary allowances have been established for only six (calcium, phosphorus, magnesium, iron, zinc, and iodine). The major or macrominerals include calcium, potassium, magnesium, sulfur, sodium, and chloride. The trace or microminerals are iron, iodine, copper, zinc, fluorine, selenium, manganese, molybdenum, and chromium. The

RDA levels for minerals are shown in Table 39–6. Table 39–7 lists the main functions and good food sources of minerals.

Supplementation is generally not necessary except for calcium (see below), iron, and zinc. Women of childbearing age, infants, young children, adolescents, and athletes often suffer from iron deficiency and may require supplements. Good sources of iron include red meat, organ meats, shellfish, eggs, beans, peas, green leafy vegetables, and whole grains. Iron absorption is tripled if iron is consumed with vitamin C. Consuming spinach with tomatoes, or steak with red peppers, for example, maximizes iron absorption. Table 39–8 illustrates how to increase dietary iron.

Osteoporosis

This condition exists when bone mass decreases excessively. It afflicts one of every

Table 39–6. Food and Nutrition Board, National Academy of Sciences—National Research Council Recommended Dietary Allowances,[a] Revised 1989 Designed for the Maintenance of Good Nutrition of Practically All Healthy People in the United States

Category	Age (years) or Condition	Weight[b] (kg)	Weight[b] (lb)	Height[b] (cm)	Height[b] (in)	Protein (g)	Vitamin A (µg RE)[c]	Vitamin D (µg)[d]	Vitamin E (mg α-TE)[e]	Vitamin K (µg)	Vitamin C (mg)	Thiamin (mg)	Riboflavin (mg)	Niacin (mg NE)[f]	Vitamin B6 (mg)	Folate (µg)	Vitamin B12 (µg)	Calcium (mg)	Phosphorus (mg)	Magnesium (mg)	Iron (mg)	Zinc (mg)	Iodine (µg)	Selenium (µg)
									Fat-Soluble Vitamins				**Water-Soluble Vitamins**						**Minerals**					
Infants	0.0–0.5	6	13	60	24	13	375	7.5	3	5	30	0.3	0.4	5	0.3	25	0.3	400	300	40	6	5	40	10
	0.5–1.0	9	20	71	28	14	375	10	4	10	35	0.4	0.5	6	0.6	35	0.5	600	500	60	10	5	50	15
Children	1–3	13	29	90	35	16	400	10	6	15	40	0.7	0.8	9	1.0	50	0.7	800	800	80	10	10	70	20
	4–6	20	44	112	44	24	500	10	7	20	45	0.9	1.1	12	1.1	75	1.0	800	800	120	10	10	90	20
	7–10	28	62	132	52	28	700	10	7	30	45	1.0	1.2	13	1.4	100	1.4	800	800	170	10	10	120	30
Males	11–14	45	99	157	62	45	1,000	10	10	45	50	1.3	1.5	17	1.7	150	2.0	1,200	1,200	270	12	15	150	40
	15–18	66	145	176	69	59	1,000	10	10	65	60	1.5	1.8	20	2.0	200	2.0	1,200	1,200	400	12	15	150	50
	19–24	72	160	177	70	58	1,000	10	10	70	60	1.5	1.7	19	2.0	200	2.0	1,200	1,200	350	10	15	150	70
	25–50	79	174	176	70	63	1,000	5	10	80	60	1.5	1.7	19	2.0	200	2.0	800	800	350	10	15	150	70
	51+	77	170	173	68	63	1,000	5	10	80	60	1.2	1.4	15	2.0	200	2.0	800	800	350	10	15	150	70
Females	11–14	46	101	157	62	46	800	10	8	45	50	1.1	1.3	15	1.4	150	2.0	1,200	1,200	280	15	12	150	45
	15–18	55	120	163	64	44	800	10	8	55	60	1.1	1.3	15	1.5	180	2.0	1,200	1,200	300	15	12	150	50
	19–24	58	128	164	65	46	800	10	8	60	60	1.1	1.3	15	1.6	180	2.0	1,200	1,200	280	15	12	150	55
	25–50	63	138	163	64	50	800	5	8	65	60	1.1	1.3	15	1.6	180	2.0	800	800	280	15	12	150	55
	51+	65	143	160	63	50	800	5	8	65	60	1.0	1.2	13	1.6	180	2.0	800	800	280	10	12	150	55
Pregnant						60	800	10	10	65	70	1.5	1.6	17	2.2	400	2.2	1,200	1,200	320	30	15	175	65
Lactating	1st 6 months					65	1,300	10	12	65	95	1.6	1.8	20	2.1	280	2.6	1,200	1,200	355	15	19	200	75
	2nd 6 months					62	1,200	10	11	65	90	1.6	1.7	20	2.1	260	2.6	1,200	1,200	340	15	16	200	75

[a] The allowances, expressed as average daily intakes over time, are intended to provide for individual variations among most normal persons as they live in the United States under usual environmental stresses. Diets should be based on a variety of common foods in order to provide other nutrients for which human requirements have been less well defined. See text for detailed discussion of allowances and of nutrients not tabulated.

[b] Weights and heights of Reference Adults are actual medians for the U.S. population of the designated age, as reported by NHANES II. The median weights and heights of those under 19 years of age were taken from Hamill et al. (1979) (see pages 16–17). The use of these figures does not imply that the height-to-weight ratios are ideal.

[c] Retinol equivalents. 1 retinol equivalent = 1 µg retinol or 6 µg β-carotene. See text for calculation of vitamin A activity of diets as retinol equivalents.

[d] As cholecalciferol. 10 µg cholecalciferol = 400 IU of vitamin D.

[e] α-Tocopherol equivalents. 1 mg d-α tocopherol = 1 α-TE. See text for variation in allowances and calculation of vitamin E activity of the diet as α-tocopherol equivalents.

[f] 1 NE (niacin equivalent) is equal to 1 mg of niacin or 60 mg of dietary tryptophan.

Source: Recommended Dietary Allowances 1989, permission obtained.

Table 39–7. Minerals

Mineral	Main Function	Good Sources
Calcium	Formation of bones, teeth, nerve impulses, and blood clotting	Cheese, sardines, dark green vegetables, clams, and milk
Phosphorus	Formation of bones and teeth, acid-base balance	Milk, cheese, meat, fish, poultry, nuts, and grains
Magnesium	Activation of enzymes and protein synthesis	Nuts, meats, milk, whole-grain cereal, and green leafy vegetables
Sodium	Acid-base balance, body water balance, and nerve function	Most foods except fruit
Potassium	Acid-base balance reactions, body water balance, and nerve function	Meat, milk, many fruits, cereals, vegetables, and legumes
Chloride	Gastric juice formation and acid-base balance	Table salt, seafood, milk, meat, and eggs
Sulfur	Component of tissue, cartilage	Protein foods
Iron	Component of hemoglobin and enzymes	Meats, legumes, eggs, grains, and dark-green vegetables
Zinc	Component of enzymes, digestion	Milk, shellfish, and wheat bran
Iodine	Component of thyroid hormone	Fish, dairy products, vegetables, and iodized salt
Copper	Component of enzymes, digestion	Shellfish, grains, cherries, legumes, poultry, oysters, and nuts
Manganese	Component of enzymes, fat synthesis	Greens, blueberries, grains, legumes, and fruit
Fluoride	Maintenance of bones and teeth	Water, seafood, rice, soybeans, spinach, onions, and lettuce
Chromium	Glucose and energy metabolism	Fats, meats, clams, and cereals
Selenium	Functions with vitamin E anti-oxidant	Fish, poultry, meats, grains, milk, and vegetables
Molybdenum	Component of enzymes	Legumes, cereals, dark-green leafy vegetables

four elderly women. As a natural part of the aging process, the body takes calcium from the bones more easily than it can be replaced. After menopause, calcium is removed at an even more rapid rate because of decreased quantities of estrogen. The bones then become porous and thin, and are susceptible to fracture. Lack of exercise and smoking may contribute to osteoporosis, as may excessive intake of vitamins A and D, caffeine, and alcohol.

The average intake of calcium is 550 to 600 mg/day. In postmenopausal women, this quantity should increase to 1000 to 1200 mg/day. Any of the following foods provides about 300 mg of calcium, or approximately 1/3 of the RDA: 8 oz of milk, 1 cup of yogurt, 1 oz of Swiss cheese, 2.5 oz of sardines, and 1.5 cups of ice cream. If an insufficient quantity of calcium is consumed in the diet, supplementation may be necessary. Many supplements are available, but they vary widely in elemental calcium.

The best supplement is one that supplies the highest concentration of calcium, is inexpensive, and is free from toxins, like those found in dolomite and bone meal. By these guidelines, calcium carbonate is the best choice.

Fluids

Water serves the following functions in the body: it is a solvent for chemical reactions; it maintains the stability of body fluids; it enables the transportation of nutrients to cells, provides a medium for excretion of waste products, acts as a lubricant between cells, and regulates body temperature by evaporation of perspiration from the skin. Although an individual could live without food for approximately 30 days, the absence of water would limit survival to a few days. Water represents 50 to 60% of the total body weight of an adult; a healthy adult weighing 150 lbs has 82 lbs of water (10 gallons) in his or her body.

Table 39–8. How To Increase Iron in the Diet

Food (3 oz, cooked, lean only)	Total Iron (mg)	Available Iron (mg)*
Beef		
Chuck, arm pot roast, braised	3.22	.48
Sirloin, broiled	2.85	.42
Ground, lean, broiled	1.79	.27
Pork		
Tenderloin, roasted	1.31	.15
Ham, boneless, 5–11% fat	1.19	.14
Lamb		
Loin, roasted	2.07	.31
Chicken		
Breast, roasted	.88	.13
Fish		
Tuna, light meat, canned	2.72	.31
Shellfish		
Oysters, 6 medium, raw	5.63	.63

Food	Total Iron (mg)	Available Iron (mg)**
Cereals		
Raisin bran (enriched), dry, ½ c.	4.5	.23
Oatmeal, cooked, ½ c.	.80	.04
Grains		
Bagel, 1	1.8	.09
Whole wheat bread, 1 sl.	1.0	.05
White rice (enriched), cooked, ½ c.	.9	.05
Fruits		
Apricots, dried, 7 halves	1.16	.06
Prunes, dried, 3 med.	.84	.04
Raisins, 2 tbsp.	.38	.02
Vegetables		
Potato, baked w/skin, 1 med.	2.75	.14
Peas, cooked, ½ c.	1.26	.06
Beans/Legumes		
Kidney beans, boiled, ½ c.	2.58	.13
Chickpeas, boiled, ½ c.	2.37	.12

* Available iron for individuals with 500 mg iron stores = (heme iron × 23%) + (nonheme iron × 5%). For this calculation, a figure of 5% absorption for nonheme iron was used. The heme iron content of beef, lamb and chicken was averaged as 55% and the heme iron content of pork, liver and fish as 35%.

** Available iron for individuals with 500 mg iron stores = nonheme iron × 5%. For this calculation, a figure of 5% absorption for nonheme iron was used.

Source: Adapted with permission from *Iron in Human Nutrition* with permission of the National Live Stock and Meat Board, © 1990. D. Whitmire: Vitamins and Minerals. *Sports Nutrition for the 90s. The Health Professional's Handbook.* Edited by JR Berning and SN Steen, Gaithersburg, MD, Aspen, 1991, p. 142.

Body tissues contain various amounts of water: muscle has 80%; fat, 20%, and bone, 25%. Lean individuals who have a higher percentage of muscle have a greater percentage of body water.

DIETARY GOALS AND RECOMMENDATIONS

As evidence of the connection between diet and health mounts, government agencies have made recommendations for improving Americans' health through diet. Many of these recommendations concern appropriate intake of fat (particularly saturated fat), refined sugar, and calories to reduce the incidence of nutrition-related diseases such as obesity, cardiovascular disease, and diabetes. The recommendations made by the Committee on Diet and Health of the National Research Council in 1989 are presented in Table 39–9. Data

**Table 39–9. Diet and Health: Implications for Reducing Chronic Disease Risk
Committee on Diet and Health, National Research Council**

- Reduce total fat intake to 30% or less of calories. Reduce saturated fatty acid intake to less than 10% of calories, and the intake of cholesterol to less than 300 mg dairy. The intake of fat and cholesterol can be reduced by substituting fish, poultry without skin, lean meats, and low- or nonfat dairy products for fatty meats and whole-milk dairy products; by choosing more vegetables, fruits, cereals, and legumes; and by limiting oils, fats, egg yolks, and fried and other fatty foods.
- Every day eat five or more servings of a combination of vegetables and fruits, especially green and yellow vegetables and citrus fruits. Also, increase intake of starches and other complex carbohydrates by eating six or more daily servings of a combination of breads, cereals, and legumes.
- Maintain protein intake at moderate levels.
- Balance food intake and physical activity to maintain appropriate body weight.
- The committee does not recommend alcohol consumption. For those who drink alcoholic beverages, the committee recommends limiting consumption to the equivalent of less than 1 ounce of pure alcohol in a single day. This is the equivalent of two cans of beer, two small glasses of wine, or two average cocktails. Pregnant women should avoid alcoholic beverages.
- Limit total daily intake of salt (sodium chloride) to 6 g or less. Limit the use of salt in cooking and avoid adding it to food at the table. Salty, highly processed salty, salt-preserved, and salt-pickled foods should be consumed sparingly.

gathered by the National Institutes of Health and the Agricultural Research Services of the U.S. Department of Agriculture in 1985 indicate that fat comprises 35% of the diet, and that 13% of total calories come from saturated fat. It is encouraging that these percentages have decreased from 42% and 16%, respectively, since 1977. Complex carbohydrate consumption has also increased.

Recommended Dietary Allowances

The National Research Council of the National Academy of Sciences has determined Recommended Dietary Allowances (RDAs) that represent the levels of essential nutrients considered to be adequate to meet the needs of almost all healthy people (see Table 39–6). The RDAs are applied to population groups and should not be confused with requirements for a specific individual. Because there is a margin of safety built into the RDAs, they exceed the requirements of the majority of people. Of the approximately 50 known nutrients, the RDAs have been determined for some, and estimated safe and adequate intake ranges have been identified for others. The United States Recommended Daily Allowances (U.S. RDAs) were developed by the Food and Drug Administration to be used for nutrition labeling.

READING NUTRITION LABELS

In response to consumer demands for nutrition information, companies provide nutrition labels for most products. By law, all food labels must state the net contents in terms of weight, measure, or count and the ingredients in order of descending weight. If any nutrition statement is made, such as "supplies 100% RDA of vitamin C" or "low-fat," the following information must be given: serving size; number of servings per container; calories per serving; grams of protein, carbohydrate, and fat; milligrams of sodium; and the percentages of the U.S. RDAs for protein, vitamin A, vitamin C, thiamine, riboflavin, niacin, calcium, and iron. From this information, one can calculate the percentage of calories from fat by multiplying grams of fat by 9 (fat has 9 kcal/g) and dividing by the total number of calories.

As dietary habits change, so must labeling change to provide information vital for optimal diet and health. For example, consumer groups are advocating adding information on fiber, calories from fat and saturated fat, and percentage of calories from fat. Vitamin deficiencies are now rare, so information on vitamins and minerals other than vitamins A and C and calcium and iron, which are the most likely to be deficient in the diet, is perhaps unnecessary.

As a result of the Nutritional Labeling and Education Act passed in 1990, the FDA is evaluating current food labeling practices and several proposed new designs for food labels. The FDA is also determining standard portion sizes for foods so that manufacturers can no longer call a product "reduced calorie" simply by decreasing the portion size. Public pressure is also mounting on the U.S. Department of Agriculture to revise the labels on meat and poultry, which are regulated separately from foods regulated by the FDA.

FOOD GROUPS

A basic nutrition principle is to consume a variety of foods containing a wide range of nutrients. This is the strategy behind the four food groups, in which foods are classified on the basis of their similar nutrient content. Adequate nutrition is based on combining specified numbers of servings in each group. The four food groups, along with the number of recommended daily servings, are shown in Table 39–10.

DIETARY EXCHANGE LISTS

The exchange lists consist of six groups of foods that have been classified together because of similar caloric content and similar percentages of carbohydrate, protein, and fat. Therefore, foods within a group may be exchanged for any other food of the same group. The exchange lists are used for diabetics, and are useful for weight control, because total calories can be calculated by the number of exchanges within each group. The exchange groups and a sample 1800-kcal diet are shown in Table 39–11.

NUTRITIONAL CONSIDERATIONS FOR THE ATHLETE

Athletes must adjust their diets to meet the energy demands of their sport; energy and nutrient requirements vary depending on weight, height, age, sex, and metabolic rate, and on the type, intensity, frequency, and duration of training. All athletes should consume at least 50%, but ideally 60

Table 39–10. The Four Food Groups—Minimum Number of Servings: A Guide to Making Wise Food Choices

Food Group	Recommended Number of Servings			
	Child	Teenager	Adult	Training
Milk	3	4	2	*
Milk or yogurt, 1 cup				
Cheese, 1 oz				
Cottage cheese, ½ cup				
Ice cream, ½ cup				
Meat	2	2	2	*
Cooked lean meat, fish, or poultry, 2–3 oz				
Egg, 1				
Dried beans or peas, ½ cup				
Peanut butter, 2 tbsp				
Cheese, 2 oz				
Fruits and vegetables	4	4	4	8
Cooked or juice, ½ cup				
Raw, 1 cup				
Medium piece of fruit, 1				
Grains (whole grains, fortified, enriched)	4	4	4	8
Bread, 1 slice				
Cereal (ready to eat), 1 oz				
Pasta, ½ cup				

* Same as age group
Source: Adapted with permission from *Guide to Good Eating,* 5th ed., courtesy of National Dairy Council®. JR Berning, Eating on the Road: In *Sports Nutrition for the 90's The Health Professionals Handbook.* Edited by JR Berning and SN Steen, Gaithersburg, MD, Aspen 1991, p. 65.

Table 39–11. The Dietary Exchange Groups*

Group	Serving Size	Similar Foods	Cho (g)	Protein (g)	Fat (g)	Energy (kcal)
Milk	1 c	Skim milk Yogurt from skim milk	12	8	Trace	90
Vegetable	½ c	Broccoli Cauliflower Carrots Tomatoes	5	2	0	25
Fruit	1 serving	½ c Peaches 1 small apple ½ grapefruit ½ c orange juice	15	0	0	60
Bread (starch)	1 slice	¾ c ready-to-eat cereal ¼ c baked beans 1 Waffle ½ c corn ½ c pasta 1 small potato	15	3	Trace	80
Meat (lean)	1 oz.	Chicken meat w/out skin Fish, lean beef Low-fat cheese (<5% butterfat) ¼ c canned tuna or salmon	0	7	3	55
Fat	1 tsp.	Margarine, butter, mayonnaise, oil 1 T salad dressing 1 strip crisp bacon	0	0	5	45

* Incomplete list of foods in each exchange
Note. The Exchange Lists are the basis of a meal-planning system designed by a committee of the American Diabetes Association and the American Dietetic Association. While designed primarily for people with diabetes and others who must follow special diets, the Exchange Lists are based on principles of good nutrition that apply to everyone. Copyright 1989 by American Diabetes Association, American Dietetic Association.

1,800-Calorie Diet Utilizing the Exchange System

Breakfast
1 fruit exchange
2 starch/bread exchanges
2 fat exchanges
1 milk exchange
Free foods

Lunch
1 meat exchange
2 starch/bread exchanges
1 vegetable exchange
1 fruit exchange
1 fat exchange
Free foods

Afternoon Snack
2 fruit exchanges

Dinner
2 meat exchanges
3 starch/bread exchanges
1 vegetable exchange
1 fruit exchange
2 fat exchanges
Free foods

Evening Snack
2 starch/bread exchanges
1 milk exchange
1 fruit exchange
1 fat exchange

Note. With permission from *Meal Plan/1,800 Calories.* Lilly Leadership in Diabetes Care. Eli Lilly and Company, Indianapolis, IN 46285.

to 70%, of total calories from carbohydrate. The remaining calories should be obtained from protein (10 to 15%) and fat (20 to 30%). Calories and nutrients should come from a variety of foods on a daily basis, as shown in Table 39–11.

Carbohydrate

The major source of energy for working muscles is glucose, which is stored as glycogen in both muscles and the liver. To ensure adequate glycogen stores for training, athletes must focus on consuming both adequate calories and a carbohydrate-rich diet every day. Fasting or crash dieting, eating a high-protein diet, or limiting or omitting high-carbohydrate foods from the diet can reduce carbohydrate stores to inadequate levels. If the athlete does not consume enough carbohydrate, fatigue and weakness will result. If the athlete finds that normal exercise intensity is difficult to maintain and that performance gradually deteriorates, a lack of carbohydrate in the diet may be the cause.

How much carbohydrate the athlete should eat every day depends on the athlete's size. In general, athletes should eat 5 to 6 g of carbohydrate per kg of body weight. Consuming more than 600 grams of carbohydrate per day will not result in proportionately greater amounts of muscle glycogen. Excess carbohydrate is stored as fat.

The rate at which muscles store glycogen is increased during the first 2 hours after exercise. From a practical standpoint, an athlete should consume 100 g of carbohydrate (400 kcal) within 15 to 30 minutes after exercise, to be followed by additional 100-g feedings of carbohydrate every 2 to 4 hours afterward. Table 39–12 lists foods high in carbohydrate.

Carbohydrate loading is a technique that can increase muscle glycogen levels to above normal. For 3 to 5 days before competition, the athlete consumes a high-carbohydrate (7 to 10 g/kg) and tapers training. The final day before the event requires total rest and maintaining the same high-carbohydrate diet. Although this regimen may benefit the athlete participating in endurance sports (90 minutes or more of nonstop effort), there is no advantage to

Table 39–12. Some Foods High in Carbohydrates (By Food Group)

Foods	Grams of Cho
Milk Group	
Chocolate milkshake (10 oz)	58
Blueberry yogurt (1 c)	42
Ice milk (½ c)	14
Low-fat milk	12
Protein Group	
Pinto beans (½ c)	23
Refried beans (½ c)	23
Meatloaf (3 oz)	13
Fruit & Vegetable Group	
Baked potato	51
Cranberry juice cocktail (1 c)	37
Raisins (¼ c)	29
Grapes (1 c)	28
Banana	27
Orange juice (1 c)	26
Applesauce (½ c)	25
Pear	25
French fries (10)	20
Corn (½ c)	20
Fruit Roll-ups (1 roll)	12
Watermelon (1 c)	12
Grain Group	
Bagel	38
Rice (½ c)	28
English muffin	28
Corn Flakes (1 oz)	24
Raisin Bran (1 oz)	21
Hot dog bun	21
Commercial High-Carbohydrate Drinks	
Exceed High Carbohydrate Source (12 oz)	89
Carboplex (12 oz)	81
Gatorade (12 oz)	70

most athletes, particularly those in start-and-stop sports.

The *pre-event meal* should be consumed 3 to 4 hours before competition and should include readily digested foods and fluids that are familiar to the athlete. These requirements can be met by including foods high in complex carbohydrate and low in fat and protein. Ingestion of salty, high-fiber, or gaseous foods should be minimized before competition. Liberal intake of fluids is needed for adequate hydration.

Fat

Although fat is a valuable metabolic fuel for muscle activity during longer-term aerobic exercise, fat intake should not exceed 30% of daily calories. In addition to health reasons, athletes who consume a high-fat diet typically eat fewer calories from carbohydrate.

Protein

Although stronger muscles can improve performance, consumption of large amounts of protein does not increase muscle size. In fact, the most important factor in increasing strength is not what the athlete eats but how the athlete trains. How much strength is gained depends on the intensity and type of weight training and heredity.

Daily protein requirements vary according to the type of sport (strength versus endurance), intensity of training, stage of training, and most importantly, the energy balance of the diet. Between 1 and 1.5 grams of protein per kg of body weight is enough *if* sufficient calories are consumed. For a 145-lb (66 kg) athlete, this would be 66 to 99 grams of protein. There are approximately 10 grams of protein in 1 ounce of meat, an egg, 8 ounces of milk, 1 ounce of cheese, or 4 slices of bread.

Athletes may buy amino acids because promoters claim that they stimulate an anabolic effect, stimulate growth, and reduce body fat. Amino acids are sold individually or in "special" combinations. Arginine and ornithine are sold as "natural steroids," and arginine and lysine are touted as promoting weight loss. These claims are unfounded.

Fluids

Water is the most important nutrient for any athlete during any phase of training or competition. Water comprises approximately 60 to 70% of body weight, and as little as a 2% decrease in body weight from fluid loss can lead to a significant decrease in muscular strength and stamina. For a 125-lb (57 kg) male, this 2% water loss would translate into a 2.5-lb drop in weight. Because a substantial level of dehydration can occur before the body feels "thirsty,"

athletes must consume fluids before (8 to 12 ounces 15 minutes before), during (3 to 4 ounces every 10 to 15 minutes), and after exercise (16 ounces for every pound lost).

For exercise bouts lasting less than 60 minutes, water is recommended as a fluid replacement. However, when the workout period exceeds 60 minutes, sports drinks can be beneficial, as they also supply energy and electrolytes, which are key ingredients for maximum fluid absorption. The best fluid replacement beverage is one that tastes good to the athlete and works well in his or her individual training regimen, does not cause gastrointestinal distress when consumed in large volumes, promotes rapid fluid absorption and maintenance of extracellular fluid volume, and provides energy (8 ounces of sports drink should provide between 14 and 19 grams of carbohydrate and between 50 and 80 kg).

Salt tablets should not be taken because they can irritate the stomach lining, cause nausea, and increase the body's need for water. Sweat contains proportionately more water, sodium, and potassium than does blood plasma. Therefore, it is important to replace fluid losses first.

Supplementation

Although it has been shown that a severely inadequate intake of certain vitamins can impair performance, it is unusual for an athlete to experience such deficiencies. Even marginal vitamin deficiencies do not appear to affect to any great extent the ability to exercise efficiently. The athlete who "crash diets" in an effort to lose weight by popping vitamins and minerals does not supply the body with adequate calories.

Indiscriminate use of supplements does not guarantee a high level of performance. Overconsumption can lead to toxicity as well as a false sense of security, and may in fact alter the utilization of other nutrients. The bottom line is that megadoses of supplements do not make up for a lack of training or talent, nor do they give any athlete an edge over the competition.

For athletes who maintain a low body weight or repeatedly lose weight, consumption of a one-a-day multivitamin/mineral supplement is prudent. Iron-deficiency anemia is a problem for some athletes, particularly female athletes and long-distance runners, so supplementation under medical supervision is indicated. For the female athlete, adequate consumption of calcium is critical because low levels can lead to stress fractures and osteoporosis.

A balance of mental concentration, physical training, and a high-performance eating plan are all key components to achieving optimal conditioning. The athlete should recognize the powerful role that nutrition plays in successful training and strive to optimize a high-carbohydrate, low-fat, nutrient-balanced diet for his or her personal regimen.

ASSESSING DIETARY INTAKE

Direct observation of food intake is the most precise method of assessment, but is expensive and may influence the behavior being evaluated. Hence, a number of more cost-efficient and less reactive measures have been used. To obtain dietary information without influencing it is difficult, and the report of food intake may depend on what the person believes the professional wants to see or hear. Some individuals may have difficulty in recording or remembering types and amounts of foods eaten. In addition, data regarding the nutrient composition of foods are incomplete for certain nutrients (e.g., magnesium and B_6). To obtain an accurate description of dietary patterns, objectivity and skill on the part of a qualified health professional are required. Several techniques may be used.

A *24-hour recall* is simple and rapid, and is particularly useful for surveying large population groups. The individual is asked to recall the foods and beverages consumed within the previous 24 hours. Pertinent information concerning portion size, food preparation, alcohol consumption, and vitamin and mineral supplementation are obtained.

A more complete picture can be obtained from a *food intake record* in which the individual records types and amounts of all foods and beverages consumed during a specified length of time, usually 3 or 7 days. The 3-day food record, which includes two weekdays and one weekend day, is representative for most people. The individual

is instructed to carry the food record at all times and to record food items immediately after eating. To increase the accuracy of the data, respondents should be advised about portion sizes by use of plastic food models, utensils, and a description of household measures.

A *food frequency record* evaluates the number of times per day, week, or month an individual consumes particular foods and beverages. This information can be used as a cross-check for the 24-hour recall and helps to clarify patterns of food consumption. The food frequency analysis may include questions about all foods, or it may be selective for specific foods suspected of being deficient or excessive in the diet (e.g., foods high in fat or sodium). The food frequency typically provides only qualitative data and relies upon the individual's memory.

A *diet history* is a more complete assessment that includes a 24-hour recall and food frequency. In addition, individuals supply information about economic status, physical activity, ethnic background, appetite, dental and oral health, gastrointestinal function, chronic disease, medications, supplements, and recent weight changes.

Interpreting Dietary Intake

In general, interpretation of intake should be performed by a nutritionist or registered dietitian. Two methods can be used to evaluate dietary intake for nutrient adequacy. The first method is a fast, crude estimate that involves estimating the number of servings from the four foods groups that were consumed during the day recorded, and comparing them to what is recommended (see Table 39–6). Low intake of protein, iron, calcium, riboflavin, and vitamins A and C can be detected in this way. The dietary goals can be used for rough evaluation of nutrients consumed in excess, such as fat, cholesterol, sugar, and sodium.

The second method is more accurate and involves calculating the nutrients present in every food consumed. This process can be done by hand, with the use of USDA food composition books and information from manufacturers and food labels, or with a computerized nutrient data bank or computer software program. (The sources used for nutrient composition vary for computer programs, and each should be evaluated carefully before a choice is made for analysis.)

After determining the nutrient composition for each food, the composition of the total diet can be calculated. A comparison can be made to a desired standard such as that of the RDA. The assumption cannot be made, however, that if an individual has an inadequate intake of a certain nutrient that they are deficient in that nutrient. The individual must give a thorough history, be examined for clinical signs of a deficiency, and undergo biochemical tests before a deficiency can be confirmed.

FACILITATING CHANGES IN DIETARY BEHAVIOR

Professionals tend to believe that providing nutritional information changes eating behavior. This assumption is probably faulty. Dietary habits in the United States would be altered dramatically if individuals simply practiced what most of us learned before we were teenagers—that we should eat a balanced diet from the four food groups.

There is clear evidence of dietary change occurring because of large-scale educational efforts. Per capita consumption of whole milk and red meat has declined, and the rate of consumption of skim milk and chicken has increased; in fact, in 1990, per capita consumption of chicken was higher than that of beef for the first time. Millions of people are concerned about what they eat, read food labels, and seek out restaurants with lighter foods, salad bars, and the like. The climate is right for encouraging even broader changes. What skills are necessary?

General Principles of Behavior Change

Specific steps can aid an individual in changing general dietary practices or in altering specific nutrient intake (e.g., salt, fat). The first step is to assess motivation for change. Some individuals are ready to change and can be guided through certain steps. Other individuals may require more encouragement.

Analyzing Eating Patterns

Dietary change is facilitated by an analysis of eating patterns. Methods for assessing the types and amounts of food were discussed previously. This information can identify how the diet compares to the recommended diet. Other patterns, such as time of eating, association of eating with certain moods, and problems with specific foods can be highlighted with a diet diary. The person records what he or she eats, the time, location, mood, and other relevant information. Patterns typically emerge from keeping such a record for several weeks. The information can be motivational and can provide targets for change.

Instruction

Relevant information can be provided on a healthy diet. The information could be general or specific, depending on the individual. For someone with no special dietary needs, general information can be provided. For persons with known problems, such as diabetes, hypercholesterolemia, or hypertension, more detailed aid is needed. Special meal plans, focused cookbooks, and food preparation classes may be helpful.

Goal Setting

The establishment of reasonable goals is important. A person suddenly motivated to eat a healthier diet because of pressure from family, doctor's orders, or social pressure may begin with a burst of motivation. Wholesale changes in the diet are the rule for such people, but the changes tend to be transient. A man told by his physician that his family history of heart disease is a reason to reduce dietary fat may hear tales of dramatic improvement in people on strict diets such as the Pritikin plan. He may forsake his favorite foods and begin eating foods he may not enjoy, a difficult plan to follow. A more sensible plan for him might be to drop his fat consumption in 5% increments until compliance begins to suffer.

Altering the Eating Environment

Structuring the eating environment can take several forms. Keeping healthy foods available and problem foods out of the house can reduce temptation and curb automatic or compulsive eating. The individual can benefit from instruction about how to shop for food in a careful and planned manner and to store, prepare, and serve food in ways that promote better eating.

SUMMARY

Adequate nutrition is essential for health and well-being. Much is known about specific types and amounts of food for optimal health, but eating behavior does not change easily. Applying current knowledge on assessing and modifying dietary behavior, and combining this with principles of nutrition education, can be instrumental in changing eating habits, and hence improving public health.

SUGGESTED READING

General Nutrition

1. Committee on Dietary Allowances, Food and Nutrition Board: *Recommended Dietary Allowances.* 9th Ed. Washington, DC: National Academy of Sciences, 1989.
2. Shils ME, Young VR: *Modern Nutrition in Health and Disease.* 7th Ed. Philadelphia: Lea & Febiger, 1988.
3. Guthrie HA: *Introductory Nutrition.* 7th Ed. St. Louis: Mosby Yearbook, 1988.
4. Krause ME, Mahan LK: *Food, Nutrition, and Diet Therapy.* 7th Ed. Philadelphia: WB Saunders, 1984.
5. Willett W. *Nutritional Epidemiology.* New York: Oxford University Press, 1990.
6. U.S. Department of Health and Human Services. *Surgeon's General's Report on Nutrition and Health.* Washington, DC: U.S. Government Printing Office (DHHS Pub. No. 88-50210), 1988.
7. National Research Council, National Academy of Sciences. *Diet and Health: Implications for Reducing Chronic Disease Risk.* Washington, DC: National Academy Press, 1989.

Sports Nutrition

1. Berning JR, Steen SN (eds.): *Sports Nutrition for the 90s: The Health Professional's Handbook.* Gaithersburg, MD: Aspen, 1991.
2. Clark N: *Nancy Clark's Sports Nutrition Guidebook: Eating to Fuel Your Active Lifestyle.* Champaign, IL: Leisure Press, 1990.
3. Coleman E: *Eating for Endurance.* Palo Alto, CA: Bull Publishing, 1988.
4. Katch FI, McArdle WD: *Nutrition, Weight Control, and Exercise,* 3rd Ed. Philadelphia: Lea & Febiger, 1988.
5. Peterson M, Peterson K: *Eat to Compete.* Chicago: Mosby, Yearbook Medical Publishers, 1989.

Chapter 40

SMOKING CESSATION

Andrew M. Gottlieb, David P. L. Sachs, and Barbara R. Newman

HEALTH RISKS OF SMOKING

Cigarette smoking is one of the key risk factors for premature death from heart disease, lung disease, and cancer. Of the 50 million Americans who smoke regularly, approximately 420,000 die of premature illness each year. Although most people are aware of the link between smoking and cancer, far fewer individuals understand the causal relationship between smoking and heart disease.

The risk of heart disease is directly related to the number of cigarettes smoked. Smoking one pack per day doubles the risk compared to nonsmoking; smoking more than one pack per day triples the risk. The main mechanisms that affect the development of heart disease are the effects of carbon monoxide. Nicotine in tobacco smoke causes increases in heart rate and blood pressure, which lead to increased work for the heart. It also may increase platelet adhesiveness, changing blood viscosity inside blood vessels. Carbon monoxide interferes with the ability of red blood cells to carry oxygen, thereby reducing the oxygen supply delivered to the heart muscle.

HEALTH BENEFITS OF QUITTING SMOKING

The health benefits of quitting smoking are immediate and substantial. They extend to the young and the old, to those with and without smoking-related disease. Smoking cessation represents the single most important step that smokers can take to enhance the length and quality of their lives.[1]

Although the risks from smoking are cumulative, the increased risk of cancer and heart disease drops rapidly after stopping smoking, even when the person has smoked for many years.[2,3] After 2½ years of nonsmoking, the risk of lung cancer is reduced by 50%. Within 3 to 5 years of nonsmoking, the risk of a heart attack is that of a nonsmoker, and within 5 to 10 years, the risk of major health problems decreases to levels only slightly greater than those of people who have never smoked. Besides the obvious major health benefits, many other benefits result, including increased energy, improved sense of smell, the ability to exercise more easily, and higher self-esteem.

WHY PEOPLE SMOKE

To counsel smokers effectively, it is useful to understand that both physical and psychologic components drive smoking behavior.[4,5] Physical dependence on nicotine is one major factor. Each cigarette puff delivers a "hit" of nicotine to the brain within 7 seconds, making smoking one of the most effective drug delivery systems known. The average smoker may self-administer 50,000 to 70,000 nicotine doses a year. Nicotine appears to have both stimulating and tranquilizing effects, depending on dosage. Evidence exists that nicotine may increase the production of brain hormones, such as beta-endorphins. This effect may explain why nicotine can reduce the perception of pain and increase feelings of well-being. The smoker can "fine-tune" emotional responses by varying the puff rate and puff depth to control the amount of nicotine delivered to the brain. Thus, the smoker literally has fingertip control of the emotional and physical responses, reducing the need for other coping techniques. Once a person becomes dependent on these effects of smoking to function normally, quitting becomes extremely difficult.

The other major component is conditioned psychologic dependence. The thousands of nicotine doses received each year are linked to situations and emotional states. Each of these situations and emotional states then becomes a cue to the smoker that it is time for a cigarette puff. Situational cues include such things as drinking coffee or an alcoholic beverage, talking on the phone, watching TV, finishing a meal, or driving. Other cues are negative emotions, such as anger, frustration, stress, or boredom.

CESSATION

The Quitting Process

The experience of quitting smoking varies a great deal among smokers. Some smokers quit "easily" and report their surprise at how much easier quitting was than they had expected; some report that quitting was the most difficult thing that they ever attempted; and others report some degree of difficulty between these two extremes. Some report the physical factors being the primary difficulty, some the psychologic factors, and others report both.

Withdrawal from nicotine can produce a variety of effects, including craving for tobacco, increased anxiety, increased irritability, increased restlessness, difficulty in concentrating, headache, drowsiness, and gastrointestinal disturbances. These symptoms are generally most intense for the first 2 to 3 days after cessation, decrease but then increase again around day 10, finally to decrease gradually thereafter. The acute phase of nicotine withdrawal is generally over within 2 to 4 weeks, although some withdrawal symptoms, such as the urge to smoke, can continue for months or even years. The number of withdrawal symptoms reported varies from none to many, and severity varies from mild to severe. Nearly 90% of smokers experience at least one withdrawal symptom.

Most smokers quit smoking a number of times before achieving long-term abstinence. The majority of smokers who relapse do so within the first 6 months after quitting; some relapse years after cessation, but they are the exception. As the duration of abstinence increases, relapse becomes less likely.[1] Many smokers are able to quit for short periods, but *maintaining* smoking cessation is a major challenge.

Approaches to Smoking Cessation

The large majority of people who have quit smoking report that they have done so on their own, without the help of a formal program or a health professional. Formal smoking cessation programs can be helpful to smokers who cannot quit on their own, often those who smoke more heavily and are more addicted.[6,7]

To guide a smoker to appropriate assistance for smoking cessation, it is important to know the options available, their effectiveness, and potential barriers to participation (cost, location, time, and cultural biases).[6] The appropriateness of a group program versus individual sessions with a health professional needs to be considered. When examining effectiveness, it is important to look at the long-term quit rate of a strategy or program because relapse is common. Some programs boast high initial quit rates, but fail to report long-term relapse rates. There is no "magic bullet" available, at any cost, that can guarantee long-term quitting. However, there is help in various forms to assist any smoker who would like to quit.

Smoking cessation techniques include: (1) pharmacologic interventions; (2) behavioral interventions; and (3) other strategies such as acupuncture and hypnosis. Stop-smoking programs are available in various formats: self-help materials (with or without minimal contact), group meetings, and individual sessions with a health professional. Many studies have been conducted evaluating various behavioral and pharmacologic smoking cessation approaches, allowing us to identify with some confidence the approaches that work.

Pharmacologic Interventions

Early pharmacologic interventions included Pronicotyl, a spice tablet, and silver acetate, which were supposed to make cigarettes taste foul when inhaled. They were generally ineffective, or only minimally effective. Lobeline, a nicotine analogue sold as CigArrest, Bantron, and Nicoban, has no advantage over placebo. More recently, some researchers have reported that clonidine hydrochloride reduces tobacco withdrawal symptoms and facilitates smoking cessation. Research findings to date, unfortunately, have been mixed regarding clonidine's effectiveness.

The most promising pharmacologic interventions currently in widespread use are nicotine replacement by nicotine polacrilex (Nicorette) and transdermal nicotine patch (Habitrol, Nicoderm, Nicotrol, and Prostep). Both are available by prescription and designed to provide a partial substitute for the nicotine obtained from cigarettes, to make the initial phase of tobacco withdrawal less unpleasant, allowing the person to learn new ways of coping with the behavioral aspects of smoking cessation (unlinking smoking-related cues from actual cigarette smoking). Nicotine replacement treatment should be used for *at least* 10 weeks following quitting; most smokers need 6 months of treatment, and some need treatment for 1 to 2 years before being able to successfully taper off nicotine medication.

Nicorette (nicotine polacrilex), 2 mg available since 1984, has nicotine bound to a resin base. When the medication is chewed, nicotine is released and is absorbed through the oral mucosa. Nicorette, 4 mg should be available in the United States by late 1992 or early 1993. It is currently available in Canada and Europe. Most researchers have reported impressive improvements in quit rates, but this has not been the case consistently. Researchers are continuing to examine ways to increase the effectiveness of nicotine polacrilex. It is necessary that clear chewing instructions and a behavioral change component accompany a Nicorette prescription.[8,9] When advising a smoker, it is important to steer the individual to either a behavioral program in which nicotine polacrilex use is an integral part or to a physician who will provide good follow-up care along with this medication.

Studies show that the effectiveness of nicotine polacrilex, 2 mg is influenced by the behavioral intervention component that accompanies it.[4,5] When there is no behavioral component, with a physican simply phoning in a prescription to a pharmacy, nicotine polacrilex can be expected to be no more effective than placebo at the one year follow-up; however, if the behav-

ioral intervention is even minimal, a significant effect can be expected. With addition of nicotine polacrilex to physician advice, studies have shown the 1-year quit rate going from approximately 5% to 9%; with addition of physician advice plus follow-up, from 15% to 27%; and with addition of a comprehensive group counseling program, from 16% to 38%. Studies in which investigators combined behavior modification approaches with nicotine polacrilex use have produced 1-year quit rates of over 40%.

The nicotine patch was approved for use in the United States by the FDA in late 1991, and has been available since then. Smokers and health professionals alike are happy to have the patches available because they provide a much easier route for nicotine delivery than does nicotine polacrilex. However, the patch is not the "magic bullet" for which many smokers were hoping. Patches come in three sizes, $30cm^2$, $20cm^2$, and $10cm^2$, delivering nicotine for 24 hours a day (Habitrol, Nicoderm and Prostep) or 16 hours a day (Nicotrol). The 24-hour patches deliver 21, 14, and 7 mg of nicotine a day depending upon the size; the 16-hour patches deliver 15, 10, and 5 mg of nicotine a day. Nicotine patches are applied once a day. Most smokers who use the 24-hour patches start out with the 21 mg patch and then go down to the 14 and 7 mg patches for nicotine tapering. Most smokers who use the 16-hour patches start with the 15 mg patch and then go down to the 10 and 5 mg patches. In a study of 935 participants, 6-month sustained abstinence rates for those receiving the nicotine patch were significantly higher than for those receiving placebo (26% versus 12%). One year abstinence rates are not available. The researchers concluded that the transdermal systems show considerable promise as an *aid* to smoking cessation.[10] A behavioral component should accompany the patch during a smoking cessation attempt. As with nicotine polacrilex, more needs to be learned about increasing the effectiveness of the nicotine patch.

Behavioral Interventions

Behavioral interventions, which include components such as self-monitoring, contracts, and assertiveness skills training, are often included in stop-smoking programs.

One of the most effective techniques is rapid smoking; when properly administered, this approach has had long-term abstinence rates of 64 to 70%. Rapid smoking is a multicomponent treatment that involves several different elements, including relapse prevention training (see subsequent discussion) and rapid smoking, in which the patient inhales smoke from his own cigarette every 6 seconds until he no longer wants to take another puff. The procedure creates an aversion to smoking that, when combined with skills training, leads to good cessation outcomes. This technique must not be attempted without proper support and guidance from a health professional.

Relapse prevention is a behavioral approach to maintaining smoking cessation. Relapse prevention teaches people to anticipate situations in which they will be tempted to smoke, and to develop new coping methods for avoiding relapse in these situations.[11] Simple questionnaires developed by Edward Lichtenstein at the University of Oregon can be used to measure a smoker's confidence in his ability to resist smoking during exposure to high-risk situations.[12] These questionnaires can be helpful in determining the types of coping skills on which to focus attention.

The relapse prevention approach is particularly valuable in smoking cessation. As Mark Twain said, "Quitting smoking is easy; I have done it many times." "Staying quit" is difficult.

Other Techniques

Smokers are often attracted to acupuncture or hypnosis as "the magic bullet"—an easy way to achieve long-term smoking cessation. Controlled studies have failed to show any positive correlation between acupuncture and smoking cessation.[13] Hypnosis can be provided individually or in groups, for one or multiple sessions. Often hypnosis is combined with other behavioral techniques. Study methodology has made it impossible to evaluate the effectiveness of hypnosis as an aid to long-term cessation.

Stop-Smoking Programs

Programs are available in a variety of formats. In a self-help/minimal intervention format, a smoker works on his or her own to quit smoking without the continued assistance of health professionals, trained leaders, or organizations. The smoker devises ways to quit and stay off cigarettes using a self-help book or guide. A study using the American Lung Association's *Freedom From Smoking in 20 Days*, one of the manuals available, reported a 1-year quit rate of 5% (versus 2% for controls). Generally, self-help programs report substantially lower quit rates than more formal programs, but they are low-cost and generally available to many smokers. Efforts are under way to maximize the effectiveness of self-help programs.[14]

Programs using a group format provide a support group that some smokers find helpful. The content, cost, and providers of these programs vary. Health organizations, as well as commercial groups, typically offer these programs. Few well-designed studies have been done to evaluate any of these programs. When specific programs boast of high success rates, it is important to ask about long-term (ideally 1 year, but at least 6 months) rates, and how they were determined.

Some smokers prefer working with a health professional on an individual basis. When choosing this format, it is important to check on the approaches used and the qualifications of the health professional.

Research studies at medical schools and other medical facilities provide another source of help for smokers. Some smokers like being a part of a research endeavor because this is often somewhat different from what they have tried during past quitting attempts.

How To Help Someone Stop Smoking

Exercise leaders are often asked to help someone stop smoking. The following guidelines have been found useful as aids to promote successful quitting.

1. Advise the smoker to quit.

Advice to quit from a health professional with good rapport with the patient or participant may have substantial impact. For example, studies show that 60 seconds of definitive advice from a physician have substantial impact on long-term (1 year) quit rate, increasing it 17-fold in one study.[15] Advice should be clear, succinct, and unequivocal regarding the dangers of smoking and the benefit of quitting for that individual. If you can, time your discussion to occur when your client is experiencing symptoms caused by, attributed to, or exacerbated by smoking, such as coughing, shortness of breath, or angina. Avoid being moralistic or punitive. Emphasize the benefits your client will experience after quitting. Advise the client to completely eliminate tobacco products. There are NO healthy tobacco products, and virtually no smokers can smoke in a limited way.

2. Work with the smoker to develop a specific plan for cessation. HELP THE SMOKER CHOOSE A SPECIFIC QUIT DATE.

A specific quit date will help the smoker prepare for nonsmoking. Review prior quit attempts to evaluate what was helpful and identify the problems. Reframe past relapses in a positive light by emphasizing that past attempts can teach something useful. Tell the smoker that most successful long-term quitters have made more than one quit attempt.

Inform the smoker about sources of help in the community such as self-help/minimal contact programs, group programs, and individual health professionals who work with patients. A list of the programs, with names and phone numbers for additional information is available, as well as information about the components of the program, format, cost, and the effectiveness of the interventions used. Good sources of information concerning local programs include local universities, medical groups, hospitals, and agencies such as the American Cancer Society, American Lung Association, and American Heart Association.

3. Encourage the smoker's efforts to quit and provide support during difficult times.

Help to motivate the client by asking about any positive health benefits or other positive things that have occurred as a result of quitting, such as increased stamina, better breathing, less coughing, and improved sense of smell. Reassure the person that withdrawal symptoms are temporary, and that they are a sign that the body is learning to get along without the nicotine. Because relapse is very common after quitting, you can ask the person about difficult times and help him or her identify ways to handle those situations.

Some of the smokers with whom you talk might not be ready to quit immediately but will change their minds at a later date. The smoker who is not ready to quit may be concerned about the negative impact of quitting or his or her ability to succeed. If you can determine these factors, you can address them. Gentle but firm reminders about the importance of quitting can also influence motivation to make the attempt to quit.

4. Respond to concern about weight gain accompanying smoking cessation.

Smokers might express concern about weight gain, either as a reason not to quit or after they have stopped smoking. Approximately 80% of smokers who quit gain weight after cessation. The average weight gain is about 5 pounds. Increases in food intake and/or decreases in energy expenditure may be at least partially responsible for postcessation weight gain. The health benefits of smoking cessation far exceed any risks from the average weight gain.[1] Suggestions such as increasing physical activity, eating low-fat sweets in response to an increased desire for sweet foods, and having low-calorie snacks available might be helpful.

SUMMARY

Cigarette smoking is the leading preventable cause of death. Smoking cessation has major and immediate health benefits for all smokers. Advice to quit smoking from you, a health professional with good rapport with your clients, may have substantial impact.

Millions of smokers have quit. For some smokers, quitting is difficult. Both physical and psychologic factors contribute to maintaining cigarette smoking behavior. There is no "magic bullet," but there is help. Most smokers quit on their own; most successful long-term quitters have made a number of short-term attempts to quit before achieving long-term abstinence.

A variety of techniques are available to help smokers who want to quit but are unable to do so on their own. Programs that include nicotine replacement in conjunction with behavioral interventions currently provide the best results. It is important to encourage smokers to quit, and to reframe past quit attempts in a positive light, providing information to help with the next attempt to quit.

REFERENCES

1. U.S. Department of Health and Human Services: *The Health Benefits of Smoking Cessation*. Public Health Service, Centers for Disease Control, Center for Chronic Disease Prevention and Health Promotion, Office on Smoking and Health. DHHS Publication No. (CDC) 90-8416, 1990.
2. Sachs DPL: Cigarette smoking: Health effects and cessation strategies. *Clin Geriatr Med*, 2:337, 1986.
3. Schuman LM: The benefits of cessation of smoking. *Chest*, 59:421, 1971.
4. Sachs DPL, Leischow SJ: Pharmacologic approaches to smoking cessation. *Clin Chest Med*, 12:769, 1991.
5. Sachs DPL: Advances in smoking cessation treatment. *Curr Pulmonol*, 12:139, 1991.
6. Fiore MC, Novotny TE, Pierce JP, et al.: Methods used to quit smoking in the United States. Do cessation programs help? *JAMA*, 263:2760, 1990.
7. Glynn TJ: Methods of smoking cessation—Finally some answers (editorial). *JAMA*, 263:2795, 1990.
8. Pomerleau OF, Pomerleau CS (eds.): *Nicotine Replacement—A Critical Evaluation. Progress in Clinical and Biological Research.* Volume 261. New York: Alan R. Liss, Inc., 1988.
9. Sachs DPL: Nicotine polacrilex: Practical use requirements. *Curr Pulmonol*, 10:141, 1989.
10. Transdermal Nicotine Study Group: Transdermal nicotine for smoking cessation. Six-month results from two multicenter controlled clinical trials. *JAMA*, 266:3133, 1991.
11. Marlatt GA, Gordon J: *Relapse Prevention: Maintenance Strategies in the Treatment of Addictive Behaviors.* New York: Guilford Press, 1985.
12. Condiotte MM, Lichtenstein E: Self-efficacy and relapse in smoking cessation programs. *J Consult Clin Psychol*, 49:648, 1981.
13. Ter Riet G, Kleijnen J, Knipschild P: A meta-analysis of studies into the effect of acupuncture on addiction. *Br J Gen Pract*, 40:379, 1990.
14. Glynn TJ, Boyd GM, Gruman JC: Essential elements of self-help/minimal intervention strategies for smoking cessation. *Health Educ Q*, 17:329, 1990.
15. Russell MAH, Wilson C, Taylor C, et al.: Effect of general practitioners' advice against smoking. *Br Med J*, 2:231, 1979.

Chapter 41

STRESS MANAGEMENT AND CORONARY HEART DISEASE: RISK ASSESSMENT AND INTERVENTION

Wesley E. Sime, Mike McGahan, and Robert S. Eliot

The topic of stress management is extremely popular as indicated by the large number of books and articles published on the subject. It is estimated that emotional stress accounts for nearly 50% of all physician visits, with a substantial number of these being related to cardiac symptoms. It is not surprising, perhaps, that populist opinion exceeds the scientific data supporting several areas of stress research.

The evidence that stress is an important risk factor for coronary heart disease (CHD) is modest in contrast to the data on smoking, lipids, and hypertension. However, ample evidence demonstrates an interaction between emotional stress and other risk factors or atherogenic markers of disease. Specifically, chronic psychologic stress in the presence of elevated cholesterol induces endothelial injury and advances the development of atherosclerosis.[1] Furthermore, the pathophysiologic route by which stress influences CHD is similar to that of smoking and hypertension.[2,3] Coronary vasoconstriction, arterial wall hardening, and atherosclerotic plaque have been observed outcomes of stress imposed on laboratory animals.[4] These vascular changes are particularly conducive to myocardial ischemia under conditions of anger and fear, as noted in laboratory studies on dogs.[5] Furthermore, these vascular changes are commonly associated with vasospasm and a higher incidence of cardiac arrythmias[6,7] as well as sudden death.[8]

At the tissue level, one mechanism by which stress may influence atherogenesis involves endothelial injury. Specifically, hypothalamic stimulation has been shown in laboratory studies to cause vasospasm, which ultimately results in severe endothelial damage with cell loss and denudation in the aorta and coronary arteries.[9] Other physiologic changes caused by stress expo-sure include increased blood pressure, which in turn can have pathophysiologic consequences through increased shearing forces on the arterial wall; increased circulating catecholamine levels, which can damage the arterial wall and the myocardium; and increased incidence of ventricular arrhythmia, a known risk factor for sudden coronary death.[10-12] In addition, such stress leads to increased levels of free fatty acid and serum cholesterol related to sympathetic activation of the liver, as well as increased platelet adhesion and aggregation in the arteries, because of elevated catecholamine levels.[13,14] Such a combination could set the stage for the development of atheromatous plaques in the coronary arteries, which in turn may potentiate CHD. Emotional stress of this type can also lead to increases in sodium levels and thus fluid retention in humans; in addition, release of epinephrine leads to loss of plasma potassium.[15,16] This combination of sodium retention and plasma potassium loss could lead to important ion imbalances, which set the stage for the aforementioned ventricular arrhythmias.

Although the evidence from laboratory animal studies and selected clinical studies is encouraging, a need remains to identify a higher-order mechanism that may demonstrate a behavioral variable that predisposes the stress-CHD link. One prominent theory is that the cardiac pathophysiology originates partly from excessive cardiovascular reactivity caused by sympatho-adrenal responses.[17] Support for this theory has been shown in studies in which high levels of cardiovascular reactivity in the presence of a high fat diet are clearly associated with the development of atherosclerosis.[18] In addition, heart rate reactivity to stress has been shown to be directly related to increased levels of cholesterol in humans.[19]

Type A individuals with elevated cholesterol also had larger cortisol secretion in response to a math test.[20] These results provide further support for the interactive role of psychologic stress in CHD risk factors.

DEFINITION AND THEORIES OF EMOTIONAL STRESS

To help patients understand these concepts, we suggest that stress be defined as any physical, psychologic, or cognitive event of either a negative (adverse) or positive (exhilarating) nature, which elicits a physiologic response requiring significant homeostatic adaptation. When this adaptation is either excessive or prolonged, the deviation from baseline levels can be referred to as "strain." In addition, these strain responses, resulting from stressful stimuli, may yield pathophysiologic consequences if they are experienced with great intensity and/or high frequency over time. The nature of the pathophysiologic findings is determined primarily by individual factors that predispose a person to one or more of various stress-related illness.

The relationship of stress to illness has been shown to include a critical role for cognitive appraisal as described by Lazarus.[21] It is the foundational element in his specificity model of illness, which illustrates that any person-environment stressor is first mediated by individual appraisal, thus determining the extent to which physiologic disturbance and possible illness occur. Because emotional stress is the appropriate distinctive label for this discussion (as opposed to environmental or exertional stress), it should be noted that Lazarus's cognitive-motivational-relational theory of emotion is an outgrowth of the appraisal model.[22] Lazarus has shown that emotions result from the way an individual constructs and evaluates events or relationships in light of his or her goals and expectations. Conflicts and untoward events have an effect only to the degree that one allows according to the cognitive interpretation. This theory is the basis for several stress management techniques presented later in this chapter.

Lazarus has suggested that stress may emanate from the reaction to change (cataclysmic and cumulative) or hassles and that temporal dimensions of stress range from acute to chronic with sequential or intermittent onset.[21] However, it is the individual difference in vulnerability that determines risk of illness.

Stress can also be viewed in terms of the response elicited by certain standardized events within any one individual. In this manner, stress or the reaction to stress can be measured and quantified for comparison of individual differences or for the analysis of change caused by intervention. For example, individual differences in stress tolerance can be observed from the presentation of simple tasks such as quizzes, mental arithmetic tasks, and cold pressor tests, which cause dramatic changes in the cardiovascular functioning in some individuals.[23-27] Furthermore, these changes are reflective of the activation of various neuroendocrine mechanisms that are known to have pathophysiologic consequences. A more complete analysis of the relationship among stress, reactivity, and CHD is found elsewhere.[28]

PHYSIOLOGIC MECHANISMS LINKING STRESS TO CORONARY HEART DISEASE

Failure to identify a single clearly defined causal mechanism for the link between emotional stress and CHD has been a major concern. Sympathetic nervous system activation and cardiac reactivity have been studied extensively in this regard. Encouraging evidence has been found in studies where cardiac reactivity in the presence of a high-fat diet is associated with the development of atherosclerosis.[18,29]

In one study focusing on stress-induced myocardial ischemia in patients with coronary heart disease, systolic blood pressure reactivity to stress was highest for the severely ischemic group, lowest for the control group and in-between for the mild to moderate ischemic group.[30] However, even for patients with minimal to moderate atherosclerosis, stress has been shown to vasocontrict coronary arteries by 25%.[31] These data, together with other similar results, suggest that level of cardiovascular reactivity, as a pathophysiological manifestation of emotional stress, is directly related to the severity of the ischemic condition.[32]

It is also recognized that elevated sympathetic activity leads to abnormal heart rate variability and the possibility that emotional upset is a trigger for acute myocardial infarction.[33,34] The level of sympathoadrenal reactivity and catecholamine response varies across individuals exposed to psychologic stresses, and tolerance to stress can be enhanced according to a physiological toughness model.[35,36]

The specific mechanisms leading to reactivity and to sudden cardiac death[37,38] have been studied extensively by these authors, who have also demonstrated a method for measuring mental or emotional stress (Table 41–1) based on noninvasive recording of cardiac output and blood pressure.[39] These measures, which include continuous recording of stroke volume by impedance cardiography, have been shown to be valid at rest and during exercise.[40] These procedures, defined as psychophysiologic stress testing, have also been predictive of mean daily blood pressure as recorded by 24-hour ambulatory monitoring in accordance

with the "hot reactor" model.[41] Abnormal cardiovascular reactivity has been found in borderline hypertensives[42] and in postinfarct patients.[43] Specifically, blunted beta-adrenergic reactivity and a predominance of alpha-adrenergic vascular reactivity was found in hypertensives. This is particularly important because systolic blood pressure has been shown to be highly predictive of fatal coronary events.[44]

Others who have examined the clinical outcomes of the hot reactor model have not found confirmatory evidence to support the theory.[45] In particular, regarding the adrenoreceptors, no differences were found between normotensives and hypertensives at rest or after mental stress,[46] leaving the issue as yet unresolved.

PSYCHOSOCIAL FACTORS LINKED TO CORONARY HEART DISEASE

Socioeconomic status, social support, and employment factors have been linked to CHD. Social dominance was associated

Table 41–1. Psychophysiological (Emotional) Stress Testing for Assessing Coronary Risk*

Psychophysiologic Stressors	
Cognitive Stressors	**Somatic Stressors**
Mental arithmetic	Cold pressor test ⎱ Both conducted with
Competitive contest	Isometric handgrip ⎰ high challenge to endure
Vigilance task	
Word/color conflict task	
Shock-avoidance task	
Ego-threatening IQ test	
Viewing traumatic disaster films	
Interview of emotionally-charged events	
Structured interview for Type A behavior	

Physiologic Measures of Emotional Stress	
Cardiovascular and Pulmonary	**Autonomic and Skeletal Muscle**
Heart rate	Electrodermal skin response
ECG	Electromyography (muscle tension)
Cardiac output	
Stroke volume (by impedance cardiography)	
Blood pressure (systolic, diastolic, and mean)	
Peripheral resistance (computed from pressure and cardiac output)	
Respiration rate and respiratory sinus rhythm	
Peripheral blood flow (pulse volume or skin temperature)	

* Adapted with permission from Sime, WE, et al.: Psychophysiological (emotional) stress testing for assessing coronary risk. *J Cardiovasc Pulm Tech*, 8:27–31, 1980.

with increased coronary artery atherosclerosis in monkeys, but only in the presence of relevant threat.[47] A relationship between social connections and mortality from heart disease was found in a study of 13,301 men and women in Finland.[48] Men, but not women, who were in the lowest categories of social connections were at increased risk of heart disease compared to those with high social connections.

Social support and job strain were studied in a large sample of 13,779 Swedish male and female workers, wherein it was discovered that individuals with jobs involving high demand, low control, and low social support experienced approximately two times greater cardiovascular disease prevalence than those individuals with low demand, high control, and high social support, especially among blue-collar workers.[49]

Corroborating data were noted in a large study of job characteristics in relation to prevalence of myocardial infarction in the United States Health Examination Survey (HES) and the Health and Nutrition Examination Survey (HANES). Employed men with jobs that were simultaneously low in decision latitude and high in psychologic workload had a higher prevalence of myocardial infarction.[50] A meta-analysis of a large number of work stress studies revealed a significant inverse relationship between job decision latitude and systolic blood pressure, which illustrates a direct link to one mechanism of the major coronary risk factors.[51]

A surprising outcome was observed in one study of 8000 men of Japanese ancestry in Hawaii in which there was an inverse relation between job strain and heart disease. This is one of the few examples of confounding results which may be accounted for by noting the unique cultural factors compounded by migrant status of the population on the island of Hawaii.[52] Similarly, another study showed that high-stress workers exhibited lower maximum heart rate and blood pressure elevations.[53] In summary, it appears that cardiovascular reactivity is attenuated by an individual's experience of chronic occupational stress, which seems to account for why reactivity has not been associated with level of work stress in some studies.

If work stress is relevant in CHD, then, perhaps, the fatigue associated with work is a factor also. One study has shown that burnout is a risk factor for coronary heart disease in a cohort of 3877 men.[54] These data show that a high level of exhaustion is a predictor for myocardial infarction. Exhaustion appears to be a factor because it accumulates over a period of time during which the patient fails to make adequate adaptation to stress.

Some dimensions of human emotional affect seem to be related to CHD. For example, in the Harvard mastery of stress study with 35-year follow-up, severe anxiety was a reliable marker for increased susceptibility, not only for CHD but also for overall future illness.[45] Anxiety was also linked to conflict with hostile impulses. Surprisingly, neither expressed nor unexpressed anger was found to be associated with higher incidence of CHD. By contrast, it should be noted that depression has not been routinely studied prospectively as a risk factor and that as many as 40% of all patients with CAD have depression disorders.[55] For example, among 560 male survivors of acute myocardial infarction, levels of depression were highly predictive of cardiac deaths and nonfatal arrhythmic events.[56]

TYPE A CORONARY-PRONE BEHAVIOR PATTERNS AND CORONARY HEART DISEASE

The initial evidence on the relationship between Type A behavior pattern and CHD were found in the Western Collaborative Group Study.[57,58] Type A is also a risk factor for other physical disorders, including accidents, violence, and cerebrovascular and peripheral atherosclerosis,[59] as well as angina pectoris,[60] peptic ulcers, thyroid problems, asthma, and rheumatoid arthritis.[61] However, in a recent follow-up study on the Western Collaborative Group, Type A was no longer significantly associated with all causes of mortality, although there was a significant relationship to morbidity.[62,63] The debate continues, however, as evidence from the Caerphilly Study on 1956 men revealed that Type A was found to be positively associated with increased risk of myocardial infarction though not related to angina.[64]

Over the past two to three decades, debate has prevailed on the question of whether Type A is causally related to CHD and whether modification of Type A behaviors would decrease coronary risk and/or cardiac mortality by reduction of the stress/arousal manifestations of Type A character. A summary of the current status of Type A research can be found in several elegant but succinct review articles that portray a balanced perspective on the Type A controversy.[65–67]

Although interest in Type A may be waning because of the negative outcome results of some recent research,[63] there is reason to believe that sampling bias may account for the negative results. Specifically, a disease-based spectrum bias occurs when studies rely on referred patients to study predictors of disease. The result is a set of statistical problems that reduce the likelihood of obtaining statistically significant results, even when a substantial relationship is present between a risk factor and a disease. The results of this research indicate that this unique bias has reduced the association between Type A behavior and CHD in reported studies.[68] Of parallel concern regarding the defense of the Type A concept, Meyer Friedman has vehemently voiced his view that the negative outcome studies emanate from misdiagnosis of the Type A medical disorders.[69]

When confounding results began to appear for the initial Western Collaborative Group Study, Dembroski, Williams, and others began to explore other salient elements of Type A phenomena that might be more singularly predictive of CHD, as noted in the subsequent section.

BEHAVIORAL MECHANISMS LINKING STRESS TO CORONARY HEART DISEASE

A recent development in Type A coronary-prone research has been the attempt to isolate unique characteristics of Type A that are specifically related to incidence of CHD. Hostility as an attitude and a behavioral manifestation has been the focus of this effort. The antagonistic form of hostility observed during personal interaction appears to be the most promising element for research in this area.[70] The specific mechanism by which this relationship exists has been postulated in several research

studies. Specifically, there appears to be exaggerated reactivity in systolic blood pressure in individuals who have negative, hostile reactions toward people but disavow these feelings and inhibit their aggression so as not to alienate others.[71] Hostility, in addition to vigorous voice stylistics, was found to be more prevalent in untreated, mildly hypertensive employed individuals than among occupationally matched normotensive subjects.[72] Some evidence also suggests that cynical hostility is especially predictive of greater diastolic blood pressure reactivity during interpersonal conflict.[73] High-hostility people reported less social support, more negative life events, and more daily irritants than the low-hostility group. Last, patients with acute myocardial infarction reported significantly lower levels of relaxation and income as well as higher levels of suppressed hostility, illustrating a behavioral mechanism for the impact of hostility.[74]

By contrast, other researchers have been unable to replicate the hostility studies with such success. In one long-term follow-up study of 35 years on a cohort of 1399 men, no relationship was found between hostility and CHD.[75] Two other studies also showed nonsignificant relationships for hostility, although each of these used several types of self-report measures, such as the Cook-Medley Hostility Inventory[76] and the Hostility Score from the MMPI,[77] which are subject to bias because people tend to deny the existence of socially undesirable behaviors.

If hostility is, in fact, related to heart disease, the mechanism underlying this relationship might be found in studies of genetic as well as family-environment sources. Results of one study[78] indicated that a less supportive and positively involved family climate was associated with attributes of potential coronary heart disease risk in children. Early signs of hostility are also found among adolescents and are thought to be one essential precursor to reactivity in the complicated etiology of cardiovascular disease.[79] Definitive evidence on environment versus genetic links is available from research on twins reared separately or together. Two studies demonstrate existence of a genetic relationship between reactivity and heart disease, perhaps mediated by sympathetic nervous system reactivity.[80,81] Both indicate that Type A behavior pattern was modestly heritable, especially for pressure, hard driving, ambitiousness, hostility, and assertiveness.

RESEARCH ON STRESS MANAGEMENT INTERVENTION IN CARDIAC REHABILITATION

The intervention strategy that has been studied most extensively in CHD is targeted directly toward the primary risk factor, i.e., Type A behavior pattern.[82] Commonly used techniques include group-administered behavioral therapy, cognitive restructuring, problem-solving, and relaxation techniques, which are all designed to improve stress-coping skills.[83] Common elements include group support, personal disclosure, values clarification, anger management, and reducing time urgency. Some have included adjunctive activities such as biofeedback and exercise.

A meta-analysis of the literature has shown that reducing Type A behavior pattern may improve the clinical outcome of CHD.[84] The research having the greatest impact regarding Type A intervention includes a long series of studies by Friedman showing that Type A behavior can be altered in postinfarct patients and that such changes are associated with a significant reduction in nonfatal myocardial infarction.[85] Subsequent reports 2 years later on the same cohort revealed that cardiac mortality rates were also reduced.[86] Even 1 year after cessation of intervention, the benefits were retained.[87] Later it was observed that the subgroup of infarct patients who benefited the most from Type A intervention counseling were those for whom the biologic effects were not yet advanced.[88] The most recent report on this large cohort revealed that the addition of Type A counseling to standard cardiac counseling resulted in decreased Type A behavior as well as 44% reduction in reinfarction.[89]

The outcome measures that were significantly changed as a result of Type A intervention were decreased anger, hostility, impatience, time urgency, depression, and increased social support, well-being, and perceived control.[90] Surprisingly, one benefit of a regular exercise program appears to be a reduction in the characteristics of Type A behavior. Fifty men and women suffering from cardiovascular disease engaged in a 10-week supervised aerobic exercise program.[91] At the end of the program, those subjects scored significantly lower on the Jenkins Activity Survey, primarily because of a reduction in their hard-driving tendencies. In this study, Blumenthal and colleagues showed simultaneously decreased blood pressure and weight with exercise, as well as a marginally significant increase in HDL. Although the typical cardiac rehabilitation patient might be characteristically more Type A and less amenable to change, these results are certainly encouraging and add support to the use of exercise as an adjunct to stress management intervention. In addition, however, counseling should be considered, given results of a randomized study involving postinfarction patients for whom Type A counseling was more effective than traditional cardiac rehabilitation in reducing the risk of recurrent infarction.[92]

Absence of social support has been identified as a risk for CHD and increased social support is one serendipitous outcome of Type A intervention.[93] Therefore, it appears to be desirable to examine the intervention efforts specifically focused upon social support. One large study conducted on 461 male postinfarct patients showed that an Ischemic Heart Disease Life Stress Monitoring Program featuring emotional support (administered as needed by nurse contacts) yielded a 50% reduction in 1-year cardiac deaths.[94] The follow-up results on this study 2 years later confirmed the previous findings and also showed that only individuals who were assessed as high stress patients were also at greater risk and subsequently benefited substantially from the intervention.[95]

Other studies provide parallel findings, which suggest that hardiness and stress resistance factors are predictive of long-term psychosocial adjustment.[96,97] Social support was found to be effective as a buffer to stress (less depression) for the spouses of the patients, particularly when the patient's illness worsened over time. Thus, it is not surprising that some cardiac rehabilitation programs have adopted social work strategies to deal with issues of family support and other socioeconomic problems.[99]

STRESS MANAGEMENT, BIOFEEDBACK, AND RELAXATION TRAINING RESULTS

The benefits of relaxation therapy have been documented generically for medical disorders including headache, insomnia, and hypertension.[100] More specific research related to CHD shows that Benson's relaxation technique produced a significant reduction in diastolic blood pressure; however, no effect was observed for behavior pattern, as might be expected.[101,102] Two other studies focusing upon either stress management[103] or a comparison of stress management with Type A counseling[104] revealed that the former was effective in reducing systolic pressure and anxiety, but it was not as effective as Type A counseling to reduce anger and hostility.

Another study compared the effect of cognitive therapy and heart rate biofeedback.[105] Not surprisingly, the former reduced anger while the latter was more effective in decreasing blood pressure. Presumably, the biological outcome of reduced pressure is a more salient and therapeutically beneficial outcome of intervention.

Last, one study included a meta-analysis of 12 independent randomized treatments of behavioral intervention for hypertension focused upon various combinations of relaxation and biofeedback.[106] The meta-analysis revealed a significant decrease in blood pressure across studies. Because most cardiac patients are electrocardiographically monitored during exercise, it is technically feasible to include heart rate biofeedback training in most cardiac rehabilitation programs. Biofeedback has been a particularly effective intervention for individuals with exaggerated Type A behavior pattern.[107,108]

INTERVENTIONS ALIGNED WITH EXERCISE THERAPY

Previous research has shown that chronic hyperventilation may be a risk factor for ischemic CHD.[109] Thus, it is remarkable to note a series of seminal clinical research studies that include systematic breathing therapy as a critical element in a cardiac rehabilitation study comparing exercise and relaxation therapy.[110] These results showed that relaxation training, together with exercise, was more beneficial for long-term outcome than was exercise alone. Subsequent follow-up reports showed that exercise training alone is not successful in all postinfarct patients and that relaxation training and behavior therapy benefit the program by decreasing failure rates by 50%.[111] Furthermore, the outcome of relaxation therapy was more beneficial for psychologic variables than was the exercise therapy[112] and these outcomes were predictable in advance by measures of Type A, well-being, and depression.[113] In addition, however, one serendipitous benefit of exercise therapy is the metabolic workload demand, which precipitates increased ventilatory volume incurred by increased rate and/or depth of breathing. Improvements in breathing efficiency are known to reduce muscle tension precipitated by emotional stress.

Comparative studies of different interventions in this area are rare. However, Roskies conducted studies on four separate interventions. She found that group therapy and behavioral therapy had similar outcomes in reducing Type A behaviors, whereas stress management versus exercise training produced different outcomes, although both were beneficial.[114]

This brings up the important consideration of the reciprocal relationship between exercise and relaxation. Although exercise seems to have a facilitating effect on the relaxation experience, a reciprocal benefit from the relaxation also occurs during exercise. Benson and other investigators demonstrated that oxygen consumption at a fixed workload was significantly lower (4%) when subjects used a relaxation response technique during exercise on a bicycle ergometer.[115]

Other elements that link stress management to exercise testing or training include the following reports. Previous research has shown that Type As tend to deny their physical symptoms during exercise tolerance testing.[116] However, one study has shown that Type As report more symptoms than Type Bs and, in addition, were shown to experience more silent ischemia than Type Bs.[117] Furthermore, patients who undergo routine diagnostic testing (treadmill test or catheterization) commonly experience some performance anxiety. Cognitive restructuring and simple relaxation are helpful techniques to alleviate this form of anxiety. In addition, one study has shown that modeling and coping skills training were effective in reducing anxiety before catheterization in 60 adult patients.[118] It should be noted that cold pressor testing, which is predictive of CHD risk, is a variant of exercise testing based upon the challenge and the sympathetic response that results.[119] The variable responses emanating from the cold pressor test are linked to individual stress tolerance and/or vulnerability.

Last, it is apparent that fitness as a result of regular aerobic exercise provides a cross-training effect so that heart rate, blood pressure, and epinephrine response to psychological testing are attenuated.[120] In addition, there may be pathologic significance to the so-called "additional responses" to stress occurring by means of these sympathetic effects on heart and vessels. Measures of total peripheral resistance and diastolic blood pressure revealed a much stronger vascular reactivity in the low fit group.[121] These results seem to confirm the importance of taking into account the effects of fitness level when comparing a patient's individual cardiovascular stress responses. Essentially, this means that an assessment of fitness level may serve additionally as an indicator of ability to tolerate cardiovascular stress response.

Exercise itself produces a paradoxic opportunity for stress reduction when it is conducted at a leisurely pace that facilitates the relaxation experience in postexercise recovery. Evidence is considerable in documenting the role of aerobic exercise of moderate intensity and duration in reducing muscle tension acutely.[122-125] Thus, exercise is an excellent facilitating prelude for relaxation training in individuals who are particularly tense. Relaxation training can be conducted effectively if it is scheduled immediately after each exercise session. Morgan has shown that exercise also reduces anxiety[126] and increases self-esteem.[127] The added advantage, of course, is safety. Because a large proportion of exercise-related cardiac complications occur in the postexercise period (during the shower or on the way home), the longer the cardiac rehabilitation staff can monitor patients after exercise (without simply wasting their time), the more efficacious the safety element in rehabilitation.

STRESS MANAGEMENT GUIDELINES BASED ON A STANDARDIZED BODY OF KNOWLEDGE

Stress management techniques are used in educational as well as broad clinical applications. It is important to include a comprehensive overview of the essential elements to be understood by qualified practitioners in the field. A recent validation study has defined the essential elements of a comprehensive, multidisciplinary approach for stress management education.[128] See Table 41-2. The guidelines for stress management education identified in this study were developed with the input of over 700 professionals from the United States and 26 foreign countries who are recognized for their educational, clinical, and/or research work in stress management.

Training and skill development in stress management education for instructors can be obtained through many college and university programs. Guidelines regarding the essential content to be covered in a suitable comprehensive education program are included in Table 41-2. The material found in this table was obtained from a study designed to provide the knowledge base for an international certification program in stress management education, currently being administered by the Biofeedback Certification Institute of America, an established national health certifying agency.[128] This program provides both a method of standardization for minimum training, experience, and knowledge criteria necessary for individuals providing stress management education and a means of quality control in this rapidly growing field within health education. The credential is comparable by parallel standards and criteria to the Health/Fitness Instructor Certification offered by the American College of Sports Medicine.

SPECIFIC STRESS MANAGEMENT TECHNIQUES FOR CARDIAC REHABILITATION

Progressive Relaxation

Procedures for teaching progressive relaxation, according to Jacobson, involve the

Table 41–2. Measuring Mental or Emotional Stress

I. Basic Concepts in Stress Management

A conceptual understanding of stressors and stress responses
Personality, perception, and sources of stress
The physiology of stress and relaxation
Stress pathophysiology and stress-related disorders
The relationship between lifestyle behavior patterns and stressors/stress responses

II. Strategies for Enhancing Stress Management Skills

Social and Environmental Change Strategies
  Assertiveness training
  Time management
  Decision-making
  Social support
  Problem-solving
  Conflict resolution
  Social engineering
  Environmental engineering
Cognitive and Behavioral Interventions
  Behavioral rehearsal
  Cognitive restructuring/reframing
  Stress inoculation
  Systematic desensitization
  Anger management
  Thought stopping techniques
  Control and perception of control
  Self-esteem enhancement
  Goal setting
  Active (reflective) listening
  Strategies for coping with deprivational stress
  Modification of lifestyle (nutrition, sleep, etc.)
Strategies to Achieve a Relaxation Response
  Progressive muscle relaxation
  Autogenic training
  Diaphragmatic breathing
  Quieting reflex
  Imaging/visualization
  Meditation
  Exercise/yoga

III. Application of Learning Theory, Measurements and Ethics in Stress Management

Application of learning theory to the teaching of stress management
Measurement of stress reactions and relaxation responses
Knowledge of experimental design and research related to stress management
Professional conduct and ethical practices

Material in I and III above is abbreviated in this table. For a more complete summary of the Blueprint of Knowledge for Stress Management Education, contact Wesley E. Sime or obtain the following: Raymer KS: Stress Management Education: Defining the Knowledge Base. Dissertation Abstracts International, 1991.

use of muscle contraction instructions for isolated muscle groups at varying levels of intensity for the purpose of enhancing sensory perception therein.[129] The patient is instructed to contract a specific, isolated muscle or muscle group and to hold that contraction until a clear and distinct sensation of effort can be distinguished in the belly of the muscle, not in the surrounding joints or in the antagonist muscle. With the instruction to stop the contraction, the patient is expected to notice the clear distinction between tension and the relative absence thereof after ceasing the contraction. A residual level of tension remains temporarily, but should decline over time. Initially, patients are often not able to perceive these signals of tension and/or relaxation accurately and need to repeat the process to gain recognition of these relatively subtle sensations. Once the sensations associated with contractions of higher intensity are perceived accurately, the patient is asked to produce tension at progressively lower levels of intensity, thus developing a more discriminating awareness of tension. Even without observable movement in the selected muscle or joint, the motivated patient can learn to recognize very low levels of tension. With this newly acquired awareness of small changes in muscle tension, the patient presumably becomes much more efficient in utilizing tension only by choice (not by emotion or by anxiety) and also uses only the minimal required level of tension for a given task. The goal is to develop skills in "differential relaxation," whereby the driver of a car can hold the steering wheel relaxed and efficiently with modest effort rather than grip it excessively tight in the misguided attempt to be overly cautious. Learning this technique requires regular practice in a systematic program focusing on each of the major muscle groups progressively from day to day.

Autogenic Training

Luthe and Schultz founded autogenic training in the same era as Jacobson, but with a completely different psychophysiologic basis.[130] Their premise was that man has an inherent homeostatic mechanism to regulate all physiologic functions. When one or more of these functions goes awry in a pathologic state, it is possible to use self-suggestion to achieve self-regulatory neutralization. Six basic exercises cover the areas of heaviness, warmth, heart, respiration, solar plexus, and forehead. In each case, the patient is instructed to use subvocal suggestive phrases to achieve the desired physiologic changes. Examples of the phrases include "my right arm is very heavy" . . . "my right arm is very warm," and so forth. In an autogenic training session, the patient is asked to repeat one of the phrases over and over subvocally. Subsequently, these individual phrases may be combined into consecutive and more lengthy phrases. Progression to new exercises occurs only after the patient has successfully achieved the outcome (sensation of heaviness, warmth). Thermal biofeedback is often used in conjunction with autogenic training to provide reinforcement and objective assessment of progress in increasing peripheral blood flow, which coincides with the increased hand temperature.

In addition to group or individual training sessions with an instructor, the patient is asked to repeat the autogenic experience in shorter periods several times throughout the day in home practice. The instructor may seek guidance from one of several instructional manuals.[130,131]

Breathing Strategies

Inherent in most relaxation techniques is the attention paid to efficient breathing strategies. Patients who have tension problems almost always exhibit disrupted breathing patterns.[132] Cardiac patients also are known to have dysfunctional breathing problems.[109] Usually, a form of reverse breathing is noted, wherein chest breathing prevails over abdominal breathing. The patient may even suck in the abdominal area while taking in a breath, thus exhibiting the most inefficient form of breathing.

In a relaxed state, the patient should breathe in a regular pattern of 8 to 12 breaths per minute. The abdomen should rise (when the patient is supine) with each inhalation and fall with the exhalation. The patient's chest should barely move, and then only after the abdominal shift appears. Patients often err by trying to breathe too deeply and, in so doing, they tend to hold the air in for a short period while at the peak of inhalation. The pause,

if any, should occur at the end of exhalation in a short rest period. Patients also tend to hold their breath or restrict breathing drastically during periods of excitement or anxiety. This pattern can be observed particularly during conversation, interview, or other test procedures. The classic signs appear in a patient who "sighs" frequently. The sigh is a homeostatic recovery phenomenon associated with periodic breath-holding behavior. Additional information on dysfunctional breathing and appropriate breathing strategies is available.[132]

Benson's Relaxation Response

This technique emanates from the structural framework of eastern meditation but is presented with objective documentation of physiologic benefits, thus satisfying western world opinion.[133] Following the Transcendental Meditation format, the instructions to participants state that it should be practiced twice daily for 10 to 20 minutes. The four basic components are:

1. Find a quiet environment with minimal distractions.
2. Focus upon a sound, word, or phrase repeated aloud or fix the gaze at an object.
3. Maintain a passive attitude to allow the relaxation process to occur.
4. Choose a comfortable position to minimize undue muscle tension.

This technique has been used commonly in studies of blood pressure control,[134] and serves a useful purpose as a simple, straightforward technique that requires little instructional training and literally no equipment or resources. The disadvantage lies in its fundamental strategy, which is inextricably aligned with eastern meditation techniques which sometimes raise concerns about religious or cult influence.

Cognitive Restructuring

Cognitive restructuring is a stress management procedure aimed at identifying and changing self-defeating and self-destructive thinking. It is based on the general principles of rational emotive therapy as outlined by Ellis,[135] and has been popularized in several books, including an excellent text by Maultsby.[136] Cognitive appraisal, according to Lazarus,[21] is an essential element in this technique and provides a useful foundation. The essence of the technique is to promote emotional control by attacking the negative self-talk of the patient. One important concept is to bring the patient to acknowledge, "I upset myself." The natural tendency is for patients to claim that "It upsets me." The "It" is usually a stressful event such as a divorce, death of a loved one, or loss of job. Although these events may be real stressors, too often the "it" is conceived and embellished in the mind of the patient. "Making mountains out of molehills" is a common experience that exacerbates the stress response. The end product of cognitive restructuring is to change a thin-skinned (easily disturbed) person into a more thick-skinned (emotionally stable) person who can better cope with the perceived reality of any stressor.

Quieting Reflex Training

The quieting reflex technique is an eclectic procedure originated by Charles Stroebel that involves a combination of progressive relaxation, autogenic training, cognitive restructuring, and a therapeutic breathing strategy in a simplified, quick exercise.[137] The patient is taught to initiate the six-second procedure upon stimulus cueing at numerous times throughout the day. The six-second technique is a basic four-step procedure that may be individually tailored to the prescribed stress and tension needs of the patient. The four basic elements include:

1. Smile inwardly and say to yourself, "alert mind, calm body."
2. Take an easy, natural abdominal breath and let all the air flow out, followed by several more smooth, regular breaths.
3. As you exhale, let jaw, tongue, and shoulders go loose.
4. As you exhale, imagine a wave of warmth and heaviness flowing from head to toes.

This technique is most effective when the patient has learned all four of the foundational procedures (progressive muscle relaxation, autogenic training, cognitive restructuring, and breathing). Its greatest strength lies in the option of being repeated hundreds of times daily in the face of mild and intensely stressful situations, thus averting the progressive buildup of residual tension and mental fatigue. Regular practice of the quieting reflex can provide a refreshing break from the stressful demands of work or home issues and a substantial reduction in arousal.

Biofeedback-Assisted Relaxation Training

We believe that all patients should be offered one or two sessions of biofeedback. Ideally, an individual biofeedback program could be initiated simultaneously or consecutively with the group stress management program. Some additional cost is involved for equipment and technician time, but the advantages far outweigh the costs. The health professional can illustrate vividly, with digital displays, auditory feedback, and possibly graphic representations, the tremendous impact that even small bouts of emotional arousal have on physiologic functions such as heart rate, blood pressure, skin temperature, and palmar sweating.[138] Many cardiac patients are hard-driving and somatically imperceptive. Although their perception of exertion may be somewhat vague, their perception of emotional response is often totally absent. The use of biofeedback equipment to demonstrate the patient's unique responsiveness to stress can be invaluable as a motivational tool and a reinforcer for the lifestyle behavior changes that are conjointly needed with any of the other stress management techniques.

Technically, biofeedback is a tool to facilitate learning to control voluntary and involuntary physiologic functions.[138] In simplest terms, it involves the transfer of analogue signals of recorded physiologic functioning into a visual or auditory mode. Thus, by a trial-and-error process, patients develop cognitive strategies for controlling physiologic functions.

The most relevant biofeedback parameters for cardiac rehabilitation are heart rate, electromyography (EMG), electrodermal response (palmar sweating), and peripheral blood flow (skin temperature). Continuous blood pressure (BP) feedback is feasible but complicated (constant cuff pressure, or indirect estimate with a pulse-wave velocity system), both of which involve considerable additional cost and compromise in accuracy.[139,140] Electroencephalographic (brain wave) feedback and stroke volume feedback procedures are technically feasible but are not commonly used in cardiac rehabilitation programs.

Biofeedback is commonly used in conjunction with one of several other self-regulation strategies discussed herein. Sessions are 20 to 30 minutes in duration and are repeated one or two times weekly for a period of 4 to 12 weeks, depending on the individual needs of the patient. Patients with hypertension and cardiac arrhythmias are especially good candidates for biofeedback.[38,41] This method of treatment can be the core of a comprehensive stress management program because the objective measurement of individual progress can be documented.

Practical Aspects of Stress Management and Relaxation Training

Table 41–3 shows a model program that documents how stress management can be

Table 41–3. Model Program Integrating Stress Management with Exercise Therapy in a Cardiac Rehabilitation Program

---

Didactic Program in Stress Management Education

Length: 8 weeks   *Duration:* 1.5 hour weekly session
Average Number of Participants: 15-20
Leader Qualification: Nurse or Master's Level
   Education
Type of Presentation: Lecture/Discussion
Sample Content:

Physiology of Stress	Assertiveness Training
Lifestyle Modification	Type A and Hostility
Cognitive Restructuring	Humor and Health
Self-Esteem	Social Support, Connectedness, and Spirituality

Relaxation Training = Skill development to follow each didactic session

Duration: 20- to 30-minute sessions held once a week for 8 weeks
Mode of Presentation: Instructions by qualified leader or tape-recorded session
Location: Specially-designed quiet room, sound-attenuated, and equipped with soft cushions, bean bags, pillows, and adjustable low lighting
Content of Relaxation Sessions:
   Progressive relaxation
   Autogenic training
   Meditation, etc.
Environmental Factors: Room temperature = 72°-74°F
Preparation: Wear loose clothing and adjust coverage according to room temperature; remove gum, glasses, contacts, and shoes; find comfortable position sitting or lying; adopt a passive attitude to allow relaxation to occur; minimize daydreaming; focus upon the process; void before starting the session; and ask questions before the session, if feeling apprehensive about relaxation
After the Session: Encourage discussion about the relative changes in tension and stress level; make adjustments for individual problems, such as temperature, mind chatter, and head, back, and leg support
Home Practice Training: Encourage daily practice for 10-20 minutes with taped instructions

On-Going Relaxation and Stress Management in Phase III Rehabilitation

Following each exercise session on Monday and Friday, the participants go directly to the quiet room for 10-20 minutes of relaxation similar to the skills training above.
On Wednesdays following exercise, the participants meet with the leader for a 10- to 20-minute lecture/discussion on topics like: time management, communication, conflict, etc.

This model program is based on an existing program at Bryan Memorial Hospital in Lincoln, Nebraska. It has been in operation for the past 13 years and was designed at the outset as a comprehensive Exercise Therapy, Relaxation, and Stress Management program by the first author. For further information, contact Dr. Wesley E. Sime at the University of Nebraska-Lincoln.

integrated with exercise therapy in a cardiac rehabilitation program. It includes a description of both the didactic program in stress management education and the specific details involved in conducting structured relaxation training in a suitable environment. Stress management intervention can be conducted on either a group or individual basis over 6 to 12 weeks (20- to 40-minute sessions, 3 times per week) for optimal benefits in the typical cardiac population with relatively deep-seated stress and tension habit patterns. Relaxation training sessions should be held at least twice a week, immediately after the exercise session, and a third session should be scheduled for support group discussion and/or lecture presentations on sources of stress and action-oriented solutions (Table 41–3). Some patients are inclined to fall asleep during the relaxation session. These individuals are probably short on sleep and should be encouraged to improve the quality or quantity of sleep. Another appropriate step is to move patients from a recumbent to a sitting position to avert the tendency to fall asleep, as well as to provide further challenge as the patient's relaxation skills develop. A more comprehensive review and evaluation of the various relaxation techniques used in stress management is available.[141]

The health professional in cardiac rehabilitation or in a health/fitness center should coordinate all stress management activities with the exercise component to achieve integration with the overall cardiac rehabilitation program. Contraindications for stress management are few, but routine precautions are advisable for high-risk patients. Prescriptive recommendations for stress management are much like those for exercise therapy, i.e., the frequency should be at least three times a week, with home exercises daily; the duration of each session should be 20 to 40 minutes; and the intensity (quality) of each session will be determined by the motivation of the patient to "allow" the relaxation experience to occur and by the skill of the instructor (therapist) in facilitating a high-quality experience.

REFERENCES

1. Schneiderman NS: Psychophysiologic factors in atherogenesis and coronary artery disease. *Circulation, 76:*41, 1987.

2. Epstein LH, Perkins KA: Smoking, stress, and coronary heart disease. *J Consul Clin Psychol, 56:*342, 1988.

3. Perkins KA, Dubbert PM, Martin JE: Cardiovascular reactivity to psychological stress in aerobically trained versus untrained mild hypertensives and normotensives. *Health Psychol, 5:*407, 1986.

4. Manuck SB, Henry JP, Anderson DE: Biobehavioral mechanisms in coronary heart disease: Chronic stress. *Circulation, 76:*158, 1987.

5. Verrier RL, Dickerson LW: Autonomic nervous system and coronary blood flow changes related to emotional activation and sleep. *Circulation, 83:*II81, 1991.

6. Rozanski A, Krantz DS, Bairey CN: Ventricular responses to mental stress testing in patients with coronary artery disease. *Circulation, 83:*II137, 1991.

7. Coumel P, Leenhardt A: Mental activity, adrenergic modulation, and cardiac arrhythmias in patients with heart disease. *Circulation, 83:*58, 1991.

8. Kamarck T, Jennings JR: Biobehavioral factors in sudden cardiac death. *Psychol Bull, 109:*42, 1991.

9. Gutstein WH: The central nervous system and atherogenesis: Endothelial injury. *Atherosclerosis, 70:*145, 1988.

10. Raab W, Stark E, MacMillan WH, Gigee WR: Sympathetic origin and anti-adrenergic prevention of stress-induced myocardial lesions. *Am J Cardiol, 8:*203, 1961.

11. Eliot RS, Buell JC, Dembroski TM: Biobehavioral perspectives on coronary heart disease, hypertension and sudden cardiac death. *Acta Med Scand, 660:*203, 1982.

12. Todd GL, Pieper GM, Clayton FC, Eliot RS: Histopathologic animal correlates of clinical sudden cardiac death and acute myocardial infarction. *Fed Proc, 36:*1073, 1977.

13. Dimsdale JE, Herd JA: Variability of plasma lipids in response to emotional arousal. *Psychosom Med, 44:*413, 1982.

14. Glass DC: Stress, behavior patterns, and coronary disease. *American Scientist, 65:*177, 1977.

15. Light KC, Koepke JP, Obrist PA, Willis PW: Psychological stress induces sodium and fluid retention in men at high risk for hypertension. *Science, 220:*429, 1983.

16. Limm M, Linton RAF, Bard DM: Continuous intravascular monitoring of epinephrine-induced changes in plasma potassium. *Anesthesiology, 57:*272, 1982.

17. Krantz DS, Manuck SB: Acute psychophysiologic reactivity and risk of cardiovascular disease: A review and methodologic critique. *Psychol Bull, 96:*435, 1984.

18. Clarkson TB: Personality, gender, and

coronary artery atherosclerosis of monkeys. *Arteriosclerosis, 7:*1, 1987.

19. Jorgensen RS, Nash JK, Lasser NL: Heart rate acceleration and its relationship to total serum cholesterol, triglycerides, and blood pressure reactivity in men with mild hypertension. *Psychophysiology, 25:*39, 1988.

20. Williams RB Jr, Suarez EC, Kuehn DM, et al.: Biobehavioral basis of coronary prone behavior in middle-aged men. Part II: Serum cholesterol the Type A behavior pattern, and hostility as interactive modulators of physiological activity. *Psychosom Med, 53:*528, 1991.

21. Lazarus R, Folkman S: *Stress, appraisal, and coping.* New York: Springer, 1984.

22. Lazarus R: Progress on a cognitive-motivational-relational theory of emotion. *Am Psychol, 46:*819, 1991.

23. Shiffer F, Hartley LH, Schulman CL, Abelman WH: The quiz electrocardiogram: A new diagnostic and research technique for evaluating the relation between emotional stress and ischemic heart disease. *Am J Cardiol, 37:*41, 1976.

24. Brod J, Fencl V, Hejl Z, Jirka J: Circulatory changes underlying blood pressure elevation during acute emotional stress (mental arithmetic) in normotensive and hypertensive subjects. *Clin Sci, 78:*269, 1959.

25. Williams RB Jr: Type A behavior and elevated physiological and neuroendocrine responses to cognitive tasks. *Science, 218:*483, 1982.

26. Hines EA, Brown GE: The cold pressor test for measuring the reactibility of blood pressure: Data concerning 571 normal and hypertensive subjects. *Am Heart J, 11:*1, 1936.

27. Lovallo W: The cold pressor test and autonomic function: A review and integration. *Psychophysiology, 12:*268, 1975.

28. Contrada RJ, Krantz DS: Stress, reactivity, and Type A behavior: Curent status and future directions. *Ann Behav Med, 10:*64, 1988.

29. Manuck SB, Kaplan JB, Clarkson TB: Behaviorally induced heart rate reactivity and atherosclerosis in cynomolgus monkeys. *Psychosom Med, 45:*95, 1983.

30. Krantz DS, Helmers KE, Bairey CM. Cardiovascular reactivity and mental stress-induced myocardial ischemia in patients with coronary artery disease. *Psychosom Med, 53:*1, 1991.

31. Yeung A, Vekshtein V, Krantz D. The effect of atherosclerosis on the vasomotor response of coronary arteries in mental stress. *N Engl J Med, 325:*1551, 1991.

32. Williams RB Jr, Suarez EC, Kuehn DM, et al.: Behavioral basis of coronary prone behavior in middle-aged men. Part I: Evidence for Chronic SNS activation in Type A's. *Psychosom Med, 53:*517, 1991.

33. Pagani M, Mazzuero G, Ferrari A, et al.: Sympathovagal interaction during mental stress. *Circulation, 83:*43, 1991.

34. Tofler GH, Stone PH, Maclure M, et al.: Analysis of possible triggers of acute myocardial infarction (The MILIS Study). *Am J Cardiol, 66:*22, 1990.

35. Dienstbier RA: Behavioral correlates of sympathoadrenal reactivity: The toughness model. *Med Sci Sports Exerc, 23:*846, 1991.

36. Sothman MS, Hart BA, Horn TS: Plasma catecholamine response to acute psychological stress in humans: Relation to aerobic fitness and exercise training. *Med Sci Sports Exerc, 23:*860, 1991.

37. Todd GL, Eliot RS: Cardioprotective effects of diltiazem when given before, during, or delayed after infusion of orepinephrine in anesthetized dogs. *Am J Cardiol, 64:*25G, 1988.

38. Eliot RS: Detection and management of brain-heart inter-relations. *J Am Coll Cardiol, 12:*1101, 1988.

39. Sime WE, et al.: Psychophysiological (emotional) stress testing for assessing coronary risk. *J Cardiovasc and Pulm Tech, 8:* 27, 1980.

40. Wilson MF, Sung BH, Pincomb GA, Lovallo WR: Simultaneous measurement of stroke volume by impedance cardiography and nuclear ventriculography: Comparisons at rest and exercise. *Ann Biomed Eng, 17:*475, 1989.

41. Morales-Balljo H, Eliot RS, Boone JL: Psychophysiological stress testing as a predictor of mean daily blood pressure. *Am Heart J, 116:*673, 1988.

42. de Champlain J, Petrovich M, Gonzalez M, et al.: Abnormal cardiovascular reactivity in borderline and mild essential hypertension. *Circulation, 17:*22, 1991.

43. Sime WE, Buell JC, Eliot RS: Cardiovascular responses to emotional stress (quiz interview) in post-myocardial infarction patients and matched control subjects. *J Hum Stress, 6:*39, 1980.

44. Menotti A, Seccareccia F, Giampaoli S, Giuli B: The predictive role of systolic, diastolic and mean blood pressures on cardiovascular and all causes of death, *J Hypertension, 7:*595, 1989.

45. Russek LG, King SH, Russek SJ, Russek HI: The Harvard mastery of stress study 35-year follow-up: Prognostic significance of patterns of psychophysiological arousal

and adaptation. *Psychosom Med, 52:*271, 1990.

46. Graafsma SJ, van Tits LJ, van Heijst P: Adrenoreceptors on blood cells in patients with essential hypertension before and after mental stress. *J Hyperten, 7:*51, 1989.

47. Kaplan JR, Manuck SB, Clarkson TB, et al.: Social status, environment, and atherosclerosis in cynomolgus monkeys. *Arteriosclerosis, 2:*359, 1982.

48. Kaplan GA, Salonen JT, Cohen RD: Social connections and mortality from all causes and from cardiovascular disease: Prospective evidence from eastern Finland. *Am J Epidemiol, 128:*370, 1988.

49. Johnson JB, Hall EM: Job strain, work place social support, and cardiovascular disease: A cross-sectional study of a random sample of the Swedish working population. *Am J Public Health, 78:*1336, 1988.

50. Karasek RA, Thorell T, Schwartz JE: Job characteristics in relation to the prevalence of myocardial infarction in the U.S. Health Examination Survey (HES) and the Health and Nutrition Examination Survey (HANES). *Am J Public Health, 78:*910, 1988.

51. Pieper C, LaCroix AZ, Karasek RA. The relation of psychosocial dimensions of work with coronary heart disease risk factors: A meta-analysis of five United States databases. *Am J Epidemiol, 129:*483, 1989.

52. Reed DM, LaCroix AZ, Karasek RA, Miller D, MacLean CA. Occupational strain and the incidence of coronary heart disease. *Am J Epidemiol, 129:*495, 1989.

53. Siegrist J, Klein D: Occupational stress and cardiovascular reactivity in blue collar workers. *Work and Stress, 4:*294, 1990.

54. Appels A, Schouten E: Burnout as a risk factor for coronary heart disease. *Behav Med, 17:*53, 1991.

55. Carney RM, Rich MW, Friedland JE: Major depressive disorder predicts cardiac events in patients with coronary artery disease. *Psychosom Med, 50:*627, 1988.

56. Ladwig K, Kieser M, Konig J, et al.: Affective disorders and survival after acute myocardial infarction. *Eur Health J, 12:*959, 1991.

57. Friedman M, Rosenman RH: *Type A behavior and your heart.* New York: Alfred A Knopf, 1974.

58. Rosenman RH, Brand RJ, Jenkins CD, et al.: Coronary heart disease in the Western Collaborative Group Study: Final follow-up experience of 8½ years. *JAMA, 233:*872, 1975.

59. Feld J, Sanders GS: Type A behavior as a general risk factor for physical disorders, *J Behav Med, 11:*201, 1988.

60. Eaker ED, Abbott RD, Knell WB: Frequency of uncomplicated angina pectoris in Type A compared with Type B persons (the Framingham Study). *Am J Cardiol, 63:*1042, 1989.

61. Rime B, Ucros CG, Bestgen Y, Jeanjean M: Type A behavior pattern: Specific coronary risk factor or general disease-prone condition? *Br J Med Psychol, 62:*229, 1989.

62. Ragland D, Brand R: Type A behavior and mortality from CHD. *N Engl J Med, 318:*65, 1988.

63. Shoham-Yakubovich I, Ragland DR, Brand RJ, Syme SL: Type A behavior pattern and health status after 22 years of follow-up in the western collaborative group study. *J Epidemiol, 128:*579, 1988.

64. Gallagher JE, Yarnell JW, Butland BK: Type A behavior and prevalent heart disease in the Caerphilly study: Increase in risk or symptom reporting? *J Epidemiol Commun Res, 42:*226, 1988.

65. Haynes SG, Matthews KA: Review and methodologic critique of recent studies on Type A behavior and cardiovascular disease. *Ann Behav Med, 10:*47, 1988.

66. Matthews KA, Woodall KL: Childhood origins of Type A behaviors and cardiovascular reactivity to behavioral stressors. *Ann Behav Med, 10:*71, 1988.

67. Dembroski TM, Costa PT: Assessment of coronary-prone behavior: A current overview. *Ann Behav Med, 10:*60, 1988.

68. Miller TQ, Turner CW, Tindale RS, Posavec EJ: Disease based spectrum bias in referred samples and relationship between Type A behavior and coronary artery disease. *Am J Clin Epidemiol, 41:*1139, 1988.

69. Friedman M: Type A behavior: A frequently misdiagnosed and rarely treated medical disorder. *Am Heart J, 115:*934, 1988.

70. Dembroski TM, MacDougall JM, Costa PT, Grandits GA: Components of hostility as predictors of sudden death and myocardial infarction in the multiple risk factor intervention trial. *Psychosom Med, 51:*514, 1989.

71. Houston BK, Smith MA, Cates DS: Hostility patterns and cardiovascular reactivity to stress. *Psychophysiology, 26:*337, 1989.

72. Irvine J, Garner DM, Craig HM, Logan AG: Prevalence of Type A behavior in untreated hypertensive individuals. *Hypertension, 18:*72, 1991.

73. Hardy JD, Smith TW: Cynical hostility and vulnerability to disease: Social support life stress and physiological response to conflict. *Health Psychol, 7:*447, 1988.

74. Wielgosz AT, Wielgosz M, Byro E: Risk factors for myocardial infarction the im-

portance of relaxation. *Br J Med Psychol,*
*61:*209, 1988.

75. Hearn MD, Murray DM, Lupker RV: Hostility, coronary heart disease and total mortality: A 35-year follow-up study of university students. *J Behav Med, 12:*105, 1989.

76. Helmer DC, Ragland DR, Syme SL: Hostility in coronary heart disease. *Am J Epidemiol, 33:*112, 1991.

77. Leoon GR, Finn SE, Murray D, Bailey JM: Inability to predict cardiovascular disease from hostility scores or MMPI items related to Type A behavior. *J Consul Clin Psychol, 56:*597, 1988.

78. Woodall KL, Matthews KA: Familial environment associated with Type A behavior and psychophysiological responses to stressed children. *Health Psychol, 8:*403, 1989.

79. McCann BS, Matthews KA: Influence of potential for hostility, Type A behavior and parental history of hypertension on adolescents' cardiovascular responses during stress. *Psychophysiology, 25:*503, 1988.

80. Turner JR, Hewitt JK: Twin studies of cardiovascular response to psychological challenge: A review and suggested future directions. *Ann Behav Med, 14:*12, 1992.

81. Pederson NL, Lichtenstein P, Ploman R: Genetic and environmental influences for Type A-like measures and related traits: A study of twins reared apart and reared together. *Psychosom Med, 51:*428, 1989.

82. Levenkron JC, Moore G: The Type A behavior pattern: Issues for intervention research. *Ann Behav Med, 10:*78, 1988.

83. Roskies E: *Stress management for the healthy Type A: Theory and practice.* New York: The Guilford Press, 1987.

84. Nunes EV, Frank KA, Kornfeld DS: Psychologic treatment for the Type A behavior pattern and for coronary heart disease: A meta-analysis of the literature. *Psychosom Med, 48:*159, 1987.

85. Friedman M, Thoreson CE, Gill JJ, et al.: Alteration of Type A behavior and reduction in cardiac recurrences in postmyocardial infarction patients. *Am Heart J, 108:*237, 1984.

86. Friedman M, Thoresen CE, Gill JJ, et al.: Alteration of Type A behavior and its effect on cardiac recurrences in post myocardial infarction patients: Summary results of the recurrent coronary prevention project. *Am Heart J, 112:*653, 1986.

87. Friedman M: Behavioral modification and MI recurrence. *Prim Cardiol, 11:*37, 1985.

88. Powell LH, Thoresen CE: Effects of Type A behavioral counseling and severity of prior acute myocardial infarction on survival. *Am J Cardiol, 62:*59, 1988.

89. Mendes de Leon C, Powell LH, Kaplan BH: Change in coronary-prone behaviors in the recurrent coronary prevention project. *Psychosom Med, 53:*407, 1991.

90. Shapiro DH, Friedman M, Piaget G: Changes in mode of control and self-control for post myocardial infarction patients evidencing Type A behavior: The effects of a cognitive/behavioral intervention and/or cardiac counseling. *Internat J Psychosom, 38:*1, 4, 1990.

91. Blumenthal JA, Williams S, Williams RB Jr, Wallace AG: Effects of exercise on the Type A (coronary prone) behavior pattern. *Psychosom Med, 42:*289, 1980.

92. Friedman M: Behavior modification and MI recurrence. *Prim Cardiol, 11:*37, 1985.

93. Orth-Gomer K, Unden A: Type A behavior social support and coronary risk interaction and significance for mortality in cardiac patients. *Psychosom Med, 52:*59, 1990.

94. Frasure-Smith N, Prince R: Long-term follow-up of the ischemic heart disease life stress monitoring program. *Psychosom Med, 51:*485, 1989.

95. Frasure-Smith N: In-hospital symptoms of psychological stress as predictors of long-term outcome after acute myocardial infarction in men. *Am J Cardiol, 67:*121, 1991.

96. Drory AY, Florian V: Long-term pscyhosocial adjustment to coronary artery disease. *Arch Phys Med Rehabil, 72:*326, 1991.

97. Brandhagen DJ: Long-term psychologic implications of congenital heart disease: A 25-year follow-up. *Mayo Clin Proc, 66:*474, 1991.

98. Revenson TA, Magerovitz SD: Effects of chronic illness on the spouse: Social resources as buffers. *Arthritis Care Res, 4:*63, 1991.

99. Robbins B: Social work and the psychosocial issues of cardiac rehabilitation, *J Cardiopulm Rehabil, 11:*240, 1991.

100. Hyman RB, Feldman HR, Harris RB, Levin RF, Malloy GB: The effects of relaxation training on clinical symptoms: A meta-analysis. *Nurs Res, 38:*216, 1989.

101. Munro BH, Creamer AM, Haggerty MR, Cooper FS: Effect of relaxation therapy on post-myocardial infarction patients' rehabilitation. *Nurs Res, 37:*231, 1988.

102. Benson H: *The Relaxation Response.* New York: Avon Books, 1975.

103. Bosley F, Allen TW: Stress management training for hypertensives: Cognitive and physiological effects. *J Behav Med, 12:*77, 1989.

104. Bennet P, Wallace L, Carroll D, Smith N: Treating Type A behaviours and mild hy-

pertension in middle-aged men. *J Behav Med, 35:*209, 1991.

105. Achmon J, Granek M, Golomb M, Hart J: Behavioral treatment of essential hypertension: A comparison between cognitive therapy and biofeedback of heart rate. *Psychosom Med, 51:*152, 1989.

106. Kaufman PG, Jacob RG, Ewart CK: Hypertension intervention pooling project. *Health Psychol, 7:*209, 1988.

107. Chen W, Coorough R: Effect of EMG-biofeedback training in reduction of muscle tension for individuals displaying Type A behavior patterns. *Percept Mot Skills, 62:* 841, 1986.

108. Stoney CM, Langer AW, Sutterer JR, Gelling PD: A comparison of biofeedback-assisted cardiodeceleration in Type A and B men: Modification of stress-associated cardiopulmonary and hemodynamic adjustments. *Psychosom Med, 49:*79, 1987.

109. Weiner H: Stressful experience and cardiorespiratory disorders. *Circulation, 83:*II2, 1991.

110. Van Dixhoorn J, Duivenvoorden HJ, Staal JA, Pool J, Verhage F: Cardiac events after myocardial infarction: Possible effect of relaxation therapy. *Eur Heart J, 8:*1210, 1987.

111. Van Dixhoorn J, Duivenvoorden HJ, Staal HA, Pool J: Physical training and relaxation therapy in cardiac rehabilitation assessed through a composite criterion for training. *Am Heart J, 118:*545, 1989.

112. Van Dixhoorn J, Duivenvoorden HJ, Pool J, Verhage F: Psychic effects of physical training relaxation therapy after myocardial infarction. *J Psychosom Res, 35:*327, 1990.

113. Van Dixhoorn J, Duivenvoorden HJ, Pool J: Success and failure of exercise training after myocardial infarction: Is the outcome predictable? *J Am Coll Cardiol, 15:* 974, 1990.

114. Roskies E, Seraganian P, Oseasohn R: The Montreal project: Major findings. *Ann Behav Med, 5:*45, 1986.

115. Benson H, Dryer T, Hartley H: Decreased V0₂ consumption during exercise with elicitation of the relaxation response. *J Hum Stress, 4:*38, 1978.

116. Schlegal R, Wellwood J, Coops B, et al.: The relationship between perceived challenge and early symptoms reporting in Type A vs. Type B post-infarct subjects. *J Behav Med, 3:*191, 1980.

117. Siegal WC, Mark DB, Lhlatky MA: Clinical correlates in the prognostic significance of Type A behavior and silent myocardial ischemia on the treadmill. *Am J Cardiol, 64:*1280, 1989.

118. Anderson KO, Masur III FT: Psychological preparation for cardiac catheterization, *Heart Lung, 18:*154, 1989.

119. Menkes MS, Matthew KA, Krantz DS: Cardiovascular reactivity to cold pressor test as a predictor of hypertension. *J Hypertension, 14:*524, 1989.

120. Blumenthal JA, Fredrikson M, Kuhn CM: Aerobic exercise reduces levels of cardiovascular and sympathoadrenal responses to mental stress in subjects without prior evidence of myocardial ischemia. *Am J Cardiol, 65:*93, 1990.

121. Vandorrnen JP, DeGeus EJC: Aerobic fitness and the cardiovascular response to stress. *Psychophysiology, 26:*17, 1989.

122. DeVries H, Hams G: Electromyographic comparison of single doses of exercise and meprobamate as to effects on muscular relaxation. *Am J Phys Med, 51:*130, 1972.

123. Sime W: Acute relief of emotional stress. *Proceedings of the American Association for the Advancement of Tension Control.* Blacksburg, VA: University Publications, 1978.

124. Brown DR: Exercise, fitness, and mental health. In *Exercise, Fitness, and Health.* Edited by C Bouchard et al. Champaign, IL: Human Kinetics Books, 1990, pp. 597–626.

125. Sime WE: Discussion: Exercise, fitness, and mental health. In Bouchard C, Shephard RJ, Stephens T, Sutton JR, McPherson BD (Eds.), *Exercise, Fitness, and Health.* Edited by C Bouchard et al. Champaign, IL: Human Kinetics Books, 1990, pp. 627–633.

126. Morgan WP: Affective beneficence of vigorous physical exercise. *Med Sci Sports, 17:* 94, 1985.

127. Sonstroem R, Morgan W: Exercise and self-esteem: Rationale and model. *Med Sci Sports Exerc, 20:*329, 1989.

128. Raymer KS: Stress management education: Defining the knowledge base. *Dissertation Abstracts International,* 1991.

129. Jacobson E: *Self-Operations Control: A Manual of Tension Control.* Chicago: National Foundation for Progressive Relaxation, 1964.

130. Luthe W, Schultz J: *Autogenic Therapy: Medical Applications.* New York: Grune and Stratton, 1970.

131. Luthe W: *Introductions to the Methods of Autogenic Therapy.* Wheat Ridge, CO: Biofeedback Society of America, 1979.

132. Fried R: *The Hyperventilation Syndrome.* Baltimore, MD: Johns Hopkins University Press, 1987.

133. Benson H: *Beyond the Relaxation Response.* New York: Berkley Publishing, 1985.

134. Everly GS, Benson H: Disorders of

arousal and the relaxation response. *Int J Psychosom, 36:*15, 1989.

135. Ellis A, Harper R: *A Guide to Rational Living.* Hollywood: Wilshire Books, 1979.

136. Maultsby MC Jr.: *Help Yourself to Happiness Through Rational Self-Counseling.* New York: Institute for Rational Living, 1975.

137. Stroebel C: *QR: The Quieting Reflex.* New York: GP Putnam, 1982.

138. Schwartz MS: *Biofeedback: A Practitioner's Guide.* New York: Guildford Press, 1987.

139. Tursky B, Shapiro D, Schwartz GE: Auto-mated constant cuff-pressure system to measure systolic and diastolic blood pressure in man. *IEEE Trans Biomed Eng, 19:* 271, 1972.

140. Steptoe A: Blood pressure control: A comparison of feedback and instructions using pulse wave velocity measurements. *Psychophysiology, 13:*528, 1976.

141. Woolfolk RL, Lehrer PM (Eds.): *Principles and Practice of Stress Management.* New York: The Guilford Press, 1984.

Section IX

ADMINISTRATIVE CONCERNS

Chapter 42

MANAGEMENT SKILLS

Larry R. Gettman

This chapter provides general information on the management skills required for the administration of exercise programs in a variety of settings. This information supplements the guidelines for program administration published in Chapter 9 of the ACSM Guidelines for Exercise Testing and Prescription, Fourth Edition.[1]

Administrator, manager, and director are interchangeable terms used to refer to a person who has the primary responsibility for an entire program. This responsibility includes the (1) macro view (how the program fits into the organization as a whole), (2) program development, (3) program planning, (4) day-to-day operation, and (5) program evaluation.[1]

Effective managers are good leaders, and leadership is the real key to a successful program. Too often, organizations consider facilities and equipment as first priorities and staff as secondary in importance. The priorities for a successful program should be exactly the reverse; qualified health and fitness professionals should be carefully selected first. The professional staff can then help plan and implement appropriate programs for the design and capabilities of the facilities and equipment.

The director of a program plays many roles at the same time: manager, planner, supervisor, educator, exercise leader, motivator, counselor, promoter, assessor, and evaluator.[2] These 10 roles are delineated in Table 42–1. Ideally, all staff members of an exercise program should possess the qualities of all 10 roles. In addition to these qualities, good management is characterized by several other special attributes described subsequently.

CHARACTERISTICS OF GOOD MANAGEMENT

Good administrators inspire their staff members to perform positively for the good of the program and the organization. Good management is characterized by concentration on result-producing activities, intelligent delegation, high performance personal leadership, team building, motivating employees, effective communication, organized planning, time management, competent decision-making, and appraising employee performance.

Concentration on Result-Producing Activities

This is also called management by objectives. Effective managers know exactly what they want to accomplish. They establish goals and objectives for the program and then concentrate on result-producing activities. The goals and objectives are prioritized so that staff efforts are not fragmented.

Goals and objectives for the program are reviewed by the entire team and a list of priorities is established. The priority list is translated into an action plan using the first-things-first principle.

The manager must respect the importance of each staff member and be sensitive to individual needs and interests when achieving the goals and objectives set for the program. The manager should strive to maintain an atmosphere in the program in which staff members can achieve their individual goals and aspirations along with those of the entire group. Individuals accomplish most when they care the most. If employees feel that managers really care about them, the employees will care more about the organization and its goals and will strive to perform at high levels.

Intelligent Delegation

Good managers motivate their employees by giving them meaningful work to do and then recognizing them for a job well done. Giving people credit encourages

Table 42–1.   Characteristic Duties of the Health/Fitness Practitioner

Manager
Administer daily operation
Design program activities
Control program
Guide and direct staff
Purchase equipment
Maintain facilities
Regulate budget
Schedule activities
Communicate with staff and participants
Cooperate with other departments

Planner
Assess organization needs
Establish goals for program
Design program
Organize resources
Arrange schedule

Supervisor
Hire and dismiss staff
Oversee program and staff
Coordinate staff and program
Motivate staff
Evaluate staff

Educator
Train staff
Instruct participants
Evaluate learning
Develop curricula

Exercise Leader
Guide participants
Conduct classes
Use safe techniques
Provide a role model

Motivator
Give impetus to program
Persuade participants
Influence participants
Induce changes in participants
Incite action

Counselor
Advise participants
Suggest changes
Express opinions
Judge effectiveness of actions
Recommend action
Consult with participants

Promoter
Design marketing techniques
Encourage participation
Use sales techniques
Advance program advantages

Assessor
Conduct participant tests
Interpret test results
Follow safe procedures

Evaluator
Design program-evaluation procedures
Perform statistical analyses
Interpret results
Analyze program trends
Convey reports to management

(With permission from Patton RW, Corry JM, Gettman LR, Graf J: *Implementing Health/Fitness Programs.* Champaign, IL: Human Kinetics, 1986.)

them to work harder. Employees have an inherent need to achieve and should be given the opportunity to experience that achievement when they complete a task. Most employees are inspired and motivated when they feel that they have been given work that is important.

Intelligent delegation can free the direc-

tor from mounds of work and the exhaustive feeling that comes with checking every detail of the operation. Delegation is an art that applies good psychology, good judgment, and the recognition of strengths and shortcomings for both employee and manager.

To implement intelligent delegation, managers should select employees who deserve more responsibility and authority. Good managers let employees know exactly what is expected (manage by objectives). Delegated work should be challenging and interesting and employees should be given the power to make decisions that will keep them involved and satisfied. Managers should keep track of employee progress and be accessible to answer questions, give feedback, and provide guidance. Managers should trust their employees enough to "let go" and then provide rewards for jobs well done (give credit where credit is due).

High-Performance Personal Leadership

A good leader is a role model to others. Effective managers have personal leadership qualities and value systems that influence others in a positive direction. A good administrator focuses on employees' strengths rather than weaknesses and appreciates an individual's needs and interests. A high-performance leader uses open and honest communication and turns job stresses into challenges and opportunities for employees rather than oppressive threats. A successful director listens attentively to employees and praises positive behavior.

Team Building

Committed teams have a positive effect on productivity and bottom-line results. A skill required of management is to make each employee feel that he or she is part of a dynamic team working together for a common good. Teamwork means that each employee understands his or her role in the program and how that role fits into the overall operation of the organization.

Understanding and Motivating Employees

An administrator should have a good understanding of basic motivational concepts.

A positive compliment on a job well done goes a long way in preparing for future tasks. The "one-minute-manager" concept of supervision is an effective motivational technique.[3] It separates the performance from the performer and emphasizes that performance can be criticized but the performer should always be praised. The one-minute-manager concept has three parts:

1. One-minute goal setting. Have regular staff meetings and delineate short, simple goals. Review these often and analyze accomplishments, problems, and strategies to solve problems.
2. One-minute praising. Praise staff immediately for doing things right, and be consistent.
3. One-minute reprimand. First, confirm the facts. Then, state the reprimand firmly, and attack the mistake, not the person. Conduct the reprimand in private.

Effective Communication

Good communication motivates people, whether they are conferring with a co-worker, conducting a meeting, or writing a report. An effective manager is open and sensitive to the needs of others, listens attentively with understanding, and then expresses himself or herself clearly, assertively, and convincingly.

Successful communication means understanding the other person as well as being understood. Two-way communication takes more time, but is much better than one-way communication. In two-way communication, the sender solicits a response and feedback from the receiver. Tools to improve two-way communication include:

1. Active listening. Focus attention on what the other person is saying. Attempt to understand what is being said and what is meant by the other person.
2. Paraphrase. Check for understanding of what is being said by paraphrasing what is heard.
3. Check feelings. Ask the other person how he or she feels. This step helps to improve your understanding of the other person's communication.
4. Describe behavior. Tell the other person what you see.

5. Give constructive feedback. Express constructive feedback positively, even if it concerns a negative situation. Feedback provides information to help the other person improve performance in achieving goals.
6. Close with clarity. End the communication session with a good understanding of what was said and why.

Organized Planning

Planning means that you decide today what you want to do in the future. The use of organized, formal planning systems leads to better coordination of efforts and better performance. It helps managers and employees understand their interactive responsibilities and prepare for sudden developments.

Organized planning includes setting up action steps, getting the plan adopted, anticipating problems, measuring the processes of a program and its outcomes, and reporting the results.

Time Management

Because time is a valuable asset, it is important to make the best possible use of it every day. If employees complain about spending a lot of time doing things but never accomplish anything, it is time for a time management plan. The above situation can lead to negative stress, anxiety, tension, and low work productivity.

Time control is a habit that can be learned and changed. Essentially, tasks should be prioritized and carried out on a "first things first" basis. Some helpful techniques to make better use of work time include:

1. Design your own priority system by deciding what is urgent and what is important. Make a plan for future work and stick to the schedule.
2. Complete the first priority before proceeding to the second (finish the project that was started).
3. Schedule your activities (make a "to do" list) and keep a log of your time. Design a filing system so that information can be retrieved quickly.
4. Recognize the difference between managing your time and just doing

things. Delegate tasks (if appropriate) for an efficient work plan.

5. Develop a simple and reliable management information reporting system to keep everyone informed of work tasks and to avoid duplication.
6. Avoid time wasters such as useless meetings and interruptions and say "no" to excessive demands on your time.
7. Anticipate problems with contingency plans.
8. Use an uninterrupted "quiet hour" each day to review the schedule and priorities and to plan for the next day.

Competent Decision Making

Making the right decisions is critical to management success. Solving problems creatively requires the ability to first recognize a problem and second find the best solution. Steps in competent decision making include:

1. Find the real problem and define it in detail. Get the facts.
2. Use group participation to find the best solution and then plan how to implement it within acceptable time frames. Develop alternate solutions and be willing to compromise.
3. Sell your decision by getting employee acceptance and ensure that the organization's approach is represented.
4. Evaluate the success of the solution.

Appraising Employee Performance

The purpose of evaluating staff members is to improve their performances. The employee performance appraisal is one of the most demanding and continuing responsibilities facing a manager. It determines the results an employee has produced and compares them to the goals and objectives set in the work plan. It compares employee performance with standards and is used to set future performance standards. The manager must be adequately prepared for the performance appraisal meeting and ready to handle performance problems.

Managers should be positive and objective in their evaluations, and each evaluation should be personal and confidential.

Table 42–2. Areas for Assessment through Staff Performance Evaluations

Job knowledge, training, and experience
Willingness to accept responsibility
Planning and organization of work
Quality and quantity of work
Cost consciousness and control
Relationships with others
Leadership qualities
Initiative and resourcefulness
Originality and creativeness
Soundness of judgment
Dependability
Personal appearance, speech, habits
Attendance and punctuality
Support for organization goals and policies
Career objectives

(From Patton RW, Corry JM, Gettman LR, Graf J: *Implementing Health/Fitness Programs*. Champaign, IL: Human Kinetics, 1986.)

Promoting, coaching, counseling, transferring, and firing are key decisions made in the performance appraisal. Each employee's dignity and sense of worth must be preserved during the appraisal.

The performance appraisal, when conducted properly, improves efficiency and boosts morale. It rewards performance and reinforces the employee's work standards. If performance is unsatisfactory, the performance appraisal is used to guide the employee to more acceptable behavior.

Areas covered in staff performance evaluations are listed in Table 42–2.

THE MACRO VIEW

How the program fits into the organization as a whole describes the management plan from a macro view.[1] This consists of four distinct aspects:

1. Mission statement. The mission statement of the program is a clearly defined and concise statement of the primary reason for existence of the program. It should harmonize with the overall mission statement of the organization.
2. Strategic plan. Top management develops a strategic plan as a course of action laid out to achieve the mission statement within a specified time period.
3. Goals, objectives, and action plans.

These are short-term strategies and actions designed to achieve the overall strategic plan and mission statement.

4. Managerial role. Administrators, managers, and directors are individuals who manage themselves and the people who report to them. A major responsibility of managers is to develop effective action plans to meet the goals and objectives of the overall strategic plan and mission statement. A manager's exact role within an organization depends on whether the organization uses a centralized or decentralized management system.

Both systems have advantages and disadvantages. Centralized management is characterized by having several layers of managers. Advantages of the centralized management system include the following:

a. More control over operations
b. More planning.
c. Highly supervised coordination of staff

However, because the centralized management system involves several layers of managers, it is expensive to the program in terms of salaries and benefits. Also, with few lower-level employees in this system, only a limited number of program components can be offered.

Decentralized management has few layers of managers, and more responsibility is given to lower level employees. Its advantages include:

a. Less expense in salaries
b. Wide variety of program components possible
c. Entrepreneurship encouraged among staff

The disadvantages of the decentralized management system include less control over operations, less supervision of staff, and more difficulty in coordinated planning by the entire organization.

PROGRAM DEVELOPMENT

Structure and Organization

Organizational relationships identify the lines of authority, responsibility, and accountability in a program. A typical organizational structure for an exercise program is illustrated in Figure 42–1.

Medical supervision and advice in a program may be provided in several different ways. Physicians may be directly involved in the organizational structure as medical directors or they may act as advisors to the program as shown in Figure 42–1. The advisory committee or advisory board usually is comprised of health fitness professionals who contribute collective knowledge toward development and operation of the program.

The exercise program staff, all under the supervision of the program director, may consist of various professionals. Support staff of the program includes receptionists, secretaries, clerical workers and custodians.

The mission and setting of the organization direct the exact composition of the professional staff. Commercial/community programs, clinically based programs, and business or industry programs may require different mixes of professional staff.

Personnel

As mentioned previously, the success of a program is closely tied to the selection of qualified personnel. Expertise in the program may vary widely. When staffing an exercise program with professionals of various specialties, a manager should follow prudent selection procedures, have written job descriptions, and establish staff training and development programs.

Selecting the right person for the right job helps avoid many potential problems in the development of a program. Some personnel problems that do arise result from poor selection of staff. Sometimes personnel are "set up for failure" by being placed in the wrong position. Effective personnel selection involves:

1. Defining the needs of the program
2. Identifying the qualifications needed for the position that will meet the needs of the program
3. Reviewing and ranking the candidates for the open position
4. Interviewing the top candidates

When evaluating a candidate, the manager should use (1) written information

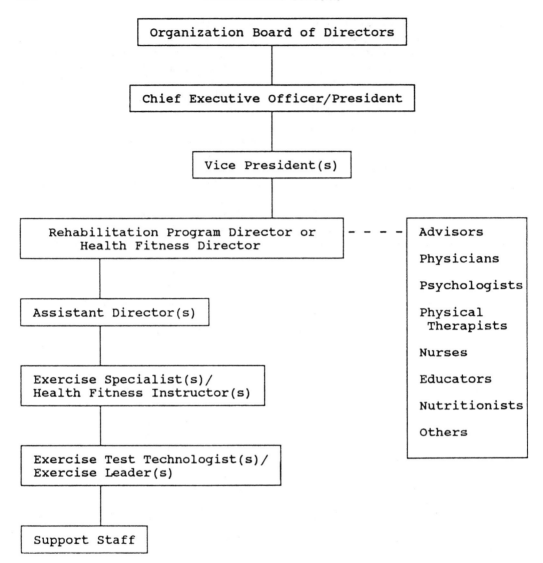

Fig. 42–1.   Sample organizational structure.

from the candidate, (2) references listed by the candidate, and (3) information obtained during a personal interview with the candidate. The skills and level of knowledge of the candidate can be determined from these sources.

The manager should carefully examine the written information from the candidate to assess communication skills. The manager should contact references listed by the candidate to discuss job qualifications and personal attributes.

The personal interview conducted with the candidate should allow discussion of program objectives from the candidate's point of view. This permits the applicant to have some input into the selection process. The interview validates the information on the candidate's application form.

The manager should avoid questions that require "yes" or "no" answers during the interview. Job expectations should not be revealed by the manager from the outset because the candidate will simply agree with those expectations without exploring them creatively. By asking questions carefully, the manager can have the candidate describe his or her qualifications and talent and explain exactly how those attributes fit into the organization. Interrupting or cutting off a response by the candidate should be avoided. It is recommended that the interview process be practiced among existing staff members. Examples of some questions to ask during an interview are listed in Table 42–3.

Compatibility of the candidate with the manager and the organization is an important consideration, but so is objective job performance. The manager should glean the opinions of co-workers by having other members of the staff interview the candidates. Use of the team approach in the selection process yields the greatest likelihood of revealing the best candidate.

Good administrative policy includes hav-

Table 42–3. Sample Questions for Job Interview

1. What interests you about the announced job opening?
2. Why are you making a change from your present position?
3. What are some of your more important accomplishments?
4. What part of your job do you like the best?
5. What duties do you like the least?
6. How would you apply what you have learned in past jobs to the current position?
7. How would you lead an exercise program under the following circumstances? (Interviewer should list some common characteristics of the current program to determine how the candidate would handle the situation.)
8. Do you have examples of how you attempt to communicate and motivate?
9. What have you done to develop your skills and experience in the past few years?
10. Describe your relationship with your past three supervisors.
11. What are your strengths in relating to other people?
12. Do you have an example of a situation in which you might not have been effective in relating to others? What would you do differently?
13. Some people are quick-tempered and impatient. How would you describe yourself?
14. Have you encountered any health problems?
15. Would you describe one or two new ideas, projects, or innovations of which you are particularly proud?
16. How do you feel about your career progress?
17. What are your future aspirations?
18. Are there any conditions that would limit your ability to take the new job?

ing job descriptions for each position, including management, in a program. The program director should define what positions exist in the program and then have descriptions written cooperatively by existing staff, if any, and the director. This process establishes, in writing, the responsibilities of each staff member so that each person knows what to expect and what is expected by management. A useful job description should be specific and should detail what the person in the job should accomplish. The job description should reflect a complete range of duties and responsibilities. Job descriptions should be reviewed and updated every 1 to 2 years. The job description is also a good tool for staff performance evaluation.

Program managers may have to coordinate several people including professional and support staff, advisory board members, student interns, consultants, subcontractors, and volunteers. Written job descriptions for all of these positions helps the program director delineate the responsibilities of each team member and blend this variety of expertise into an efficient and effective program. Written job descriptions also help the staff members to understand their own responsibilities in relation to those of other individuals. The written descriptions are also excellent guides in the orientation and training of new staff members.

Regardless of the quality of the staff selection process, some training of staff members is usually necessary. The training process involves orientation of new staff members to the new work environment, to other staff members, to the policies and procedures of the organization, to the job responsibilities of staff members, and to the staff reporting relationships.

The Business Plan

A start-up business plan differs from the annual business plan in that it: (1) requires significant allocation of resources (capital), (2) provides an evaluation of the risks/benefits of the proposed new program, and (3) contains more detailed analysis and more speculative projections.[1] The annual business plan contains the tactics of the long-range strategic plan that can be accomplished in one year with the purpose of achieving the organization's prime objective.

The most important function of a business plan is to identify areas that require further analysis and modification of strategies. An example of a business plan format is listed in Table 42–4.[1]

Business plans may be presented in many different formats depending on the form of the business enterprise. It is important to be familiar with the four forms of business enterprise.

1. Sole proprietorship—A single person owns all of the assets of the business. The single person bears all liabilities of the business and reaps all of the profits.
2. Partnership—Two or more persons share ownership of the business in a partnership. The business is not a legal entity separate from the partners. Partners are both individually and jointly liable for all debts of the business.

    In a general partnership, all partners share in the profits and losses of the business according to a previously agreed proportion.

    In a limited partnership, the liability of each partner depends on the extent of the capital contribution of each partner.
3. Corporation—A legal entity that is recognized as being separate and distinct from its owners. As a separate entity, it can acquire, hold, and convey property, sue and be sued, and generally act in its own name. It follows state statutes and bylaws.
4. S-corporation—A corporation that has elected to be taxed as if it were a partnership. Profits and losses flow directly to individual shareholders. The shareholders must report the gains and losses on their individual tax returns.

Two of the most important concerns in the business plan are the sources of revenue and the amount of cash needed for operations. Sources of revenue vary by setting:

Clinical setting: Participant fees
                    Budget from organization

Table 42–4. Components of a Business Plan[1]

1. Summary
    Business Description
        Name and location
        Product/services
        Market and competition
        Management expertise
    Financial Needs Summary
    Operation Projections Summary
2. Description and History of Current Business
    Brief history
    Identification of need
    Corporate mission and long-range goals
    Strengths, weaknesses, opportunities, and threats
3. Market Assessment
    Description
    Competition
    Industrial trends
    Market potential and customer base
    Market strategy
4. Management
    Key management personnel/experience
    Board structure and role
    Organizational chart
5. Technical and Operation Plan
    General operating plan/policies
    Costs/pricing
    Critical risks and problems
6. Facilities
    Rationale for location
    Description
    Leased/owned
    Occupancy costs
7. Financial Plan
    Capitalization plan
    Explanation of financial structure
    Summary/highlights of projected performance
    Financial requirements/potential sources
    Financial management
    Financial Statements (3-year projections)
        Profit and loss statement forecasts
        Proforma cash flow projections (by month)
        Proforma balance sheets
        Sources and uses of funds
    Explanation of financial projections
        Best and worst case scenarios
        Capital expenditure estimates
        Strengths of plan
8. Appendix (optional)
    Letters of support for concept
    Market studies
    Resumes of management team

Grants from foundations or government

Community setting: Participant fees

Budget from municipal taxes

Budget from social service agency

Budget from organization

Grants from foundations or government

Commercial setting: Personal funds

Banks

Government

Venture capital

Participant fees

Corporate setting: Annual budget

Participant fees (?)

A special note is made here with regard to reimbursement fees as sources of revenue. Each discipline is unique in its education, certification process, and means of receiving payment from third party carriers. Payment guidelines for various services differ between carriers and between states. Public payment for outpatient services is defined by the Health Care Financing Administration (HCFA). The following areas used by HCFA are general guidelines to determine coverage:

1. Compliance with state and local laws
   a. Licenser of facility
   b. Licenser of personnel
2. Governing body and administration
   a. Ownership
   b. Administration
   c. Professional personnel
3. Patient services
   a. Scope of services
   b. Patient assessment
4. Clinical records
   a. Content
   b. Protection of information
5. Safety and comfort of patients
   a. Emergency procedures
6. Sanitary environment
   a. Cleaning standards
7. Equipment maintenance
8. Physical access for the handicapped
   a. Toilet facilities
   b. Doorways, passageways, elevators
   c. Parking

9. Utilization review
   a. Admissions
   b. Treatment plan
   c. Clinical practice
   d. Discharges

The capital needs identified in the business plan are described in three categories:

1. Initial start-up capital—Initial capital may be needed for feasibility study, architectural, facility, equipment, legal, accounting, licenses, permits, marketing, advertising, and financing costs.
2. Operating capital—Variable operating capital may be needed for marketing, advertising, maintenance, repairs, supplies, printing, postage, utilities, payroll, fringe benefits, legal, and accounting fees. Fixed operating capital may be needed for insurance, taxes, interest/debt service, depreciation, and leases.
3. Reserve capital—Reserve capital may be needed for unexpected costs, low income, or operating the program for one year with no income.

PROGRAM PLANNING

Evaluation of Need

Planning involves the use of objective information from the evaluation process combined with industry trends and economics to determine the need for change, growth, or decline. Input information defines where the organization is now and where it wants to be in the future.

Input data should be collected from clients (participants) and employees within the organization to accurately assess needs and interests. Several methods may be used to gather input information. These methods may include interviews with current participants, upper management, advisors, and staff; and surveys of potential participants.

When interviews are used to evaluate need in the planning process, a structured approach should be used. This approach is much like conducting a written survey, but the personal interview format is used. The purpose of the personal interview is to determine what the clients really want and need.

Input information is also obtained by meeting with the organization's upper management to clarify the general philosophy of the program and what the management considers as needs. Questions to be answered include:

1. How does management view the program?
2. How does the exercise program fit with the goals and mission of the sponsoring organization?
3. Does management's philosophy of the organization match with the philosophy of the exercise program?

Another channel for information input is to form a program advisory committee. Meeting with the committee provides a forum to obtain their ideas on how they view the program, what should be offered, and how it should be conducted. The advisors may be representatives from the organization's staff and participants and/or outside professionals who have an interest in helping the program.

Meetings with program staff and employees of the organization are also important sources of input information. If the program is new, prospective staff members may be interviewed to get their ideas on program concepts. Staff and employee ideas are sources of information that should not be overlooked.

The Planning Process

After the needs of the program have been identified through the evaluation process, objectives for the program, and the tasks necessary to meet those objectives should be placed in order of priority. Some questions to answer in the planning process include:

1. What are your resources?
2. What are your staffing needs?
3. What are your options?
4. What are the anticipated obstacles?
5. What programs can be offered within the budget?
6. How will you keep the participants motivated?
7. How will you ensure participant safety?
8. How will you document the program's effectiveness?
9. How will records be kept?

Objectives for the program should be established on short-term, medium-range, and long-term bases. Guidelines for establishing objectives based on time include the following:

Short-term	3–12 months
Medium-range	12–24 months
Long-term	24–48 months

Implementation

The implementation stage of the management process involves four steps:

1. Review the planned objectives and tasks
2. Assign the tasks to staff members
3. Implement the tasks
4. Supervise the implementation of the tasks

This series is initiated on the assumption that the program staff members have been hired and are available to implement the tasks assigned to them. Reviewing the planned objectives and tasks with the staff members helps to increase communication between management and staff and improves the understanding that everyone is working for the same goals.

DAY-TO-DAY OPERATIONS

Managerial Responsibilities

The manager is responsible for all aspects of the program[1]:

1. Development and implementation of program protocols
2. Development and implementation of operating policies
3. Coordination of services
4. Hiring, supervising, and evaluating staff
5. Staff development and training programs
6. Budget assessment and management of expenses
7. Recommendations to the Board of Directors for capital improvements/investments
8. Coordination and approval of all promotional plans, marketing projects, and public relations efforts
9. Program evaluation and planning for growth
10. Development of research projects and funding

11. Administration of testing and evaluation of participants
12. Orientation and counseling of program participants

Resources

Several resources surrounding a program are available to help the program accomplish its operational tasks. Some of the resources include part-time consultants, subcontractors, student interns, and volunteers. Consultants and subcontractors may be available to provide certain aspects of the program, such as medical/fitness testing, exercise class leadership, or educational seminars. The use of outside consultants and services may reduce the compensation and overhead costs of having permanent staff on the payroll. Use of outside resources may also free in-house staff to spend more time counseling participants and preparing for other aspects of the program.

In some instances, participant volunteers may help to recruit, encourage, and motivate other participants. Volunteers are usually used to help with special events, such as fun-runs, fitness days, tournaments, and seminars. Volunteers represent a tremendous source of talent to help the program achieve some of its objectives. Volunteers may be located by word of mouth, newsletters, or in-house announcements.

Marketing

Prompting consumers to use the program involves not only good management processes and staffing but also good marketing and implementation procedures. Regardless of the quality of the staff and programs, they will not be used unless the consumer knows about their availability.

Although marketing methods have gained a certain mystique, the definition of marketing is simple: determine the wants and needs of the people and satisfy them. For commercial exercise programs, an additional statement can be made—make a profit doing it. There are eight guidelines for effective marketing:

1. Define and concentrate on the best market (called market segmentation)
2. Position your organization and programs in a market niche

3. Keep the price credible, then make it affordable
4. Find the right distribution channel
5. Help sellers sell
6. Make advertising a faithful extension of the product itself
7. Keep your marketing innovative
8. Never betray the customer's trust

Successful marketing of an exercise program must serve a consumer need or desire and must do so in an honest, reliable way. Otherwise, the program will not win repeat participants and referrals. Ultimately, the participant-provider relationship lives or dies on the basis of mutual respect and trust.

In providing a credible exercise program, the staff, program, and facilities must be professional and well organized. Separate staff should be hired to market the exercise program if the purpose is to expand widely and/or to make a profit. It is difficult for technical personnel in a program to also be the marketing staff; there simply is not enough time in the day to be effective at both tasks. If marketing is of prime importance to the program, full-time marketing personnel should be hired. Marketing staff should have full knowledge of all details of the program, with familiarity of technical aspects of the program as well.

A good marketing system for an exercise program involves development of a marketing strategy, implementation of that marketing plan, and evaluation of the results. The development phase requires a description of the marketplace in terms of the geographic, demographic, and economic characteristics of the potential users. The marketing plan should include a description of the competition, with a comparison of their services to those of the current program. The needs of the users should be identified in the marketing plan by surveying the market.

After the market has been described thoroughly, special groups should be targeted to begin the promotional plan outlined for the exercise program. The initiation of market trials before a full market plan is implemented is advisable. Market trials could first include program employees and spouses. Volunteers from the program can also be used. As feedback is received from the market trials, the marketing plan is adjusted to provide the most effective strategy for obtaining program participants.

The effectiveness of a full marketing plan should be evaluated. Strengths and weaknesses of the plan are identified and the results are used to design new marketing plans for the future. The concept of product life-cycle should be clearly understood. Most products and services grow initially in sales and profitability due to their uniqueness and newness. After a certain period of time (which varies considerably by product), profitability plateaus and then starts to decrease. The decrease may be due to stagnation in marketing the product. The manager should be aware of product life cycles and plan new and exciting marketing strategies to maintain or increase profitability.

A good marketing plan includes some form of advertising. The purposes of advertising are to announce programs, establish need, upgrade image, and draw potential buyers. Examples of pertinent advertising techniques include:

Word of mouth
Media releases
Print advertising
Radio announcements
Staff speaking engagements
Direct mail
Brochures
Audio and video tapes
Free memberships

One major function of marketing is to build a good relationship with clients (potential participants). A good relationship with the media (radio, TV, newspaper) may also help to promote programs. Good public relations is a foundation for soliciting program participants and building a referral network. Public relations strategies should coincide with the company's objectives.

Another important managerial responsibility is office administration. Clerical and secretarial details, maintenance, and custodial services are often overlooked or taken for granted in a program. These positions are important to the success of a program. For example, receptionist or secretary is often considered a low-paid, low-priority position. Yet, in an exercise program, this person is often the first line of communication with the participants. This person is therefore an important key to the program. The receptionist or secretary should have good "people" skills and should be friendly, courteous, and personal. This person should be efficient when making appointments, have good typing and word processing skills, be careful about keeping accurate files, and be well organized.

Maintenance and custodial personnel are responsible for keeping the facilities and equipment clean and operating safely. The manager should place special emphasis on these responsibilities. A successful health fitness program requires a sanitary environment for the participants.

Legal Concerns

Because the health fitness field is unregulated and nonstandardized at the present time, the director must rely on professional associations for guidelines and standards that are reasonable and take into account that which is being done in similar settings. In the absence of specific regulations, litigation will be based on that which is reasonable, prudent, and consistent with policies and procedures in similar facilities.[1]

To minimize legal problems, the manager should utilize risk management procedures such as[1]:

1. Careful screening and monitoring of participants
2. Properly obtained informed consent
3. Written policies and procedures
4. Regular in-service and continuing education activities
5. Informing participants of program policies and procedures
6. Thorough, real-time documentation of incidents (Fig. 42–2)

To minimize legal problems specifically regarding emergency procedures and informed consent:

1. Select certified professionals to lead classes and supervise exercise on equipment
2. Require current CPR certification of all staff members
3. Provide written guidelines of emergency procedures

Step 1. Name of participant _____
Date of incident _____

Step 2. Describe the nature of the injury or health problem.

_____
_____

Step 3. Describe how the injury/accident occurred.

_____
_____

Step 4. Describe the staff's response to the incident.

_____
_____

Step 5. Describe any problems encountered in the situation.

_____
_____

Step 6. List the names of witnesses to the injury/accident or emergency procedures.

_____
_____

Step 7. Where and to whom was the participant referred?

_____
_____

Step 8. Other comments.

_____
_____

Staff Signature _____
Date _____

Figure 42-2. Sample Accident/Injury Form.

4. Rehearse the emergency procedures
5. Inform participants about the risks and dangers of exercise and obtain informed consent
6. Require medical clearance before allowing participants to exercise
7. Instruct staff to limit their advice to their own area of expertise and not to "practice medicine"
8. Provide a safe environment by following building codes and a regular maintenance schedule for equipment
9. Purchase adequate liability insurance for the staff

PROGRAM EVALUATION

Evaluation of the exercise program involves two methods: process evaluation and outcome evaluation. Process evaluation verifies that the assigned tasks have been accomplished. Outcome evaluation determines if the objectives of the program were met. Both types can be used to evaluate short-term, medium-range, and long-term objectives.

During process evaluation, the manager should monitor the program activities to ensure that:

1. Operation of the program was efficient
2. Tasks assigned were reasonable
3. Time schedule was realistic
4. Staff members were prepared to perform and actually did complete the tasks
5. Staff members were dependable and enthusiastic
6. Proper resources were available for effective programming
7. Budget was adequate
8. Program was fun, accessible, and personalized

The facts collected for outcome evaluation include:

1. Number of participants starting a program
2. Number of participants completing a program
3. Survey of participants and management to determine if the program objectives were met
4. Cost/benefit or cost-effective analysis

The findings of the process and outcome evaluations are then combined and the overall effectiveness of the program is determined. If the program is effective, the participants should exhibit positive changes in:

1. Exercise behaviors—increased activity levels
2. Health—more energy, disease risks reduced, health care costs reduced
3. Fitness—improved cardiovascular endurance, fat to lean body weight ratio, flexibility, and strength
4. Knowledge—health and fitness concepts understood
5. Attitudes—improved morale and self-confidence

Financial Accountability

The director of a program must have a thorough understanding of how to prepare a budget and monitor revenue and expenses. Planning and controlling a budget helps:

1. Analyze the program's cost effectiveness
2. Determine the importance of each program component
3. Reveal high-quality results of some program components
4. Evaluate the overall financial health of the program

A well-designed budget is a good decision-making guide. Components for future programs are selected on the basis of best participation and/or revenue. The program budget must be flexible so that managers can transfer monies to areas of need or best use.

Documentation

Careful record keeping is an important responsibility of the manager. In this age of accountability, the administrator can not rely solely on participant testimonies to justify a program's existence. The manager must be able to show a program's accomplishments through written documentation and evidence.

The computer has become a very practical tool for storing large amounts of information in a very small space. The personal computer continues to get smaller in size, more powerful in operation, and faster in speed. Wise use of a computer can save the manager valuable time.

Very extensive software systems have been developed for personal computers, local area networks, minicomputers, and mainframes. Software systems available for health fitness programs include[4]:

- Health risk appraisals
- Health screening variables
- Medical records
- Fitness test results
- Exercise prescriptions
- Nutrition evaluations and diet plans
- Educational reports
- Activity participation and caloric expenditure
- Check-in control

- Tournament scheduling
- Equipment utilization
- Inventory
- Traffic flow
- Membership status
- Accounting and billing
- Club management
- Data base analysis (research, statistics, etc).

The overall documentation plan involves collecting information on membership, staff, and program operations. With regard to participant membership, the following information should be documented[4]:

- Name, sex, age, height, weight
- Marital status, children
- Address, telephone (home and office)
- Membership contracts, program registration
- Health information, needs and interests
- Medical clearance records
- Fitness test results, fitness goals
- Exercise records, club usage
- Services purchased, amenities desired
- Injury reports

Documented information about the staff includes a report of each person's personnel evaluation[4]:

- Job knowledge, training, experience
- Willingness to accept responsibility
- Planning and organization of work
- Quality and quantity of work
- Cost consciousness and control
- Relationships with others
- Leadership qualities
- Initiative and resourcefulness
- Originality and creativeness
- Soundness of judgment
- Dependability
- Support for organization goals and policies
- Career objectives

Departmental documentation includes[4]:

- Program/class registrations
- Facility attendance records
- Equipment usage patterns
- Equipment maintenance records
- Supply inventory
- Pro shop operations
- Laundry service

Cost/Benefit and Cost-Effectiveness Analyses

A cost/benefit analysis (or more accurately a benefit/cost analysis) is used to analyze the savings (benefits) of a program relative to the costs incurred. It is used most appropriately in an employee health promotion program to determine if the calculated savings in medical claims, insurance, absenteeism, turnover, and productivity exceed the costs of the program designed to impact those variables. The benefit/cost results of various health promotion programs have been summarized by the Association for Fitness in Business.[5] The benefit range per employee for health promotion programs has been found to be $51 to $610 in lower medical costs, 1 to 2 days fewer absences, and 4 to 25% increased productivity.

The costs of a program are usually obvious and easy to document. Those costs generally involve[4]:

- Facility
- Construction
- Amortization
- Depreciation
- Rent
- Utilities
- Maintenance
- Equipment
- Supplies
- Contract services
- Salaries and fringe benefits
- Insurance
- Publications and dues
- Travel
- Special events and awards
- Printing
- Advertising and promotion
- Office
- Miscellaneous

The benefits of programs are less obvious and may be difficult and sometimes impossible to document. Benefits claimed by many health promotion programs include[4]:

- Reduced health care costs
- Lower absenteeism
- Lower turnover
- Higher morale
- Lower risk of cardiovascular disease
- Lower risk of incurring injuries
- Faster recovery time from injury or illness
- Increased energy and stamina
- Increased mental alertness
- Increased self-confidence and self-esteem
- Less tension and anxiety
- Increased productivity

A cost-effectiveness analysis is used to compare the effectiveness of two or more programs relative to the cost incurred in each program. For example, the group stop-smoking program in the following analysis is the most cost-effective.

Stop-Smoking Program	Success Rate	Cost/ Person
Individual Self-Help	40%	$75
Support Group	80%	$40

REFERENCES

1. American College of Sports Medicine: *Guidelines for Exercise Testing and Prescription.* Fourth Edition. Philadelphia: Lea & Febiger, 1991.
2. Patton RW, Corry JM, Gettman LR, Graf JS: *Implementing Health Fitness Programs.* Champaign, IL: Human Kinetics, 1986.
3. Blanchard K, Johnson S: *The One Minute Manager.* New York: Berkley Books, 1982.
4. Patton RW, Grantham WC, Gerson RF, Gettman LR: *Developing and Managing Health Fitness Facilities.* Champaign, IL: Human Kinetics, 1989.
5. Opatz J, Chenoweth D, Kaman R: *Economic Impact of Worksite Health Promotion.* Indianapolis, IN: Association for Fitness in Business, 1991.

Chapter 43

BUDGET CONSIDERATIONS

Ami M. Drimmer and Jeffrey L. Roitman

BUDGET CONSIDERATIONS

Professional advancement requires assumption of a leadership role, which usually requires expanded knowledge and skills. One of the new, major responsibilities is often the formulation and control of the budget. The scope and depth of this responsibility can vary and will depend on the overall organizational structure and its financial orientation. However, regardless of the organizational structure, an understanding of the budget and the budgetary process is important for the successful fulfillment of a leadership role.

Because many professionals in health and fitness are not prepared in the area of budget and finance, it can be an uncomfortable responsibility. The first section of this chapter addresses the issue of budget from the basic concepts. Learning objectives include an understanding of:

The limitations of a budget
The benefits of a budget
How to construct a budget
The difference between a capital and operating budget
Utilization of a budget
Budgeting terminology

A budget should be thought of as a plan. Planning and allocating time and use of facilities is also budgeting. Program directors are responsible for a business, perhaps a large business such as an independent center, or a smaller business such as a program within a department. The business goal is to create or increase profit. "Profit" is the lifeline of any business. The profitability of a center or a program will offer fiscal stability and provides for expansion of existing programs and development of new programs and projects. One of the major aspects of business planning is the budget, which in this case represents a fiscal plan.

A budget is a blueprint that reflects management assumptions, commitment, and expectation. It is a detailed description of all expected revenues and expenses.

Benefits and Limitations

Because the proper preparation of a budget is a detailed and time-consuming activity, it makes sense that the first step following the understanding of a budget is to examine its benefits and limitations. The benefits of a budget are summarized in the following paragraphs.

The budget is a plan. Following its preparation, the budget is reviewed and approved by upper management. The management approval formalizes the planning activities and the budget becomes an action plan representing management commitment and expectations. For example, a pilot who flies from New York to San Francisco must have a flight plan. The formal plan that the pilot is following ensures that the flight reaches a specific destination at a specific time. Budgets function similarly by organizing activities so that the results will match management objectives.

A budget is a tool and a basis for performance evaluation. The person responsible for a professional activity center or program has the responsibility to manage the day-to-day operation within the given plan. The budget becomes one criterion for evaluation. Review and analysis of the budget will provide answers to questions such as:

Does each program meet its fiscal goals?
Was projected revenue accurate?
Were projected expenses accurate?
How does this program compare to previous programs
Is this activity cost-effective?

It can be seen from this analysis how the budget can become a tool used to evaluate performance. This tool can help the administration evaluate programs and staff performance. It should be, however, only one of several tools used in the evaluation process. In addition to being part of the performance appraisal of the department or program director, regular reviews of the budget provide management with a "yardstick" to evaluate the progress of the program or center toward set objectives. This review can provide the program director and management with an opportunity for early intervention, if necessary, to keep the action plan on track toward the business objectives of the operation.

A budget is also a method for coordination and communication. Any organization with different functions and programs must coordinate its activities to allow progress toward the achievement of stated goals and objectives. A budget requires coordination and communication among divisions within the organization.

This coordination and communication starts when the budget is constructed and continues throughout the budget period. For example, the number of participants in a weight management program affects the revenue side of the budget. This number is partly dependent on the promotion of the programs which, in turn, affects the expense side of the Marketing Department budget. For the objectives of the weight management program to be met, it is clear that coordination and communication between those who deliver the program and those who are responsible for program promotion are required.

From the above discussion, it is clear that there is a value in a budget and the budgetary process, but as with any other process, there are some limitations.

A budget is only as good and complete as the effort and attention to details put forth in its preparation. If incorrect data were used or unrealistic assumptions were made, the budget is of little value. A budget must be based on accurate and realistic projections of both revenue and expenses. If it is not, its usefulness is limited.

All budgets affect employees and, therefore, human relations. Employees may perceive the budget to be a negative evaluation tool. However, all employees should understand that the budget not only discloses weakness, but is used by management to help identify strengths and opportunities. The budget is used to assist in achieving the business goals of the organization.

Budgeting and budgets cannot replace effective day-to-day management. A budget is a tool, a plan, and not an end product.

Developing a Budget

The process of budget development differs between institutions and industries. The differences may be caused by size, goals, and objectives of the operation, or any number of other reasons. At the same time, some factors and steps should be considered regardless of the specific budgetary process.

The process of constructing a budget can occur in one of two ways: the *top-to-bottom* or *bottom-to-top* approach. These two concepts are simple, but can have a profound effect on the acceptance of the budget and the way it is carried out.

The *top-to-bottom* approach means that the budget is developed and prepared by top management with little or no input from other staff. This approach has the advantage of a relatively short preparation time, limited discussions, and it reflects the organizational goals and objectives as defined by top management. The limitation of this approach is that the middle and lower level management and personnel do not have ownership in this budget and may lack the commitment for its implementation.

The *bottom-to-top* approach starts at lower levels of staff or management and works its way up the organizational chart. It usually starts with a specific budgetary guideline issued by upper management. Then, various management and employee levels have the opportunity for input. The benefit of this approach is that it reflects the experience of all levels within the "real world" of this specific organization. The result is a budget formulated by those who will manage it, which gives stronger incentive for its implementation. This method, however, has shortcomings. It can be time-consuming, more-labor intensive, and, therefore, more expensive. When considering the direction of budget development, the question is, "Do the benefits of a specific approach outweigh the limitations?" Based on the answer to this question, the proper process can be chosen. Some budgets are developed using a combination of these methods. Regardless of the method, the development of the budget should follow the general steps described below.

Establish Budget Period Goals

Because the budget is a plan, setting specific fiscal or other operational goals for the year will define the outcomes. These goals might be revenue from a specific program, the number of patients in a rehabilitation program, or a specific health-related cost reduction for a given organization. The goals should be specific and measurable.

Assemble All of the Information

Determine such things as the feasible, reasonable, and payable fee for services. Project noncollectible revenue and the cost of all the supplies and materials needed. Estimate salaries and benefits of employees, as well as the number of employees required to provide the service. Information such as hours of operation, inflation allowances for supplies and labor, other expenses, and costs of professional development should be considered.

List All Capital Expenses

It is important for the budget to be realistic. For any budget to be realistic, one must consider capital expenses (equipment, facilities, etc.) as well as operational expenses. Capital expenses are different during the early years of operation, when the capital expenditures are greater, than in the later years, when such expenses include replacement of equipment and, perhaps, facility renovation.

Determine Whether the Budget Is Realistic

Despite the fact that a budget "looks good on paper," take the time to compare it with previous budgets. Compare it to specific data from the appropriate geographic location and industry. It may be useful to allow an "expert" consultant to examine the details of the budget, especially in new

organizations. A budget can be useful only if it is functional, and to be functional it has to be realistic.

Operational versus Capital Budgets

The terms "operational budget" and "capital budget" are defined as follows. The operational budget reflects all the costs of operating the center and of operating the program. This includes direct and indirect costs. Direct costs are directly related to the activity or production of a product. For example, in a human performance laboratory, ECG electrodes and paper are items that directly relate to testing. Their usage is related to testing; therefore they are in the direct-cost category. On the other hand, the rent and the electricity for the facility, which include the testing laboratory, are indirect costs because they are not related to the specific performance of the test. The capital budget, on the other hand, reflects the cost of facility and equipment needed to provide the service. For example, in the laboratory, the equipment, e.g., treadmill, bike, ECG monitor, and recording system, are considered capital expenses and should be part of the capital budget.

Constructing the Budget

The purposes, processes, and steps for formulating a budget have been presented. To illustrate this step in the process, a budget for a Phase III community-based cardiac rehabilitation program is developed. The first step is to identify the goal, in this case the addition of a Phase III community-based program. The next is to project the revenue and expenses of this program.

Revenues include program fees and testing fees. Program fees should be structured considering competitors, financial status of patients, and the economic status of the community, as well as the expenses of the program. Method of payment is another factor that should be considered. Monthly or yearly payments are two of the possibilities. The importance of this factor is that payment structure will determine "cash flow" for the program or center. Cash flow relates to the amount of revenue collected on a regular basis that is available to pay operating expenses. In this illustration, a membership fee of $35 per month is set. The fee for evaluation, which includes exercise testing, risk factor analysis, etc. which is required for all patients entering the Phase III program is established at $150. The final step in projecting the revenue is estimating patient referrals and participation. The projected members are multiplied by the appropriate fee and units of service to determine the total revenue.

Once all revenues are projected, all forseeable expenses for the program should be listed and total program cost determined. These include both capital and operational expenses, direct and indirect. Staffing, supplies, rent, utilities, etc. are listed. Salary allocation should be determined by the time of operation of the program allowing for preparation and administrative time. Educational materials, towels, charts and notebooks, ECG paper, electrodes, electrode gel, and other miscellaneous expenses are determined.

Table 43–1 is a "line item budget" associated with the proposed program divided into appropriate categories or items (often called "lines" or "line items" in a budget). These line items and categories may differ from institution to institution. The budget is an annual budget spread evenly by month; thus only "Month" and "Annual" columns appear. Some programs spread the budget by expected monthly expenses and revenue; thus it may not spread evenly over the 12 month period.

Is the Budget Realistic?

After the development of the budget, some assessment should be performed. To do this, examine the items in the budget lines to determine their accuracy. The costs, pricing, and fee structure should be consistent with the principles discussed and the facts dictated by the situation.

In this case, salaries are based on a 4-hour-per-day program operating 3 days per week for a total of 12 hours per week per staff member. It appears that this program will take two staff members about 100 hours per month. Because this staff is already employed at the center, no administrative or preparation time is allotted because it will be allowed elsewhere. Benefits are structured at 15% of salary (specific to this institution). Other expenses within the operationing budget are relatively simple and straightforward. The portion of the towel service can be estimated from the number of patients, as can the medical supplies for testing ($7.50 per test) and the materials for patient education ($24.75 per patient). Miscellaneous expense is an estimate for such items as copies, flyers, and expenses unaccounted for in other lines. Overhead, maintenance and utilities are based on a prorated cost of expenses already known for the facility.

Revenue is based on volume projections, which are estimates formulated from present Phase II volumes and results of a physician survey. Based on eight new entries per month, a total of 96 patients are projected to enter during the year. Allowing for a 20 to 25% dropout, approximately 74 patients will finish the year in the program (see Table 43–2). The revenue from those patients can be projected. The testing revenue is based on eight entries per month. "Total Revenue" on Table 43–2 is the combination of testing and membership fees.

The review of the budget and the projections is considered to be realistic and workable. This review process should be duplicated with all budgets formulated by the staff, especially for new programs.

Table 43–1. Line Item Budget

Expenses	Month	Annual
Salary	$1560	18,720
Benefits	234	2808
Supplies		
Educational Materials	198	2376
Towels	150	1800
Medical Supplies	36	432
Miscellaneous	100	1200
Overhead		
Rent	150	1800
Utilities	80	960
Maintenance	120	1440
Total Expenses	2628	31,536
Revenue		
Membership Fees	1435	17,220
Evaluation Fees	1200	14,400
Total Revenue	2635	31,620
Net Profit/(Loss)	7	84

Table 43–2. Revenue Projection

Month	Evaluation* # Tests	Revenue	Membership† # Part	Revenue	Total Revenue	Dropouts	Revenue Loss	Net Revenue
Jan	8	1200	8	280	1480	2	0	1480
Feb	8	1200	14	490	1690	2	70	1620
Mar	8	1200	20	700	1900	2	70	1830
Apr	8	1200	26	910	2110	2	70	2040
May	8	1200	32	1120	2320	2	70	2250
Jun	8	1200	38	1330	2530	2	70	2460
Jul	8	1200	44	1540	2740	2	70	2670
Aug	8	1200	50	1750	2950	2	70	2880
Sep	8	1200	56	1960	3160	2	70	3090
Oct	8	1200	62	2170	3370	2	70	3300
Nov	8	1200	68	2380	3580	2	70	3510
Dec	8	1200	74	2590	3790	2	70	3720
Total		14,400		17,220	31,620			30,850

* Evaluation = $150/test
† Membership = $35/month

Utilization of a Budget

Using the budget on an ongoing basis, as previously described, is simple. The budget can, and should, be used as a tool for monitoring the program and its productivity. If, on a monthly basis, the projections are not met, analysis and action may be required.

A comparison of the Net Revenue from actual budget activity in Table 43-3 with the projected monthly expenses in Table 43-1 shows a shortfall in every month except January, September and October.

Dropouts exceed projections in the months of April, May, July, October, November, and December. Seasonality may account for some of this activity. Action at two levels may be considered. An effort to increase enrollment in the preceding and/or succeeding months may be helpful. Planning for the next budget year should include decreasing volume projections and changing staff time allocations. This will provide a more realistic picture of the actual revenue and expenses expected during those months.

Table 43–3. Budget Summary, Actual Annual Activity

Month	Evaluation* # Tests	Revenue	Membership† # Part	Revenue	Total Revenue	Dropouts	Revenue Loss	Net Revenue
Jan	16	2400	16	560	2960	0	0	2960
Feb	8	1200	24	840	2040	0	0	2040
Mar	8	1200	30	1050	2250	2	70	2180
Apr	8	1200	33	1155	2355	5	175	2180
May	8	1200	33	1155	2355	8	280	2075
Jun	8	1200	40	1400	2600	1	35	2565
Jul	6	900	38	1330	2230	8	280	1950
Aug	5	750	41	1435	2185	2	70	2115
Sep	8	1200	47	1645	2845	2	70	2775
Oct	8	1200	49	1715	2915	6	210	2705
Nov	8	1200	47	1645	2845	10	350	2495
Dec	5	750	47	1645	2395	5	175	2220
Total		14,400		15,575	29,975			28,210

* Evaluation = $150/test
† Membership = $35/month

Analysis of the budget can also identify a break-even point. Table 43–2 is a detailed, annual revenue projection of a budget for a new project. This revenue projection, together with projected expenses, is often presented to upper management for justification of new programs or projects. When approved, it becomes the budget and the action plan for the program. It also becomes, as previously stated, a tool for evaluation of progress towards stated goals for that program. If the goals are met and exceeded, the budget can be used to justify expansion of the program. In this case, the revenue projection (Table 43-2) identifies July as the first month where projected revenue (either "total" or "net") exceeds expenses of the program. It also reveals a deficit for the first year (net revenue from Table 43-2 less total annual expenses from Table 43-1). The total first-year deficit is projected to be $686. If projections are accurate, the program should be profitable in the second year and collect enough revenue to make up for the first-year loss. When projecting second-year budgets, making allowances for growth in both revenue and expenses is important.

Finally, comparison of the pro forma (Table 43–2) with the actual annual budget activity (Table 43–3) assists in the next year's budget projections. Growth should be part of the plan if it is expected. Allowances for the exceptions to the plan for this year should be included in any projection for the coming year, as previously stated. Using the present-year actual financial activity as well as any other past data should make future projections more accurate.

General Considerations

In addition to the specific information regarding the steps and actions needed to construct and control a budget, some general, budget-related concerns are required for in-depth knowledge of the budgetary process. These considerations include the following.

1. *Seasonality*: These are changes in activity level based on a calendar cycle. The Phase III illustration indicates the decrease in new participants and activity levels in certain months. These changes in number of participants that are predictable need to be part of the budget process.

2. *Cash Flow*: One of the major concerns of any business is cash flow. Departments or programs within a large organization may not be directly affected by cash flow. However, free-standing centers and small businesses may be directly affected and cash flow is of major importance. A cash flow budget should reflect all expenses as they come due so that cash is available to pay them. Posting all expenses when due, projecting revenue when collected, and accounting for other variables such as seasonality are essential for good cash management.

3. *Other Expenses*: There may be other general expenses in some budgets. These may be more applicable to a free-standing facility or indendent operation and may include such line items as liability or other insurance coverage and taxes such as property or FICA (often included in the salary line).

4. *Master Budget*: In some situations, a final step in the budget process is the aggregation of several program or departmental budgets, such as described earlier, into one comprehensive, institutional budget. This "master budget" reflects all of the operational requirements and expectations of each program and of the center as a whole.

Summary

The purpose of this chapter was to introduce the principles of the budget and finance, the construction of a budget, and using budgets as tools for evaluation in businesses. A budget is a plan of action that represents specific assumptions, commitment and expectations by management and staff. The benefits of careful budget planning and analysis were described as well as the limitations of the budget process. The principles and specific actions required to construct a budget were reviewed in detail together with the definition and explanation of the differences between capital and operational budgets. Some general considerations that are part of understanding a budget and its construction and control were reviewed.

REIMBURSEMENT FOR CLINICAL EXERCISE PROGRAMS*

One of the major factors contributing to the revenue side of the budget in clinical programs (and thus, to the Center) is the reimbursement of clinical exercise therapy by third party payors—health insurance. Some understanding of the rules and regulations governing reimbursement is necessary to understand reimbursement in general and to budget for these revenues. The rules and regulations usually delineate the medical indication for therapy, the diagnosis that will be covered, the amount that will be paid for any given service, and the allowable length and frequency of service. Furthermore, the current state of health care makes reimbursement an issue of major importance for clinical programs. This part of the chapter discusses some aspects of reimbursement for clinical exercise programs.

Preventive and rehabilitative exercise programs can, and do, encompass various clinical disciplines that either individually or collectively include physical therapy, occupational therapy, recreation therapy, respiratory therapy, exercise physiology, athletic training, nursing, nutrition, behavioral medicine, and physician services. Each discipline is unique in its education/certification process and requirements for receiving payment from third-party carriers. As a result, the various disciplines have developed their own means to secure reimbursement.

Insurance Company Review

Millions of Americans are protected by one or more forms of health care insurance. Health insurance organizations can be classified into two distinct parts: the private sector and the public sector. The private sector is primarily composed of the Blue Cross/Blue Shield, private commercial insurance companies, health maintenance organizations (HMOs) and preferred provider organizations (PPOs).

Most of the private sector companies offer basic coverage, with major medical coverage provided at an additional cost. The public sector encompasses government-administered insurers such as Medicare, Medicaid, Civilian Health and Medical Program of the Uniformed Services (CHAMPUS), Indian Health Services, Worker's Compensation Medical Care, and the Bureau of Vocational Rehabilitation (BVR).

Reimbursement for Prevention of Chronic Disease

At the present time, reimbursement of preventive health services is uncommon, but some trends suggest that portions of these programs may become reimbursible. Many employers play an important role in programs that are designed to reduce absenteeism, improve productivity, and lower health claims and workmen's compensation costs by increasing the well-being of the working population and society. There are many obstacles to reimbursement of "prevention programs" in the insurance industry, not the least of which is a primary concern for cutting the cost of health care.

Reimbursement for Rehabilitative Programs

Most rehabilitative programs focus on the restoration of physical functional capacity along with secondary prevention of chronic disease. Treatment through rehabilitative medicine usually includes one or more of the disciplines mentioned at the beginning of this chapter.

Public payment for outpatient services is well defined through the regulation of the Health Care Financing Administration (HCFA) and through the Civilian Health and Medical Program of the Uniformed Services (CHAMPUS). These organizations are the two largest public health insurance providers. The HCFA standards and criteria are relatively strict and should be carefully reviewed and followed by rehabilitative programs to ensure appropriate reimbursement. Because HCFA administers its program by using regional intermediaries, there are some variations in the interpretation and execution of HCFA regulations. This will affect pay-

---

* Parts of this section directly quoted and/or adapted from Meyer G: Reimbursement for Clinical Exercise Programs, in *Resource Manual for Guidelines for Exercise Testing and Prescription*. First Edition. Philadelphia: Lea & Febiger, 1988.

ment for services. It is advisable to identify the regional Medicare intermediary and to clarify their interpretation of the HCFA guidelines.

Payment for Services

The various services, payors, and standards for reimbursement make diagnosis, utilization review guidelines and professional personnel primary concerns for those delivering the service and requesting reimbursement. For example, specific diagnoses are often required for reimbursement of cardiac rehabilitation or pulmonary rehabilitation services. Utilization review guidelines often require a plan of treatment and documentation of progression toward measurable outcomes. These are essential for continuing reimbursement. "Maintenance programs" are generally not reimbursible. Program staff should be congnizant of the rules and regulations as set forth by the third-party carrier.

The current state of health care makes reimbursement an issue of major importance. Changes in reimbursement policies of third-party carriers can (and do) occur frequently and quickly. Different group and individual policies issued by the same company often have different criteria, standards, and reimbursement practices. Programs requesting reimbursement must develop and maintain ongoing relationships with third-party carriers to stay abreast of the changes and practices.

TERMINOLOGY

accounts payable: money owed by the business to vendors, suppliers, and providers of service

accounts receivable: money owed to the business for services or goods

accrual basis: an accounting system that records all expenses and revenues at the time they occurred, not at the time they are paid

assets: everything a business owns with monetary value; can be divided into current assets (can be converted into cash quickly) and fixed assets (for long term use)

balance sheet: a report showing the balance of all assets, liabilities, and equity for a particular date or period

collection period: the number of days elapsing before accounts receivable are actually collected

deficit: when expenses exceed revenue

depreciation: a systematic way to account for the expense of an asset over a fixed number of years; usually applies to fixed assets

expenses: the costs of operating a business; can be divided into fixed expenses (do not fluctuate with business activity) and operating expenses (generally do fluctuate with activity)

liability: the total of all goods, services, or cash that business owes a creditor; can be divided into current liabilities (expected to be paid within 1 year) and non-current liabilities (with longer term due dates, often more than 1 year)

line item: a budget line showing a particular expense or revenue item

net income: excess of total revenues over total expenses

net loss: excess of total expenses over total revenue

pro-forma budget: a projection of expenses and revenue for a new program

BIBLIOGRAPHY

American College of Sports Medicine: *Guidelines for Exercise Testing and Prescription*. Fourth Edition. Philadelphia: Lea & Febiger, 1991.

Meyer GC: Reimbursement for clinical exercise Programs. In *Resource Manual for Guidelines for Exercise Testing and Prescription*. First Edition. Philadelphia: Lea & Febiger, 1988.

Needles BE Jr, Anderson HR, Caldwell JC; *Principles of Accounting*. Fourth Edition. New York: Houghton Mifflin Co., 1990.

Patton RW, Grantham WF, Gerson RF, Gettman LR: *Developing and Managing Health and Fitness Facilities*. Champaign, IL: Human Kinetics Books, 1989.

Solomon L, Vargo D, Walther L: *Accounting Principles*. West Publishing Co., 1990.

Wilson PK, Fardy PS, Froelicher VF: *Cardiac Rehabilitation, Adult Fitness and Exercise Testing*. Philadelphia: Lea & Febiger, 1981.

Chapter 44

LEGAL CONSIDERATIONS

William G. Herbert and David L. Herbert

Legal considerations abound for professionals who provide exercise testing, prescription, and physical training programs for adults. These concerns encompass the professional-patient relationship and the activities performed within the legal confines of that relationship; the setting within which program activities are conducted; the purpose for which such activities are performed; and the procedures employed by the professional in providing services to the exercise client. The law influences exercise personnel in each of these domains. Despite the fact that jurisdictional variations exist, some principles in law have broad application to exercise testing, prescription, and leadership. Preventive and rehabilitative exercise program personnel should be cognizant of these principles and endeavor to develop practices to reduce risk of negligence-type litigation and, concomitantly, to maintain safe care of their clientele.

Although statistical data indicate a rather low risk of serious cardiovascular accidents among adults who participate in moderate-vigorous exercise, untoward events can and do occur, especially with diseased or high-risk patients.[1] Only a small fraction of these cases have ever resulted in legal claims against exercise professionals, but such claims are decidedly being processed through the legal system and thus forecast an ever increasing risk of claim and suit.[2,3]

TERMINOLOGY AND CONCEPTS

Almost invariably, legal claims against exercise professionals center on either alleged violations of contract law or tort principles. These two broad legal concepts, along with written and statutory laws, define and govern most legal relationships between individuals.

Contract Law

The law of contracts defines undertakings that may be specified among individuals. A legal contract is simply a promise or performance bargained for and given in exchange for another promise or performance, all of which is supported by adequate consideration, i.e., something of value. In examining exercise testing and prescription activities, the law of contracts affects the relationship established between exercise professionals and their clients. In effect, the conditions of the contract are satisfied in that both parties bargain for performance, which is supported by something of value. The client may receive physical fitness information and recommendations on exercise training; likewise, the professional may perform exercise testing services in exchange for payment, reimbursement, or some other valuable consideration. This contract relationship also encompasses any related activities that occur before and after exercise testing, such as health screening and exercise prescription. If expectations during this relationship are not fulfilled, lawsuit for breach of contract *may* be instituted. At the core of such a suit is alleged nonfulfillment of certain promises or alleged warranties, including implied warranties that the law sometimes imposes on many contractual relationships.

Informed Consent

Aside from breach of contract claims arising from a lack of promise fulfillment, claims against exercise professionals can also be based on breach of contract for failure to obtain adequate informed consent from exercise participants. Although claims based on lack of informed consent, which are founded upon contract principles, are somewhat archaic, suits promulgated upon such failures can still be put forth in some jurisdictions. More frequently, however, such claims are brought forth in connection with negligence actions rather than breach of contract suits. To subject another individual to a specific exercise procedure both properly and lawfully, the client must give *informed* consent to the procedure with full knowledge of the material risks and benefits associated with that activity. This consent can be express (written) or implied by law arising out of the conduct of the parties. To give consent validly to a procedure, the individual must be of lawful age; not be mentally incapacitated; know and fully understand the importance and relevance of the material risks; and give consent voluntarily and not under any mistake of fact or duress.[4]

In many jurisdictions, programs are required to provide enough information on the informed consent process to ensure that the participant knows and understands the risks and circumstances associated with the procedure. In such states, a so-called subjective test is utilized to determine whether the particular person involved (as opposed to a reasonable man) understood and comprehended the risks and the procedures associated with the matter at hand. Other states have adopted a less rigid rule and provide an objective test to determine an individual's consent to a procedure or treatment. Under this test, the legal determination centers on whether this participant, as a reasonable and ordinary person, understood the facts and circumstances associated with the procedure so as to give a voluntary consent. In any case, exercise personnel must give special attention to the legal requirements of the informed consent process so that participants may freely decide whether to proceed with any particular test or programmatic activity.

Suits arising from the informed consent process can also occur, in which an injured party claims that a professional was negligent in the explanation of the procedure including the risks, and that the participant would not, but for the negligence of the professional, have undergone the procedure. These cases are often decided upon the testimony of expert witnesses who determine whether the professional engaged in substandard conduct in securing the informed consent. These informed-consent cases can involve claims related to contract law, warranties, negligence, and malpractice. Suits arising from alleged deficiencies in the informed consent process related to testing, exercise prescription, or activity are becoming more commonplace. The law is moving toward a requirement for ever-broadening risk disclosure for participants. Some courts have even gone so far as to require the disclosure of all possible risks as opposed to those which are simply material.[5] Such a requirement imposes substantial burdens on programs and raises substantial medicolegal concerns.[6] These concerns need individualized analysis and response.

Tort Law

A tort in law is simply a type of civil wrong. Most tort claims affecting the exercise professional are based on allegations of either negligence or malpractice.

Negligence

Negligence, although incapable of precise legal definition, may be regarded as a failure to conform one's conduct to a generally accepted standard or duty. A legal cause of action for negligence may be established given proof of certain facts, namely, that one person failed to provide *due care* to protect another person to whom the former owed some duty or responsibility, and that such failure proximately caused some injury to this latter person.[4]

Malpractice

Malpractice is a specific type of negligence action involving claims against professionals arising from the course of their relationship with a patient or client. Malpractice actions generally involve claims against certain *statutorily defined* professionals for alleged breaches of professional duties and responsibilities toward patients or other persons to whom they owed a particular standard of care or duty.[4] Historically, malpractice claims have been confined to actions against physicians and lawyers. By statute or case law, however, some states have expanded this group to include nurses, physical therapists, dentists, psychologists, and other health professionals.

DEFENSES TO NEGLIGENCE/ MALPRACTICE ACTIONS

If properly given, consents can sometimes be used as legal defenses to claims based on either tort or contract principles. In such cases, defense counsel may seek to characterize a consent as an *assumption of the risks by the plaintiff*. Assumption of the risks of a procedure, however, is often difficult to establish without an explicit written statement or clear conduct that demonstrates such an assumption. In addition, an assumption of the risks never relieves the exercise professional of the duty to perform in a competent and professional manner. Even when a valid informed consent/ assumption of the risks is obtained, a participant's spouse, children, and/or heirs can sometimes independently file suits against the exercise professional for loss of consortium-type claims (even when the participant could not have asserted those claims because of his or her own assumption of the risks.[7] Recent trends in this area may indicate a need to obtain a consent from a participant, the participant's spouse, and perhaps, in a limited number of states, to make it binding on any children. Certainly such consents should be binding on the patients' estates if certain of these negligence/ malpractice claims are to be avoided successfully from those quarters.

Informed consents are often confused with so-called "releases." Releases are statements sometimes written into consent documents that contain exculpatory language professing to relieve a party from any legal responsibility in the event of a participant's injury or death due to the professional's negligence. These releases are prospective waivers of responsibility and in some states may be disfavored. Moreover, in a medical setting, the use of such releases has, with certain exceptions, been declared invalid as being against public policy. In nonmedical settings, however, particularly with certain ultrahazardous as well as other activities (e.g., auto racing and sky diving), and with some exercise-related activities, the use of such releases can be valid in some jurisdictions and under certain circumstances if properly drafted and utilized by a program.

Several other defenses to claims of negligence or malpractice are also available. In some states, for example, proof of a participant's negligence, referred to in law as *contributory negligence*, can preclude any recovery of damages from the defendant. In many states, however, this rule has been modified by adoption of a so-called system of *comparative negligence*. Under this latter rule, the negligence of the injured party is compared with the negligence of all defendants in the case. Then, if the negligence of the injured party is found to be less than that of all defendants in the case or in some states in any case, the plaintiff is allowed to recover, although in an amount that is reduced by the sum of the injured party's own negligence.[4]

OPERATING ENTITIES FOR EXERCISE PROGRAMS

Many operating entities typically provide exercise-related services. Basically, "there are three relevant choices: corporate, partnership or sole proprietorship."[19] A sole proprietorship is simply a business entity operating through a person under either that person's name or under an assumed or fictitious name. [T]his structure is the easiest and least complex to organize and operate . . . [but] it also leaves its owner open to claims of personal liability arising out of business operation—for both contracts and negligence."[8]

"A partnership quite simply is 'an association of two or more persons to carry on, as co-owners, a business for profit,' UNIFORM PARTNERSHIP ACT Para. 6(1). Partners share equally in the profits of the business unless the parties expressly stipulate and agree upon a different share of the profits. Unless otherwise agreed, partners also share equally in the management rights and obligations of the partnership, and are each jointly and severally liable for partnership debts and liabilities, and for the acts of the other parties which may lead to injury and liability . . . Partnerships are creatures of state statutes. All states have adopted in some shape or form the Uniform Partnership Act (UPA) . . . to govern the relationship of partners. Like the sole proprietorship, parties are taxed individually in such proportions as they have previously agreed as to the profits of the firm. Since partnerships are governed by state statutes, a greater degree of liability is required to organize the business structure than is required of the sole proprietorship."[8]

Unlike either a sole proprietorship or a partnership, a corporation is a separate legal entity that exists independently of its owners, the shareholders. "Since a corporation is a separate legal entity, it can sue and be sued, enter into contracts, own property and so forth just the same as an individual. One of the main advantages of the corporate form is that it offers its shareholders/owners limited personal liability for the corporation's debts and liabilities. The shareholders are only at risk to the extent of their capital contributions as to these obligations, unless they personally guarantee such debts."[8]

"The main drawback of the corporate form of business is the complexity in establishing and operating the business as well as being subject to double taxation. Corporations like partnerships are created and governed by state statutes. The corporation must operate in accordance with its charter and bylaws. The corporation must also elect and appoint directors and officers to oversee and run the business. A court of law might 'pierce the corporate veil' and impose liability upon shareholders directly if a corporation is not operating within the law and pursuant to the formalities that govern corporations. If that is the case, the corporate form will be disregarded and the shareholders/owners would become personally liable."[8]

"Corporations, unlike partnerships and sole proprietorships, are subject to double taxation. Profits are taxed once at the corporate level, then again when any money is distributed to the shareholders in the form of dividends or salaries. An alternative solution to the problem of double taxation . . . [is the formation of] an "S" CORPORATION. An "S" corporation is taxed like a partnership or sole proprietorship inasmuch as all profits or salaries are taxed directly to the shareholders with the corporation filing information returns only.

Despite this comparison, this form of business entity still retains the other benefits of the corporate form such as limited liability."[8] While there are certain restrictions and formalities for the formation and operation of an "S" corporation, it is used by many in the field to conduct exercise business activities. The advantages and disadvantages of any form of operating entity should be reviewed with a program's legal counsel and tax advisors before commencing operation.

STANDARDS OF PRACTICE FOR EXERCISE PROFESSIONALS

Standards of practice have been promulgated by several prominent professional associations that should be regarded as benchmarks of competency that would certainly be used in a court of law to assess a professional's performance in given situations. In fact, the use of these standards in certain cases dealing with exercise testing and exercise leadership has already occurred.[3] The standards developed by the American College of Sports Medicine, the American Heart Association, the American College of Cardiology, the American Association of Cardiovascular and Pulmonary Rehabilitation, the American Medical Association, the National Council of YMCAs, the American Physical Therapy Association, and the Aerobics & Fitness Association of America, among others, provide guidelines of professional conduct for persons engaged in exercise programs for healthy adults as well as patients.[9-19] Unfortunately, these guidelines are not entirely uniform and in the event of participant injury or death, may create confusion rather than provide a solution as to the benchmarks of professional behavior to be applied in a particular exercise setting. For example, in the area of exercise testing, the standards of the American Heart Association (AHA) and those of the American College of Sports Medicine (ACSM) are somewhat inconsistent in that the former imply that the physical presence or significant involvement of a physician is necessary during any graded exercise test, especially with diseased patients or individuals at risk.[10,12] In contrast, the ACSM guidelines are more liberal and do not mandate the presence of a physician except when testing higher risk or diseased individuals.[9]

The AHA guidelines and those of ACSM are also at variance relative to some aspects of professional authority for exercise prescription. The AHA guidelines reserve exercise prescription activities exclusively for physicians, particularly if the participant is at a higher-risk level or has heart disease.[10] The movement toward the adoption of written standards and guidelines for various provider areas is sure to continue. For example, new standards for health and fitness facilities have been developed by the ACSM and were published in 1992 by Human Kinetics, Publishers of Champaign, Illinois (ACSM's Health/Fitness Facility Standards and Guidelines). This statement is sure to have a rather dramatic effect upon the industry and should be among the materials reviewed by professionals. In the ACSM guidelines, the emphasis for prescription is clearly with the qualified and certified Exercise Specialist or Program Director.[9]

UNAUTHORIZED PRACTICE OF MEDICINE AND OTHER ALLIED HEALTH PROFESSIONAL STATUTES

The modern trend in medicine is to utilize certain paraprofessionals in ever-increasingly important and expanded treatment roles. In fact, various states have undertaken efforts to expand nursing practice and other medical practice laws beyond mere observation, reporting, and recording of patient signs/symptoms. Various physician assistant or similar paraprofessional laws allow more nonphysicians expanded treatment authority when dealing with patients. Until this ongoing process is completed, however, some nonphysicians who engage in certain practices that might be characterized as the practice of medicine or some other statutorily defined and controlled allied health profession, run the risk of engaging in unauthorized practices. This practice could lead to both criminal and civil sanctions. Many states have defined the practice of medicine broadly so that persons engaged in exercise testing and prescription activities could, under some circumstances, fall within the ambits of such statutes. Thus, without the presence or assistance of a li-

censed physician or other allied health professional for certain aspects of these exercise services, claims as to the unauthorized practice of medicine could be put forth. Under some of these state statutes, such practices are often classified as crimes, usually misdemeanors, punishable by imprisonment for less than 1 year and/or a fine.

In addition, a person found to have engaged in the unauthorized practice of medicine or some other allied health profession faces (after the fact) the legal expectation to provide an elevated standard of care in the event of participant injury or death. Under this rule, the exercise professional's actions are compared to an assumed standard of care of a physician or other allied health professional acting under the same or similar circumstances. In the event that the professional's actions do not meet this standard (which the nonphysician or allied health professional cannot meet because of inadequacies of knowledge, skill, authorization and experience), liability may result.

COMMON AREAS OF POTENTIAL LIABILITY AND EXPOSURE

In the course of conducting exercise programs, certain common claims seem to be the most likely sources of litigation. A summary follows:

1. Failure to monitor an exercise test properly and/or to stop an exercise test in the application of competent professional judgment
2. Failure to evaluate the participant's physical capabilities or impairments competently, factors that would proscribe or limit certain types of exercise
3. Failure to prescribe a safe exercise intensity in terms of cardiovascular, metabolic, and musculoskeletal demands
4. Failure to instruct participants adequately as to safe performance of the recommended physical activities or the proper use of exercise equipment
5. Failure to supervise properly the participant's exercise during program sessions or to advise individu-

als regarding any restrictions or modifications that should be imposed in performing conditioning activities during unsupervised periods

6. Failure to assign specific participants to an exercise setting with a level of physiologic monitoring, supervision, and emergency medical support commensurate with their health status

7. Failure to perform or render performance in a negligent manner in a variety of other situations

8. Rendition of advice to a participant that is later construed to represent diagnosis of a medical condition or is deemed tantamount to medical prescription to relieve a disease condition and that subsequently and/or proximately causes injury and/or deterioration of health and/or death

9. Failure to refer a participant to a physician or other appropriately licensed professional in response to the appearance of signs or symptoms suggestive of health problems requiring medical or other professional attention

10. Failure to disclose certain information in the informed consent process or failure to maintain proper and confidential records documenting the informed consent process, the adequacy of participant instructions with regard to performance of program activities, and the adequacy of their physical responses to physical activity regimens[4]

11. Failure to respond adequately to an untoward event with appropriate emergency care.

This discussion is but an overview of the potential legal problems that face the exercise professional. As more and more participants are exposed to organized exercise programs, the actual number of untoward, as well as avoidable, events will inevitably rise. Increased numbers of these occurrences will result in negligence-type claims that will ultimately find resolution in court. The probabilities of such traumatic actions are low, particularly for individuals and organizations that operate programs in a

manner commensurate with professional standards. Awareness of the areas of special legal vulnerability and the adoption of legally sensitive practices in response, however, will keep the risks of litigation low and concurrently lead to safer and more efficacious programs. Professionals would be well advised to keep up to date and current as to developments in this ever-changing medicolegal field.[20]

REFERENCES

1. Rochmis P, Blackburn H: Exercise tests: A survey of procedures, safety and litigation experience in approximately 170,000 tests. *JAMA, 217:*1061–66, 1971.
2. *DeRouen vs. Holiday Spa Health Clubs of California.* Superior Court of County of Los Angeles, Case No. C346987 (Dismissed upon settlement 1985).
3. *Tart vs. McGann.* U.S. District Court, Southern District of New York, Case No. 81-CIV-IL-3899 (ELP 1981). *Cited* in 697 F. 2d 75 (2d Cir. 1982).
4. Herbert DL, Herbert WG: *Legal Aspects of Preventive and Rehabilitative Exercise Programs.* Second Edition, Canton, OH: Professional Reports Corporation 1989.
5. *Hedgecorth v. United States,* 618 F.Supp. 627 (E.D. Mo. 1985).
6. Herbert DL: Informed Consent Documents for Stress Testing to Comport With *Hedgecorth v. United States. Exercise Standards and Malpractice Reporter, 1:*81, 1987.
7. Child Sues for "Loss of Consortium." *Lawyers Alert, 3:*249, 1984.
8. Koeberle D: *Legal Aspects of Personal Fitness Training,* Canton: Professional Reports Corporation 1990, pp. 35–38.
9. American College of Sports Medicine: *Guidelines for Exercise Testing and Prescription.* 4th Ed. Philadelphia: Lea & Febiger, 1991.
10. American Heart Association, Special Report; Exercise Standards, A Statement for Health Professionals, *Circulation, 82:*2286, 1990.
11. American College of Cardiology: Recommendations for cardiovascular services. *Cardiology, 15:*4, 1986.
12. American Association of Cardiovascular and Pulmonary Rehabilitation: *Guidelines for Cardiac Rehabilitation Programs.* Champaign, IL: Human Kinetics, 1991.
13. American Medical Association, Committee on Exercise and Physical Fitness: Evaluation for exercise participation: The apparently healthy individual. *JAMA, 219:* 900–901, 1972.
14. American Medical Association, Council on

Scientific Affairs: Indications and contraindications for exercise testing (A council report). *JAMA, 246:*1015–1018, 1981.

15. American Medical Association: Standards and Guidelines for Cardiopulmonary Resuscitation (CPR) and Emergency Cardiac Care (ECC). *JAMA, 244:*453–509, 1980.

16. Golding L, Myers C, Sinning W (eds): *The Y's Way to Physical Fitness (revised): A Guidebook for Instructors.* Rosemont, IL: Program Resources Office for the National Board of YMCA of the USA, 1982.

17. American Physical Therapy Association, Cardiopulmonary Specialty Council: *Specialty Competencies in Physical Therapy: Cardio-pulmonary.* Manhattan Beach, CA: Board for Certification of Advanced Clinical Competence, American Physical Therapy Association, 1983.

18. Cooper PG (ed): *Aerobics Theory & Practice.* Sherman Oaks, CA: Aerobics and Fitness Association of America, 1985.

19. Herbert WG, Herbert DL: Exercise testing in adults: Legal and procedural considerations for the physical educator and exercise professionals. *JOHPER, 46:*17–18, 1975.

20. *See* The Exercise Standards and Malpractice Reporter (Published 6 times a year by Professional Reports Corporation, Canton, Ohio 44718-3629).

Chapter 45

FACILITY DESIGN, EQUIPMENT SELECTION, AND CALIBRATION

William C. Grantham and Edward T. Howley

This chapter provides an overview of the various processes involved in the planning and designing of health and fitness facilities. In addition, information concerning equipment purchasing, selection, and calibration is discussed. This information complements the guidelines established for program administration published in Chapter 12 of the ACSM Guidelines for Exercise Testing and Prescription (4th Ed.).[1]

FACILITY DESIGN

The process of planning and designing a health and fitness facility can vary from a small renovation project to the building of a large multipurpose center. The procedure must consider user efficiency, budgetary issues, maintenance considerations, and program features. Unfortunately, many health/fitness professionals have little experience or knowledge in the architectural or construction field. Often, the general manager of a commercial fitness center or the program director of a wellness center is placed in the position of project manager for the construction of a new multimillion dollar complex. Unless the person has been a part of a team of professionals that has previous experience in the development of facilities of this nature, difficulties can arise.

A sequential process must be established and followed to ensure that the proper planning, design, and construction of a health and fitness facility are accomplished. Included in this procedure is a series of steps beginning at the conceptual stage of defining the purpose of the project, establishing the needs and desires of the community, and finalizing all aspects of the construction phase. Although some variations of this approach can be taken, depending on the extent and complexity of the program, most projects follow a similar format to verify that all aspects of facility planning and design considerations have been addressed.

The Facility Design Process

The facility design stage incorporates four phases[2]:

1. Predesign
2. Design development
3. Construction
4. Preoperations

A major benefit of the design stage is that all phases are compatible with any type of health/fitness facility: community, corporate, wellness, or clinical. The project manager must simply decide which factors of each phase are necessary so that they can be applied to a particular setting. Although each of these phases has specific functions, they often overlap during the course of a project. For example, any facility or program information obtained in the predesign phase (i.e., market analysis) is also used in design development so that the facility will reflect the needs of the public. However, the overlap does not mean that the sequence of phases should be taken out of order. The facility design process is a series of steps that are continually influenced by outside factors.

It has been estimated that the average length of time to complete a well-planned facility is 6 months to 2 years, depending upon the size of the project. The approximate percentage of time for each phase of the project is:

1. Predesign — 25% or 6 months
2. Design development — 12% or 3 months
3. Construction — 50% or 12 months
4. Preoperation (start-up) — 13% or 3–4 months

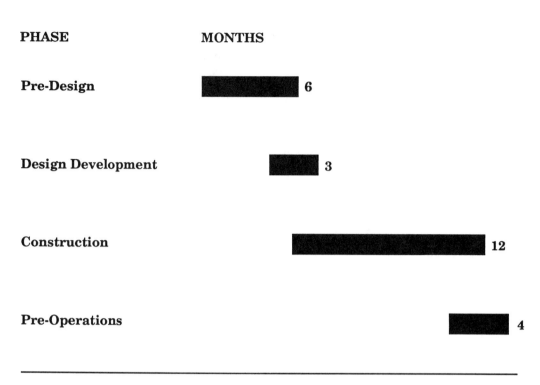

Fig. 45–1. The facility design process. With permission from Patton RW, Grantham WC, Gerson RF, Gettman LR: *Developing and Managing Health/Fitness Facilities.* Champaign IL: Human Kinetics Publishers, Inc., 1989.

The overlapping and sequential aspects of the facility design process are illustrated in Figure 45–1.

Predesign Phase

The predesign phase is the planning stage of the project. Data collected from an assortment of meetings, surveys, and studies are evaluated by a team of professionals who decide upon the eventual concept, design, and construction of the facility.

The steps involved in the predesign phase include:

1. Defining the project
2. Selecting the "project team"
3. Program analysis
4. Feasibility study
5. Site selection
6. Cost analysis

Defining the Project. The idea for a building project may result from discus-sions among staff, colleagues, members, and associates. During these meetings, a true "need" is established for a new facility, or a decision to upgrade an existing plant is made. Once the idea has been approved in concept, a planning committee or a spec-ified individual is given the responsibility to define its scope and feasibility. In addition, the goals and objectives of the proposed project are established during this time. It is recommended that both short-term (1-month) and long-term (5-year) goals be identified.

Some questions to answer in determin-ing the goals and objectives include:

1. Will the project improve the overall appearance of the existing facility?
2. Are there enough members or indi-viduals who would use the facility if it were built?
3. What programs could be offered with this addition?

4. Will the expansion increase revenues?
5. Does the scope of the project coincide with the mission statement?

Once this process has been completed, a final definition of the project should be prepared and agreed upon. This document is called the "program statement" and is used to describe the project to everyone involved.

Selecting the Project Team. Depending on the size and scope of the project, various forms of team planning are needed at each phase. Seldom do positive results occur from one person doing the planning. The individuals who can represent the project team are shown in Figure 45–2.

The primary role of the project team is to translate the "program statement" into reality. This is accomplished by hiring professionals who not only have experience in facility development and construction, but have also planned and designed facilities similar in size and scope to the proposed project.

It is beyond the scope of this chapter to discuss the procedures involved in hiring consultants, architects, and contractors. However, it is recommended that further analysis be made regarding these procedures because they result in some of the most important decisions associated with the building process.

Program Analysis. The programs to be offered by the proposed facility (i.e., special events, physical activities, and specialty services) are often determined by means of questionnaires or interviews during a feasi-

bility study. Program information is crucial in the development of a well-planned facility to ensure that the design of the facility will accommodate the programs, rather than limit their delivery.

Feasibility Study. The primary purpose of a feasibility study is to answer one question: is it feasible to build a health/fitness facility in a particular location so that its maximum potential can be achieved? The answer can be determined only by conducting a study to obtain information on the following:

1. Facility location
2. Program offerings
3. Revenue estimates
4. Financial data
5. Potential target markets
6. Estimated usage
7. Competitors
8. Pricing structures

This information is used for the business plan and marketing, and forms the basis for the overall master plan of the project.

Site Selection. Selecting the proper site for a new facility is as important as the design and construction process itself. Data collected in the feasibility study is used to ensure that the proposed site is acceptable to the target population. If the consumers do not perceive the location to be convenient, aesthetically pleasing, and compatible with the existing surroundings, they will choose not to attend, even if the complex is well designed.

Cost Analysis. During the predesign phase it is important to obtain early esti-

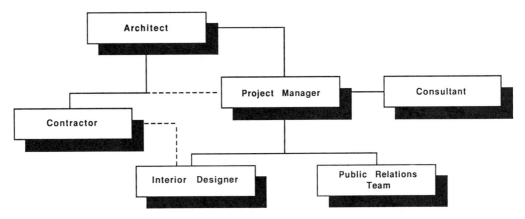

Fig. 45–2. The project team.

mates on land and construction costs. Rarely do building projects cost less than what is originally proposed. Consequently, it is best to perform a cost analysis before entering into the design phase, which can be both expensive and time-consuming. Most architectural firms have cost estimators who can prepare a fairly accurate bid from early program statements, initial drawings, and other pertinent information. The overall purpose of the cost analysis is to adjust the owners' desires to the financial constraints associated with real estate and construction prices.

Design Phase

The design stage allows the architect to take what has been proposed and begin to shape and define the facility. Much of the information used by the architect is obtained from written guidelines submitted by the project team members. These guidelines include a general description of the various facility uses, a prioritized facility "wish list," and any special concerns or features which the architect should consider during the design phase.

Once the predesign planning is completed, the architect begins preparing a series of drawings that ultimately lead to the final set of blueprints used for construction. The three-stage process used by architects to obtain final approval of the design plans is:

Schematic Design → Design Development
→ Construction Documents

Schematic Design. The schematic design process consists of analyzing the spacial relationships of various aspects of the facilities, taking into consideration member

Table 45–1. Sample Space Requirements for a Multiuse Fitness Center*

Ground Floor	Square Footage	% of Total Footage	Second Floor	Square Total Footage	% of Total Footage
Lobby	1124	2.0	Gymnasium	6980	13.0
Auditorium	2170	4.2	Racquetball	1848	3.5
Play area	939	2.1	Aerobics	2673	5.1
Women's kit lockers	440	0.8	Storage	440	0.8
Women's lockers	3408	6.6	Offices	1045	2.2
Pool area	4876	9.4	Weight lifting	3393	6.6
Lounge	1232	2.4	Fire stair	250	0.5
Electrical	160	0.3	Chase	250	0.5
Toilets	483	0.9	Toilets	160	0.3
Juice bar	260	0.5	Stairs	352	0.7
Cardiovascular	196	0.4	Elevator	50	0.1
Mechanical	468	0.9	Check-in	176	0.3
Men's lockers	4564	8.8	Waiting	196	0.4
Men's kit lockers	745	1.0	Subtotal	17,793	34.0
Laundry	840	2.0	Circulation	714	1.0
Storage	150	0.3	Total	18,507	35.0
Offices	527	1.0	Mezzanine:		
Administration	315	0.6			
Pro shop	252	0.5	Running track	6798	13.1
Check-in	300	0.6	Warm-up & stairs	308	0.6
Elevator/basement	80	0.1	Total	7106	13.7
Stair/basement	223	0.4			
Stair/fire	223	0.4	Grand total:		
Stair activity	352	0.7			
Elevator/activity	50	0.1	Ground floor	26,219	50.0
Subtotal	24,377	47.0	Second floor	18,507	36.3
Circulation	1842	3.0	Mezzanine	7106	13.7
Total	26,219	50.0	Gross Sq. Ft.	51,832	100.0

* With permission from Patton RW, Grantham WC, Gerson RF, Gettman LR: *Developing and Managing Health/Fitness Facilities.* Champaign IL: Human Kinetics, 1989.

access, traffic patterns, and crowd control. Evaluate the site plan by discussing how the new building interrelates with the new site or an existing facility. Review building codes to determine what effect, if any, they will have on the structural, mechanical, and electrical systems. Finally, obtain an early estimate of construction costs for budgetary purposes.

Design Development. Once the schematic phase is approved by the client, the plans are prepared on a larger scale. The following are areas that are completed during the design development phase:

1. Floor plan design
2. Building elevations
3. Specifications development
4. Equipment and furniture arrangements
5. Detailed building costs

Construction Documents. After receiving final approval of the design plans, the architect begins preparing detailed working drawings and construction specifications. The drawings provide the graphic design of the facility and written specifications which accompany the project. The construction documents ensure a coordinated effort between the general contractor, subcontractors, and engineers.

The final drawings are used to project final cost estimates and ensure that the plans are acceptable to the client. The architect then assists the owner in obtaining construction bids and awarding contracts.

Construction Phase

Once the construction bid has been approved, the architect and project manager meet with the contractor to clarify procedures that will be followed during the construction process. When these matters are cleared, construction begins and the architect becomes involved with:

1. Issuing bulletins and change orders
2. Making periodic visits to the job site
3. Providing to the client certificates of payment
4. Serving as mediator between client and contractor on construction-related matters
5. Retaining the right to reject inferior workmanship.

Table 45–1 provides a list of multiuse facilities and their size requirements. In addition, Table 45–2 provides a list of facility design measurements, which are considered to be industry standards for recommended building sizes and space allocations.

Preoperation Phase

The preoperation phase consists of planning and organizing all operational matters associated with the "start-up" of a facility. Before this, the major emphasis has been on the design and construction aspects of the building. The design team must now concentrate on the business-related areas, which are essential to ensure a successful operation.

The object of the preoperation phase is to take the information obtained from the market analysis and predesign sessions, and begin applying them to a management and business format. Because a wide variety of topics (i.e. organizational structure,

Table 45–2. Facility Design Measurements*

Square footage per member for the building (excluding tennis courts):
  10–15 square feet—average
  6–8 square feet—high density (8–10 square feet preferred)
  8–10 square feet—medium density (10–12 square feet preferred)
  10–12 square feet—low density (12–14 square feet preferred)

Square footage per participant:
  36–40 square feet—for aerobics
  40–50 square feet—for floor work or weight training

Space allocations as percentage of total space:
  40% for exercise and activity areas
  35% for locker room and shower facilities
  25% for administration and service areas

Locker room space per member during peak usage:
  10–20 square feet; 8–10 feet between locker rows

Number of lockers: Peak usage number plus 10%, or one locker per 10 users.

Peak usage: 10% or total member population

---

* With permission from Patton RW, Grantham WC, Gerson RF, Gettman LR: *Developing and Managing Health/Fitness Facilities.* Champaign IL: Human Kinetics, 1989.

staffing, operational issues, etc.) are discussed during this time, the preparation of a checklist is recommended. Once the major topics have been established, a detailed outline with time goals should be prepared for each area. Although this phase is scheduled to take approximately 3 to 4 months, managers often underestimate the importance of this phase and are not properly prepared when construction is completed.

EQUIPMENT CONSIDERATIONS

The proper selection, purchasing, maintenance, and operation of fitness equipment has become an arduous process to many individuals in the health and fitness field. The wide assortment of vendors and varied types of products on the market today can confuse even the seasoned buyer. Although anyone involved in equipment purchasing is subject to this frustration, those who have become successful have established criteria to assist them through the decision-making process. A checklist of features to look for when purchasing equipment includes:

1. Function
2. Cost
3. Space
4. Durability
5. Safety
6. User appeal
7. Maintenance contracts
8. Versatility
9. Life expectancy
10. Equipment features

Although there is a variety of equipment to choose from when designing a health and fitness facility, the intended user must find the equipment appealing or it may not be used. Evaluating the type of equipment necessary to attract interested users involves many factors. These factors include such things as name recognition, color, size and shape, convenience, single versus co-ed setting, and intimidating/massive appearance versus a "user-friendly" design. Including these considerations with the factors mentioned will ensure that the equipment will follow the initial philosophy and image of the organization.

When deciding upon the types of equip-

Table 45–3.   List of Cardiovascular and Resistance Training Equipment

Cardiovascular Equipment	Resistance Training Equipment
Treadmills	Free weights
Stationary cycles	Multi-station machines
Recumbent cycles	Single-station
Rowing machines	machines
Stair machines	Machine circuit
Hand climbers	systems
Arm ergometers	Handicapped
Swimming ergometers	equipment
Wall climbing	Youth fitness
Mini-tramps	equipment
Jump ropes	Outdoor circuit
Ski simulators	systems

ment to purchase, managers or owners must decide what mix of cardiovascular, resistance training, rehabilitation, or special-use equipment (e.g., handicapped, youth, performance testing, etc.) will be needed. There are advantages and disadvantages in selecting each type of equipment. The final decision should be based on the mission statement, which defines the type of facility you represent to the public. When reviewing the corporate, community, commercial, and clinical settings, the most popular types of equipment purchased are for cardiovascular and resistance training. A review list of some of the most common cardiovascular and resistance training equipment available in today's market can be found in Table 45–3.

Liability Concerns

Involvement in the health and fitness industry creates its own unique form of liability problems. For example, allowing various age groups to use a wide assortment of exercise equipment in a highly active and competitive atmosphere can increase the risk of an accident. To reduce this risk and the associated liability, employees must pay close attention to all facets of the fitness setting, with the emphasis on preventive safety measures. The responsibilities of the staff should include:

1. Making thorough daily inspections of all equipment
2. Inspecting all equipment when received and installed

3. Posting full instructions of how to use all equipment
4. Instructing participants and supervising their daily use of all equipment
5. Repairing broken equipment immediately, or posting signs warning that equipment is out of order.

Exercise leaders responsible for supervising participants need to be made aware that negligence claims against exercise specialists and fitness instructors depend on one question: "Did the professional meet his or her expected duty of care toward the participant?"[3] In other words, were personnel acting in a "prudent" fashion when the incident occurred? If the necessary safety precautions are in place and being followed daily by the exercise leader, the potential for legal action should be reduced.

Purchasing Equipment

Purchasing of exercise equipment necessitates a systemized approach that will guarantee the best product for the best price. The first step in accomplishing this goal is to become familiar with the current policies for equipment procurement by your organization. Some businesses may have established procedures that must be followed to meet federal or state laws. Others may use a process that has been developed over the years and is being implemented through a centralized purchasing division. Whether an existing system is currently in place or new equipment is being purchased for the first time, there are recommended purchasing guidelines that should be followed. A list of these recommendations is presented in Table 45–4.

Used or Leased Equipment

Paying full price for new equipment may be difficult for some organizations. After building expenses are paid, equipment represents the largest single expense for health and fitness facilities. Considering that the average cost of a single piece of new equipment ranges from a few hundred dollars to several thousand dollars, outfitting a weight room, cardiovascular area, or stress testing laboratory could

Table 45–4. Equipment Order Recommendations

Investigate the Equipment Market
- Field-test equipment
- Hire a consultant to assist
- Perform a personal investigation
- Obtain input from vendors and staff

Write Specifications
- List clear and precise specifications (e.g., brand, model, color, size)
- Provide 2 or 3 alternative models
- Contact preferred manufacturer for assistance in preparing specifications

Obtain Bids
- Provide adequate time for all vendors to bid
- Establish a reliable vendor list
- Ask for bidder assistance with installation, on-site repair, and warranty period
- Let all vendors know that you are bidding the equipment
- Don't always accept lowest bid

Purchasing Suggestions
- Understand all payment requirements (i.e. shipping costs, taxes, 50% down and 50% on receipt of equipment, etc.)
- Consider used, leased, or lease to buy options, if money is a problem
- Consider withholding 10% of total payment for leverage

Consult with Other Facilities
- Obtain vendor recommendation list
- Call clients and obtain equipment performance information
- Ask if vendor has provided adequate warranty coverage

quickly surpass a pre-established budget. If cost-cutting is necessary, there are four options to consider:

1. Purchase used equipment
2. Refurbish used equipment
3. Lease new equipment
4. Lease/purchase new equipment

Certain companies specialize in restoring old equipment. These companies can save 30 to 50% off the cost of new equipment, provide a reduction on sales tax, and save on depreciation.[4] In addition, some vendors of used equipment pay 35 to 65 cents on the dollar for trade-ins.[5] However, before purchasing equipment from these companies, it is recommended that a manufacturer's warranty, which includes parts and labor, be discussed in detail.

CALIBRATION OF EQUIPMENT

This section deals with the calibration of two of the most common instruments used in exercise testing, the treadmill and the cycle ergometer. The equipment selected for exercise testing must be reliable, and allow for routine calibration. The resulting quality control allows one to evaluate the effectiveness of an exercise program, or simply to establish the fitness levels of those beginning an exercise program. It is assumed that the various kinds of equipment used during the tests, i.e., sphygmomanometers, gas analyzers, ventilation meters, or electrocardiographs, are also calibrated. This section is meant to be instructive and not a replacement for the specific procedures recommended by the manufacturer.

Treadmill

The treadmill is one of the most common pieces of equipment used to study exercise responses. The intensity of the exercise can be altered by changing the speed and/or grade. Reasonable estimates of the oxygen requirements for walking or running on the treadmill depend on accurate grade and speed settings.[1]

Speed Calibration

Method 1. In some older treadmills, a mechanical counter is attached to the rear of the treadmill with a microswitch suspended over the treadmill belt. As the belt moves around the drums, an elevated surface on the outside edge of the belt triggers the switch. If the belt length (in meters) and the number of times the belt moves past the switch per minute are known, belt speed can be calculated in meters per minute ($m \cdot min^{-1}$). It is possible to use the same procedure on any treadmill by doing the following:

1. Using a meter stick, measure exact length of the belt, and record the value.
2. Place a small piece of tape on the belt surface near the edge, or mark the surface with a pen.
3. Turn on the treadmill to a given speed, using the speed control.
4. Count the number of belt revolutions in one minute by counting the number of times the piece of tape on the belt passed a fixed point. (Note: start counting with "zero" and start your watch as the tape first moves past the fixed point.)
5. Convert the number of revolutions to revolutions per minute. For example, if the belt made 33 complete revolutions in 58 seconds:

   $58 \text{ sec} \div 60 \text{ sec} \cdot min^{-1} = .967 \text{ min}$.
   So, $33 \text{ rev} \div .967 \text{ min} = 34.14 \text{ rev} \cdot min^{-1}$

6. Multiply the calculated $rev \cdot min^{-1}$ (step 5) times the belt length (step 1). The product is the belt speed in $m \cdot min^{-1}$. For example, if the belt length were 2.532 m:

   $34.14 \text{ rev} \cdot min^{-1} \times 2.532 \text{ m} \cdot rev^{-1} = 86.4 \text{ m} \cdot min^{-1}$.

7. To convert $m \cdot min^{-1}$ to miles per hour ($mi \cdot hr^{-1}$), divide the answer in step 6 by 26.8 $m \cdot min^{-1}$ per $mi \cdot hr^{-1}$:

   $86.4 \text{ m} \cdot min^{-1} \div 26.8 \text{ m} \cdot min^{-1} \text{ per } mi \cdot hr^{-1} = 3.22 \text{ mi} \cdot hr^{-1}$

8. The value obtained in step 7 is the actual treadmill speed in $mi \cdot hr^{-1}$. If the speed indicator does not agree with this value, adjust the dial or display to the proper reading using directions in the manual that accompanied the treadmill.
9. Repeat for a number of different speeds to ensure accuracy across the speeds used in test protocols.

Method 2. If your treadmill is equipped with a device to count the revolutions of one of the drums, the counter may be used to check the accuracy of the speedometer. Simply set the counter to zero, set the treadmill to the desired speed, and operate the counter for exactly 1 minute. Check the instruction manual for your treadmill to make sure of the relationship between the $rev \cdot min^{-1}$ and speed in $mi \cdot hr^{-1}$. Adjust the speedometer to the correct setting. This method is accurate only if the treadmill belt is properly adjusted and does not slip.

Elevation Calibration

The manual that comes with the treadmill describes how to calibrate the grade with a simple "carpenter's level" and a "square." This calibration procedure is shown below.

1. Use a carpenter's level to make sure that the treadmill is level and check the "O" on the grade dial under these conditions (with the treadmill electronics "on"). If the dial does not read "O," follow instructions to make the adjustment.
2. Elevate the treadmill so that the grade dial reads approximately 20%. Measure the exact incline of the treadmill as shown in Figure 45–3. When the level's bubble is exactly in the center of the tube, the "rise" measurement is obtained. Calculate the grade as the "rise" over the "run" (tangent θ), and adjust the treadmill meter to read that exact grade. For example, if the "rise" were 4.5 inches to the "run's" 22.5 inches, the fractional grade would be:

Grade = tangent θ = rise ÷ run = 4.5 in ÷ 22.5 in = 0.20 × 100% = 20%

3. Repeat this process at grades between 0 and 20° (0–34%) to make sure the meter is correct.

This "Rise" over the "Run" method is a typical engineering method for calculating grade—the vertical rise divided by the horizontal run. This method gives the tangent of the angle (the opposite side divided by the horizontal distance, as shown in Fig.

Table 45–5. Table of Natural Sines and Tangents

Degrees	Sine	% Grade	Tangent	% Grade
0	0.0000	0.0	0.0000	0.0
1	0.0175	1.7	0.0175	1.7
2	0.0349	3.5	0.0349	3.5
3	0.0523	5.2	0.0524	5.2
4	0.0698	7.0	0.0699	7.0
5	0.0872	8.7	0.0875	8.7
6	0.1045	10.4	0.1051	10.5
7	0.1219	12.2	0.1228	12.3
8	0.1392	13.9	0.1405	14.0
9	0.1564	15.6	0.1584	15.8
10	0.1736	17.4	0.1763	17.6
11	0.1908	19.1	0.1944	19.4
12	0.2079	20.8	0.2126	21.3
13	0.2250	22.5	0.2309	23.1
14	0.2419	24.2	0.2493	24.9
15	0.2588	25.9	0.2679	26.8
20	0.3420	34.2	0.3640	36.4
25	0.4067	40.7	0.4452	44.5

45–3). Although this tangent method is not exactly correct, it is a good approximation for grades less than 20% or 12° (see Table 45–5).

The "correct" method expresses grade as the sine of the angle (sin θ), where sin θ equals the vertical rise (opposite side) over the hypotenuse [sin θ = rise ÷ hypotenuse (see Fig. 45–3)]. This method should be used to calculate steep grades (above 20%). The vertical rise can be calculated simply for a treadmill with a fixed rear axle. Simply measure the change in the height of the front axle above the horizontal (rise). When you divide this by the axle length (hypotenuse), you have the grade, expressed as a fraction (Fig. 45–4).

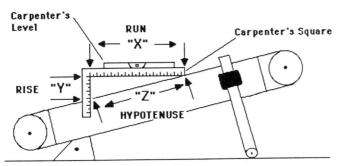

Grade = Tangent θ = Rise ("Y") ÷ Run ("X")

Grade = Sine θ = Rise ("Y") ÷ Hypotenuse ("Z")

Fig. 45–3. Calibration of grade by tangent method (rise run) with carpenter's square and level.

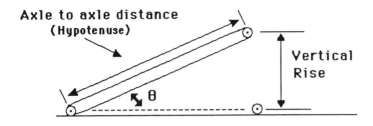

Axle to axle distance
(Hypotenuse)

Vertical
Rise

Fig. 45–4. Calibration of grade for fixed rear axle treadmill by sine method (rise hypotenuse).

Fixed rear axle treadmill

Grade = Sine θ = Rise ÷ Hypotenuse

For a treadmill with movable rear and front axles, the vertical rise is equal to the sum of the rise of the front axle and the drop of the rear axle (Fig. 45–5). When this total is divided by the axle-to-axle length, the quotient is the grade, expressed as a fraction. For example, if the front axle height is 0.327 m on the level (0% grade) and 0.612 m at the unknown grade, the front axle rise is 0.612 − 0.327 = 0.285 m. Similarly, if the rear axle height is 0.324 m at 0% grade and 0.299 m at the unknown grade, the drop is 0.025 m. The total vertical rise is then equal to the "rise" plus "drop" or 0.285 + 0.025 = 0.31 m. If the axle-to-axle length (hypotenuse) is 2.095 m, the grade can be calculated as:

Grade = total rise ÷ hypotenuse = 0.31 m ÷ 2.095 m = 0.148 × 100% = 14.8%

Note: For low grades (below 20%), the sine method gives a value that is nearly equal to the tangent method, so the method does not matter (see Table 45–5). For steep grades, one can also use the "rise" over the "run" method (using the carpenter's square) to obtain the tangent value and then look across the table to obtain the correct sine value to set on the treadmill dial. For example, if the "rise" over the "run" method yielded 0.268 or 26.8% (tangent), the "correct" setting would be 25.9% (sine). The latter value is set on the grade dial of the treadmill.

Cycle Ergometer

Work rate or power output is expressed in a variety of ways. To make some sense out of this, the basic units of measurement are presented. Mechanics involve three "undefinables" or measures that cannot be defined in any other units. These are length, time, and mass. In the metric system, length is measured in meters (m), time in seconds (sec), and mass in kilograms (kg).

Work is equal to force times the distance through which the force acts: $W = F \cdot d$.

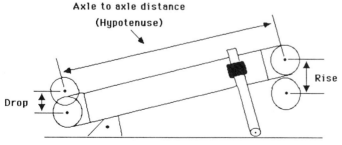

Axle to axle distance
(Hypotenuse)

Rise

Drop

Fig. 45–5. Calibration of grade for movable rear axle treadmill by sine method (rise hypotenuse).

Total Vertical Rise = Rise + Drop
Grade = sine θ = Total Vertical Rise ÷ Hypotenuse

Force is equal to the product of the mass of an object and its acceleration: $F = m \cdot a$. The basic unit of force is the newton (N); it is that force that, when applied to a 1 kg mass, gives it an acceleration of 1 m·sec^{-2}.

Although mass is a measure of the quantity of matter an object contains, its weight is the *force* with which it is attracted toward the center of the earth. Weight is appropriately expressed in newtons (N). If we return to our formula for work: $W = F \cdot d$ (with distance in meters), then Work = F (N)· d(m) = Nm. One Nm (Newton meter) is equal to one joule (J), which is the basic unit of work. A common unit used to express force is the kilopond, not the kilogram (mass unit). The kilopond is defined as the force acting on the mass of 1 kg at the normal acceleration of gravity, and is equal to 9.80665 N.

On the Monark cycle ergometer, a force (kp) is moved through a distance (meters), so work is expressed in kpm. Because work is accomplished over some period of time (minutes), the proper term is work *rate*, not workload. Another name for work rate is *power*. In the preceding example, work rate is expressed in kpm·min^{-1}.

The wheel on the Monark cycle ergometer travels 6 meters per pedal revolution; therefore, at 50 rev·min^{-1}, the wheel travels 300 m·min^{-1} (i.e., $6 \text{ m·rev}^{-1} \times 50 \text{ rev·min}^{-1} = 300 \text{ m·min}^{-1}$). If a force of 1 kp hangs from that wheel, the work rate or power output would be 300 kpm·min^{-1} (i.e., $1 \text{ kp} \times 300 \text{ m·min}^{-1} = 300 \text{ kpm·min}^{-1}$). The distance that the wheel travels per minute is easy to measure because you can count pedal revolutions. However, the pedal rate must be maintained and monitored for the test to be a valid representation of the power output. For example, if a subject is pedaling at 55 rev·min^{-1} instead of 50 rev·min^{-1}, 10% more work is being done than specified in the protocol. The estimated oxygen cost of the activity would be underestimated.[1] As a consequence, a person's estimated cardiovascular fitness would also be underestimated.

Although the force exerted on the wheel is easily set and maintained, calibration of the force values on the scale is necessary to ensure that the work rate is accurate. In addition, the load setting must be monitored to adjust for any "drift" that occurs during a test. The following steps outline the procedures to follow in the calibration of the Monark cycle ergometer scale.[6]

Calibration of the Monark Cycle Ergometer

1. With a carpenter's level, adjust a table to ensure that it is *level* and put the ergometer on it.
2. Disconnect the "belt" at the spring.
3. Adjust the set screw on the front of the bike against which the numerical scale rests, so that the vertical mark on the pendulum weight is matched with "0" kp on the force scale. The pendulum must be free-swinging. Lock the adjustment screw.
4. Suspend a 0.5 kg weight from the spring so that no contact is made with the flywheel and see if the pendulum moves to the 0.5 kp mark. If not, place tape over the scale and make a mark in line with the pendulum. Suitable calibration weights (#9102-26 [1 kg], −27 [0.5 kg], −28 [0.25 kg], −30 [100 g], −25 [0.5 kg weight pan]) can be obtained from Quinton Instrument Company, 2121 Terry Ave., Seattle, WA 98121.[7]
5. Systematically add weight to the spring. The pendulum mark should match the weight scale mark for each weight. If the marks do not match, put tape over the marks and numbers on the force scale, and label the taped scale appropriately. Note: Be sure to calibrate the ergometer through the range of values to be used in your tests.
6. Reassemble the cycle ergometer.

REFERENCES

1. American College of Sports Medicine: *Guidelines for Exercise Testing and Prescription*, 4th Edition. Philadelphia: Lea & Febiger, 1991.
2. Penman KA: *Planning Physical Education and Athletic Facilities in Schools*. New York: Wiley, 1977.
3. Herbert DL, Herbert WG: *Legal Aspects of Preventative and Rehabilitative Exercise Programs*. Canton: Professional and Executive Reports and Publications, 1984.

4. Strock RE: Step up the savings. *Club Business International*, October, 1990.

5. Patton RW, Grantham WC, Gerson RF, Gettman LR: *Developing and Managing Health Fitness Facilities*. Champaign, IL: Human Kinetics Publishers, Inc., 1989.

6. Åstrand PO: *Work Test with the Bicycle Ergometer*. Varberg, Sweden: Monark-Crescent AB.

7. Quinton Instruments Instruction Manual—Model 24-72. Quinton Instruments, Seattle, Washington, 1970.

Chapter 46

EVALUATION OF PREVENTIVE AND REHABILITATIVE EXERCISE PROGRAMS

Paul J. Lloyd, Steven N. Blair, and Brenda Mitchell

The evaluation of preventive and rehabilitative exercise programs asks two basic questions. First, did the program work? Second, can any observed impact be attributed to the program intervention? Participants and prospective clients want to know whether the program is worth their time and effort. Health fitness directors and administrators want to know if their programs are effective. This chapter describes the process of program evaluation associated with answering these two questions and specifically addresses the following questions: Why evaluate? What questions help to clearly focus the evaluation process? What are the advantages and disadvantages of different designs for various stages of the evaluation process? What are different data collection and analysis procedures? What is the standard format of an evaluation report? What pertinent issues are involved in the management of evaluation activities? Although anyone who needs information regarding the merits of a program is a potential user of evaluation findings, the major purpose of this overview of planning and conducting evaluations of health and fitness preventive and rehabilitative exercise programs is to equip health fitness directors and rehabilitative program directors and their staff with the rudimentary skills necessary for successful program evaluation. As noted by Cronbach,[1] the best evaluation is that which has a positive effect on program improvement. From this perspective, we hope to encourage program coordinators to both increase their understanding of the principles of program evaluation and become producers and consumers of evaluation studies.[2]

EVALUATION: WHAT IS IT? WHY DO IT?

Program evaluation helps to determine whether or not a program is effective. For most programs (or products), evaluation provides a framework for answering questions about goals, objectives, activities, outcomes, and costs. For example, effectiveness can be determined by comparing a person's improved health and fitness to expenditures in terms of human and other resources. The board of directors of a cardiac rehabilitation program may want to know how effective the programs are in returning patients to work. A company president may be interested in the extent of employee participation in a preventive exercise program. A program manager may want to decide which behavioral intervention to use to accomplish a specific objective for a client.

Evaluation is an essential component in the development and maintenance of a comprehensive and current state-of-the-art exercise program. The evaluation process provides the necessary information for rational decision making. It is mandated in rehabilitation settings, but is equally important in everyday clinical practice, corporate and community settings. Evaluation is **not** an additional duty and responsibility for a program director, but part of a daily routine. Performance evaluation in both personal and professional settings is part of a daily routine, as is ongoing, informal evaluation of effectiveness and efficiency of health promotion and/or rehabilitation programs. However, systematic program evaluation is often not the case in such programs. Inadequate evaluation procedures may lead to poor problem solving and decision making and make few contributions to program enhancement.

One example of a popular evaluation procedure that may lead to poor decision making is the one-group pre-post design. Because of the absence of a comparison (control) group, the interpretation of results suffers from a lack of attention to systematic, controlled evaluation procedures. Interpretation of results in this type of situation is questionable. However, systematic evaluation can make the case for future, better-designed evaluation studies. As is the case with integrating exercise into daily activities, some well-designed program evaluation procedures are better than none at all.

PROGRAM EVALUATION IN ACTION

Plans for program evaluation should be made during the planning stage of program development. At its best, program evaluation is a form of ongoing action research. However, it is common for evaluation procedure to be designed after the start of the program or even requested after the completion of the program. An evaluator may find it helpful to be an external, impartial observer of a program such as an exercise-based health promotion, sports medicine, or cardiac rehabilitation program. From this viewpoint, the best strategy for evaluation can be determined.

The development of the procedure is influenced by several factors. Primary factors include basic information required for all evaluations as well as the point of entry for starting the evaluation process. Money, time, available resources, program priorities, and program complexity are all factors that determine the approach to program evaluation.

The first step in the evaluation process is to formulate a subset of questions to help focus the evaluation process clearly. These are generally derived from the exercise program's goals and objectives. What are the intended immediate and long-term effects of the program? All evaluation activities must be organized so that this subset of questions can be answered directly and accurately.

The next step is locating and gathering information with an informal needs assessment. This can be facilitated by planning meetings with program managers, staff, organizational administrators, and current or prospective participants. These meetings can take the form of group conferences, individual interviews, or both. Each participant in the planning process should be given the opportunity to reflect on the

most important parts of the program for purposes of evaluation and to discuss the positive impact of the program on participants. How the program meets organizational and/or accreditation standards should also be considered. Specific components that reflect areas of concern for program improvements should be discussed. The meetings should produce anecdotal statements that will prove invaluable in developing more systematic procedures. These discussions should also address the history of the exercise program and its purposes, organizational structure, and long range plans.

Another source of information is a more formal needs assessment for the initial program planning phase. This is a formal survey of the attitudes, beliefs, and intentions of administrators, staff, and participants, and it provides important information concerning the interest and reasons for participation and objectives for the program. A representative sample of all current or prospective program administrators and participants is desirable. Each person who dropped out of present or past programs, as well as people outside of the program purview, can give additional helpful perspectives for program evaluation.

The qualitative data gathered through both informal and formal needs assessment form the basis for a thorough description of the program, its goals, and its objectives. The goals and objectives must be formalized before the evaluation questions can be meaningfully stated. The goals of preventive and rehabilitative exercise programs should address such major concerns as the type of program, assessments and screening, staffing and professional development, equipment facilities, planning and evaluation, and marketing and promotion. These goals statements define processes and outcomes in broad terms and are not quantifiable or measurable. Ideally, the goals relate to a program mission statement and provide a basis for smooth program implementation.

Written objectives that are measurable are an important part of a program evaluation. Objectives should answer the questions: who, what, when and how much? A measurable objective has numbers in it. If it does not, it is probably a goal. Examples from *Healthy People 2000: National Health Promotion and Disease Prevention Objectives*[3] of both process and outcome objectives include the following:

> *Process Objective*: By the year 2000, increase to at least 30% the proportion of people aged 6 and older who engage regularly, preferably daily, in light to moderate physical activity for at least 30 minutes per day.
>
> *Outcome Objective*: Reduce coronary heart disease to no more than 100 per 100,000 people.

Additional information about the program may be obtained from written proposals, annual reports, brochures, products produced by the program, organizational structure, and staff members. This will help formulate the list of questions for the evaluation and supplement the data base.

A program description (example in Table 46–1) should be prepared that states the program's goals and activities and provides some means for measuring program activities and goals. This information can be easily translated into questions. Examples of evaluation questions might include:

1. How many individuals complete the entire program?
2. What is the change in physical work capacity (PWC) in program participants after 6 months of exercise conditioning?
3. What percentage of hypertensive subjects have their blood pressure under control?

The evaluation may include process-oriented questions relating more to the success of program implementation and based on general considerations that are not derived directly from the program description. For example, what factors control exercise participation and adherence? What affects whether a participant joins an exercise program, stays in the program, or changes behavior after the formal program intervention has been completed?

Once a preliminary draft of the questions that help to closely focus the evaluation process is prepared, the program staff should meet to establish priorities for the questions, add or delete questions, and ensure that all questions can be answered within the time period, given the resources available, time-line for the implementation of evaluation procedures including program monitoring and assessment of program effectiveness should be accessible. This preliminary stage of locating, gathering, and organizing information prepares the evaluator to select the evaluation design and develop an evaluation plan.

EVALUATION PLAN AND DESIGN SELECTION

Developing an evaluation plan is the next step in the process. The plan summarizes information about the degree of scientific validity acceptable for an evaluation. Based on the evaluation questions, the plan should specify the variables, the sampling procedures and address concerns to scientific validity so that the evaluation questions will be satisfactorily answered.

The evaluation design is a systematic procedure that specifies the ways in which participants are grouped and what variables are manipulated and measured to an-

Table 46–1. Example of a Program Description

Goal*	Activity	Evidence of Merit
Improve physical work capacity (PWC)	Exercise program	Increased PWC
Weight control	Weight loss counseling	Weight loss in overweight participants
Blood pressure control	Nutrition counseling, exercise program, drug therapy	Improved blood pressure in participants
Return to work (post-myocardial infarction)	Total rehabilitation program	Return to work by most patients

* For all goals, additional evidence of merit is provided by behavior change or adherence to therapeutic regimens.

swer one or more evaluation questions. In some evaluations, a single design is used to answer all questions, whereas in other evaluation several designs are required.

Systematic observation procedures can efficiently produce accurate estimates of all participants using information from only a subset, thus reducing costs. The ways in which participants are selected for an evaluation vary. Three common methods for obtaining representative samples are:

1. Random sample—A lottery system is used to select an appropriate number of subjects from the total population. Each person in the target population has an equal opportunity to be selected.
2. Stratified random sample—The total population is divided into subgroups (e.g., sex or age categories) and a certain number of subjects is randomly selected from each subgroup.
3. Purposive sample—Individuals or groups are deliberately selected to provide a focus on specific subgroups.

Evaluation designs can be one of three types: experimental, quasi-experimental, and pre-experimental designs. The type of design depends upon whether participants are randomly assigned to groups and whether a comparison or control group is included. A summary of each of several designs to be used to evaluate preventive and rehabilitative exercise programs follows.[4-6] These designs are illustrated, using the following conventions:

1. The letter "R" means random assignment to control and experimental groups (a design in which equivalent groups are created)
2. A broken straight line ("------") indicates non-random assignment to groups (nonequivalent groups)
3. The letter "O" indicates an observation (a set of measurements)
4. The letter "X" indicates the intervention (treatment variable)

Common methodologic problems in program evaluation are low participation rate, small sample size, selection bias, lack of comparable control group, no means to monitor adherence, poor generalizability, lack of specific and consistent definitions of risk factors or interventions, poor definition of outcome measures, self-selection of program participants, and inappropriate techniques. Examples of these problems and other threats to scientific validity are included in the description of the following designs.

Experimental Design

Experimental design is composed of equivalent groups with randomized assignment of participants to groups. Participants are assigned to treatment groups by random selection so that the groups are essentially the same at the start of the program.

This design is the theoretical "standard" against which alternative evaluation designs can be judged. An evaluation design such as this should be selected when possible to offset the most likely threats to validity. The classic true experimental designs are the pretest and post-test control group and the post-test only control group designs.

PRETEST AND POST-TEST CONTROL GROUP DESIGN

$$R\ O_1\ X\ O_2\ -\ \text{Experimental Group}$$

$$R\ O_3\ \ \ \ O_4\ -\ \text{Control Group}$$

POST-TEST ONLY CONTROL GROUP DESIGN

$$R\ X\ O_1\ -\ \text{Experimental Group}$$

$$R\ \ \ \ O_2\ -\ \text{Control Group}$$

Note that the Experimental Group is the group in which the intervention or treatment is used and the Control Group is the group in which no treatment or intervention is utilized. Experimental designs are the most likely to help determine whether to reject alternative explanations for the program outcomes. If so, it can be stated that the program intervention had a significant effect on the outcome measures. Evaluation data could include measurements (observations) of body fat composition, strength, and general well being. One method to accomplish randomization of participants when withholding treatments is unethical or unfeasible is to have program applicants randomly assigned to a waiting list to serve as the control group.

Quasi-Experimental Design

Quasi-experimental design is appropriate when it is not feasible to have random assignment of subjects to groups. In many evaluation settings, the demand simply does not exceed the supply of prospective participants, which precludes random sampling as a necessary prerequisite for true experimental designs. Three frequently used designs are the time series, nonequivalent control group and multiple time series designs.

The use of quasi-experimental designs in program evaluation is widespread. The major advantage of a time series design over a single group pre- and post-design comes from obtaining a series of measurements at equal intervals over time before and after the implementation of the program. It is an excellent way to monitor program performance to see if the program is being implemented in the way it was designed. This design has the advantage in that a "criterion reference" can be used to determine whether the outcome is clinically significant. This allows interpretation of the numbers within the setting in which they will be used. With a one-group design, it is still difficult to know for certain if changes in the observed measures after the treatment can be attributed to the intervention or some alternative explanation.

TIME SERIES DESIGN

$$O_1 \; O_2 \; O_3 \; O_4 \; X \; O_5 \; O_6 \; O_7 \; O_8$$

The nonequivalent control group design can be useful when evaluating exercise programs if the difference between groups attributable to selection bias is avoided. Simply stated, a selection bias is present when the groups are different to begin with because of the criteria used for selecting them. Using a comparison group permits the analysis of the differences between the effects of the program and other plausible explanations.

NONEQUIVALENT CONTROL GROUP DESIGN

$$\frac{O_1 \; X \; O_2}{O_3 \; X \; O_4}$$

The multiple time series design combines the features of the time series design and the nonequivalent group design. Observations are made at different points in time for a treatment and a comparison group. This design is appropriate for retrospective and prospective data that are easily accessible or when an organization already has archival data for program participants. This design yields a greater certainty of interpretation, and comparisons are possible with a control group over intervals of time.

MULTIPLE TIME SERIES DESIGN

$$\frac{O_1 \; O_2 \; O_3 \; O_4 \; X \; O_5 \; O_6 \; O_7 \; O_8}{O_9 \; O_{10} \; O_{11} \; O_{12} \; O_{13} \; O_{14} \; O_{15} \; O_{16}}$$

The one-group, pretest and post-test design, with respect to scientific validity, is a weak design because there is no comparison group. Even with its shortcomings, however, this design is useful for some evaluation questions in health and fitness programs. It is essential to use extreme care when interpreting results. An example is pretest and post-test measures of $\dot{V}O_{2max}$ without a control group.

Pre-experimental Design

Pre-experimental designs are useful when a legitimate comparison or control group cannot be found. Four of these designs are the one-group, pre-post, one-shot case study, static group comparison, and content validation studies.

ONE-GROUP PRETEST AND POST-TEST DESIGN

$$O_1 \; X \; O_2$$

The one-shot case study can be used as a record-keeping procedure for post-program follow-ups. For example, attitudes can be evaluated by such a post-test-only measure. It is the most frequently used evaluation design and is essentially an exit

Table 46–2. Example of an Evaluation Design Strategy

| Evaluation Questions | Design Strategy | | | |
	Type	Independent/ Dependent Variables	Sampling	Threats to Validity
Change in physical work capacity (PWC)	One group pretest-post-test	$\dot{V}O_{2max}$ or PWC (dependent): age, sex, disease state, smoking status; body weight (independent)	Purposive (all participants)	History, maturation, mortality
Return to work	Nonequivalent controls	Employed rate (dependent); demographics/ health status (independent)	Random sample of controls and participants	Selection, reactive effects, multiple program interference

polling procedure that is humanitarian and cheap.

ONE-SHOT CASE STUDY

X O

This design permits comparison of results of a particular program with results of other programs or well-established norms. The outcomes of a particular group are compared with those of other programs or groups which are similar but may be better established or larger.

Additional evaluation procedures include observation and assessment by outside experts (consultants), program participants and program administrators. Depending on the background of the evaluator, it may be wise to seek advice of an expert in program evaluation and/or a biostatistical consultant because of the complexity of determining sample size and selecting appropriate research designs and

data analysis techniques. A design strategy for answering a sample of two evaluation questions is provided in Table 46–2.

STATIC-GROUP COMPARISON

$$\frac{X\ O_1}{O_2}$$

MANAGEMENT OF A DATA BASE

Close attention must be paid to ensure that all evaluation questions are answered. Each evaluation question, together with the data collection techniques and a list of any limitations imposed by the schedule of the evaluation design, or sampling procedures should be listed. Specific data about the instruments, time and place for data collection, who is included in the sample, and who will collect the data should be in the list. An example of a data collection plan is provided in Table 46–3.

The following are common techniques for data collection.[7] Some advantages and

Table 46–3. Example of an Information Collection Plan

Evaluation Questions	Collection Technique/ Instruments	Time/Place	Limitations	Who Will Collect
Improve physical work capacity	Exercise tests	Baseline and follow-up care	Expense of testing	Laboratory staff
Return to work	Questionnaire	1–2 years after program	Difficulty in tracking, subjective response	Program administrative staff

disadvantages of each technique are explained.

1. Performance test: An individual or group performs an activity or task and the quality of the performance is assessed. Examples include exercise tests, laboratory values, and weight loss.
   Advantage:
   It relies on objective data.
   Disadvantage:
   It is usually time-consuming and expensive.
2. Rating and ranking scales: These scales can be used for self-assessment or to assess other people, events, or products for a given dimension or variable. Examples include feelings of well-being and life satisfaction.
   Advantages:
   They are relatively inexpensive to construct and administer, they are usually easily understood, and the data they provide readily lends itself to analysis.
   Disadvantage:
   They are subject to many types of bias.
3. Existing record: This technique refers to collecting evaluation data from program-related documents. Examples include reviewing patient charts for data that are not included in the computer data base or reviewing past medical or employment records.
   Advantage:
   It does not interfere with the program being evaluated and it is relatively inexpensive.
   Disadvantages:
   Participants' rights of privacy prohibit access to many records, and the possibility that program documents may be disorganized, unreliable, or unavailable.
4. Observations: Data collected by observers can be reported by check lists, rating scales, narrative records, and summary reports. Examples include rating program staff on communications skills.
   Advantages:
   a. They help the data collectors become familiar with and sensitive to the program.
   b. They are often the only feasible and economical way to gather certain kinds of data.
   Disadvantages:
   a. It is costly to train data collectors.
   b. The people observed may not behave normally because of the presence of the observer.
   c. Several observations may be needed to obtain consistent results.
5. Interviews: In an interview, a person talks with another person or group and records data on narrative records, structured interview forms, summary reports, or other related forms. Examples include diet recalls, exercise histories, or family issues and problems.
   Advantage:
   They permit in-depth probes of sensitive subjects, such as attitudes and values.
   Disadvantages:
   They are usually time-consuming and costly, and interviewers must be specially trained.
6. Questionnaires: Self-administered survey forms consist of a set of questions for which answers may be either free responses or forced choices. Examples include health behavior inventories, medical histories, and psychological factors.
   Advantages:
   They are less expensive to construct and administer than most measures, and the resulting data are relatively easy to analyze.
   Disadvantage:
   The kind of data obtained is sometimes limited.

COLLECTING EVALUATION DATA

The five major activities related to the collection of evaluation data are:

1. Identifying appropriate indicators of program objectives
2. Developing data collection instruments and procedures
3. Training data collectors
4. Making observations

5. Organizing evaluation data for analysis.

Developing Data Collection Instruments

Selecting an instrument for collecting data involves reviewing currently available measure and then choosing or adapting the most appropriate choice. Advantages of selecting an existing data collection instrument are that it is less expensive than developing a new one, and technical data about the validity, reliability, and applicability of the instrument are usually available. The disadvantage is that instruments appropriate for answering the evaluation questions are not always readily available.

New data collection tools may be developed by combining the features of several instruments. This approach can save time and money, but may require obtaining permission for use and a study to validate the hybrid instrument. Designing and validating an evaluation instrument are the best guarantee for obtaining the necessary data, but this process requires considerable skill and time.

Training Data Collectors

Before beginning the data collection activities, data collectors should learn as much as possible about the program, the evaluation questions, and the specific data collection activities they will conduct. They should receive detailed training about how to obtain, record, and communicate data.

Many data collection activities are subject to legal restrictions and may require clearance or approval from an Institutional Review Board or other supervisory groups. Matters of confidentiality and informed consent must be incorporated into the data collection plan. These issues should be considered an integral part of the training of data collectors.

Pilot Study

Because it takes additional time and effort, program managers may be tempted to omit this step. Thorough pilot testing is ideal and may not always be possible, but problems can be avoided if time is allotted for a pilot study. Pilot testing of the instruments and procedures can answer questions such as:

1. Are certain words or questions used in the instruments redundant or misleading?
2. Are the instruments appropriate for the audience?
3. Can the data collectors administer, collect, and report data in a standardized manner using the written directions and special coding forms?
4. How consistent are the data obtained by the instruments (reliability)?
5. How accurate are the data obtained with the instruments?

The ideal pilot test should be conducted following these guidelines:

1. Conduct all activities under conditions that are identical to those followed in the evaluation.
2. Include a representative sample of the participants in the pilot study.
3. Omit participants in the pilot study from any subsequent evaluation activities because they will be familiar with the evaluation measures (threat to internal validity).
4. Have experts review the data collection plan, the instruments, and other evaluation guidelines.
5. Revise the instruments and procedures if necessary.
6. Repeat the pilot testing until you are confident that the evaluation instruments and procedures are feasible and yield credible data.

PLANNING AND CONDUCTING DATA ANALYSES

Even before the data collection begins, preferably as part of the evaluation planning activities, the analyses should be planned so that the evaluation questions can be answered directly. The evaluation design and data collection plan must be coordinated with the data analyses. Choices of analyses are always guided by the evaluation design to be used.

The methods used to set up a data base and file management are important considerations. Using a computerized format such as machine-readable forms for gathering data makes the data entry easier. Noting treatment group and data collection date in the file name help in the organization and retrieval of files.

The results of analyses are numbers, descriptions, explanations, justifications of events, and statistical statements. Interpreting the results means using the findings of the analyses to answer each of the evaluation questions. When all questions have been answered, the results may discussed in perspective to evaluate the program as a whole and to provide recommendations and offer suggestions concerning the merits of the program and methods to improve the program.

When making interpretations, important precautions are as follows: (1) Be sensitive to personal bias; (2) Do not extrapolate beyond the limits of the data; and (3) Report only data that are related to the evaluation questions or the evidence of program merit.

THE PROGRAM EVALUATION REPORT

A program evaluation report explains the procedures used to obtain the answers and provides the answers to the evaluation questions. Sometimes reports serve as the sole information base for decision makers. Therefore it is extremely important to take into consideration the purpose of the report and the intended audience. Written and oral reports should include the following components:

1. Title Page
2. Executive Summary (abstract)
3. Table of Contents
4. Program Description
   a. Historical Background
   b. Rationale for the Evaluation
   c. Goals and Objectives
   d. Description of Participants and Setting
   e. Evaluation Questions
5. Design Strategy
   a. Sampling Procedures
   b. Evaluation Design
   c. Limitations
6. Data Collection Procedures
   a. Instruments
   b. Schedule of Activities
7. Data Analysis
8. Results
9. Costs of the Program
10. Conclusions
11. Recommendations

MANAGEMENT OF EVALUATION PROJECT

It is important that evaluation activities be coordinated so that the information is ready when needed for decision making. Directors of evaluation studies must give attention to establishing schedules, assigning staff and monitoring their activities, and budgeting. Establishing evaluation schedules requires attention to the specific evaluation activities, deadlines for completing activities and reports, and the total amount of time to be given to each activity. The evaluator should decide the skills needed to perform each activity so that the staff members with those skills can be assigned appropriately. These tasks are usually addressed during the planning stages and are incorporated into the original proposal.

Managing an evaluation also means monitoring the efficiency of the staff in performing the evaluation activities. Data collected should describe the amount of time spent on each activity, how thoroughly each activity has been accomplished, and any problems encountered. Frequent informal meetings or reports to the project staff are helpful.

Evaluation budgets vary in form and detail; they are usually part of the planning process. An evaluation usually has a given amount of money and must be accomplished without exceeding the amount. A thorough understanding of the available resources (staff, time, equipment, and money) must be considered when making decisions about the overall program and evaluation plan. Programs planned well in advance with appropriate evaluation activities generally have a higher likelihood of success than unplanned evaluation activities.

Two approaches to economic assessment that are logical extensions of evaluation procedures are cost-benefit analysis and cost effectiveness analysis.[8,9] Cost-benefit analysis measures the economic efficiency in monetary units of a program as a relationship of costs and benefits. For example, measure of productivity expressed in units produced/hours worked for staff productivity. This is a measure of resource consumption in dollars. Often cost-effectiveness analysis is an easier approach in measuring the value or merit of a program. It measures program success in nonmonetary units. For example, an improved sense of well-being and a high level of wellness lead to an improved ability to handle stress and help meet an organizational objective of reducing the number of sick days. This type of evaluation is limited because it does not allow the comparison of programs with different outcomes.

CONCLUSION

The importance of networking with other program directors through personal contact and professional associations such as the American College of Sports Medicine (ACSM) cannot be overemphasized. Staying up to date and sharing information helps sharpen your evaluation skills. If this is an early attempt at program evaluation, keep it neat and simple. Indeed, this is a basic rubric for most program evaluation projects. Be certain that the program objectives are specific, measurable activities that are relevant and technically feasible.

REFERENCES

1. Cronbach LJ, et al.: *Toward Reform of Program Evaluation.* San Francisco: Jossey-Bass, 1980.
2. Blair SN, et al.: *Resource Manual for Guidelines for Exercise Testing and Prescription.* Philadelphia: Lea & Febiger, 1988.
3. *Healthy People 2000: National Health Promotion and Disease Prevention Objectives.* U.S. Department of Health and Human Services. DHHS Publication No. (PHS) 91-50212.
4. Campbell DT, Stanley JC: *Experimental and Quasi-Experimental Designs for Research.* Chicago: Rand McNally, 1966
5. Cook TD, Campbell DT: *Quasi-Experimentation-Design and Analysis Issues for Field Settings.* Boston: Houghton Mifflin, 1979.
6. Green LW, Lewis FM: *Measurement and Evaluation in Health Education and Health Promotion.* Palo Alto: Mayfield, 1986
7. Blair SN: How to assess exercise habits and physical fitness. In Matarazzo, JD: *Behavioral Health: A Handbook of Health Enhancement and Disease Prevention.* New York: John Wiley & Sons, 1984.
8. Posavac EJ, Carey RG: *Program Evaluation: Methods and Case Studies,* 3rd ed. Englewood Cliffs, NJ: Prentice-Hall, 1989.
9. Rossi PH, Freeman HE, Wright SR: *Evaluation—A Systematic Approach.* Beverly Hills: Sage, 1979.

SUGGESTIONS FOR FURTHER READING

1. Altman DG: A framework for evaluating community-based heart disease prevention programs. *Soc Sci Med, 22:*4, 1986
2. Brinkerhoff RO, et al.: *Program Evaluation: A Practitioner's Guide for Trainers and Educators.* Boston: Kluwer-Nijhoff Publishing, 1982.
3. Conrad KM, Conrad KJ, Walcott-McQuigg J: Threats to internal validity in worksite health promotion program research: Common problems and possible solutions. *Am J Health Prom, 6:*2, 1991.
4. Cronbach LJ: *Designing Evaluation of Educational and Social Programs.* San Francisco: Jossey-Bass, 1982.
5. Daniel WW: *Biostatistics: A Foundation for Analysis in the Health Sciences.* New York: John Wiley & Sons, 1974.
6. Fink A, Kosecoff J: *An Evaluation Primer Workbook: Practical Exercises for Health Professionals.* Beverly Hills: Sage, 1978.
7. Fink A, Kosecoff J: *An Evaluation Primer.* Beverly Hills: Sage, 1978.
8. Fitz-Gibbon CT, Morris LL: *How to Design a Program Evaluation.* Beverly Hills, Sage, 1978.
9. Guttentag M, Struening EL: *Handbook of Evaluation Research.* Beverly Hills: Sage, 1975.
10. Hawkridge, DG, Campeau, PL, Trickett, PK: *Preparing Evaluation Reports: A Guide for Authors.* Pittsburgh: American Institutes for Research, 1970.
11. Herman JL, Morris LL, Fitz-Gibbon CT: *Evaluator's Handbook,* 2nd Ed. Beverly Hills: Sage, 1978.
12. Kerlinger F: *Foundations of Behavioral Research.* 2nd Ed. New York: Holt, Rinehart, and Winston, 1973.
13. McCuan RA, Green LW: Multivariate analysis in health education and promotion research. In *Advances in Health Education and Promotion,* Volume III. Edited by W Ward and FM Lewis. London: Jessica Kingsley, 1990.
15. Morris LL, Fitz-Gibbon CT: *Evaluator's Handbook.* Beverly Hills: Sage, 1978.
16. Morris LL, Fitz-Gibbon CT, Lindheim E: *How to Measure Performance and Use Tests.* Beverly Hills: Sage, 1987.
17. Nunnally JC: *Psychometric Theory.* 2nd Ed. New York: McGraw-Hill, 1978.
18. Patton MQ: *Practical Evaluation.* Beverly Hills: Sage, 1982.

19. Schulberg HC, Baker F: *Program Evaluation in the Health Fields.* New York: Human Sciences Press, 1979.
20. Ward WB (Ed.): *Advances in Health Education and Promotion.* Volume 1, Part B. Greenwich, CT: JAI Press, 1986
21. Windsor RA: The utility of time series designs and analysis in evaluating health promotion and education programs. In *Advances in Health Education and Promotion.* Volume 1, Part B. Edited by WB Ward. Greenwich, CT: JAI Press, 1986
22. Windsor RA, Baranowski T, Clark N, Cutter G: *Evaluation of Health Promotion and Education Programs.* Palo Alto: Mayfield, 1984.

Chapter 47

POLICIES AND PROCEDURES IN P&R PROGRAMS

Linda K. Hall and Larry R. Gettman

It is inherent within any human to compare what he or she is doing against a standard and give it a rating. We do it on a regular basis in rating food, movies, performances in sports, and any number of things, with questions such as "On a scale of 1 to 10, how did you like that movie?" The operation of a cardiopulmonary rehabilitation program and/or a fitness or health enhancement program involves regular quality control examinations, certifications, licensure, and review. Several agencies have established review procedures for health care organizations: The Joint Commission On Accreditation of Healthcare Organizations (JCAHO), the American Public Health Association (APHA), and the Commission on Accreditation of Rehabilitation Facilities (CARF). Now others, the American College of Sports Medicine (ACSM) for example, have established certification procedures for fitness centers and health clubs. Because of these review and certification processes, it is necessary for the program to establish an operational design that sets standards for performing the business of the organization.

OPERATIONAL DESIGN

The first time the concept of developing a program or fitness center is discussed is at the beginning of establishing the operational design. It is at this initial meeting that the "mission of the program" is verbalized, shaped, and finally established.

Mission Statement and Philosophy

A mission statement is a combined statement of purpose and philosophy of operation. The purpose explains why the program, department, or center was or is to be developed and continues to exist. The philosophic statements reflect the beliefs that are held with regard to achieving the purpose.

Example: "The cardiac rehabilitation department (CRD) supports the parent organization in its mission to serve the charitable purpose of the communities it serves. This is accomplished through the delivery of a comprehensive range of services to patients, the education and training of health professionals, and the conduct of research. The CRD strives to achieve excellence in all of its patient care, education and research activities."[1]

As the program, department, or organization changes, becomes larger, or accepts different types of participants, this mission statement may be reviewed and rewritten. The statement must truly reflect the philosophy of the current operation of the organization. The basic premise on which the philosophy should be formulated is the process of delivering quality service with expectation of positive outcomes.

Policies and Procedures

Once the mission and philosophy of the organization are developed, all other areas fall into place. A physical setting is designed, staffing requirements are delineated, programs for carrying out the mission are developed, and a process for evaluating all of these components is put into place. During each of these steps, as specifics are established, a policy and procedure manual (PPM) evolves. The PPM establishes policies and rules or directives for carrying out the policies. Policies may be defined as general guidelines of operational procedures.

Example: Equipment shall be operated within the guidelines provided by the manufacturer's operating manual and in a manner to ensure the safety of the participants.

Rules and directives provide specific details relative to carrying out the policies.

Example:

1. All treadmills should be returned to a speed of 1.5 mph and a 0% grade before being turned off.
2. All treadmills should have an emergency stop button immediately visible on the console.

The PPM then becomes the staff member's guide to standard operating procedure (SOP). Several things are inherently implied in carrying out the SOP on a daily basis:

1. Staff are trained according to the descriptions which are found in the policy and procedure manual.
2. If the staff know the appropriate thing to do, but do not do it, some form of discipline is necessary.
3. If staff have been taught the standard and are unable to do it, the standard needs to be revised.
4. The most important thing in PPM development is to define the correct thing to do, teach staff to do the correct thing, and teach them well enough so that they do the correct thing the first time.[2]

POLICIES AND PROCEDURES IN CLINICAL SETTINGS

The ultimate goal of the clinical rehabilitation facility is delivery of a high quality level of care for individual patients and/or patient groups. Three major variables act and interact with program management and patient care considerations. They are structure, process, and outcomes related to management and patient care.

STRUCTURE

It is fitting that structure be the first section to be considered as the policy and procedure manual is formed; usually the physical setting is structured before programs are actually designed and patients are treated. The first consideration under structural concerns is that the physical setting in which patient care will be undertaken is built according to safety, building, fire, and health care codes. When building

a clinical office, exercise area, and/or health fitness facility, it is critical that all fire safety, state building, public health, and Joint Commission on Accreditation of Healthcare Organizations (JCAHO) regulations be addressed.

Structure Related to Patient Care

The PPM should address specific issues other then general building code, fire safety code, and emergency exit code regulations. Some examples of these are the following:

1. In all modes of undress, examination, and verbal interviews, the patient's privacy is ensured.
2. Chart and medical record confidentiality is ensured
3. Storing, locking, or protecting patient valuables is ensured
4. Structured emergency plans are made for the following:
   a. Fire and evacuation
   b. Cardiac arrest and related problems
   c. Anatomic injury and related problems
   d. Infection control and barriers to infection
   All staff are familiar with the plans and regularly practice "mock" trials.
5. Operation manuals are provided, with notebooks recording and documenting service calls, repair and calibration, and clinical engineering data for all exercise equipment, mechanical equipment, and electrically powered devices.

Structure Related to Program Management

In structuring the program, it is important to start with a well-formed series of written statements. These written documents are accumulated in several manuals and are reviewed semi-annually, revised any time there are changes, initialled, and dated. These written documents include, but may not be limited to, the following:

1. National Guidelines, Federal and State Guidelines. The department PPM should not have a standard that is less than that established by the Na-

tional, Federal, and/or State guidelines.

2. Mission statements from the parent organization and department.

3. Comprehensive job descriptions of each position in the department. Each staff member should have a current resume on file in the department, and the resume for the specific job and the job description requirements should match.

4. All personnel certifications, licenses, and registration numbers. These should be current.

5. A policy and procedure relative to staff scheduling and staffing patient ratios.

6. A written record of department meetings, stating that problems have been identified, followed, and resolved.

7. Documentation of regular inservices, opportunity for educational pro-

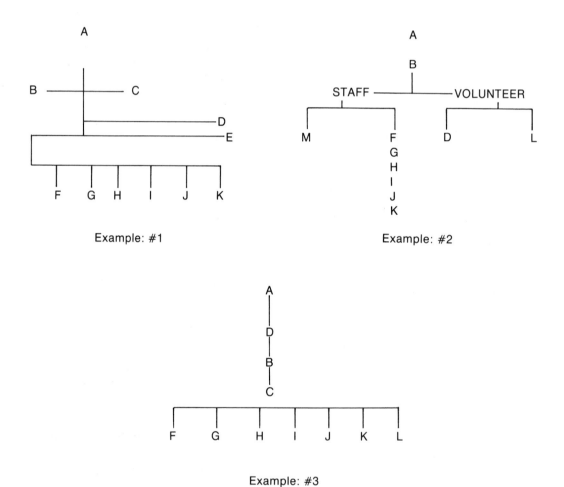

Example: #1

Example: #2

Example: #3

A = Hospital Administration
B = Medical Director
C = Program Director
D = Advisory Board
E = Assistant Director
F = Clinical Nurse CR Specialist

G = Exercise Physiologist
H = Secretary
I = Dietary Consultant
J = Intern
K = Social Worker
L = Other

Fig. 47–1. Types of organizational grids for management of cardiopulmonary rehabilitation programs.

grams, training programs, and new procedure training. Dates, times, and attendance for each staff and each program are documented.

8. Performance objectives and an annual performance review of all staff.
9. Public notification of patient rights and right to treatment in English and Spanish.

It is in this area of program management and structure that consideration needs to be given to a chain of command management grid. Where do physician medical directors and program directors fit, and who does what?

Figure 47–1 presents three different models of program management. The favored schematic for most clinical programs is number one. It allows each person to work within the area of his or her primary responsibilities and appropriate decision-making chain of command. Daily interaction with physicians in a clinical setting demands a certain courtesy and professional demeanor. The medical director of the department is responsible for all medical decisions in the clinical application of the department's business. Patients in the clinic should not become a part of the medical director's private practice unless they were originally. However, the medical director should act in the patients' best interest at all times when they are at the clinic. The medical director may direct management of emergency procedures, provide standing orders, approve all exercise prescriptions, approve disposition of patients when untoward response to therapy occurs, and in general oversee all medical decisions. A supervising physician may act on the medical director's behalf.

The role of the referring (primary care) physician is important to program design and the PPM. The primary care physician initiates the patient referral to the hospital, surgery, or special procedures unit, and he or she is the one to whom the patient returns when the consultation, surgery, or special procedure is done. The PPM should define and outline this physician's role in the program and should also define the communication required between the program and the referring physician.

The program director is the "orchestra"

leader with the physicians. The PPM defines the roles of the physicians and ensures that their role in the patient's program is well defined. Communication and reports outline patient progress and maintain the role of each physician. Additionally and critically, the PPM defines documentation guidelines for the program staff and physicians. One of the most frequent citations from JCAHO is for incomplete physician documentation on patients' medical records.

PROCESS

Process is concerned with the way in which you deliver the program. It should be:

1. systematic and timely
2. appropriate
3. reflecting standards in the field
4. accessible to the patient
5. ensuring continuity of care.

Patient Care Considerations

The essentials of the process of organizing a department concerning patient care are in a descriptive flow chart of what is done with or to the patients from the moment they are referred into the program until they are discharged. A review of the mission statement, philosophy, and general guiding principles upon which the department was designed is the initial step in formulating this chart. Once that is complete, the following are policy needs that define the process:

1. Referral and admission procedures:
   a. Referral forms
   b. Required documents, e.g.: patient history, graded exercise test results, catheterization reports, etc.
   c. Patient interview form
2. Risk stratification:
   a. Utilization of risk stratification[3]
   b. Requirements for continuous ECG telemetry[4,5]
3. Exercise training process:
   a. Exercise prescription principles
   b. Modality selection
   c. Projected goals and expected outcomes
   d. Vocational requirement retraining

4. Risk factor status:
   a. Educational components
   b. Behavioral interventions
   c. Specific and special classes
      (1) Smoking cessation, diet, cooking, etc
5. Discharge planning and instructions
   a. When is the program completed?
   b. Where, when, and how do they go after the program?
   c. Exit paperwork

Process Related to Program Management

This is specifically related to the writing of the policies and procedures as they relate to the patient care considerations. In writing the policies and procedures and reviewing them regularly, it is important that they:

1. Match and are in consort with the facility mission statement and the parent organization statement, and are complete.
2. Are reviewed and revised regularly. Current management theory challenges workers and managers to learn to apply the policy and the procedure to the point where it is operating smoothly. At that time, they are challenged to ask and experiment with how it may be done better. Once that is accomplished, the policy and procedure are rewritten. Continuous quality improvement, according to Imai,[6] is constant and change occurs as soon as something is done well. This ensures better delivery of patient care and results in high levels of patient satisfaction.
3. Reflect the standards in the field. Currently, three sets of guidelines are available for implementation of clinical programs: those of the American Heart Association,[5] the American College of Sports Medicine,[3] and the American Association of Cardiovascular and Pulmonary Rehabilitation.[7] Additionally, the American College of Cardiology has a published position stand relative to clinical programs for cardiac rehabilitation.[4] All staff members should be familiar with these documents, and the policies should not be less than the minimal

standard of practice defined in composite form from these documents. The guidelines of the four organizations and the PPM should be immediately available for reference. The standards implied in the PPM should be implemented by each staff member consistently.

OUTCOMES

The PPM should ensure continuous quality improvement (CQI) through management by outcomes (both expected and achieved). The PPM defines outcomes through policies, delineating methods of documentation, and measurement of objective outcome criteria.

Outcomes Related to Patient Care Considerations

When the patient enters the program, a specific therapeutic intervention is designed, based on past history, the nature of the disease process, and what the patient wishes to accomplish. The program is applied, testing the goals, resetting the goals and measuring the goals that were mutually established by the staff member and the patient. A comprehensive patient care plan takes into account the following:

1. Past medical, social, and work history
2. Physical, mental, and physiologic capacity, past and present
3. Analysis of patient risk factors
4. Patient's goals and objectives
5. Projected outcomes and timeline for completion.

As the program is applied, informal assessments are made, perhaps even on a daily basis, and problems are identified and addressed. Goals are reviewed regularly and reset as necessary. The patient is involved in all of the plans, goals, objectives, and determined outcomes. Objectives should be based on what the patient wants to achieve, learn, and change relative to the improvement of the clinical aspects of their disease process. Weekly logs should be kept on progress, setbacks, and new goals.

Once the program is complete, a final assessment of all goals and objectives should be made, with a comparison to entry levels and the differences documented. If

Performance will be monitored in general by the Clinical Department Chairman, the Division director, and the Department Director/Manager and will at least specifically examine performance relative to the following criteria. It is the goal of the institution that there be no avoidable deviation from the stated criteria. Whenever a deviation from one of these criteria occurs, a detailed review will be undertaken to determine the cause. The review process will assist in minimizing avoidable deviations. Whenever it is determined that a deviation was avoidable, appropriate corrective action will be initiated.

1. All inpatients with appropriate physician orders will exhibit functional improvement and become fully ambulatory as established by their Cardiac Rehabilitation treatment plan, unless precluded by medical conditions.

2. All outpatients will achieve or make progress toward expected outcomes as established by their Cardiac Rehabilitation treatment plan, unless precluded by medical conditions or patients' ability to comply.

3. All Cardiac Rehabilitation Staff medically responsible for patients during dynamic activities will review emergency treatment procedure on a monthly basis.

4. There will be no evaluation of inpatient and outpatient programs by the patient which shall score lower than satisfactory (Bi-annual Review).

5. All cardiac rehabilitation staff will exhibit participation in professional education enhancement activities, e.g., in-service education programs, professional meetings, grand rounds, staff development.

6. A quarterly random review of charting by each staff member in inpatient and outpatient programs will demonstrate compliance to program charting guidelines.

Fig. 47–2. Quality assurance objectives of cardiac rehabilitation department.

there is no change, reasons for no change should be sought and stated. This report remains in the patient chart or file, and a copy is sent to the primary care physician. The PPM should provide specific directions for this activity and accompanying documentation.

Outcomes as They Relate to Program Management

It is essential, from the outset, that the program components be designed with good record keeping relative to program operations as a major goal. Such information as where the patients come from geographically, referring physicians, the primary diagnoses, the number of entries, completions versus dropouts, why the noncompliance occurred, complications and clinical emergencies, readmissions to the hospital, etc., should be tracked weekly, monthly, and annually. These data should be reviewed to note trends, marketing information, and problems to be corrected.

CQI is a program requirement by the JCAHO to ensure that written policies and procedures are applied to program management and patient care. Documentation of that process ensures compliance to a standard level of achievement. When problems are identified, they must be tracked and resolved, and this process must be documented. An example of a CQI plan for JCAHO is found in Figure 47–2.

Notice that these objectives comprehensively review most aspects of the program: application of inpatient and outpatient therapy with measured outcomes, staff training and education, patient progress notes and charting, and finally patient evaluation of the program. Any time problems are identified, they are tracked and corrected, and the documentation is included in a monthly report and CQI record keeping.

CONCLUSION

To put all of the policies and procedures necessary for running a program in a clinical setting in a chapter such as this is not feasible. It is apparent, from what is in this chapter and also all other chapters of this resource manual, that whatever a program claims to do, apply, measure, or document, must be a written policy that denotes, who, when, where, why, and how. Also, it must be aligned with current existing standards and guidelines. Additionally, the process of establishing a PPM is continuous. When staff and department operations are managed smoothly, it is then that the question, "How can it be done better?" must be asked.

DOCUMENTATION IN HEALTH AND FITNESS PROGRAMS

Most of the needs in health/fitness programs involve proper documentation of membership roles, demographic data, clearance forms if required, health information, exercise records, contracts, and other information, perhaps used by the marketing and sales department.[8] Computer technology and a multitude of software programs for health clubs make this type of record-keeping available to most clubs at reasonable costs. Larger clubs and fitness centers should attempt to keep and quantify as much of this information as possible for use in marketing, cost-effectiveness studies, and member retention efforts.

Development of specific reports and forms to track participation rates in various programs and areas of the center is useful. Rates of adherence to specific exercise programs, visit rates, high use times, etc. can all be used by club managers and directors. Figure 47–3 is an example of a form that can be used to record attendance for adherence and member retention data collection. Figure 47–4 is a further example of a form that might be used in a member retention and adherence "campaign." It is a contract form for a participant and a professional staff designed to stimulate progression.

Cost-benefit records are most appropriate and important in corporate settings, but can be used in almost any health and fitness environment. Although costs are relatively easy to document and accumulate, the benefit may not be as easy or available without a significant amount of effort in collection and maintenance of those records.

Every program should have a written manual containing the policies and procedures of the program. These policies and procedures should include input of all employees or their representative in its development. In health/fitness environments,

Participant Adherence & Retention—Weekly Report

Name _____

Activity	Number of Workouts per Week						
	Su	Mo	Tu	We	Th	Fr	Sa
_____	—	—	—	—	—	—	—
_____	—	—	—	—	—	—	—
_____	—	—	—	—	—	—	—
_____	—	—	—	—	—	—	—
_____	—	—	—	—	—	—	—

Participant Adherence & Retention—Monthly Report

Participant	Number of Workouts per Month											
	1	2	3	4	5	6	7	8	9	10	11	12
_____	—	—	—	—	—	—	—	—	—	—	—	—
_____	—	—	—	—	—	—	—	—	—	—	—	—
_____	—	—	—	—	—	—	—	—	—	—	—	—
_____	—	—	—	—	—	—	—	—	—	—	—	—
_____	—	—	—	—	—	—	—	—	—	—	—	—

Fig. 47–3. Sample attendance report.

My Responsibilities:

    To increase distance by ¼ mile each week
    for the next four weeks.

    To accept my partner's free lunch award
    at the Healthy Salads Restaurant.

My Exercise Partner's Responsibilities:

    To help me increase my distance by jogging with me.

    To pay for my lunch at the Healthy Salads
    Restaurant after I achieve my goal.

Signed: Date:
Me _____   _____
Partner _____ _____
Staff _____ _____

Fig. 47–4. Sample goal setting contract. Plan: To increase my jogging from one mile to two miles.

these policies generally cover safety, personnel, record keeping, and financial procedures. They may, however, be written to cover any of the various services and programs that clubs offer.

The policies should be evaluated annually, but changes can be made at any time if the need arises. The evaluation process should look for clear understanding of policies, contradictions, unclear or confusing statements, and appropriateness of procedures. Employees should be informed of policy updates or revisions as soon as possible. All manuals should be corrected accordingly.

Finally, documentation of injury and/or accident "incidents" is essential for health/ fitness environments. The legal liability involved in club activities, either supervised in programs or in unsupervised activity, is extensive. It is extremely important that the staff be well versed in the documentation of incidents and that these policies and procedures be tightly controlled and adhered to by all staff members. The chapter entitled "Management Skills" (Chap. 42) provides an example of this report form.

REFERENCES

1. Allegheny Health Systems: Mission Statement. Pittsburgh, PA: Allegheny Health Systems, 1991.
2. Deming WE: *Quality, Productivity and Competitive Position.* Cambridge, MA: Massachusetts Institute of Technology, Center for Advanced Engineering Study.
3. ACSM: *Guidelines for Exercise Testing and Prescription.* Philadelphia: Lea & Febiger, 1991, pp. 123–130.
4. American College of Cardiology Position Report on Cardiac Rehabilitation. *J Am Coll Cardiol, 7:*451, 1986.
5. Fletcher FF, Froelicher VF, Harley LH, et al.; Exercise standards: A statement for health professionals from the American Heart Association. *Circulation, 82:*2236, 1990.
6. Imai M: *Kaizen, the Key to Japan's Competitive Success.* New York: McGraw-Hill, 1986.
7. American Association of Cardiovascular and Pulmonary Rehabilitation: *Guidelines for Cardiac Rehabilitation.* Champaign, IL: Human Kinetics, 1990.
8. Patton RW, Grantham WC, Gerson RF, Gettman LR: *Developing and Managing Health/Fitness Facilities.* Champaign, IL: Human Kinetics, 1989.

ADDITIONAL READING

Health/Fitness Facility Standards and Guidelines, American College of Sports Medicine, Human Kinetics, Champaign, IL, 1992.

Appendix A

TERMINOLOGY IN EXERCISE PHYSIOLOGY

Russell R. Pate and Maria Lonnett Burgess

The following glossary provides definitions of terms that are used frequently in the field of exercise physiology. Included in this list are terms that appear in the exercise physiology sections of the behavioral objectives that must be met by candidates for the various preventive and rehabilitative exercise program certifications.

aerobic metabolism: catabolism of energy substrates with the utilization of oxygen; energy transfer resulting from involvement of glycolysis, beta oxidation, Krebs cycle and electron transport.

action potential: the momentary change in electrical potential across the cell membrane of a nerve or muscle fiber that occurs with fiber stimulation.

agility: the ability to move quickly into and out of different linear planes, e.g., to be able to move rapidly from one line of direction to another.

anaerobic metabolism: catabolism of energy substrates without the utilization of oxygen; energy transfer that does not require oxygen.

anaerobic threshold: the power output at which blood lactate concentration starts to increase during graded exercise (i.e., onset of blood lactate accumulation, OBLA); the power output at which metabolic acidosis and associated changes in respiratory gas exchange occur during graded exercise.

anemia: a condition marked by an abnormally low number of circulating red blood cells and/or hemoglobin concentration.

angina pectoris: the pain associated with myocardial ischemia (insufficient blood flow to the heart muscle); usually manifested in the left side of the chest and/or in the left arm, but sometimes in the right arm, back, and neck.

anorexia nervosa: loss of appetite for food not explainable by local disease; an eating disorder diagnosed as an intense fear of becoming obese.

apnea: a temporary cessation of breathing.

atrophy, muscular: decrease in size of muscle tissue, especially due to disease and/or disuse.

arteriovenous oxygen difference $(a - \bar{V}_{O_2})$: the difference in oxygen content between the blood entering and that leaving the pulmonary capillaries.

blood pressure: the pressure exerted by the blood against the walls of blood vessels.

body composition: relative amounts of muscle, bone, and fat in the body; often taken as the relative amounts of fat (fat mass) and fat-free mass.

body fat distribution: distribution of adipose tissue across storage sites in the body; visceral (internal) fat mass relative to total fat mass; often quantified as waist-to-hip ratio.

bradycardia: slow heart action; usually defined as a heart rate under 60 beats $\cdot$ min^{-1}.

breathing frequency: the rate of breathing cycles (inhalation and exhalation); usually expressed as breaths per minute.

bulimia: a neurotic disorder characterized by bouts of overeating followed by voluntary vomiting, fasting, or induced diarrhea.

calorimetry: determination of heat loss or gain; a means of determining energy expenditure of an animal by direct measurement of its heat production or indirect measurement of respiratory gas exchange.

cardiac output: volume of blood pumped from the left ventricle each minute; the product of heart rate and stroke volume.

cardiovascular fitness: the ability to perform moderate to high intensity exercise for prolonged periods of time; often used interchangeably with physical work capacity and maximal oxygen consumption ($\dot{V}O_{2max}$).

cholesterol: a fat that can be synthesized by the liver or ingested in the diet from animal fat; is a precursor of various steroid hormones and is used in the biosynthesis of cell membranes.

concentric muscle action: shortening of the muscle as it develops tension; sometimes referred to as "positive exercise."

coordination: the working together of various muscles in the execution of movement.

diastolic blood pressure: arterial pressure during the diastolic phase of the heart's cycle (i.e., ventricular filling).

dynamic exercise: alternate contraction and relaxation of a skeletal muscle or group of muscles causing partial or complete movement through a joint's range of motion.

dyspnea: difficult or labored breathing.

eccentric muscle action: lengthening of a muscle as it develops tension; sometimes referred to as "negative exercise."

electrocardiogram (ECG): a record of the electrical activity of the heart; shows certain waves called P-, Q-, R-, S- and T-waves. (The P-wave is caused by depolarization and contraction of the atrial muscle tissues. The remaining waves are related to depolarization and contraction of the ventricles.)

ergometer: an instrument used to measure work and power output.

ergometry: measurement of work and power; using standardized equipment to measure work and power output during exercise.

essential fat: physiologically essential fat stored in bone marrow, brain, spinal cord, and other internal organs.

fat-free body weight: the weight (or mass) of all the body's nonfat tissue (e.g., skeleton, water, muscle, connective tissue); equals body mass minus fat mass.

flexibility: range of motion possible in a joint or series of joints.

high density lipoprotein (HDL): a plasma lipid-protein complex containing relatively more protein and less cholesterol and little triglyceride; is thought to transport cholesterol from the peripheral vascular compartment to the liver, where it is catabolized and released into the small intestine as bile.

heart rate: number of contractions (beats) of the heart per unit of time; expressed as beats per minute.

heat cramps: involuntary cramping and spasm in muscle groups during exercise in the heat, often resulting from an alteration in the sodium and potassium in muscle as a result of dehydration and salt depletion.

heat exhaustion: a condition resulting from acute blood volume loss and the inability of the circulatory system to compensate for the simultaneous vasodilation of blood vessels in skin and exercising muscle in hot environments; body temperature usually <39.5° Celsius; characterized by a rapid, weak pulse, low blood pressure, fainting, profuse sweating, and disorientation.

heat stroke: a condition resulting from hypothalamic temperature-regulatory failure (specifically the sweating-center); a serious medical emergency; characterized by high body temperature (>40° Celsius), hot, usually dry skin, confusion, and/or unconsciousness.

hemodynamic: relating to the forces involved in circulating blood through the body.

hyperemia: increased amount of blood in a body part, caused by increased inflow or decreased outflow of blood.

hyperplasia: proliferation of cells (increase in the number of cells).

hyperpnea: an increase in depth and rate of breating as with exercise.

hypertension: higher than normal arterial blood pressure; often defined as a resting blood pressure greater than 140/90 mm Hg or a mean arterial pressure in excess of 110 mm Hg.

hyperthermia: increased body temperature caused by inefficient heat dissipation by any or all of the following mechanisms: radiation, conduction, convection, and evaporation; can lead to cell death, heat stroke, and brain damage.

hypertrophy: increased size of an organ or tissue, usually caused by increased size of cells or tissue elements.

hyperventilation: increased inspiration and expiration of air caused by increased rate and/or depth of respiration; can lead to respiratory alkalosis because of depletion of carbon dioxide in the blood.

hypothermia: decreased body temperature caused by inadequate heat production or storage, which depresses the central nervous system and the ability to shiver; can lead to decreased cellular metabolism, unconsciousness, and cardiac dysrhythmias.

hypoventilation: decreased inspiration and expiration of air caused by reduced rate and/or depth of breathing.

hypoxia: low oxygen content; lack of adequate oxygen in inspired air, as occurs at high altitude.

ischemia: local deficiency of blood, usually caused by the constriction or partial occlusion of arterial blood vessels.

isokinetic: referring to contraction of a muscle or muscle group so that joint movement occurs at a constant angular velocity (speed).

isometric: referring to action of a muscle in which shortening or lengthening is prevented; tension is developed but no mechanical work is performed, with all energy being liberated as heat.

isotonic: referring to muscle action in which constant tension is maintained by the muscle while the length of the muscle is increased or decreased.

kilocalorie (kcal): a measure of energy equal to the amount of heat required to change the temperature of 1 kg of water from 14.5°C to 15.5°C.

lactic acid: an acidic metabolite that is the end product of anaerobic glycolysis.

lean body weight: fat-free body mass plus essential fat stores; equals body mass minus storage fat (although not the same, fat-free weight and lean body weight are often used interchangeably).

lipoprotein: a complex consisting of fat and protein molecules bound together; cholesterol and triglycerides are transported in the blood stream as parts of the lipoprotein structure.

maximal oxygen consumption ($\dot{V}O_{2max}$): the greatest rate of oxygen consumption attained during exercise at sea level; usually expressed in liters per minute ($1 \cdot min^{-1}$) or milliliters per kilogram body weight per minute ($ml \cdot kg^{-1} \cdot min^{-1}$); represents the maximal rate of aerobic metabolism.

MET: a metabolic equivalent unit; a unit used to estimate the metabolic cost of physical activity relative to resting metabolic rate; one MET = 3.5 mL of oxygen consumed per kilogram of body weight per minute; one MET = resting metabolic rate.

minute ventilation: the volume of air inhaled or exhaled per minute; the product of tidal volume and breathing frequency.

muscular endurance: the ability of a muscle or group of muscles to contract repeatedly at a submaximal force or to sustain a submaximal force over a period of time.

muscular strength: the maximal force or tension generated by a muscle or muscle group.

myocardial: concerning the myocardium, the heart muscle.

myocardial infarction: an area of cardiac muscle tissue that undergoes necrosis (death) after cessation of blood supply through a segment of the coronary arterial system; also called a "heart attack."

obesity: accumulation and storage of excess body fat.

orthostatic hypotension: lower than normal arterial blood pressure occurring when a subject assumes an erect posture.

overweight: body weight in excess of some standard, usually the mean weight for a given height.

oxygen consumption: the rate at which oxygen is used by the body in aerobic metabolism; usually expressed as liters of oxygen consumed per minute ($L \cdot min^{-1}$) or millimeters of oxygen consumed per kilogram body weight per minute ($mL \cdot kg^{-1} \cdot min^{-1}$).

percent fat: the percentage of the total body weight that is fat tissue.

pH: the negative logarithm of the hydrogen ion concentration of a solution; 7.0 is neutral, values less than 7.0 are acidic, and values greater than 7.0 are basic. Normal arterial blood pH is 7.4; heavy exercise may reduce blood pH values.

plyometrics: a form of explosive jump training that takes advantage of the inherent stretch-recoil mechanism of skeletal muscle (i.e., the myotactic reflex); specifically, overload is applied in a manner that rapidly places the muscle on stretch immediately before concentric contraction.

power: work accomplished per unit time.

premature atrial contraction (PAC): early contraction of the atria originating at some ectopic site outside of the sinoatrial node.

premature ventricular contraction (PVC): early contraction of the ventricle resulting from initiation of an impulse either within or at some ectopic site outside of the conduction system.

progressive resistance exercise (PRE): a weight training technique in which exercises are designed to strengthen specific muscles by causing them to overcome resistances that are gradually increased over time.

reciprocal innervation: simultaneous activation of an agonist muscle group and inhibition of the antagonist muscle group.

repetition (REP): one complete cycle of a given exercise; usually used to describe cycles of weight training exercises.

RPE (rating of perceived exertion): numerical ratings assigned to the perceived effort associated with performance of an exercise task; usually, either a 0–10 or 6–20 rating scale is used (see ACSM guidelines).

respiratory exchange ratio: the ratio of carbon dioxide produced to oxygen consumed; computed as V_{CO_2}/V_{O_2}.

respiratory acidosis: lower than normal blood pH secondary to pulmonary insufficiency resulting in retention of carbon dioxide; can be caused by hypoventilation.

respiratory alkalosis: higher than normal pH of blood and other body fluids in association with reduced blood carbon dioxide level; can be caused by hyperventilation.

set: a series of repetitions of a given exercise performed continuously; usually applied to weight training exercises.

speed: the velocity at which movement is performed, usually expressed as distance per unit time.

static exercise: the contraction of a skeletal muscle or group of muscles without movement of a joint (see "isometric").

stroke volume: the volume of blood pumped from the heart with each beat.

systolic blood pressure: arterial pressure during the systolic phase of the heart's cycle (i.e., ventricular contraction).

tachycardia: abnormal rapidity of heart action, usually defined as a resting heart rate over 100 beats·min^{-1}.

tidal volume: the volume of air moved during a single respiratory cycle (inhalation or expiration).

total cholesterol/HDL ratio: the ratio between the total cholesterol concentration in plasma and the concentration of cholesterol bound to high-density lipoprotein.

triglycerides: a compound consisting of three molecules of fatty acid and one molecule of glycerol.

Valsalva maneuver: an attempt to exhale forcibly with the glottis closed; increased intrathoracic pressure, slowed pulse rate, decreased venous return, and increased venous pressure may result.

ventilatory threshold: the intensity of exercise at which a curvilinear increase in ventilation is detected.

watt: unit of power equal to work done at the rate of one joule per second.

work: the product of force and the linear distance to which an object is moved; measured in Newton-meters (N-m), kilogram-meters, or joules.

BIBLIOGRAPHY

Brooks GA, Fahey TD: *Exercise Physiology: Human Bioenergetics and its Applications.* New York: Macmillan Co., 1985.

Howley ET, Franks BD: *Health Fitness Instructor Handbook,* 2nd Ed. Champaign, IL: Human Kinetics Books, 1992.

McArdle WD, Katch FI, Katch VL: *Exercise Physiology: Energy, Nutrition and Human Performance.* 3rd Ed. Philadelphia: Lea & Febiger, 1991.

Stedman's Medical Dictionary, 25th Ed. Baltimore: Williams & Wilkins Co., 1990.

Webster's Dictionary, Encyclopedic Ed. New York: Lexicon Publ., Inc., 1989.

Appendix B

RECOMMENDATIONS FOR ROUTINE BLOOD PRESSURE MEASUREMENT BY INDIRECT CUFF SPHYGMOMANOMETRY

American Society of Hypertension Public Policy Position Paper (With permission from American Journal of Hypertension, 5:207–209, 1992)

These guidelines for measurement of blood pressure by indirect cuff sphygmomanometry should be followed whenever the blood pressure is measured, either in the office by health practitioners or in the home by the patient. Incorrect readings obtained by inaccurate equipment or faulty technique may lead to serious mistakes in the diagnosis of hypertension and in the monitoring of its course. Those who take the measurement should be adequately trained and tested with particular attention to hearing ability.

EQUIPMENT

Cuff. The cuff should be an inflatable bladder within a cloth sheath.

Bladder Length. The bladder length should nearly or completely encircle the patient's arm; too short a bladder may not transmit the pressure fully against the artery and result in falsely high readings. For many adults, the standard "adult" sized bladder (12 × 23 cm) is not long enough and the "obese" sized bladder (15 × 31 to 39 cm) is strongly recommended. For those with large obese or muscular arms, the "thigh" sized bladder (18 × 36 to 50 cm) should be used, with the cuff folded over itself if it is too wide to fit on the arm. If only short cuffs are available, the center of the bladder must be positioned directly over the artery.

Bladder Width. Bladder width is less important than length but it should be at least 40% of the circumference. In children, the widest and longest bladder that can be applied to the arm should be used.

Inflation-Deflation Bulb and Valve. The bulb should be capable of producing a bladder pressure 30 mm Hg above the systolic pressure within 5 sec of rapid inflation and should hold that pressure until the deflation valve is opened. Deflation should be possible at a rate of 3 mm/sec or pulse beat. If the pressure cannot be held or smoothly released, the deflation valve is likely faulty and should be replaced.

Manometer. *Mercury.* The column should be at zero before inflation with a clearly visible meniscus which should move freely when pressure is applied. If the meniscus is below zero, add mercury to the reservoir.

Aneroid. The needle should be at zero before inflation. The accuracy of the gauge over the entire range of pressure levels should be checked by connecting the aneroid to one limb of a **Y**-piece, the other limb to a mercury manometer, and the bottom to a bladder which can be inflated to various levels of pressure. If the needle is not at zero or the gauge is inaccurate, the device should be repaired.

Electronic Devices. These should be checked if possible with a **Y**-piece against a mercury manometer. If that is not possible, the accuracy of the device should be

This document was prepared by the American Society of Hypertension's Public Policy Committee and approved by the ASH Executive Committee. It is intended to serve as a standard for indirect routine measurement of blood pressure both in clinical research and in office practice. If these guidelines are followed, simple reference to this manuscript should suffice to document the validity of the measurements. Hopefully, the widespread use of these techniques should improve the accuracy of routine blood pressure measurements and bring much needed uniformity and comparability to the procedure.

Address reprint requests to Public Policy Committee, American Society of Hypertension, 515 Madison Avenue, Suite 2100, New York, NY 10022.

checked by simultaneous comparison against another cuff with a mercury manometer used on the other arm. Guidance in selection of suitable devices can be found in the review by Evans et al, J Hypertens 1989;7:133–142.

PATIENT

Circumstances. To establish a reasonable baseline blood pressure, office measurements of multiple sets of at least two readings each should be obtained on at least three occasions at least a week apart. Home measurements taken under varying conditions may be useful in establishing a stable level.

Extraneous variables should be minimized or, if unavoidable, noted. These include a) Food intake, caffeine-containing beverages, cigarette smoking, or strenuous exercise within 1 h prior to measurement; b) Sympathomimetic agents including eyedrops to dilate the pupils; c) Full urinary bladder; d) If patients are taking antihypertensive therapies, the time since the prior dose should be noted. It may be particularly useful to obtain readings at the end of the dosing interval, ie, 24 h after a once-a-day dose. Readings taken at or near the time of peak action, usually 2 to 6 h after intake, may not reflect the more sustained efficacy of the medication.

The patient should be allowed to sit or lie quietly in a comfortably warm place (temperature around 25°C) for 5 min with the arm supported at heart level, preferably with the cuff in place and with no restrictive clothing on the arm.

For young children, conventional sphygmomanometry may be impossible because the Korotkoff sounds cannot be heard reliably. More sensitive detection systems used Doppler ultrasound or oscillometry should be used.

Posture. Seated posture with the arm and back supported and the arm at heart level is preferable for routine measurements.

To recognize postural hypotension, the pressure should be taken immediately and 1 to 5 min after standing. If necessary, patients may hold onto something for stability, but should support their body weight.

During pregnancy, readings should be performed with the patient either seated or in the left lateral position.

At the initial exam, particularly in young hypertensive patients, pressure should be taken in one leg to rule out coarctation of the aorta. A thigh cuff (bladder size 18 × 42 cm) should be wrapped around the thigh of the prone patient and Korotkoff sounds ausculted in the popliteal fossa. With an adequate-sized bladder in the cuff, leg pressure should be equal to arm pressure.

TECHNIQUE

Number of Readings. On each occasion, at least two readings should be taken, separated by as much time as is practical but at least 1 min apart. If the two readings vary by more than 5 mm Hg, additional readings should be taken until two are similar. All readings should be recorded but the average of the last two should be taken as the level on that occasion. If the heart rate is irregular, increase the number of readings to at least five and average them.

Initially, pressure should be taken in both arms. If the pressures differ by more than 10 mm Hg (as in the presence of a subclavian steal syndrome), obtain simultaneous readings in the two arms and thereafter use the arm with the higher pressure.

Performance. The proper sized cuff should fit snugly with the lower edge 2 to 3 cm above the antecubital fossa. The tubing should come from the top of the cuff to avoid interference with auscultation.

The systolic pressure should first be estimated by palpation of the disappearance of the radial pulse in order to avoid the ausculatory gap. The pressure at which the pulse disappears or when it reappears on deflation of the cuff is taken as the systolic pressure. Deflate the cuff rapidly.

After palpation of the brachial artery in the antecubital fossa, the bladder should be inflated quickly to a pressure 20 to 30 mm Hg above the systolic pressure.

The stethoscope is placed gently over the brachial artery and the bladder deflated 3 mm Hg every second or heart beat.

The systolic pressure is taken at the first

appearance of clear, repetitive tapping sounds (Korotkoff Phase 1).

The diastolic pressure is taken at the disappearance of repetitive sounds (Phase 5). In those in whom sounds continue until the zero point, the diastolic is taken at the distinct muffling of the repetitive sounds (Phase 4), which is usually higher than the true diastolic pressure and should be clearly recorded, e.g., 140/80/0.

Both measurements should be recorded to the nearest 2 mm Hg, avoiding terminal digit preferences of 1 and 5, i.e., 80 or 85 rather than 82.

If the levels are not clearly identified, deflate the balloon to zero, and, to enhance the loudness of the sounds, have the patient close and open the fist five or six times while the arm is raised and then start again.

Special Recommendations for Home Blood Pressure Measurements. For diagnostic reasons, multiple readings under various conditions may be useful, including different times of day, after physical exercise, or in the presence of symptoms. A diary should be kept.

For long-term monitoring of therapy, readings should be taken routinely at the same time and circumstances in relation to meals and medications. When therapy is changed, a series of measurements should be obtained, starting just before and repeated throughout the dose interval.

The device should be checked against a mercury manometer at least every year. A large sized cuff (bladder length over 30 cm) should be used for those with obese or muscular arms.

CHECKLIST FOR PUBLICATION UTILIZING BLOOD PRESSURE MEASUREMENTS

Observer

1. Observers trained and tested.
2. Same or multiple observers.

Equipment

1. Size of bladder: uniform or variation by size of arm.
2. Type of manometer.
3. Accuracy of equipment checked against mercury manometer.

Patient Conditions

1. Posture and length of time at rest before measurement.
2. Arm used.
3. Time of day and relation to meals and medication.
4. Notation of unavoidable variables, e.g., arrhythmia.

Technique

1. Arm at heart level and supported.
2. Bladder inflated to above systolic, deflated at rate 3 mm Hg/sec or heart beat.
3. Korotkoff phases 1 and 5 used. If phase 4 used, indicate reason.
4. Take at least two measurements separated by more than 1 min in each posture. If more than 5 mm Hg difference, take additional readings until readings are stable and average last two.

Index

Page numbers in *italic* indicate figures; those followed by "t" indicate tables.